Dental
Treatment
of
Medically
Compromised
Patient

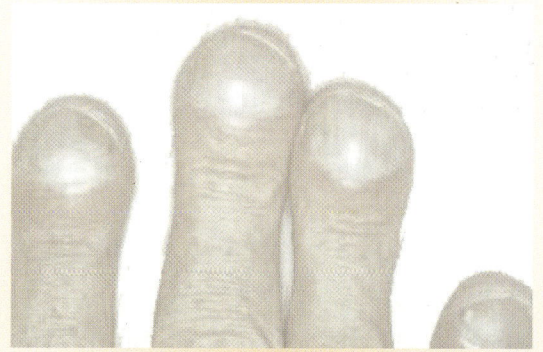

Dental
Treatment
of
Medically
Compromised
Patient

RAGAB RADWAN R. EL-BEIALY

Chairman, Department of Oral and Maxillofacial Surgery
Faculty of Oral and Dental Medicine—Cairo University

Chairman, Department of Oral and Maxillofacial Surgery
Faculty of Oral and Dental Medicine, Misr International University

Professor, Emeritus of Oral and Maxillofacial Surgery—Egyptian Military Hospitals

Member, Educational and Examination Board of the Royal College
"Specialized Military Hospital"

President (Rotatory), Egyptian Dental Association

President, Cairo Dental Syndicate

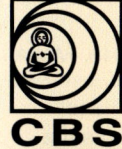

CBS

CBS Publishers & Distributors Pvt Ltd

New Delhi • Bengaluru • Chennai • Kochi • Mumbai • Pune
Hyderabad • Kolkata • Nagpur • Patna

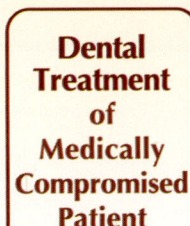

Dental Treatment of Medically Compromised Patient

CBS ISBN: 978-81-239-2343-7

Copyright 2011 © Ragab Radwan R. El-Beialy

First Indian Edition: 2014

This edition has been published by CBS P&D under special arrangement with the author/copyright holder Ragab Radwan R. El-Beialy

All rights reserved. No part of this book may be reproduced or transmitted in any form or by any means, electronic or mechanical, including photocopying, recording, or any information storage and retrieval system without permission, in writing, from the author and the publishers.

Sales territory: Indian sub-continent

Published by Satish Kumar Jain for

CBS Publishers & Distributors Pvt Ltd

4819/XI Prahlad Street, 24 Ansari Road, Daryaganj, New Delhi 110 002, India.
Ph: 23289259, 23266861, 23266867   Website: www.cbspd.com
Fax: 011-23243014   e-mail: delhi@cbspd.com; cbspubs@airtelmail.in

Corporate Office: 204 FIE, Industrial Area, Patparganj, Delhi 110 092
Ph: 4934 4934   Fax: 4934 4935   e-mail: publishing@cbspd.com; publicity@cbspd.com

Branches

• **Bengaluru:** Seema House 2975, 17th Cross, K.R. Road, Banasankari 2nd Stage, Bengaluru 560 070, Karnataka
Ph: +91-80-26771678/79   Fax: +91-80-26771680   e-mail: bangalore@cbspd.com
• **Chennai:** 20, West Park Road, Shenoy Nagar, Chennai 600 030, Tamil Nadu
Ph: +91-44-26260666, 26208620   Fax: +91-44-42032115   e-mail: chennai@cbspd.com
• **Kochi:** 36/14 Kalluvilakam, Lissie Hospital Road, Kochi 682 018, Kerala
Ph: +91-484-4059061-65   Fax: +91-484-4059065   e-mail: kochi@cbspd.com
• **Mumbai:** 83-C, Dr E Moses Road, Worli, Mumbai 400018, Maharashtra
Ph: +91-9833017933   e-mail: mumbai@cbspd.com
• **Pune:** Bhuruk Prestige, Sr. No. 52/12/2+1+3/2 Narhe, Haveli (Near Katraj-Dehu Road Bypass), Pune 411 041, Maharashtra
Ph: +91-20-64704058, 64704059, 32342277   Fax: +91-20-24300160   e-mail: pune@cbspd.com

Representatives

• **Hyderabad** 0-9885175004   • **Kolkata** 0-9831437309, 0-9051152362
• **Nagpur** 0-9021734563   • **Patna** 0-9334159340

Printed at Magic International Pvt. Ltd., Greater Noida

to

my wife
Doria K. Montasser

daughters-in-law
Nadia, Nadine and Nariman

my grandchildren
Jana, Yusuf, Karma, and

the new member
Dara Ramy El-Beialy

Preface

Writing and developing this textbook continues to be a wonderful experience for me challenging, sometimes overwhelming, exhilarating, and a great learning opportunity. A special word of thanks is due to Dr Mahmoud Talaat, Resident in Oral and Maxillofacial Surgery, Ahmed Maher Educational Hospital, for his further help and advice. I must express my sincere thanks to Dr. Ahmed Fawzy, Consultant in Oral and Maxillofacial Surgery, Pediatric Hospital of Cairo University, for his care in going through the text and pointing through the text and pointing out a number of errors and assistance in preparation of the manuscript. This endeavour would not have been possible without the continued interest, support of residents, instructors and colleagues of Misr International University, for whom I am most grateful. I am very grateful to Dr. Tamer Nasr, Lecturer in Oral and Maxillofacial Surgery, Misr International University, for his intense drive, academic precision and patient work on the typescript and proofs. A special debt is owed to Dr. Hossam A. Abd-Elhalime, Assistant Lecturer in Oral Maxillofacial Surgery, MIU. It is a pleasure to acknowledge the help received by Dr. Marwa Ragaai, Doaa Galal and M. Omar El Shawadfy, Instructors of Oral Surgery, Misr International University. I am particularly glad to have this opportunity to express my gratitude to Dr. Alaa Osama Awad. Instructor Oral and Maxillofacial Surgery, Misr International University, for her intellectual curiosity, kindness, help in preparation of diagrams, for the quality of the photographs taken over the years, and on so many occasion. I wish to thank first and foremost Professor Salah Marie and his staff, Ahmed and Mariam Marie and Mohamed Radwan who took charge of the graphic design of the colored cover. I sincerely hope that the use of modern multicolor printing has made it possible to present things more clearly and in a more uniform way. Due to constraints of time and the expanse of new knowledge, it is almost impossible for a single individual to produce a book that adequately covers the pathology of the head and neck. I have been fortunate, however, to secure the aid of several new outstanding collaborators to assist in this endeavor and wish to extend to them my sincere thanks and appreciation for lending their time and expertise.

Ragab R. El-Beialy

Author's Note

Several people have asked me why I don't retire from the classroom. The answer is that I find classroom teaching the most fulfilling aspect of my profession. I work continually at finding more and more effective ways of getting concepts across to them. The best ideas for communicating difficult medical ideas often come to mind during my face-to-face interactions with students, and may are the times that I have dashed back from the lecture room to the drawing pad or keyboard to sketch concepts for new illustrations or write down new explanations. Grading exams and homework assignments also continually gives me new impressions of whether I have effectively taught an idea through my writing. Thus, my students are my unwitting writing teachers.

This book is recommended for students studying human diseases earlier in the undergraduate curriculum and subsequently in oral and maxillofacial surgery in the clinical years. It is also of value for postgraduate dental students, dental practitioners, and residents receiving training in oral and maxillofacial surgery. However, even experienced surgeons may find valuable information in this text.

Dentists treat problems related to the teeth, gums and related structures. They look beyond the mouth and treat people as individuals. Many systemic disease processes can be identified by examination of the mouth and teeth. Dentists detect and diagnose diseases, provide for the esthetic appearance of the teeth, provide surgical restoration of teeth, and provide public information about prevention. Dentists perform surgery related to the mouth and can administer and prescribe medications as needed. The specialty of dentistry that includes the diagnosis, surgical and adjunctive treatment of diseases, injuries, and defect that involve the oral and maxillofacial region also called oral surgeons.

Being convinced that the knowledge base of medicine is of value to the dental general practitioner and the maxillofacial surgeons, so this book has been prepared as up to date as the rapid advances in knowledge allow. This book contains information obtained from authentic, recent and highly regarded sources. A wide variety of references are listed. Reasonable efforts have been made to publish reliable data and information.

This book is not a textbook of internal medicine or pharmacology however, a large portion of it deals not with drugs but with the "management of the case in the widest sense of the term". It is not concerned with surgery, but it has focused on the signs and symptoms of systemic diseases and strengthened further especially those areas of practical, often day-to-day, concern to all dental staff, such as the problems associated with a bleeding tendency, cardiac, liver, kidney, hormonal problems and other transmissible diseases including HIV, and immunosuppressive treatment.

Hoping that the directions given will suffice to enable a dentist without much previous experience to carry out the measures which have been described. As far as possible the indications, contraindications and dangers of each recommended method or drug are fully discussed. There has been an enormous amount of new information that impacts on the daily practice of surgical pathology.

Ragab R. El-Beialy

Contents

1. Selection of Patients for Treatment under Local Anesthesia   1

2. Anxiety   11

3. Cardiovascular System   17

4. Respiratory System   67

5. Liver   97

6. Kidneys   131

7. Diabetes Mellitus   145

8. Adrenal Glands   157

9. Thyroid and Parathyroid Glands   171

10. Deseases of the Immune System   189

11. Neurosensory Deficit "Facial Neuralgias"   285

12. Neuromotor Deficits   337

13. Hormonal Upsets   361

14. Hemorrhage and Bleeding Disorders   387

15. Alarming Bell   433

16. Index   467

    Suggested Reading   480

Detailed Contents

1. Selection of Patients for Treatment under Local Anesthesia   **1**

Medical History	2	Pre-anesthetic Assessment of the Patient	5
Co-operation of the Patient	4	Medical Risks (ASA Classification)	6
Type of Treatment	5	Physical Evaluations	7

2. Anxiety   **11**

Introduction	12	Stress and the Adrenal Medulla	13
Diseases Commonly Provoked by Anxiety	12	Stress Reduction Protocol	14

3. Cardiovascular System   **17**

Anatomy	19	Signs and Symptoms	41
Physiology	20	Medical Management	42
Cardiac Cycle	21	Dental Management	43
Measurements of Cardiac Function	23	Ischemic Heart Disease	45
Neurophysiology of Rhythmic		Angina Pectoris	45
Contraction of the Heart	23	Anatomy of Coronary Arteries	45
Blood Pressure	25	Pathology	47
Normal Arterial Blood Pressure	25	Risk Factors	48
Heart Sounds	26	Treatment Options	49
Regulation of Blood Pressure and		Dental Management	50
Flow	27	Myocardial Infarction	51
Postural Hypotension	31	Physiology	51
Pathophysiology	31	Pathology	51
Predisposing Factors	32	Signs and Symptoms	51
Dental Management	33	Complications	52
Hypertension	34	Management	52
Hemodynamic Mechanism		Endocarditis	54
of Hypertension	34	Physiology of Valves	54
Factors Transiently Alter the Blood		Heart Valve Diseases	55
Pressure	34	Valvular Insufficiency	55
Types	35	Mitral Valve Prolapse	56
Signs and Symptoms	36	Endocarditis	56
Complications	36	Rheumatic Heart Disease	58
Medical Management	37	Dental Procedures and	
Dental Management	38	Endocarditis Prophylaxis	60
Vasoconstrictor Ingredient of		Congestive Heart Failure	62
the Local Anesthetic Cartridge	39	Pathology	62
Drug Interaction with Epinephrine	40	Signs and Symptoms	63
Cardiac Arrhythmias	41	Dental Management	63
Cardiac Rhythm	41	Cardiac Arrest	64
Cardiac Arrhythmias	41		

4. Respiratory System   67

Anatomy	69	Types of Oral Tuberculosis	84
Pulmonary Circulation	69	Transmission and Prevalence	84
Physiology of Respiration	70	Etiology	85
Control of Respiration	71	Pathogenesis	85
Clinical Terminology of Ventilation	72	Immunologic aspect	86
Chronic Obstructive Pulmonary Diseases	73	Latent TB infection (LTBI)	86
Bronchial Asthma	76	Tuberculous Gingivitis	89
Precipitating factors	77	Jaw Bone Involvement	89
Skin Test	78	Histopathological Features	92
Medical Therapy	78	Diagnosis	92
Dental Management	79	Medical Therapy	93
Emphysema	80	Dental Management	93
Pathology	80	Aspiration	94
Signs and Symptoms	82	Common manifestation	96
Dental Management	83	Other Potential Complications	96
Tuberculosis	83	Treatment	96

5. Liver   97

Anatomy	99	Cirrhosis	111
Normal Hepatic Physiology	101	Laboratory Findings	111
Liver Function Testing	105	Medical Management	112
Hepatitis	106	Dental Management	115
Viral Hepatitis	106	Surgical Considerations in Acute and	
Hepatitis A	106	Chronic Hepatic Insufficiency	117
Hepatitis B	107	Cross-Infection	119
Hepatitis C	107	Decontamination of Instruments and	
Hepatitis E	107	Equipment	122
Delta Hepatitis	107	Infection Control Checklist	126
Signs and Symptoms	110	Prophylaxis of Viral Hepatitis	126
Phases of acute viral hepatitis	110	Practice Infection Control Policy	127

6. Kidneys   131

Anatomy	133	Bone Osteodystrophy	138
Functions of the Kidneys	133	Renal Dialysis	139
Physiology "Glomerular Filtration"	134	Hemodialysis	139
Urine Analysis	134	Peritoneal Dialysis	140
Renal Insufficiency	136	Complications of Dialysis	141
Chronic Renal Failure	136	Dental Management of Chronic	
Clinical Features	137	renal failure	142
Laboratory Findings	137	Renal transplant	143
Oral Complications	137		

7. Diabetes Mellitus   145

Pancreas	147	Physiology	147
Anatomy	147	Insulin	148

Glucagon	149	Comas	151
Somatostatin	149	Hypoglycemic Coma	151
Types	150	Hyperglycemic Coma	152
Type I	150	Management of Comas	153
Type II	150	Oral Manifestations of Diabetes Mellitus	153
Diagnosis	151	Complications of Diabetes Mellitus	153
		Dental management of Diabetes Mellitus	155

8. Adrenal Glands   157

Anatomy	159	Pathophysiology of Suppression of Adrenal Functions	164
Physiology	159	Prevention of Adrenal Crises	165
i. Adrenal Medulla	159	Management of Acute Adrenal Insufficiency	165
ii. Adrenal Cortex	161	Hyper-and Hyposecretion of Cortisol	166
Cortisol	161	i. Hypersecretion "Cushing's syndrome"	166
Pharmacological Action	161	ii. Hyposecretion "Addison's disease"	168
Prescription of Corticosteroid Drugs	162	Suggested Dental Outlines	169
Complications of Systemic Corticosteroid Therapy	163		

9. Thyroid and Parathyroid Glands   171

THYROID GLANDS	**172**	**PARATHYROID GLANDS**	**182**
Anatomy	173	Anatomy and Physiology	183
Physiology	173	Hyperparathyroidism	185
Hyperthyroidism	175	Incidence	185
Signs and Symptoms	175	Etiology/Pathophysiology	185
Laboratory Findings	178	Signs and Symptoms	185
Medical Management	178	Management	187
Dental Aspects	178	Hypoparathyroidism	187
Dental Management	179	Pathophysiology	187
Hypothyroidism	179	Dental Aspects of Hypoparathyroidism	187
Cretinism	179		
Myxedema	180		
Dental Management	181		

10. Diseases of the Immune System   189

I. THE LYMPHATIC SYSTEM	**191**	**II. THE IMMUNE RESPONSE**	**203**
Origin of Lymph	191	Introduction	204
Functions of Lymph	192	Types of Immunity	204
Components of the Lymphatic System	193	Innate Immunity	205
i. Lymphatic Vessels	193	Acquired Immunity	205
ii. Lymphatic Cells	194	Functions of the Immune System	209
iii. Lymphatic Organs	195	Components of the Immune System	209
Lymphatic Circulation	200	Properties of Immunity	217
Lymphedema	201	Immune Responses	217

III. UPSETS OF THE IMMUNE RESPONSE 221
A. Autoimmune Diseases 221
Autoimmune Disease Manifestations
and Mechanisms of Tissue Injury 224
Examples of Autoimmune Disease 224
• Rheumatoid Arthritis 224
– Pathophysiology 226
– Signs and Symptoms 227
i. Joints (other than
the Temporomandibular 227
Joint) Radiologic Features 228
ii. Rheumatoid Arthritis Involving
the Temporomandibular joint 230
Incidence 230
Clinical Feature 231
iii. Non-articular Manifestations
of Rheumatoid Arthritis 234
Progression of Rheumatoid
Arthritis 237
Laboratory Features 238
Complications of Rheumatoid
Arthritis 239
Treatment 239
B. Immune Deficiency States "Acquired
Immunodeficiency Syndrome (AIDS),
Human Immuno-deficiency Virus
(HIV)" 244
Categorization of Immuno-
deficiency 244
Diseases which Suppress the
Immune Response 244
Drugs which Suppress the
Immune Response 246
Acquired immunodeficiency
Syndrome (AIDS) 247

Introduction 247
Incidence 247
Pathology 249
Mode of Transmission 250
Signs and Symptoms 251
Oral Manifestations 252
Medical Treatment 259
Dental Treatment 260
C. Hypersensitivity (Allergy) 262
Introduction 262
Pathophysiology and Complications 262
Type of Hypersensitivity 262
Type I Hypersensitivity 264
Pathophysiology 264
Atopy 264
Clinical Examples 266
Anaphylaxis 267
Pathophysiology 267
Signs and Symptoms 267
Skin tests 267
Hay Fever 267
Angioneurotic Edema 267
Treatment 268
Allergic Reactions to Local
Anesthesia 270
Management 271
Type II Hypersensitivity 272
Pathophysiology 272
Blood Transfusion 272
Type III Hypersensitivity 277
Type IV Hypersensitivity 277
Tissue and Organ Transplant
Rejection 279
Dental Protocol for Organ
Transplant Patients 282

11. Neurosensory Deficit "Facial Neuralgias" 285

Facial Neuralgias 286
(I) TRIGEMINAL NEURALGIA 286
(A) Idiopathic Trigeminal Neuralgia 287
Etiology 288
Signs and Symptoms 289
Trigger zones 291
Diagnosis 293
Differential Diagnosis 293
Treatment 293
Medical Management 294
Surgical Management 297

Alcohol Injection 297
Indications 298
Injection of the Supraorbital
and Supratrochlear Nerves 299
Alcohol Injection of the
Infraorbital Nerve 300
Alcohol Injection of the
Inferior Alveolar Nerve 302
Alcohol Block of the Mental
Nerve 303
Alcohol Injection of the Maxillary

Nerve at the Foramen Rotundum   306
Alcohol Injection of the Mandibular
Nerve at its Exit from Foramen
   Ovale   307
Peripheral Neurectomy   308
  Indications   308
   Advantages   308
Neurectomy of the Supraorbital
Nerve   308
Neurectomy of the Infraorbital
Nerve   308
Neurectomy of the Inferior Alveolar
Nerve   312
Neurectomy of the Mental Nerve   312
  Avulsion of the Nerve by Cryoprobe   312
Major Operative Procedures   315
  Rhizotomy   316
  Percutaneous Balloon Micro-
   Compression of the Trigeminal
   Ganglion   318

Microvascular Decompression
  of the Trigeminal Ganglion   318
(B) Atypical Trigeminal Neuralgia   318
  Introduction   318
   Etiology   319
   Clinical Feature   320
   Investigations   321
   Anesthesia Dolorosa   322
II. OTHER CRANIAL NEURALGIAS   322
  i. Idiopathic Glossopharyngeal Neuralgia   322
  ii. Geniculate Neuralgia   325
  iii. Great Auricular Neuralgia   325
  iv. Occipital Neuralgia   325
III. OTHER NEUROPATHIC FACIAL PAIN   329
  A. Postherpetic Neuralgia   329
  B. Neuroma   330
  C. Burning Mouth Syndrome   330
Disorders of Taste   332

12. Neuromotor Deficits   337

Motor Unit   339
  Neuromuscular Junction   339
  Neuromuscular Blockage   341
Myasthenia Gravis   342
  Etiology   342
  Signs and Symptoms   342
  Diagnostic Tests   343
  Treatment   343
Multiple Sclerosis   344
  Incidence   344
  Etiology   344
  Pathophysiology   344
  Signs and Symptoms   344
  Dental Management   345
Facial Paralysis   346
  Pathophysiology   347

Bell's Palsy   347
  General Management   348
  Dental Aspects   349
Epilepsy   349
  Pathophysiology   350
  Types   350
  Signs and Symptoms   351
  Medical Management   351
  Dental Management   352
  Oral Complications   354
Parkinson's Disease   356
  Etiology   356
  Signs and Symptoms   356
  Pathophysiology   357
  Medical Management   358
  Dental Management   358

13. Hormonal Upsets   361

Introduction   362
Functions of the Endocrine System   363
Hormone Interactions   365
Adaptation Syndrome "Stress Response"   366

Pregnancy   367
  Physiology   367
  Treatment Considerations   372
Breastfeeding   374

Oxytocin	375
Prolactin	375
Drugs Contraindicated and Alternatives in Lactating Mothers	376
The Menopause	**376**
Osteoporosis	**377**
Etiology	378
Signs and Symptoms	380

Diagnosis	381
Treatment	383
Suggested Dental Guidelines	384
Osteopenia	384
Depression	**384**
Addictive Drugs and Mood Disorders	384
Pineal Gland	385
Treatment	386

14. Hemorrhage and Bleeding Disorders   **387**

Hemorrhage	389
Classifications of Hemorrhage	389
Physiologically Induced Hemorrhage	391
Hemostasis	392
i. Vascular Phase	392
ii. Platelet Phase	393
iii. Coagulation Phase	394
iv. Fibrinolysis	398
Blood Coagulation Tests	400
BLEEDING DISORDERS	**401**
1. Diseases due to a Defect in Coagulation	**402**
A. Hemophilia	402
i. Hemophilia A	402
ii. Hemophilia B (Christmas Disease)	404
iii. Pseudohemophilia (von Willebrand's Disease)	405
Dental Extraction in a Hemophiliac on Outpatient Basis	405
Dental Extraction in a Hemophiliac in the Hospital	407
B. Hypoprothrombinemia	408

2. Diseases due to Thrombocytopenia	**410**
i. Idiopathic Thrombocytopenia	410
ii. Secondary Thrombocytopenia	410
3. Diseases due to Abnormality of Capillaries	**411**
DRUGS INDUCED HEMORRHAGE (ANTICOAGULANTS)	**413**
Indications of Anticoagulants	413
Types of Anticoagulants	414
A. Heparin	414
B. Coumarin	415
C. Aspirin	416
D. Nonsteroidal anti-inflammatory drugs (NSAIDs)	417
Management of Patients on Anticoagulant Therapy	417
Control of Hemorrhage Following Dental Procedures	420
Local Methods for Control of Hemorrhage	420
Systemic Methods for Control of Hemorrhage	424

15. Alarming Bell   **433**

A	Adrenergic Drugs	434
	Analgesics and NSAIDs	435
	Antibiotics	435
	Anticholinergic	436
	Anticonvulsants	436
B	Bacterial Endocarditis	437
	Botulism	438
C	Coagulopathy	439
	Anticoagulant Therapy	439
D	Dementia	440
	Diabetes	442

	Drug Interactions	442
E	Steps for Assessment in Emergencies	443
	Dental Office Emergency	444
F	Fibrinolytic Therapy	445
G	Graves' Disease	445
	Goiter	445
H	Angina Pectoris	446
	Heart Failure	447
I	Adrenal Insufficiency	447
	Adrenal Medulla	448
K	Kaposi's Sarcoma	449

L Liver Disease   449
M The use of Local Anesthesia in
      Medically Compromised Patients   450
   Metabolic Rate   450
N Narcotics–Morphine   452
O Oxyhemoglobin   452
   Methemoglobinemia   453
   Carbon Monoxide Poisoning   453
P Body Planes   453
Q Quiescent Period   454

R End-stage Renal Disease   454
   Respiratory Stimulants   454
S Sialorrhea   454
T Trismus   456
   Disorders of Taste   457
U Management of Unconscious Patient   458
   Cardiopulmonary Resuscitation (CPR)   459
V Vasoconstrictors   461
W Body Weight and Energy Balance   462
X Xerostomia (Dry Mouth)   464
Y Yellow Bone Marrow   465
Z Alzheimer's Disease   465

16. Index   **467**

Medical Dictionary   468
Abbreviations   479
Equivalents   479

Domestic Measures   479
Metric Weight and Volume   479
Suggested Reading   480

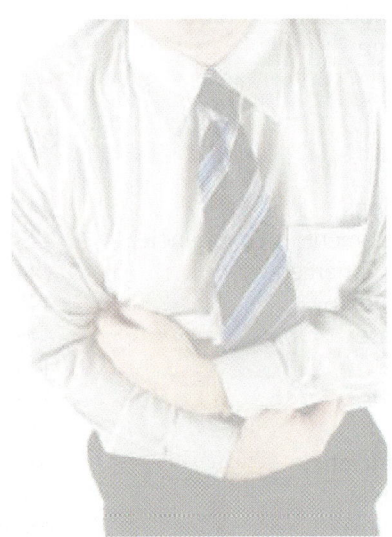

1

Selection of Patients for Treatment under Local Anesthesia

- Medical History
- Pre-anesthetic Assessment of the Patient
- Medical Risks (ASA Medical Risk Category)
- Physical Evaluation

The vast majority of dental procedures that require anesthesia are undertaken with the use of local anesthetic for the simple reason that, with very few exceptions, local anesthesia is the safest, most effective and most convenient form of anesthesia for dentistry. General anesthesia may be needed for certain types of treatment, e.g. complex surgery, or because of the patient's inability to co-operate with the treatment. However, general anesthesia carries a higher risk of complications, some of them are serious, both during the operative procedure and afterwards. It should, therefore, only be used when there are clear and specific indications.

Sedation administered either by the intravenous or the inhalational route, offers an effective and relatively safe way of assisting some patients to accept treatment under local anesthesia, and raises the threshold for requiring a general anesthetic.

The determinants of anesthetic choice are:
- The patient's medical history.
- Level of patient co-operation.
- Type of treatment to be provided.

MEDICAL HISTORY

For psychological reasons, the term "health history" is preferable to "disease history". We, therefore, ask, do you feel healthy? or "is your health disturbed in any way"? For patients with particular health risk, a thorough medical history is extremely important. The fact that patients have been able to reach the office without assistance has little to do with their health status. Targeted questions must provide information that makes it possible to anticipate the effect of any therapeutic measure on the patient's systemic well-being. A complete medical history will also include relevant information from the family history, e.g. genetic disorders, tumors, deformities, and metabolic disturbance (Box 1.1). No questionnaire, no matter how comprehensive it is, can replace a discussion between the dentist and the patient. At the start of the interview, the patient should be given the opportunity to speak freely. Do not interrupt. Do not ask several questions at the same time. Give the patient sufficient time to respond.

In general, local anesthesia is preferred to general anesthesia on grounds of safety. For most patients with complicated medical histories, this generalization is of even greater relevance. Local anesthesia, unlike general anesthesia, does not alter the patient's level of consciousness (and impinge on the ability of the patient to maintain their airway). Some factors may, for instance, complicate pre-existing respiratory disease, or require 4–6 hours fasting before treatment (so disrupting blood glucose control in diabetics).

There are few contraindications to local anesthesia on grounds of medical history. One important example, however, is that of hemophiliacs, when hemorrhage deep in the tissues around the pharynx could follow the injection of an inferior dental block, and thus threaten the patency of the airway. Treatment to replace the deficient clotting factor and/or the use of superficial infiltration injections often overcome the problem without recourse to a general anesthetic. Occasionally, a general anesthetic is still required.

All recent medications that the patient is taking need to be evaluated as to their interaction with other medications the dentist might be giving. Examples of medications the patient may be taking include antihistamines, anticoagulants, decongestants, antibiotics, immunosuppressives, psychosedatives, endocrine augmentation or suppression drugs, cardiac active drugs, and local anesthetics. All of these agents factor into the potential ability for the patient to undergo dental procedures that are being planned.

Drugs that dentists might be familiar with are the anticoagulants. The most common drug is warfarin sodium (Coumadin). Warfarin inhibits formation of certain clotting factors and, therefore, prolongs bleeding. The physiologic effect of warfarin can be evaluated by the laboratory test international normalized ratio (INR). Other medications that can affect bleeding are aspirin and nonsteroidal anti-inflammatory drugs (NSAIDs). Their mechanism of prolonged bleeding is different from that of warfarin. Aspirin and NSAIDs affect platelet function. Platelet replacement is the only effective therapy, if the bleeding is prolonged. When there is any doubt about the suitable choice of anesthetic, the patient's medical practitioner and/or hospital specialist should be consulted.

Box 1.1: Medical history

Name .... M .... F .... Date of Birth ....

Address ....

Telephone (Home) .... (Work) .... Height .... Weight ....

Today's Date .... Occupation ....

Answer all questions by circling either Yes or No and fill in blank spaces where indicated.

Answers to the following questions are for our records only and are confidential.

1. My last medical physical examination was on (approximate) ....

2. The name and address of my personal physician is ....

3. Are you now under the care of a physician?
   If so, what is the condition being treated? .... Yes   No

4. Have you had any serious illness or operation?
   If so, what was the illness or operation? .... Yes   No

5. Have you been hospitalized within the past 5 years?
   If so, what was the problem? .... Yes   No

6. Do you have or have you had any of the following diseases or problems?
   a. Rheumatic fever or rheumatic heart disease .... Yes   No
   b. Heart abnormalities present since birth .... Yes   No
   c. Cardiovascular disease (heart trouble, heart attack, angina, stroke, high blood pressure) .... Yes   No
      1. Do you have pain or pressure in chest upon exertion? .... Yes   No
      2. Are you ever short of breath after mild exercise? .... Yes   No
      3. Do your ankles swell? .... Yes   No
      4. Do you get short of breath when you lie down, or do you require extra pillows when you sleep? .. Yes   No
      5. Have you been told you have a heart murmur? .... Yes   No
   d. Asthma or hay fever .... Yes   No
   e. Hives or a skin rash .... Yes   No
   f. Fainting spells or seizures .... Yes   No
   g. Diabetes .... Yes   No
      1. Do you have to urinate more than six times a day? .... Yes   No
      2. Are you thirsty much of the time? .... Yes   No
      3. Does your mouth usually feels dry? .... Yes   No
   h. Hepatitis, jaundice or liver disease .... Yes   No
   i. Arthritis or other joint problems .... Yes   No
   j. Stomach ulcers .... Yes   No
   k. Kidney trouble .... Yes   No
   l. Tuberculosis .... Yes   No
   m. Do you have a persistent cough or cough up blood? .... Yes   No
   n. Venereal disease .... Yes   No
   o. Other (list) .... Yes   No

7. Are you taking any drugs or medications? If so, what? .... Yes   No

8. Have you had abnormal bleeding associated with previous extractions, surgery, or trauma?
   a. Do you bruise easily? .... Yes   No
   b. Have you ever required a blood transfusion? .... Yes   No
   c. If so, explain the circumstances .... Yes   No

9. Do you have any blood disorder such as anemia, including sickle cell anemia? .... Yes   No

10. Have you had surgery or radiation treatment for a tumor, cancer or other
    condition of your head or neck? .... Yes   No

11. Are you taking any of the following?
    a. Antibiotics or sulfa drugs .... Yes   No

b. Anticoagulants (blood thinners)	....	Yes	No
c. Medicine for high blood pressure	....	Yes	No
d. Cortisone (steroids) (including prednisone)	....	Yes	No
e. Tranquilizers	....	Yes	No
f. Aspirin	....	Yes	No
g. Insulin, or similar drugs	....	Yes	No
h. Digitalis or drugs for heart trouble	....	Yes	No
i. Nitroglycerin	....	Yes	No
j. Antihistamine	....	Yes	No
k. Oral contraceptive or other hormonal therapy	....	Yes	No
l. Other	....	Yes	No

12. Are you allergic or have you reacted adversely to?

a. Local anesthetics [procaine (novocaine)]	....	Yes	No
b. Penicillin or other antibiotics	....	Yes	No
c. Sulfa drugs	....	Yes	No
d. Aspirin	....	Yes	No
e. Iodine or X-ray dyes	....	Yes	No
f. Codeine or other narcotics	....	Yes	No
g. Other	....	Yes	No

13. Have you had any serious trouble associated with any previous dental treatment? .... Yes No

14. Do you have any disease condition, or problem not listed above that you
   think I should know about? If so, explain .... Yes No

15. Are you employed in any situation which exposes you regularly to X-rays
   or other ionizing radiation? .... Yes No

16. Are you wearing contact lenses? .... Yes No

Women

17. Are you pregnant or have you recently missed a menstrual period? .... Yes No

18. Are you presently breastfeeding? .... Yes No

....
Signature of patient

....
Signature of dentist

CO-OPERATION OF THE PATIENT

Most patients find most forms of dental treatment under local anesthesia acceptable. There are, however, some groups of patients with whom the use of local anesthetic alone does not ensure adequate co-operation so that the dental procedure can proceed safely and effectively. These include:
• Young children below the age of reason.
• Mentally handicapped people.
• People with dental phobia.
• Patients with extreme anxiety.

For the first two groups of patients, there may be an indication for general anesthesia but for the anxious patient, or those with a phobia of dentistry, sedation offers a preferable way of making dental treatment with local anesthesia an acceptable possibility.

TYPE OF TREATMENT

Local anesthesia is best suited for operative procedures that are limited both in time, severity, and anatomical extent. Most types of dental treatment fall into this category, but some kinds of dentistry, notably multiple extractions or complex surgical procedures, may test the boundaries of what patients will comfortably tolerate in the fully conscious state.

Here again there is an important role for the techniques of intravenous or inhalation sedation to recruit more patients to treatment without a general anesthetic. The types of treatment for which local anesthesia is less well suited include:

- Difficult or extensive surgical procedures.
- Multiple operative sites in different quadrants of the mouth.
- Anatomical sites that are difficult to anesthetize (e.g. the deep aspect of a dental cyst in the maxilla close to the antrum).
- Drainage of abscesses in deep tissue spaces.

The choice of anesthetic technique that is most appropriate for any given patient will depend on a combination of the factors discussed in this chapter. While local anesthesia is the safest option in the vast majority of cases, there are complications attributable to local anesthetic agents and the methods of their delivery.

PRE-ANESTHETIC ASSESSMENT OF THE PATIENT

Before administering any anesthetic, either local or general, the dentist should make a pre-anesthetic evaluation of the patient. The dentist bears the responsibility not only for rendering efficient and competent dental service but also for understanding the patient's general physical condition. Medical history is of value to evaluate the major systems that might affect or be affected by the dental treatment. It should be kept in mind that the dentist is securing pertinent information to evaluate and not to diagnose or treat the patient for any medical problem. While evaluating the patient, the dentist should determine the following:

1. The patient's general physical and psychological condition.
2. The need for a medical consultation.
3. The history of any previous unpleasant anesthetic experience.
4. The specific drug sensitivities of the patient.
5. The need for premedication or intraoperative sedation.
6. The time to be allotted for the procedure.
7. The technique or method to be used.
8. The choice of an anesthetic solution.
9. The need and quantity of a vasoconstrictor.

A good listener will get much more from the patient's answers.

The fundamentals involved in history taking are to:

1. Ask clear, concise questions,
2. Listen attentively,
3. Observe, and
4. Integrate.

The questions should not be confusing to the patient but should be asked in a manner that will elicit the most useful information. The patient should not be unduly cut short when answering. Listening to and integrating the answers is an art, as is asking the questions.

In general terms, the dentist should look at the patient's cardio-hemodynamic status, endocrine status, respiratory status, and neurologic status. The dentist needs to evaluate medications the patient may be taking and any allergies. The dentist should also examine past hospitalizations and past medical emergencies as well as adverse experiences the patient may have had in previous dental care.

MEDICAL RISKS

For accuracy in communication, the American Society of Anesthesiologists (ASA) has adapted a grading system for relating a patient's physical status. The system is only a relative method and does not detail specific conditions responsible for various gradations. However, it serves as a convenient method for relating the fact that impairment may exist in one or more system, assess the patient's risk category and that a degree of physiological fragility may necessitate special patient care.

The American Society of Anesthesiologists (ASA) Medical Risk Category contains five categories:

ASA I: ASA I patients are considered healthy and normal. Physiologically, the generally recognized activity measure for these patients is that they can walk up two flights of stairs or walk two city blocks without shortness of breath (Fig. 1.1), these patients are able to tolerate the stress involved in a dental treatment plan without added risk of serious complications.

ASA II: ASA II patient has a mild systemic disease or is a healthy (ASAI) patient who demonstrates extreme anxiety and fear toward dental treatment. These patients can walk up one flight of stairs or two level city blocks but may have shortness of breath after completion.

Examples of ASA II patients include the following:
• Well-controlled NIDDM.
• Well-controlled epilepsy.
• Well-controlled hyperthyroid or hypothyroid.

• Disorders in which patients are under a physician's care.
• ASAI patients with upper respiratory infections.
• Healthy pregnant women.
• Healthy patients with allergies, especially to drugs.
• Healthy patients with extreme dental fears.
• Healthy patients over 60 years of age.

Adults with blood pressures between 140 and 159 mmHg systolic and/or 90 to 94 mmHg diastolic. Generally, the ASA II patient can perform normal activities without experiencing distress (e.g. undue fatigue dyspnea).

ASA III: Patients have severe systemic disease that limits activity but is not incapacitating. These patients are able to walk up one flight of stairs or two city blocks but may stop en route because of shortness of breath or distress. At rest, ASA III patients do not exhibit signs and symptoms of distress; however, distress is exhibited when the patient experiences either physiologic or psychologic stress.

For example, an anginal patient may be normal in the waiting room but develop chest pain when seated in the dental chair. Examples of ASA III patients include the following:

• Stable angina pectoris.
• Postmyocardial infarction more than 6 months before treatment with no residual signs or symptoms.
• Well-controlled insulin-dependent diabetes mellitus (IDDM).

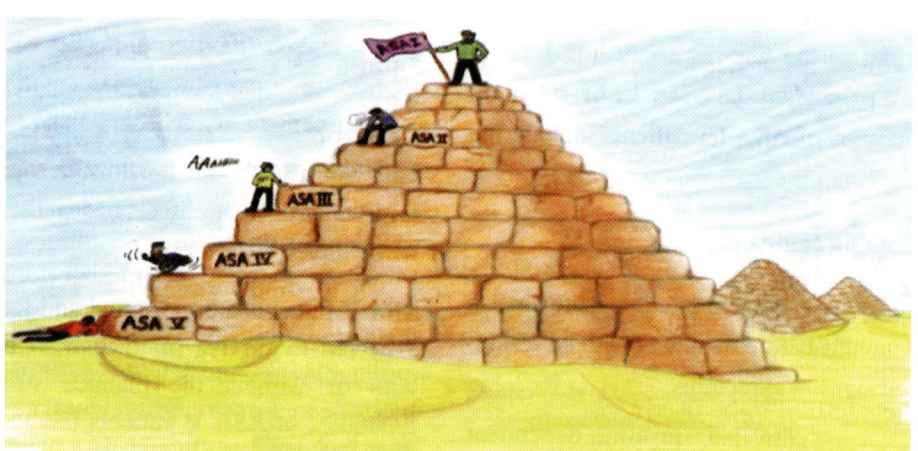

Fig. 1.1: The ASA classification for assessment of the patients

- Congestive heart failure with orthopnea and ankle edema.
- Chronic obstructive pulmonary disease: emphysema or chronic bronchitis.
- Exercise-induced asthma.
- Less well-controlled epilepsy.
- Hyperthyroid or hypothyroid disorders when patients are asymptomatic.

Adults with blood pressures between 160 to 199 mmHg systolic and/or 95 to 114 mmHg diastolic.

ASA IV: Patients have an incapacitating systemic disease that is constant threat to their lives. Examples of ASA IV patients include the following:

- Unstable angina.
- Myocardial infarction within the past 6 months.
- Cerebrovascular accident within the past 6 months.
- Adult blood pressure greater than 200 mmHg systolic or 115 mmHg diastolic.

- Severe congestive heart failure or chronic obstructive pulmonary disease (requiring oxygen supplementation or confinement in a wheelchair).
- Uncontrolled epilepsy.
- Uncontrolled insulin-dependent diabetes mellitus.

ASA V: Patients are moribund and are not expected to survive more than 24 hours with or without the planned surgery. Examples of ASA V patients include the following:

- End-stage renal disease.
- End-stage hepatic disease.
- End-stage cancer.
- End-stage infectious disease.
- End-stage cardiovascular disease.
- End-stage respiratory disease.

It is important for the dentist to be familiar with the ASA classifications because they are generally accepted way of classifying medical risk for a patient undergoing a procedure.

PHYSICAL EVALUATIONS

Physical evaluation of the patient is as important as reviewing the medical history. The fundamental physical evaluation starts with evaluating the patient's vital signs, including blood pressure, heart rate, heart rhythm, respiratory rate and quality, temperature, weight, and height.

Blood Pressure

Pressure is often measured by observing how high it can push a column of mercury(Hg) up an evacuated tube called a *manometer*. Mercury is used because it is very dense and enables us to measure pressure with shorter columns than we would need with a less dense liquid such as water. Because pressures are compared to the force generated by a column of mercury, they are expressed in terms of millimeters of mercury (mmHg). Blood pressure is usually measured with a **sphygmomanometer** (*sphygmo* + pulse, *mano* = rare, sparse, roomy) a calibrated tube filled with mercury and attached to an inflatable pressure cuff wrapped around the arm (Fig. 1.2).

Blood pressure by itself can classify the patient according to the ASA guidelines. Therefore, blood pressure taken by the dentist prior to procedure is one indication of whether a procedure can be

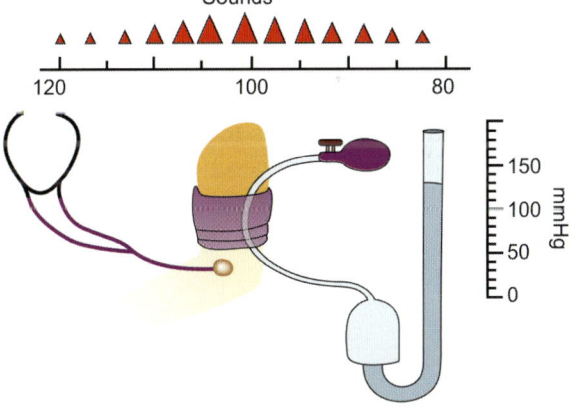

Fig. 1.2: Diagrammatic representation of the typical sound pattern obtained when blood pressure in a noromotensive adult is recoded *(From Guyton AC, Hall JE. Textbook of Medical Physiology, ed 11, Philadelphia, 2006, Elsevier Saunders)*

accomplished safely or whether medical consultation is required. A blood pressure of less than 140/90 mm Hg indicates an ASA I patient eligible for routine elective dentistry. Blood pressure of 140–160/90–95 mmHg classifies an ASA II patient whose blood pressure should be rechecked in a non-threatening, non-stressful environment in 5 minutes. If the reading exceeds the medical guidelines three times, the patient needs medical consultation prior to elective dentistry, otherwise, routine dental treatment can proceed.

A blood pressure of 160–200/95–115 mmHg classifies the patient in an ASA III category. Medical consultation is mandatory prior to elective dental care. Finally, a patient presenting with a blood pressure of 200/115 mmHg or greater requires mandatory immediate medical consultation and examination. This patient should not be merely referred to their doctor, but should be referred for an immediate evaluation.

Heart Rate

The pulse is used as an indicator of the rate and regularity of cardiac contraction. It is observed by palpating a peripheral artery and count beats per minute. Several arteries are superficial enough for this purpose. The most commonly used is the radial artery palpable on the ventral surface of the wrist just proximal to the joint (Fig. 1.3).

Other arteries that serve well are the superficial temporal felt just anterior to the tragus of the ear and the external maxillary which is just palpated as it crosses the inferior border of the mandible. The pulse in the common carotid artery in the neck is easily palpated as well, but this site should not be used routinely (Fig. 1.4). It is reserved for urgent situations where no pulse is felt elsewhere or no blood pressure is found. This site is to be avoided because digital pressure on the carotid sinus located here can cause lowered blood flow to the cerebrum with syncope-

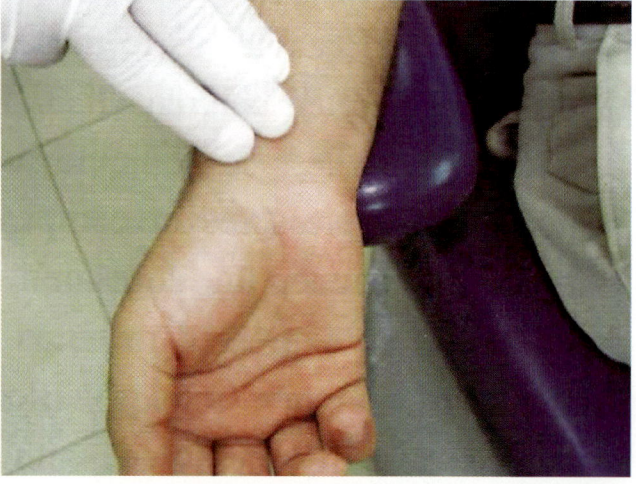

Fig. 1.3: Palpation of the radial pulse. Apply the fleshy pads of fingers (other than thumb) on the ventral surface of the wrist on the side toward the thumb and just proximal to the wrist joint

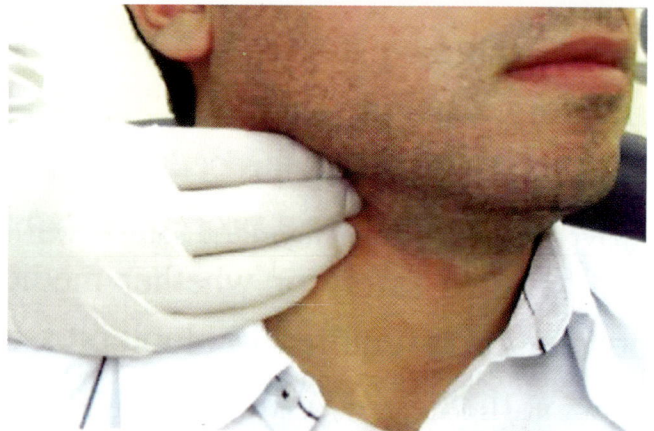

Fig. 1.4: Palpation of the carotid pulse

like results. In newborn infants, the resting heart rate is commonly 120 beats per minute (bpm) or greater. It declines steadily with age, averaging 72 to 80 bpm in young adult females and 64 to 72 bpm in young adult males. It rises again in the elderly.

Tachycardia (tachy = speed, fast, card = heart, ia = condition)

Tachycardia is a persistent, resting adult heart rate above 100 bpm. It can be caused by stress, anxiety, drugs, heart disease, or fever. Heart rate also rises to compensate to some extent for a drop in stroke volume. Thus, the heart races when the body has lost a significant quantity of blood or when there is damage to the myocardium.

Bradycardia *(brady = slow)*

Bradycardia is a persistent, resting adult heart rate below 60 bpm. It is common during sleep and in endurance trained athletes. Endurance training enlarges the heart and increases its stroke volume. Thus, it can maintain the same cardiac output with fewer beats. Hypothermia (low body temperature) also slows the heart rate and may be deliberately induced in preparation for cardiac surgery. Diving mammals such as whales and seals exhibit bradycardia during the dive, as do humans to some extent when the face is immersed in cool water.

Heart rate is also an important indicator of a patient's medical status. Heart rate is evaluated not only in beats per minute, but also the quality of both the rhythm (whether it is regular or irregular) and pulse (whether it is bounding, thready, or weak) and determined. Extra beats also are evaluated and a patient generally should have less than five PVCs per minute, otherwise the condition is pathologic.

Heart Sounds

Through the cardiac cycle, *heart sounds occur.* Listening to sounds made by the body is called **auscultation.** Each cardiac cycle generates two or three sounds that are audible with a **stethoscope.** The first and second heart sounds, symbolized S1 and S2, are often described as a "lubb-dupp"—S1 is louder and longer and S2 a little softer and sharper.

In children and adolescents, it is normal to hear a third heart sound (S3). This is rarely audible in people older than 30, but when it is, the heartbeat is said to show a *triple rhythm* or *gallop.*

If the normal rhythm is roughly simulated by drumming two fingers on a table, a triple rhythm sounds a little like drumming with three fingers.

The heart valves themselves operate silently, but S1 and S2 occur in conjunction with the closing of the valves as a result of turbulence in the bloodstream and movements of the heart wall. The cause of each sound is not known with certainty, but the probable factors are discussed in the respective phases of the cardiac cycle.

Respiratory Rate

The patient's respiratory rate is age dependent. A 1-year-old's average respiratory rate at rest is 24 breaths per minute, whereas an adult's average respiratory rate at rest is 12 to 18 per minute. Respiratory rate, however, is only used as a guideline. In addition, the quality of respirations (whether they are deep or shallow) is used to evaluate the respiratory status of the patient. Auscultation is an important adjunct: knowing whether the patient has wheezes also helps the practitioner to evaluate the patient's respiratory status.

Temperature

Temperature is also an important indicator. The normal range for oral temperature is 97 to 99.6°F. It is important for the practitioner to understand that the oral temperature is elevated after significant dentistry in the mouth, especially following soft tissue procedures. The patient and the practitioner may believe that the patient is running a fever due to inflammation in healing, therefore, after significant oral surgical procedures, rectal, axillary, or tympanic temperatures should be recorded.

Weight and Height

The patient's weight and height are general guidelines used for dosing and categorizing general risk. A physical evaluation beyond this level generally is not needed for dental procedures unless something in the medical history or presentation in the patient indicates it. Refer to Chapter 15, page 463.

2

Anxiety

- Introduction
- Stress and the Adrenal Medulla
- Stress Reduction Protocol

Introduction

Anxiety is the anticipation of an unpleasant event. Anxiety is a defense reaction, ranging from disquiet, through apprehension, to fear and downright terror. Like pain, we must accept that anxiety is a factor that may need to be measured, rather than simply noted as present. Some anxiety or fear is clearly advantageous. For example, finding one self at the edge of a cliff or having misjudged the speed of an oncoming car makes one move swiftly to reduce the danger (many people will also go out of their way to cause anxiety by bungee jumping, or fairground rides). But anxiety associated with dental treatment is often unhelpful because it not only causes great suffering but also creates barriers to dental care. It is the dental practitioners' obligation to aim to minimize their patients' suffering and anxiety. Some anxiety may even be frankly damaging. For example, in a patient with moderate to severe ischemic heart disease, the increase in work done by the heart as a result of the fear might not be matched by an increase in coronary blood flow. This can precipitate angina or worse (Fig. 2.1). Where fear of a particular thing, event or concept, is unreasonably, it may be described as phobia. The distinction between what is a somewhat exaggerated concern about dental treatment and what is a true phobia is rather blurred. The diseases precipitated by anxiety are listed in Box 2.1.

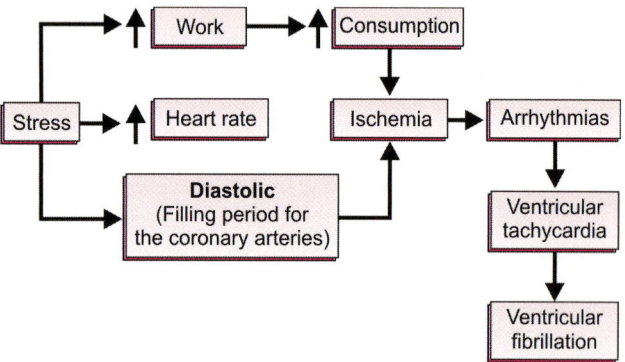

Fig. 2.1: Relationship between work and oxygen consumption. Stress increases the heart rate (HR), which in a diseased heart can cause ischemia by both the greater need of the coronary arteries for O_2 and the reduced time available for them to get it

Box 2.1: Diseases commonly provoked by anxiety

Anxiety commonly provokes or perpetuates the following medical conditions:
1. Angina pectoris
2. Thyroid crisis
3. Myocardial infarction
4. Diabetes (hypoglycemia)
5. Asthmatic bronchospasm
6. Adrenal insufficiency
7. Epilepsy
8. Severe hypertension

The patient's description is again of great value, and many people will openly discuss their concerns about dental treatment. However, embarrassment or loss of face can be experienced (particularly among men) by admitting to fear, particularly when the patients feel that their fear may be irrational. There is, therefore, an underreporting of anxiety and considerable variation in the weight that individuals place on their own fear. For this reason, it is important that you actively look for and assess the level of anxiety.

Clues can be found in body language: posture and facial expression. Overt signs of sympathetic nervous system activity such as pallor and sweating may be diagnostic.

Behavior such as failing to attend or canceling appointments, aggressive behavior or dreadful episodes may also be clues. If you need more evidence, the patient's pulse and blood pressure would show considerable increase.

Most dental procedures can prove stressful to patients. Stress may be of either a physiologic (pain or strenuous exercise) or psychologic nature (anxiety or fear).

In either case, however, one of the body's responses to stress involves an increase in the release of catecholamines (epinephrine and norepinephrine) from the adrenal medulla and other tissue storage sites into the cardiovascular system, resulting in an increase in the body's cardiovascular workload (increased heart rate, strength of myocardial contraction, and myocardial oxygen requirement) (Fig. 2.1).

The sympathetic nervous system plays a very important role in immediately preparing the individual for environmental challenges. This is commonly called the fight or flight reaction.

Harvard Medical School's physiologist Walter Cannon, who coined such expressions as homeostasis and the "fright, fight or flight reaction", dedicated his career to the physiology of the autonomic nervous system. Cannon found that an animal can live without a functional sympathetic nervous system, but it must be kept warm and free of stress; it cannot survive on its own or tolerate any strenuous exertion. The autonomic nervous system is more necessary to survival than many functions of the somatic nervous system; an absence of autonomic function is fatal because the body cannot maintain homeostasis. We are seldom aware of what our autonomic nervous system is doing, much less able to control it; indeed, it is difficult to consciously alter or suppress autonomic responses. Stress increases the heart rate (HR), which in a diseased heart can cause ischemia by both the greater need of the coronary arteries for O$_2$ and the reduced time available for them to get it.

STRESS AND THE ADRENAL MEDULLA

A stressful condition is first perceived by the brain and other sensory receptors. The hypothalamus releases corticotropin-releasing hormone (CRH), which in turn stimulates the release of ACTH from the anterior pituitary, which causes the release of cortisol from the adrenal cortex (Fig. 2.2). Increased amounts of cortisol help the body with stress in the following ways:

1. The catabolism of protein releases amino acids as an energy source and also is a means of tissue repair in case of injury.
2. Amino acids are converted into glucose by the liver (gluconeogenesis). This provides a source of energy during stress, when eating and digestion are reduced.
3. The breakdown of triglycerides into fatty acids and glycerol (lipolysis) provides another energy source.

When the individual is physically or emotionally threatened, a mass discharge of the sympathetic nervous system can occur. The result of this discharge permits the person to perform far more strenuous physical activity than would otherwise be possible. The functions of the sympathetic nervous system will be discussed later.

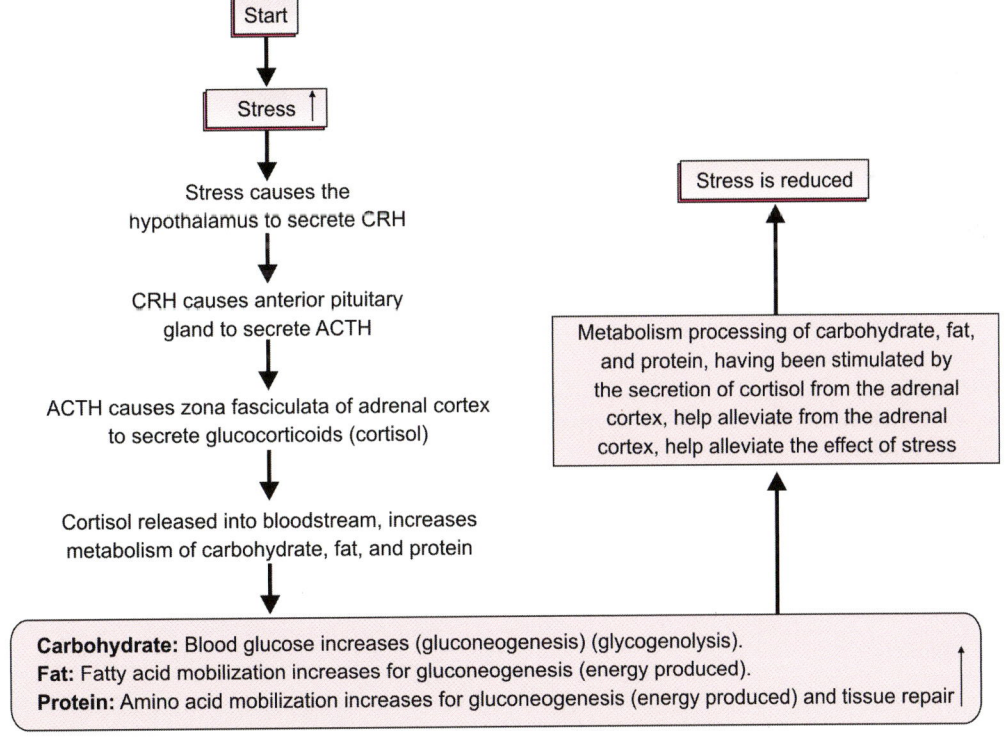

Fig. 2.2: Response to stress. Stress indirectly stimulates the adrenal cortex to secrete cortisol and directly stimulates the adrenal medulla to secrete epinephrine and norepinephrine. • *CRH: Corticotropic-releasing hormone* • *ACTH: Adrenocorticotropic hormone*

STRESS REDUCTION PROTOCOL

Anxiety and stresses may be expressed clinically as a gagging sensation. Gagging is a common clinical problem, and control is an important factor. When faced with an impression tray, many normal children and adults become quite anxious. Gagging is the most common fear of children. It can be helpful to rehearse an impression with an empty tray before proceeding. Often the patient will gain some control from helping to hold the handle of the tray and may also benefit by knowing that the tray can be removed at any time, if a signal is given, such as raising the hand. After practice with a tray, few patients request that it be removed prematurely, and the sense of safety and control over its removal is enough to accomplish the task. The patient should always be told how long the tray will be in the mouth and should be informed as the time passes.

The dental team should never leave a patient who is afraid of gagging unattended. The patient can sit up once the tray is in place and can be encouraged to hold the low-volume suction. Many patients like to hold the tray. When the patient is allowed this sense of safety, taking impressions is usually much less stressful.

The five medical risk categories reported by the American Society of Anesthesiologists (ASA) have to be considered here. Although ASA I patients may be able to tolerate such changes in cardiovascular activity, ASA II, III, and IV patients increasingly are less able to withstand them safely.

For example, patients with angina may respond to increased stress with episodes of chest pain , and various dysrhythmias may develop. Even patients with non-cardiovascular disorders can respond adversely when faced with increased levels of stress. For example, patients with asthma may develop acute episodes of breathing difficulty (bronchospasm), and epileptic patients may suffer seizures.

Unusual degrees of stress in ASA I patients may be responsible for several psychogenically-induced emergency situations such as hyperventilation or vasodepressor syncope. The stress reduction protocol listed here should be followed (Box 2.2).

Box 2.2: General anxiety (stress) reduction protocol

Before appointment

- Hypnotic agent to promote sleep on night before surgery (optional).
- Sedative agent to decrease anxiety on morning of surgery (optional).
- Morning appointment and schedule so that exception room time is minimized.

During appointment

Non-pharmacologic means of anxiety control:
- Frequent verbal reassurances.
- Distraction conversation.
- No surprises (clinician warns patient before doing anything that could cause anxiety).
- No unnecessary noise.
- Surgical instruments out of patient's sight.
- Relaxing background music.

Pharmacological means of anxiety control:
- Local anesthetics of sufficient intensity and duration.
- Nitrous oxide.
- Intravenous anxiolytics.

After Surgery

- Succinct instructions for postoperative care.
- Patient information on expected post-surgical sequel (i.e. swelling or minor oozing of blood).
- Further reassurance.
- Effective analgesics.
- Patient information on who can be contacted, if any problem arises.
- Telephone call to patient at home during evening after surgery to check, if any problem exists.

A great deal can be done to reduce anxiety without medication. Seen from the opposite perspective, there are a number of things that might make things worse: uncertainty, worries about pain and worries about being unable to control the situation. The attitude of the whole dental team to the patient can make a major contribution to the comfort of the patient.

Openness and honesty are very important. You do not need to describe unpleasant things in graphic detail, but advising your patient that he or she will feel pressure and hear noises, but should suffer no pain, is reassuring and still permits alternative outcomes. Long periods of silence are worrying; try to maintain a flow of conversation.

Avoid repeated questions as they prompt the patient into action (this can interfere with treatment) and questions such as 'are you all right?' signal to the patient that you think they might not be. It may be helpful to find a topic of conversation that in some way interests the patient. Distraction by conversation, background music, surgery decor can all contribute to a reduced level of anxiety. It may be helpful to talk through a pleasant scenario for the patient undergoing treatment. They might be asked to ongoing on the beach in the sun, it is warm and they are resting on soft sand.

MODIFYING ATTENTION AND USING DISTRACTION

People have a remarkable ability to turn their attention away from objects and events. Every student knows how to daydream, and one can drive a car to a destination and not even remember the trip. The key to using distraction is to use it appropriately. Distraction works best when it is individualized, so the patient, should be asked what is distracting. For one patient, it may be listening to a CD of rock music; for another, the dentist telling stories about his or her children may be best. Involved and complicated distractions are more effective. Soft background music does not work well. For children, stories and riddles are potential distractions. Distraction is not appropriate when a patient is upset. Distraction is not a substitute for good local anesthesia; it is best used as a complement. Distraction also enhances the effectiveness of nitrous oxide. Distraction works quite well with gaggers. It is a key element in almost every advocated technique. Simply engaging the interest of the patient in a story or one-way conversation is enough to divert attention away from concerns about choking.

Flexibility in your approach; for instance, at the patient's request performing only one or two extractions at a time, when several are required, can also give the patient a considerable feeling of control. Timing can also be important. For a new and nervous patient, it is better to start treatment with less frightening procedures. Hypnosis is thought of as a more formal psychological technique, which at its best gives the patient full control over whether they suffer pain or any other adverse effect. However, distraction is probably the most minor form of hypnosis. The depth that can be achieved is dependent upon the patient, the environment, the skill of the dentist and the amount of time and effort employed.

3

Cardiovascular System

- Anatomy
- Physiology
- Blood Pressure
- Postural Hypotension
- Hypertension
- Cardiac Arrhythmias
- Ischemic Heart Disease
- Angina Pectoris
- Myocardial Infarction
- Endocarditis
- Congestive Heart Failure

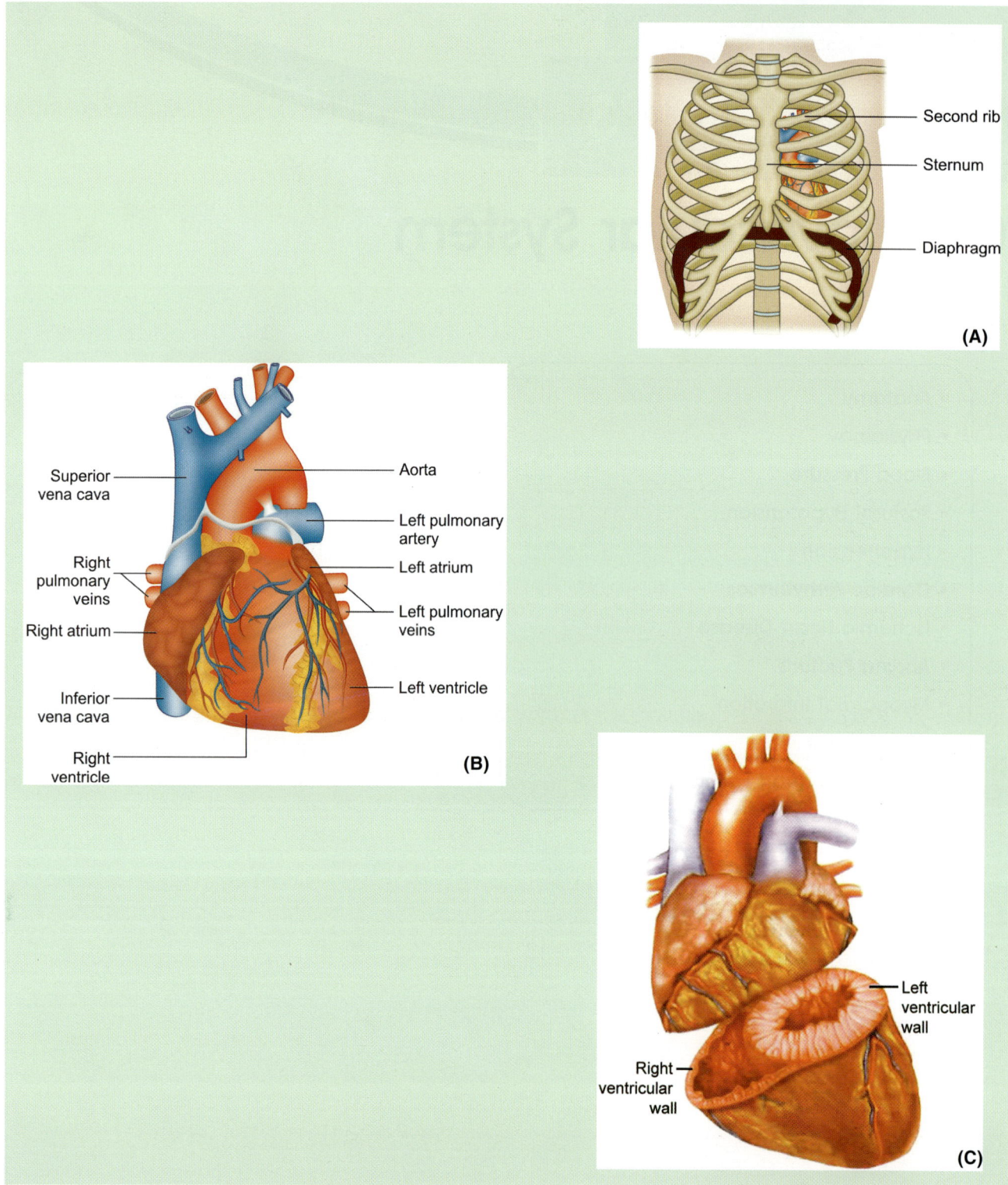

Plate I (A) Position of the heart in the thoracic cavity showing relationship to the thoracic cage. **(B)** The heart with the major arteries and veins. **(C)** Comparison of right and left ventricular wall thickness. The wall of the left ventricle is about three times thicker than that of the right ventricle, because the left ventricle must generate a force sufficient to push blood through the systemic circuit and return it to the heart *(McKliney and O'houghlin, 2006)*

The only significant advance came from **Muslim medicine, when thirteenth-century physician Ibn Al Nafis** described the role of the coronary blood vessels in nourishing the heart. The sixteenth century dissections and anatomical charts of Vesalius, however, greatly improved knowledge of cardiovascular anatomy and set the stage for a more scientific study of the heart and treatment of its disorders, the science we now call **cardiology.**

In the early decades of the twentieth century, little could be recommended for heart disease other than bed rest. Then nitroglycerin was found to improve coronary circulation and relieve the pain resulting from physical exertion, digitalis proved effective for treating abnormal heart rhythms, and diuretics were first used to reduce hypertension. Coronary bypass surgery, replacement of diseased valves, clot-dissolving enzymes, heart transplants, artificial pacemakers, and artificial hearts have made cardiology one of the most dramatic and attention-getting fields of medicine in the last quarter-century.

ANATOMY

SIZE, SHAPE, AND POSITION OF THE HEART

The heart is located in the thoracic cavity in the mediastinum, the area between the lungs. About two-thirds of it lies to the left of the median plane (Fig. 3.1, plate I (A). The broad superior portion of the heart, called the base, is the point of attachment for the great vessels described previously.

Its inferior end, the apex, tilts to the left and tapers to a blunt point. The adult heart is about 9 cm (3.5 in.) wide at the base, 13 cm (5 in.) from base to apex, and 6 cm (2.5 in.) from anterior to posterior at its thickest point—roughly the size of a fist. It weighs about 300 g (10 oz). Each side of the heart contains an elastic upper chamber called an atrium, where blood enters the heart, and a lower pumping chamber called a ventricle, where blood leaves the heart.

The systemic circulation starts in the heart, blood flows to the muscles, organs, and tissues of the body; and then returns to the heart. The pulmonary circulation flows only from the heart to the lungs and back to the heart. Oxygenated blood is red, deoxygenated blood is blue.

THE BLOOD VESSELS

The arteries, capillaries, and veins constitute a closed system for the distribution of blood throughout the body. Major blood vessels, most of which are paired left and right, are shown in Fig. 3.2.

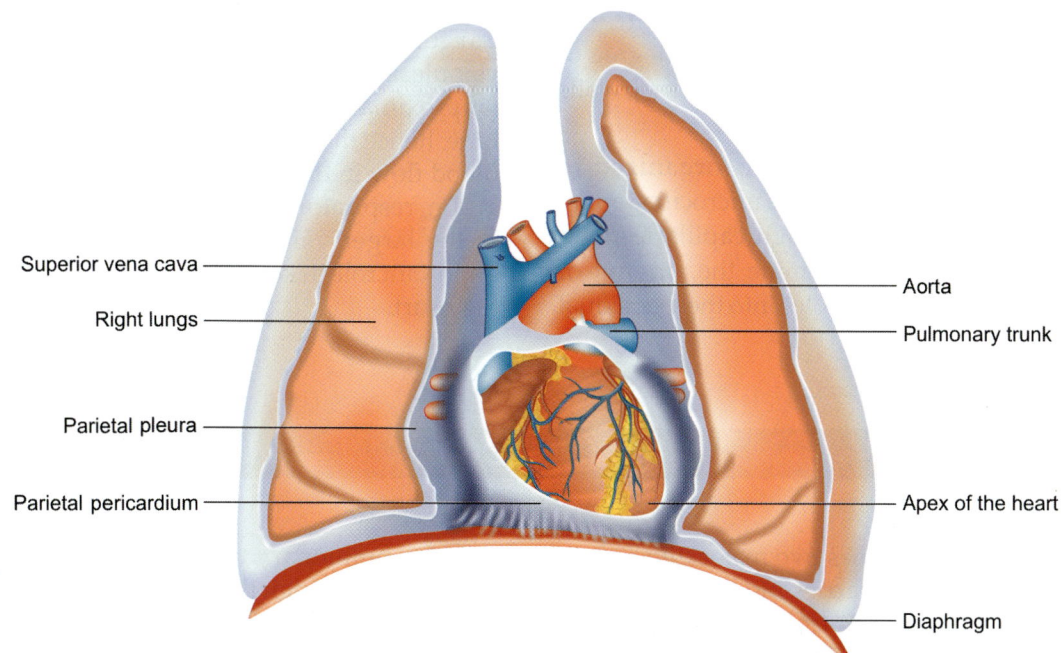

Fig. 3.1: Position of the heart in the chest with the lungs slightly retracted

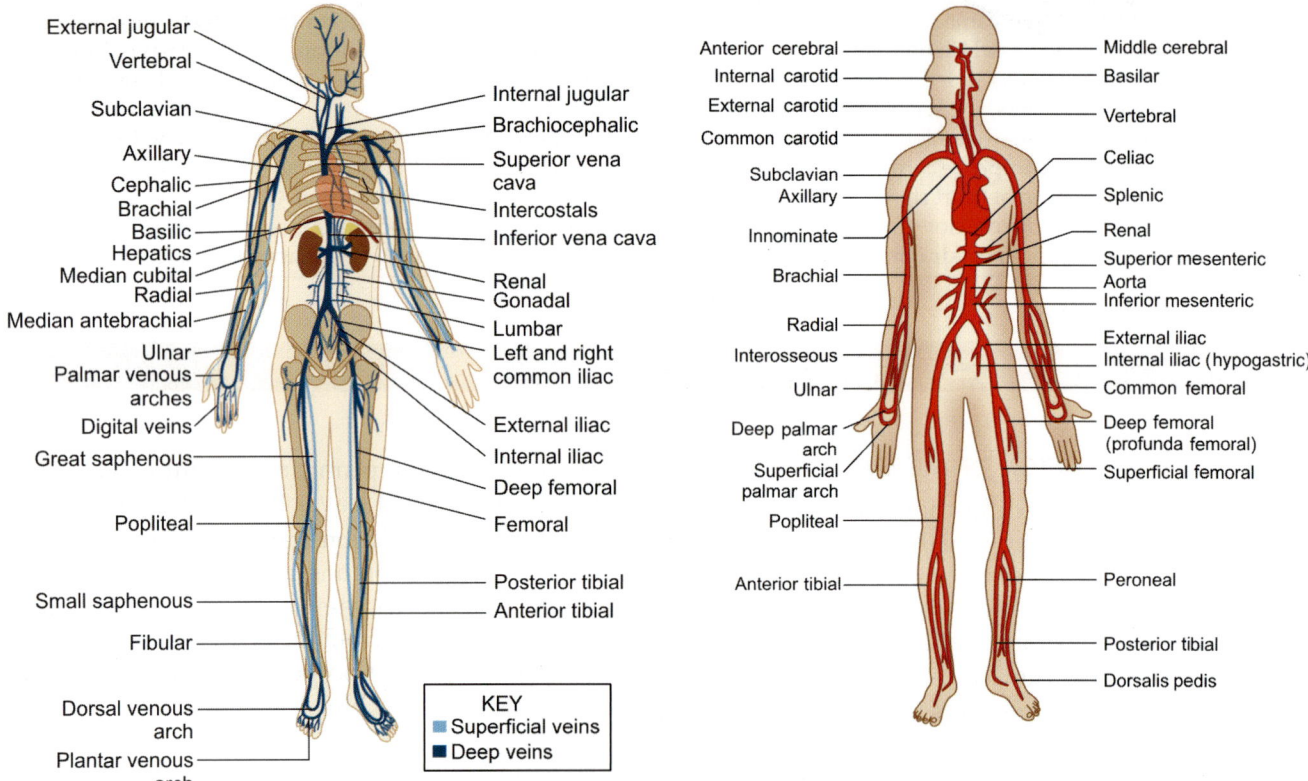

Fig. 3.2: Overview of the major arteries and veins

- Arteries transport blood away from the heart into the lungs or to body tissues.
- Arterioles are the smaller branches of arteries that control the amount of blood flowing into the capillaries in specific areas through the degree of contraction of smooth muscle in the vessel walls (vasoconstriction or dilation).
- Capillaries are very small vessels organized in numerous networks that form the microcirculation. Blood flows very slowly through capillaries, and precapillary sphincters determine the amount of blood flowing from the arterioles into the individual capillaries, depending on the metabolic needs of the tissues.
- Small veinules conduct blood from the capillary beds toward the heart.
- Larger veins collect body draining from the veinules. Normally, a high percentage of the blood (approximately 70%) is located in the veins at any time; hence the veins are called capacitance vessels. Blood flow in the veins depends on skeletal muscle action, respiratory movements, and gravity. Valves in the larger veins in the arm and legs have an important role in keeping the blood flowing towards the heart.

PHYSIOLOGY

The cardiovascular system has two major divisions; a *pulmonary circuit,* which carries blood to the lungs for gas exchange and then returns it to the heart, and a *systemic circuit,* which supplies blood to every organ of the body (Fig. 3.3). The right side of the heart serves the pulmonary circuit. It receives blood that has circulated through the body, unloaded oxygen and nutrients, and picked up a load of carbon dioxide and other wastes. It pumps the oxygen-poor blood into a large artery, the *pulmonary trunk,* which immediately

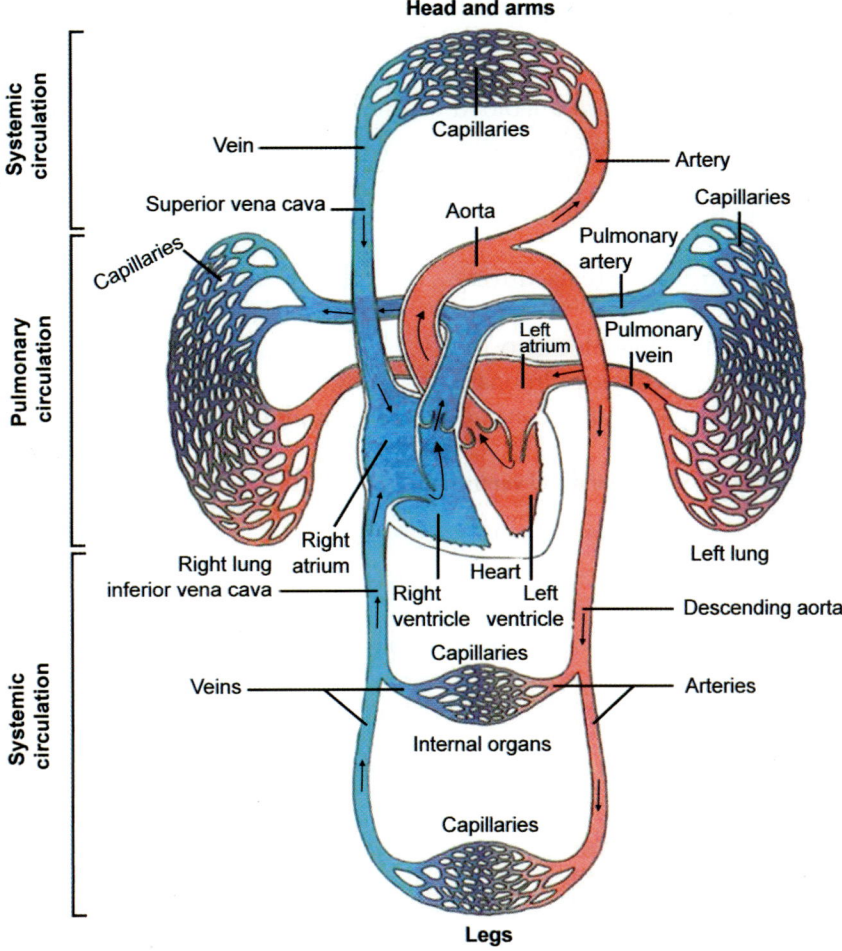

Head and arms

Systemic circulation

Capillaries

Vein

Superior vena cava

Aorta

Artery

Capillaries

Pulmonary circulation

Capillaries

Pulmonary artery

Left atrium

Pulmonary vein

Right lung

Right atrium

Left lung

inferior vena cava

Heart

Descending aorta

Right ventricle

Left ventricle

Capillaries

Systemic circulation

Veins

Arteries

Internal organs

Capillaries

Legs

Fig. 3.3: General schematic of the cardiovascular system

divides into *right* and *left pulmonary arteries*. These transport blood to lungs, where carbon dioxide is unloaded and oxygen is picked up. The oxygen-rich blood then flows by way of the *pulmonary veins* to the left side of the heart. The left side of the heart serves the systemic circuit.

CARDIAC CYCLE

The path of blood through the heart is as follows:
1. Blood enters the atria (Fig. 3.4A). Oxygen-poor blood from the body flows into the right atrium at about the same time as newly oxygenated blood from the lungs flows into the left atrium:
   a. The superior vena cava returns blood from all body structures above the diaphragm (except the heart and lungs).
   b. The inferior vena cava returns almost all blood to the right atrium from all regions below the diaphragm.

c. The coronary sinus returns about 85% of the blood from the coronary circulation to the right atrium.
d. The pulmonary veins carry oxygenated blood from the lungs into the left atrium. The blood entering the right atrium (blue) in Fig. 3.4A is low in oxygen and high in carbon dioxide because it has just returned from supplying oxygen to the body tissues.

The blood entering the left atrium **(red)** in Fig. 3.4A is high in oxygen because it has just passed through the lungs, where it has picked up a new supply of oxygen and released carbon dioxide. (This is the only time or place in the adult where oxygen-rich blood is carried by veins. All other times, oxygen-rich blood is carried by arteries.) Approximately 75% of this blood in the atria passes into the ventricles prior to atrial contraction.

2. Blood is pumped into the ventricles (Fig. 3.4B). The heart's natural pacemaker (SA node) elicits an electrical impulse that coordinates the contractions of both atria (arterial systole). Blood remaining in the atria is forced through the one-way arterioventricular valves into the relaxed ventricles. This is called the "capping off of ventricular filling.

3. The ventricles, filled with blood, relax during AV nodal delay (Fig. 3.4C).

4. The ventricles contract, sending blood to the body (systemic circulation) and lungs (pulmonary circulation) (Fig. 3.4D). The venricular contrac-

tion generates pressure that closes the atrioventricular valves between the atria and ventricles while opening the two semilunar valves leading out of the ventricles. The right ventricle forces blood low in oxygen out through the right and left pulmonary arteries to the lungs. The left ventricle pumps the newly oxygenated blood through the aortic semilunar valve into the aorta. The aorta branches into ascending and descending arteries that carry oxygenated blood to all parts of the body (Fig. 3.4D). The left and right ventricles pump simultaneously, so that equal volumes of blood

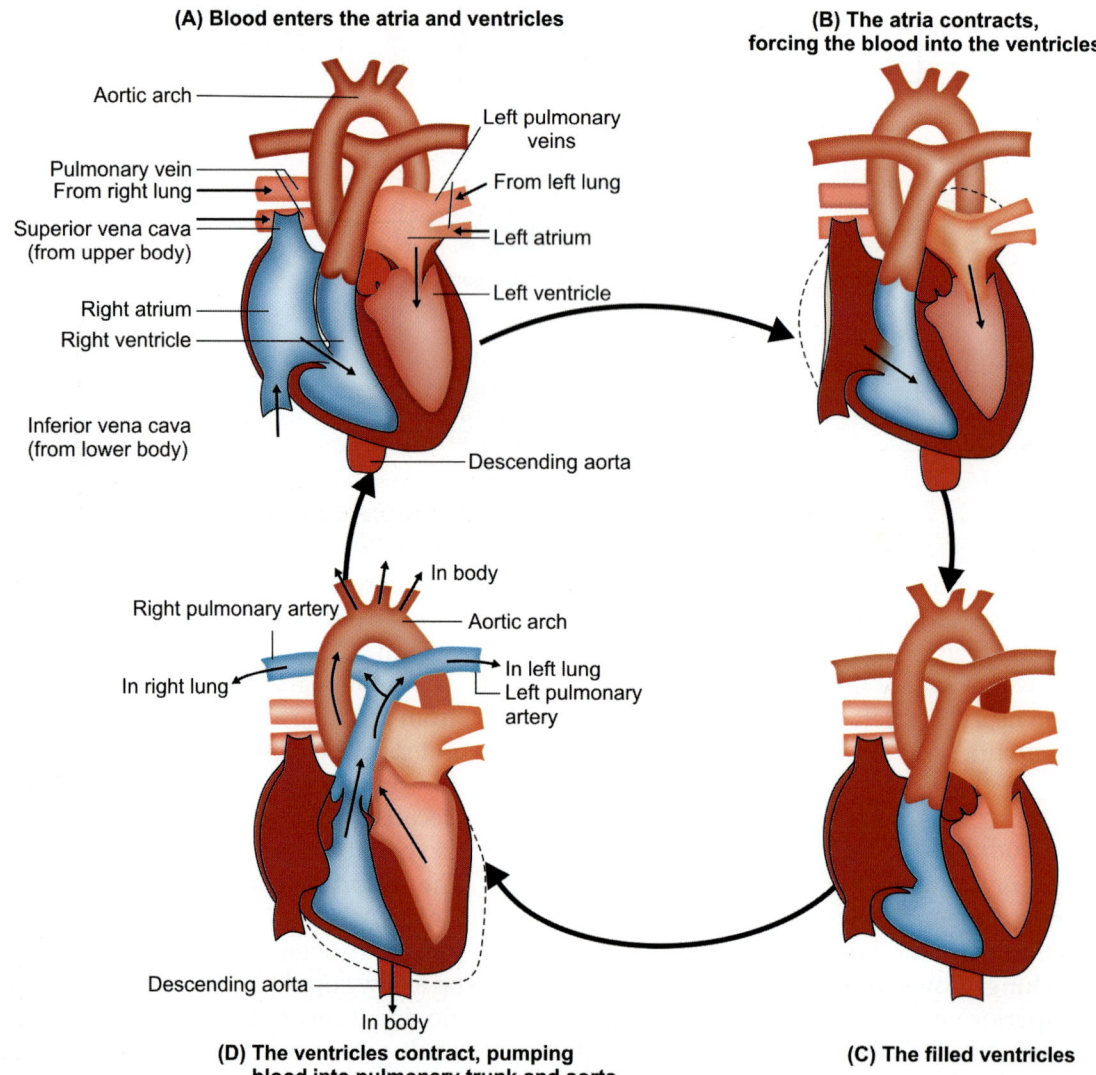

(A) Blood enters the atria and ventricles

Aortic arch

Left pulmonary veins

Pulmonary vein
From right lung

From left lung

Superior vena cava
(from upper body)

Left atrium

Left ventricle

Right atrium

Right ventricle

Inferior vena cava
(from lower body)

Descending aorta

**(B) The atria contracts,
forcing the blood into the ventricles**

In body

Right pulmonary artery

Aortic arch

In right lung

In left lung
Left pulmonary artery

Descending aorta

In body

**(D) The ventricles contract, pumping
blood into pulmonary trunk and aorta**

(C) The filled ventricles

Fig. 3.4: (A) Blood enters the atria and ventricles. **(B)** Blood is pumped into the ventricles. **(C)** The ventricles relax. **(D)** The ventricles contract, pumping blood through the pulmonary trunk and aorta to the lungs and to the rest of the body *(Wynsberghe et al, 1995)*

leave the heart. By this time, the atria have already started to refill, preparing for another cycle.

MEASUREMENTS OF CARDIAC FUNCTION

Cardiac function can be measured in a number of ways:
- *Cardiac output (CO)* is the volume of blood ejected by a ventricle in one minute and depends on heart rate (HR) and stroke volume (SV, the volume pumped from one ventricle in one contraction) (Fig. 3.5). This means that at rest, the heart pumps into the system an amount equal to the total blood volume in the body every minute, which is a remarkable feat. When necessary, the normal heart can increase its usual output by four or five times the minimum volume.
- *Stroke volume* varies with the sympathetic stimulation and venous return. When an increased amount of blood returns to the heart, as during exercise, the heart is stretched more, and the force of the contraction increases proportionately. During exercise, stress, or infection, cardiac output increases considerably.
- *Cardiac reserve* refers to the ability of the heart to increase output in response to increased demand.
- *Preload* refers to venous return.
- *Afterload* is determined by the peripheral resistance to the opening of the semilunar valves. For example, afterload is increased by a high diastolic pressure resulting from excessive vasoconstriction.

NEUROPHYSIOLOGY OF RHYTHMIC CONTRACTION OF THE HEART (CARDIAC CENTERS)

Although the nervous system does not initiate the heart beat, it modulates its rhythm and force. The cardiac center of the medulla oblongata consists of two neuronal pools, a cardioacceleratory center and a cardioinhibitory center.

The cardioacceleratory center sends signals by way of sympathetic *cardiac accelerator nerves*. These nerves secrete norepinephrine, which binds to adrenergic receptors in the heart and increases the heart rate. Cardiac output peaks when the heart rate is 160 to 180 bpm, although the sympathetic nervous system can get the heart rate up to as much as 230 bpm. This limit is set mainly by the refractory period of the SA (sinoauricular) node; it cannot fire any more frequently. At such a high rate, however, the ventricles beat so rapidly that they have little time to fill between beats; therefore, the stroke volume and cardiac output are less than they are at rest. At a heart rate of 65 bpm, ventricular diastole lasts about 0.62 seconds, but at 200 bpm, it lasts only 0.14 seconds. At that high rate, there is less time available for refilling between beats.

The cardioinhibitory center sends signals by way of parasympathetic fibers in the vagus nerves to the SA (sinoauricular) and AV (atrioventricular) nodes. The right vagus nerve innervates mainly the SA node, and the left vagus nerve innervates the AV node. The vagus nerves secrete acetylcholine, which slows down the heart rate. The vagus nerves maintain a background firing rate called *vagal tone* that inhibits the nodes. If the vagus nerves to the heart are severed, the SA node fires at its own intrinsic frequency of about 100 times per minute. With the vagus nerve intact, however, vagal tone holds the heart rate down to the usual 70 to 80 bpm. Maximum vagal stimulation can reduce the heart rate to as low as 20 bpm.

A rise in blood pressure is sensed by stretch receptors in the wall of the heart and the major arteries above it. These receptors send nerve signals to a *cardiac center* in the brainstem. The cardiac center integrates this input with other information and sends nerve signals back to the heart to slow it and lower the blood

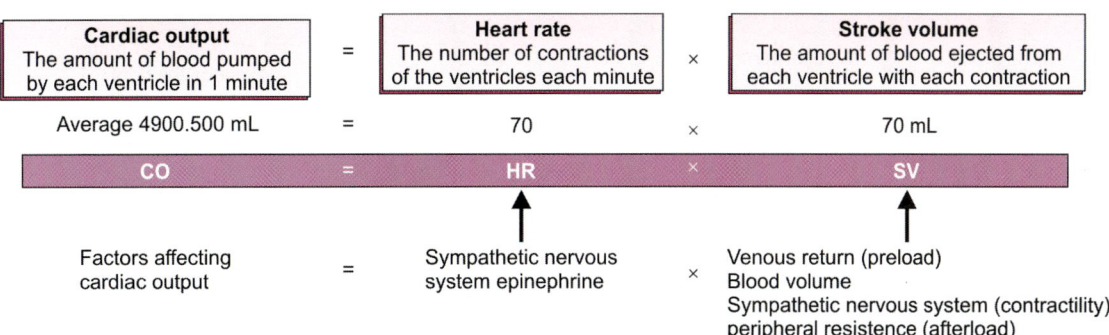

Fig. 3.5: Cardiac function and factors affecting cardiac output

pressure. Thus we can see that homeostasis is maintained by self-correcting negative feedback loops.

The cardiac center receives and integrates input from multiple sources. Sensory and emotional stimuli can act on the cardiac center by way of the cerebral cortex, limbic system, and hypothalamus; therefore, heart rate can climb even as you anticipate taking the first plunge on a roller coaster, and it is influenced by emotions such as love and anger. The cardiac center also receives input from receptors in the muscles, joints, arteries, and brainstem.

Both ventricles eject the same amount of blood even though pressure in the right ventricle is only about one-fifth the pressure in the left. Blood pressure in the pulmonary trunk is relatively low, so the right ventricle does not need to generate very much pressure to overcome it. It is essential that both ventricles have the same output. If the right ventricle pumped more blood into the lungs than the left side of the heart could handle on return, blood would accumulate in the lungs and cause pulmonary hypertension and edema (Fig. 3.6). This would put a person at risk of suffocation as fluid filled the lungs and interfered with gas exchange. Conversely, if the left ventricle pumped out more blood than the right heart could handle on return, blood would accumulate in the systemic circuit and cause hypertension and edema there. Over the long term, this could lead to aneurysms (weakened, bulging arteries), stroke, kidney failure, or heart failure. To maintain homeostasis, the two ventricles must have equal output.

Despite the complexity of cardiovascular physiology, the purpose of this system is rather simplistic; it must perfuse tissues with oxygenated blood. The blood pressure required to perfuse tissues adequately varies from patient to patient and is influenced by medical status and posture at the time of assessment. To assess perfusion of peripheral tissues, apply finger pressure to nailbeds or oral mucosa. Color should return within 3 seconds, assuming normal room temperature. Perfusion within the central nervous system (CNS) can be evaluated by the patient's response to verbal and painful stimuli or the pupil reflex when unconscious or heavily sedated. If perfusion is considered inadequate, the clinician may elect to increase systolic blood pressure, diastolic blood pressure, or both. In each case, a separate set of physiologic determinants should be considered.

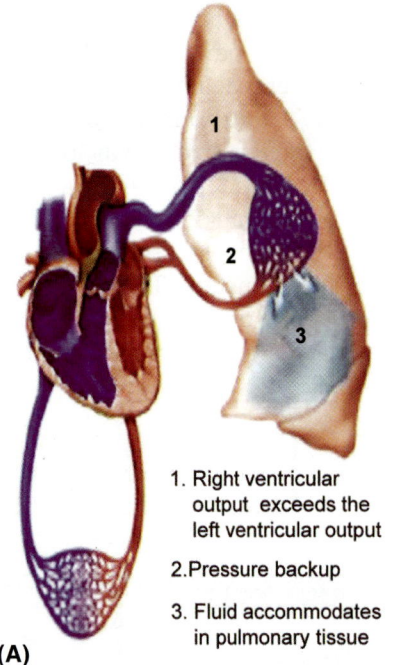

1. Right ventricular output exceeds the left ventricular output

2. Pressure backup

3. Fluid accommodates in pulmonary tissue

(A)

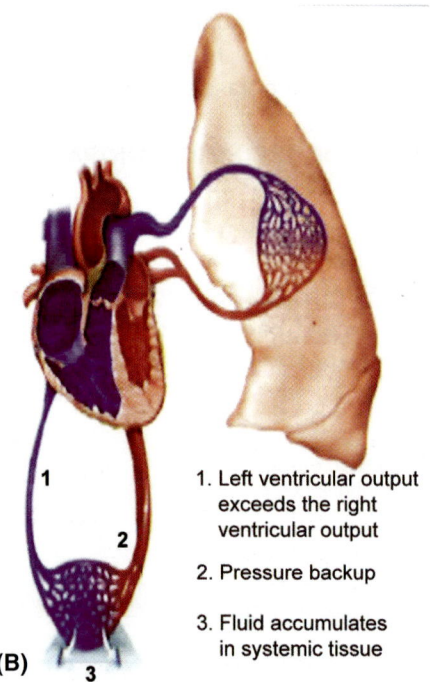

1. Left ventricular output exceeds the right ventricular output

2. Pressure backup

3. Fluid accumulates in systemic tissue

(B)

Fig. 3.6: The necessity of balanced ventricular output. **(A)** If the left ventricle pumps less blood than the right, blood pressure backs up into the lungs and causes pulmonary edema. **(B)** If the right ventricle pumps less blood than the left, pressure backs up in the systemic circulation and causes systemic edema. To maintain homeostasis, both ventricles must pump the same average amount of blood *(Saladin, 2003)*

BLOOD PRESSURE

Blood pressure refers to the pressure of blood against the systemic arterial walls. Blood pressure is usually measured with a **sphygmomanometer** (Fig. 3.7). Sphygmomanometer consists of inflatable cuff, a rubber bulb, and either a column of mercury, an air gauge, or an electronic display. The cuff is wrapped around the upper arm and inflated with the rubber bulb to a pressure above the systolic pressure. (This high cuff pressure compresses the brachial artery under the cuff, stopping the flow of blood). The pressure within the cuff is shown on the scale of the sphygmomanometer. A stethoscope is placed over the brachial artery just below the cuff, and the pressure in the cuff is slowly released until the blood begins to flow. At that point, there is a faint tapping sound in the stethoscope. When the sound is first noted, the blood pressure figure represents the systolic blood pressure. As the cuff pressure is lowered further, the sounds become progressively louder and then softer. When the sound is no longer heard, the diastolic blood pressure is noted. The absence of sound indicates that blood is flowing freely and smoothly through the brachial artery.

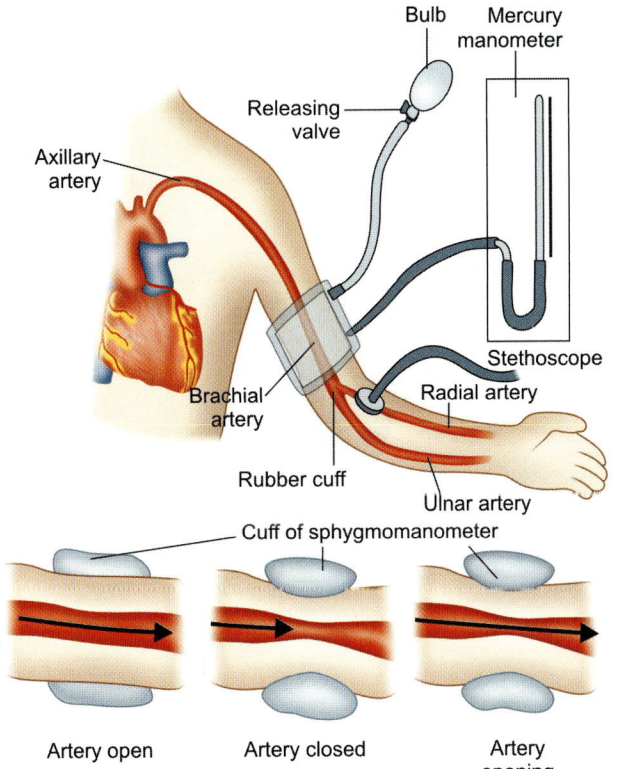

Fig. 3.7: The materials needed for measuring blood pressure. Arterial events are shown. Sounds heard through a stethoscope when the cough pressure of sphygmomanometer is gradually reduced. The first sounds indicate systolic pressure, and the cessation of blood indicates diastolic pressure *(Wynsberghe et al, 1995)*

Pressure is often measured by observing how high it can push a column of mercury (Hg) up an evacuated tube called a *manometer*. Mercury is used because it is very dense and enables us to measure pressure with shorter columns than we would need with a less dense liquids such as water. Because pressures are compared to the force generated by a column of mercury, they are expressed in terms of millimeters of mercury (mmHg).

Two pressures are recorded: **systolic pressure** is the peak arterial BP attained during ventricular systole (at the peak of ventricular contraction, i.e. the pressure exerted by the blood when ejected from the left ventricle), and *diastolic pressure* is the minimum arterial BP between heartbeats. Diastolic pressure represents the total resting resistance in the arterial system after passage of the pulsating force produced by contraction of the left ventricle, i.e. the pressure that occurs when the ventricles are relaxed. Arterial BP is written as a ratio of systolic over diastolic pressure: 120/75. For a healthy person aged 20 to 30, these pressures are typically about 120 and 75 mmHg, respectively. Blood pressure rises with age (Table 3.1) as the arteries become less distensible and absorb less

Table 3.1: Normal arterial blood pressure at various ages*

Age (years)	Male	Female
1	96/66	95/65
5	92/62	92/62
10	103/69	103/70
15	112/75	112/76
20	123/76	116/72
25	128/78	117/74
30	126/79	120/75
40	129/81	127/80
50	135/83	137/84
60	142/85	144/85
70	145/82	159/85
80	145/82	157/83

Average for healthy individuals

systolic force. Atherosclerosis also stiffens the arteries and leads to a rise in BP.

THE HEART SOUNDS

The heart sounds 'Lubb-dupp" which can be heard with a stethoscope, result from vibrations due to closure of the valves. Closure of the AV valves at the beginning of ventricular systole causes a long, low 'lubb' sound, followed by a 'dupp' sound as the semilunar valves close with ventricular diastole. Defective valves that leak or do not open completely cause unusual turbulence in the blood flow, resulting in abnormal sounds or murmurs. A hole in the heart septum resulting in abnormal blood flow would also cause a heart murmur. The pulse indicates the heart rate. Although the pulse (heart rate) can be felt by the fingers (not the thumb) placed over an artery that passes over bone or firm tissue as the wrist, however, it can be felt in the following four areas in the head and neck (Fig. 3.8):

- *Carotid pulse:* The common or external carotid artery can be palpated in the anterior triangle of the neck. This is one of the strongest pulses in the body. The pulse can be obtained either by palpating the common carotid artery posterolateral to the larynx or the external carotid artery immediately lateral to the pharynx midway between the superior margin of the thyroid cartilage below and the greater horn of the hyoid bone above.
- *Facial pulse:* The facial artery can be palpated as it crosses the inferior border of the mandible immediately adjacent to the anterior margin of masseter muscle.
- *Temporal pulse:* The superficial temporal artery can be palpated anterior to the ear and immediately posterosuperior to the position of the temporomandibular joint.
- *Temporal pulse:* The anterior branch of the superficial temporal artery can be palpated posterior to the zygomatic process of the frontal bone as it passes

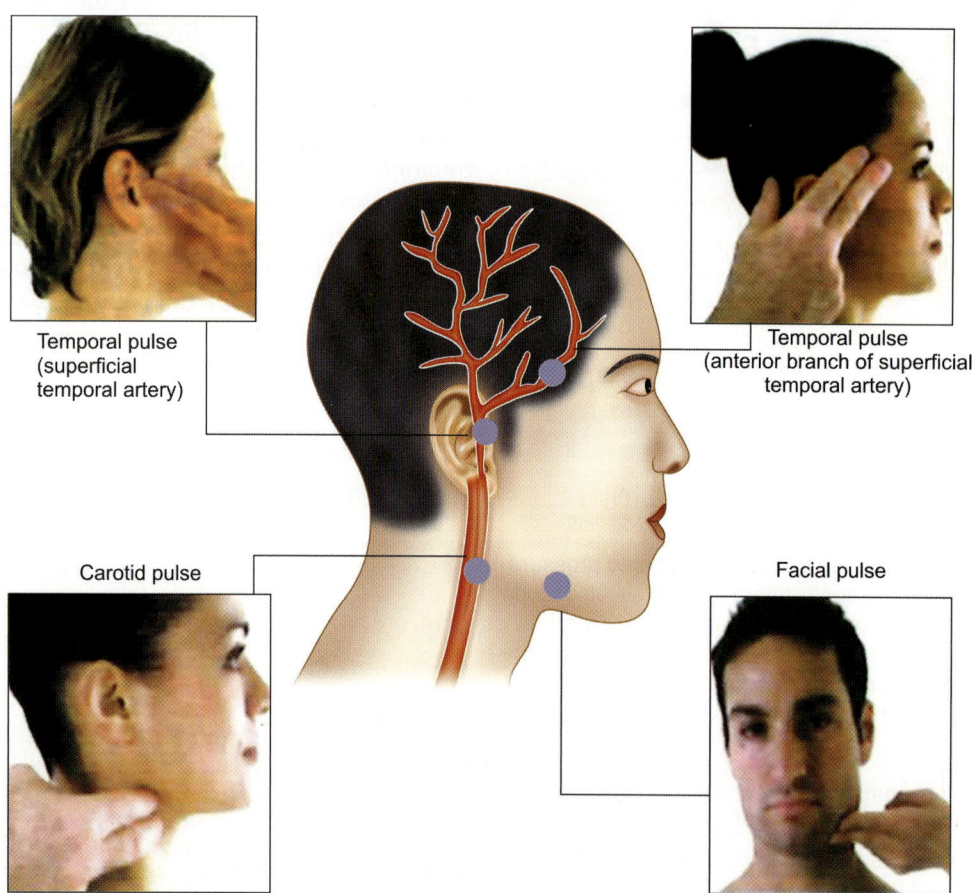

Temporal pulse
(superficial
temporal artery)

Temporal pulse
(anterior branch of superficial
temporal artery)

Carotid pulse

Facial pulse

Fig. 3.8: Where to take arterial pulses in the head and neck

lateral to the temporal fascia and into anterolateral regions of the scalp. In some individuals, pulsations of the superficial temporal artery can be seen through the skin.

The pulse indicates the heart rate. The difference between systolic and diastolic pressure is called *pulse pressure* (not to be confused with pulse *rate).* For the preceding BP, pulse pressure would be 120 – 75 = 45 mmHg. This is an important measure of the stress exerted on small arteries by the pressure surges generated by the heart.

The pulsating force is modified by the degree of elasticity of the walls of larger arteries and the resistance of the arteriolar bed. Control of vascular resistance is multifactorial, and abnormalities may exist in one or more areas. Mechanisms of control include neural reflexes and ongoing maintenance of sympathetic vasomotor tone, neurotransmitters such as norepinephrine, extracellular fluid, and sodium stores; rennin-angiotensin-aldosterone pressor system; and locally active hormones and substances such as prostaglandin, kinins, adenosine, and hydrogen ions (H^+).

REGULATION OF BLOOD PRESSURE AND FLOW (Fig. 3.9)

Blood pressure is subjected to local, neural, and hormonal controls over vasomotion. We now consider each of these three influences in turn.

Local Control

Autoregulation is the ability of tissues to regulate their own blood supply. According to the *metabolic theory of autoregulation,* if a tissue is inadequately perfused, it becomes hypoxic and its metabolites (waste products) accumulate CO_2, H^+, K^+, lactic acid, and adenosine, for example. These factors stimulate vasodilation, which increases perfusion. As the bloodstream delivers oxygen and carries away the metabolites, the vessels constrict. Thus, a homeostatic

dynamic equilibrium is established that adjusts perfusion to the tissue's metabolic needs.

Blood platelets, endothelial cells, and the perivascular tissues secrete a variety of *vasoactive chemical* substances that stimulate vasomotion. Histamine, bradykinin, and prostaglandins stimulate vasodilation under such conditions as trauma, inflammation, and exercise. Endothelial cells secrete prostacyclin and nitric oxide, which are vasodilators, and polypeptides called *endothelins,* which are vasoconstrictors.

If a tissue's blood supply is cut off for a time and then restored, it often exhibits reactive hyperemia (an increase above the normal level of flow). This may be due to the accumulation of metabolites during the period of ischemia. Reactive hyperemia can be seen when the skin flushes after a person comes in from the cold. It also occurs in the forearm, if a blood pressure cuff is inflated for too long and then loosened. In the long run, a hypoxic tissue can increase its own perfusion by angiogenesis the growth of new blood vessels, (this term also refers to embryonic development of blood vessels). Three situations in which this is important are the regrowth of the uterine lining after each menstrual period, the development of a higher density of blood capillaries in the muscles of well-conditioned athletes, and the growth of arterial bypasses around obstructions in the coronary circulation. Several growth factors and inhibitors control angiogenesis, but physiologists are not yet sure how it is regulated. Malignant tumors secrete growth factors that stimulate a dense network of blood vessels to grow into them and provide nourishment to the cancer cells. Oncologists are interested in finding a way to block tumor angiogenesis, which would choke off a tumor's blood supply and perhaps shrink or kill it.

The blood vessels are under remote control by the autonomic nervous system and hormones (Fig. 3.10).

Neural Control
(The vasomotor center and vasomotor tone)

The *vasomotor center* of the medulla oblongata (Figs 3.11 and 3.12) exerts sympathetic control over blood vessels throughout the body, (precapillary sphincters have no innervation, however, and respond only to local and hormonal stimuli). Sympathetic nerve fibers stimulate most blood vessels to constrict, but they dilate the vessels of skeletal and cardiac muscles in order to meet the metabolic demands of exercise. The

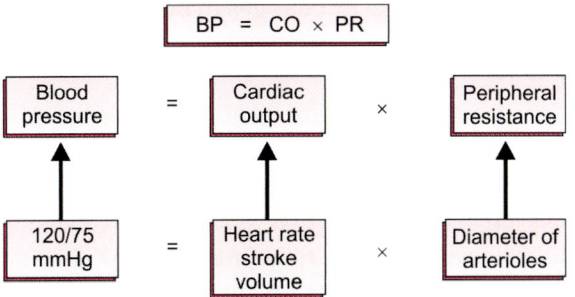

Fig. 3.9: Blood pressure *(Gould BE, 2006)*

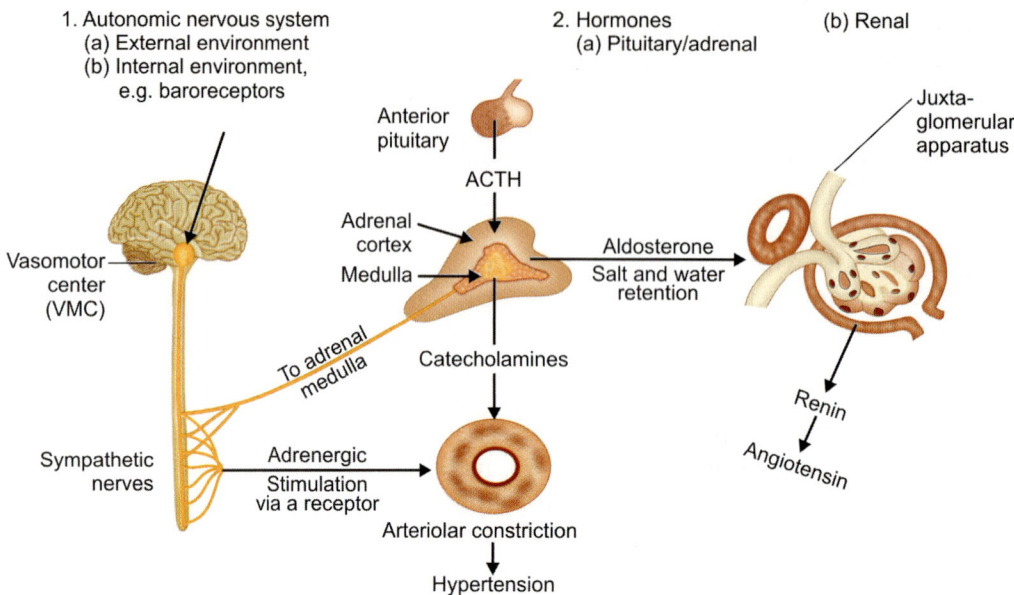

Fig. 3.10: The autonomic nervous system **(1)** and hormonal control **(2)** of blood pressure (Reid 2005). *Note:* Both nitric oxide (NO), and endothelin are produced physiologically by endothelial cells. They have powerful and opposite effects. Nitric oxide—vasodilatation (short acting), Endothelin—vasoconstriction (long acting)

role of sympathetic tone and vasomotor tone in controlling vessel diameter is illustrated in Fig. 3.13.

The sympathetic fibers to a blood vessel have a baseline sympathetic tone which keeps the vessels in a state of partial constriction called vasomotor tone. An increase in firing rate causes vasoconstriction by increasing smooth muscle contraction.

A drop in firing frequency causes vasodilation by allowing the smooth muscle to relax. The blood pressure in the vessel, pushing outward on its wall, then dilates the vessel. Thus, the sympathetic division alone exerts opposite effects on the vessels. Sympathetic control of vasomotor tone can shift blood flow from one organ to another according to the changing needs of the body. In times of emergency, stress, or exercise, the skeletal muscles and heart receive a high priority and the sympathetic division dilates the arteries that supply them. In time of emergency, stress, or exercise, the skeletal muscles and heart receive a high priority and the sympathetic division dilates the arteries that supply them.

Such processes as digestion, nutrient absorption, and urine formation can wait; thus the sympathetic division constricts arteries to the gastrointestinal tract and kidneys. It also reduces blood flow through the skin, which may help to minimize bleeding in the event that the stress-producing situation leads to injury. Furthermore, since there is not enough blood in the body to abundantly supply all the organ systems at once, it is necessary to temporarily divert blood away from some organs in order to supply an adequate amount to the muscular system.

The *medullary ischemic reflex* is an autonomic response to a drop in perfusion of the brain. Within seconds, the cardiac and vasomotor centers of the medulla oblongata send sympathetic signals to the heart and blood vessels that induce:

1. An increase in heart rate and contraction force and
2. Widespread vasoconstriction.

These actions raise the blood pressure and ideally restore normal perfusion of the brain. The cardiac and vasomotor centers also receive input from other brain centers. Thus stress, anger, and arousal can also raise the blood pressure. The hypothalamus acts through the vasomotor center to redirect blood flow in response to exercise or changes in body temperature.

Hormonal Control (Fig. 3.10)

All of the following hormones influence blood pressure:

- *Angiotensin II:* This is a potent vasoconstrictor that raises the blood pressure.
- *Aldosterone:* This "salt-retaining hormone" primarily promotes Na+ retention by the kidneys. Since water follows sodium osmotically, Na+ retention promotes

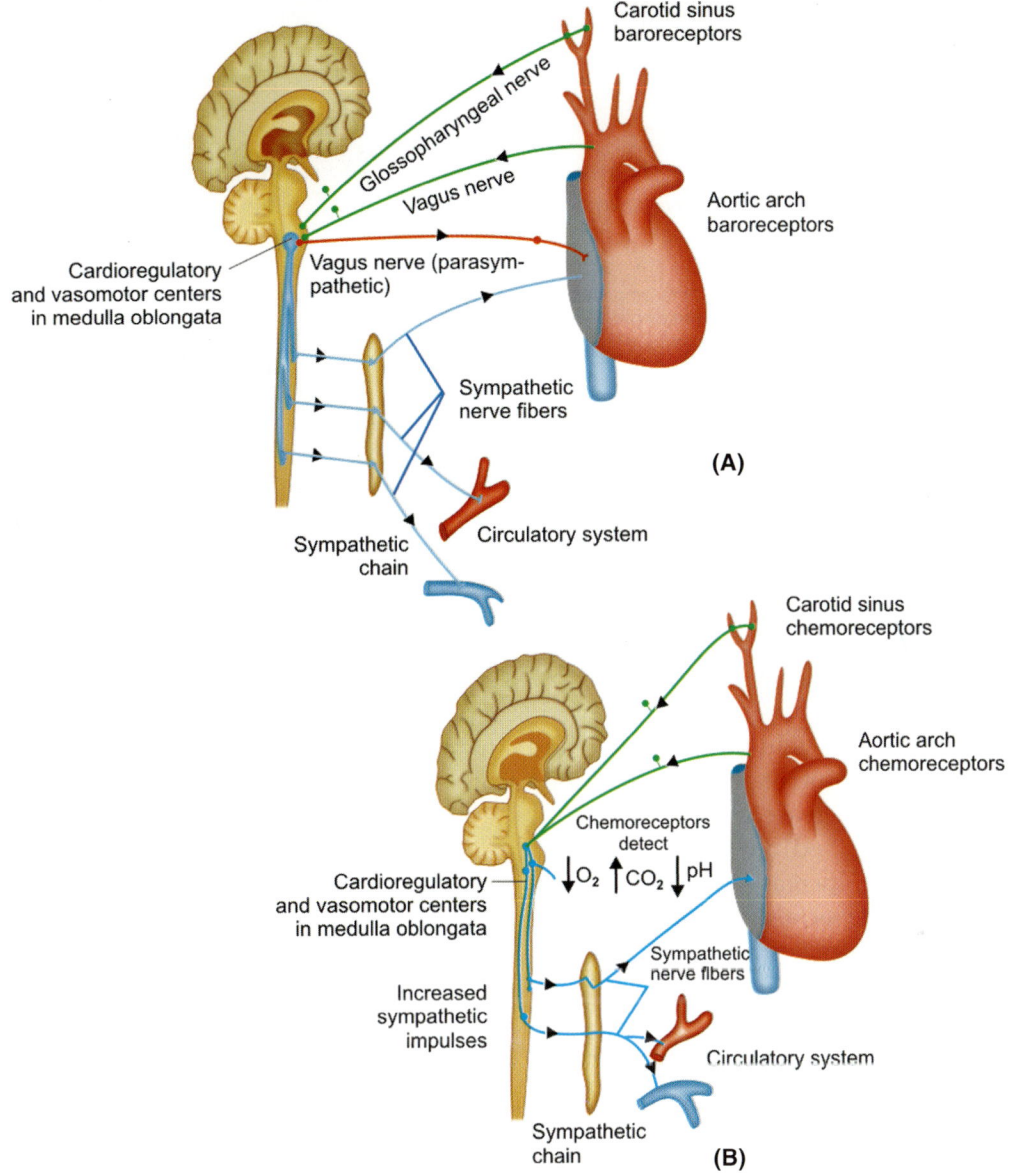

Fig. 3.11: Nervous reflex mechanisms regulating blood pressure. Essential of anatomy and physiology (*Seeley RR and Stephens, 1996*)

water retention, thus promoting a higher blood volume and pressure.

- *Atrial natriuretic peptide:* ANP, secreted by the heart, antagonizes aldosterone. It increases Na⁺ excretion by the kidneys, thus reducing blood volume and pressure. It also has a generalized vasodilator effect that contributes to lowering the blood pressure.
- *Antidiuretic hormone:* ADH primarily promotes water retention, but at pathologically high concentrations, it is also a vasoconstrictor hence its alternate name, *vasopressin.* Both of these effects raise blood pressure.
- *Epinephrine and norepinephrine:* These adrenal and sympathetic catecholamines bind to adrenergic

receptors on the smooth muscle of most blood vessels. This stimulates the muscle to contract, thus producing vasoconstriction and raising the blood pressure. In the coronary blood vessels and blood vessels of the skeletal muscles, however, these chemicals bind to adrenergic receptors and cause vasodilation, thus increasing blood flow to the myocardium and muscular system during exercise.

Many physiologic factors may have an effect on blood pressure. Increased viscosity of the blood (e.g. polycythemia) may cause an elevation in blood pressure that result from an increase in resistance to

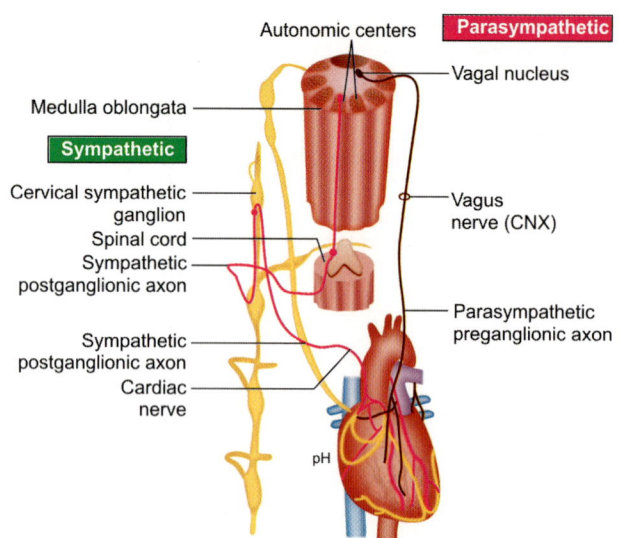

Fig. 3.12: Autonomic innervations of the heart. Cardiac output and heart rates are modified by autonomic centers in the hindbrain. (Left) Sympathetic stimulation is carried through the cardiac nerves. (Right) Parasympathetic stimulation is carried by vagus nerve *(McKliney & O'houghlin, 2006)*

flow. A decrease in blood volume or tissue fluid volume (e.g. anemia, hemorrhage) reduces blood pressure. Conversely, an increase in blood volume or tissue fluid volume (e.g. sodium/fluid retention) increases blood pressure. Increase in cardiac output associated with exercise, fever, and thyrotoxicosis also may increase blood pressure.

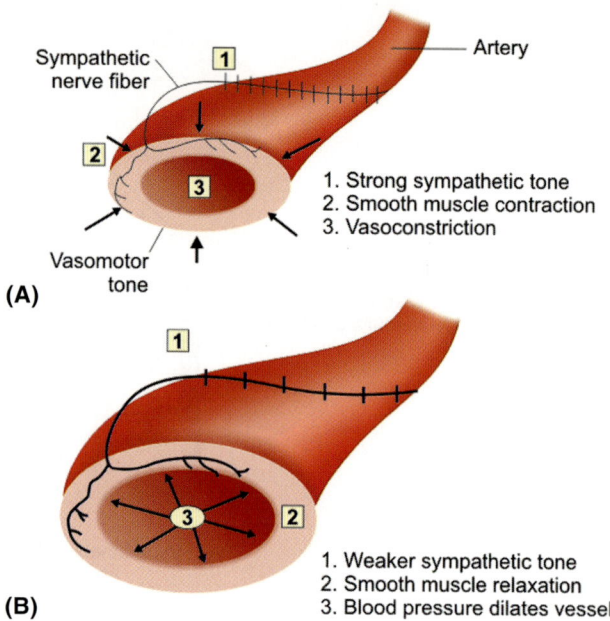

1. Strong sympathetic tone
2. Smooth muscle contraction
3. Vasoconstriction

1. Weaker sympathetic tone
2. Smooth muscle relaxation
3. Blood pressure dilates vessel

Fig. 3.13: Sympathetic tone and vasomotor tone. **(A)** Vasoconstriction in response to a high rate sympathetic nerve firing. **(B)** Vasodilation in response to a low rate of sympathetic nerve firing *(Saladin, 2003)*

Figure 3.14 illustrates the physiological mechanisms controlling blood pressure. They are presented in 2 groups but are complex and interconnected with feedback controls.

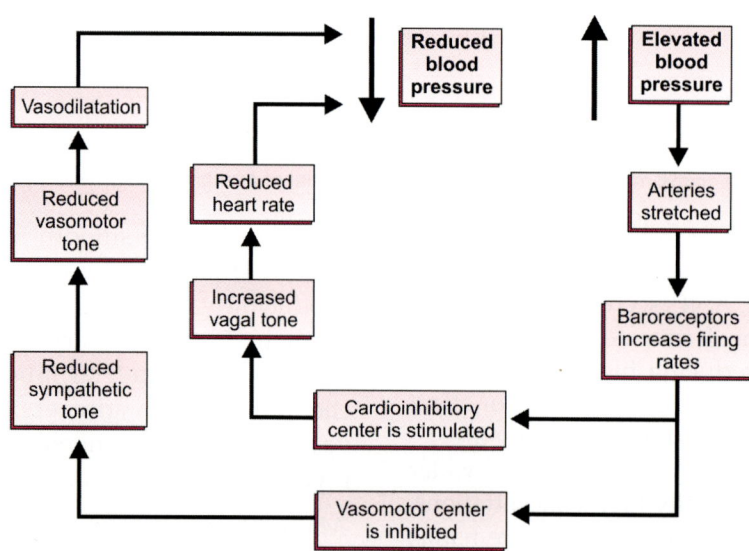

Fig. 3.14: Negative feedback control of blood pressure. The reaction here occurs in response to a rise in blood pressure *(Reid 2005)*

POSTURAL HYPOTENSION (ORTHOSTATIC HYPOTENSION)

Postural hypotension is defined as a disorder of the autonomic nervous system in which syncope occurs when the patient assumes an upright position. When the patient moves from a supine into an upright position, gravity's effect on the cardiovascular system intensifies. Blood pumped from the heart must now move upward, against the force of gravity, to reach the cerebral circulation and supply the brain with the O_2 and glucose it needs to maintain consciousness. On the other hand, when the patient is in the supine position, the force of gravity is distributed equally over the entire body and blood flows more readily from the heart to the brain. In other positions (e.g. semisupine, Trendelenburg), the effect of gravity is intensified upon the cardiovascular system. The systolic pressure decreases by 2 mmHg for each inch that the patient's head is situated above the level of the heart; while for each inch that the head is situated below the level of the heart, blood pressure increases by 2 mmHg (Fig. 3.15).

The usual (normal) reaction of the cardiovascular system when an individual is tilted from the supine into the upright sitting position is an immediate drop in systolic blood pressure from 5 to 40 mmHg and the pulse increases.

Box 3.1: Positional changes of pulse and blood pressure

Symptoms develop "when individual stand".
Standing pulse increases at least 30 beats per minute.
Standing systolic blood pressure decreases at least 25 mmHg.
Standing diastolic blood pressure decreases at least 10 mmHg.

This drop is followed by an equally rapid rise so that within 30 seconds to 1 minute, the systolic blood pressure is equal to or slightly higher than that recorded in the supine position. Thereafter, the systolic blood pressure tends to remain within 10 mmHg higher or lower (usually higher) of the supine recording. The diastolic blood pressure rises approximately 10 to 20 mmHg. Heart rate (pulse) increases approximately 5 to 20 beats per minute when the patient is standing (Table 3.2).

Pathophysiology

To maintain normal blood pressure, i.e. adequate supply of oxygen and glucose nutrient to the brain, a number of mechanisms are brought into action, these mechanisms include:

1. Arteriolar vasoconstriction. Stimulation of the pressure receptors located in the carotid sinus and aortic arch (pressure receptors) which leads to reflex arteriolar constriction.

2. Reflex increase in heart rate which occurs simultaneously with the increase in arteriolar tone.

3. An increase in muscle tone and contraction in the legs and abdomen—the so-called venous pump—that facilitates the venous return of blood of vital importance (because at least 60% of circulating blood volume at any given moment is in venous circulation).

4. A reflex venous constriction that increases the return of venous blood to the heart.

5. A reflex increase in respiration, which also aids in the return of venous blood to the right side of the heart via changes in the intra-abdominal and intrathoracic pressures.

6. The release into the blood of various neuro-humoral substances, such as norepinephrine, antidiuretic hormone, rennin, and angiotensin.

Blood pressure during the syncopal period of postural hypotension is quite low, as it is during vasodepressor syncope. Unlike vasodepressor syncope, during which individuals exhibit bradycardia, the heart rate during postural hypotension remains at the baseline level or somewhat higher (> 30 beats per minute above baseline). The patient with postural hypotension exhibits all the clinical manifestations of unconscious patients. If

Table 3.2: Cardiovascular response to positional changes

Change (at 60 seconds) after sudden elevation	Normal	Postural hypotension
Systolic blood pressure	Baseline or +\–10 mmHg	Decrease of > 25 mmHg
Diastolic blood pressure	Increase of 1–20 mmHg	Decrease of > 10 mmHg
Heart rate	5–20 beats per minute above baseline	Baseline or higher (> 30 beats per minute)

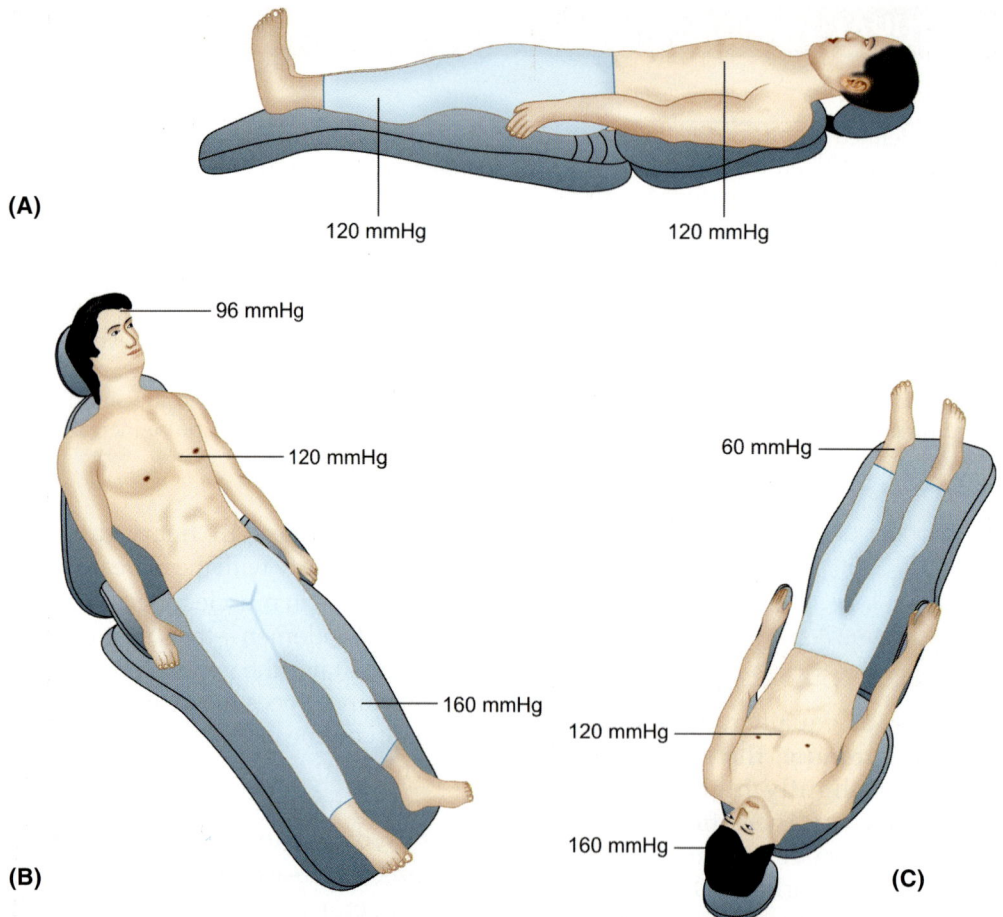

Fig. 3.15: The effect of gravity on blood pressure. **(A)** In the supine position, the effect of gravity is equalized over the entire body. The blood pressures in the legs, heart and brain are approximately equal. **(B)** In the semi-upright position, pressure is decreased by 2 mmHg for each inch the individual remains above the level of the heart. **(C)** In the Trendelenburg (head down) position, blood pressure increases to 2 mmHg for each inch the individual is situated below the level of the heart

unconsciousness persists for 10 or more seconds, the patient may exhibit minor convulsive movements. Consciousness returns rapidly once the patient is returned to the supine position.

Predisposing Factors

The factors which most commonly predispose to the development of postural hypotension are:

1. Prolonged period of recumbency or convalescence.
2. Advanced age.
3. Venous defects in the legs (e.g. varicose veins).
4. Physical exhaustion and starvation.
5. Late-stage pregnancy.
6. Recovery from sympathectomy for essential hypertension.
7. Drugs, e.g. antihypertensive drugs.
8. Addison's disease.

Postural hypotension shows a very definite increase with increasing age as hypovolemia is more common in this group, and it proves to be a major problem in the aging population.

With long appointments, e.g. the patients may remain reclined in the dental chair undergoing treatment for two or three hours. In these circumstances, postural hypotension may develop when the dental chair is returned to the upright position or the patient stands. The excessive pooling of blood in the veins of the legs in case of varicose veins predisposes to postural hypotension.

Pregnant women may demonstrate two forms of hypotension. In the first, the woman experiences postural hypotension during the first trimester, usually when she rises from bed in the morning but not recurring again during the day. The second form, known as the supine hypotensive syndrome of pregnancy, occurs late in the third trimester, if the woman remains in the supine position for more than 3 to 7 minutes. It has been demonstrated that the flaccid, gravid uterus compresses the inferior vena cava, decreases venous return from the legs to the heart with resultant syncope. Best to have the pregnant women lie more on the left side, or standing position, the weight of the uterus no longer creates this pressure on the vena cava and the clinical symptoms of syncope rapidly reverse.

Recovery from sympathectomy for high blood pressure: Surgical procedures designed to lower blood pressure and improve circulation to the legs may result in a greater incidence of postural hypotension.

Probably the most frequently encountered cause of postural hypotension in the dental office is in response to the use of drugs. The dentist may administer these drugs before, during, or after the dental treatment or the physician may prescribe them for the management of specific physical or psychologic disorders. These drugs include: antihypertensive drugs especially sodium depleting diuretics, calcium channel blockers, and ganglionic blocking agents, psychotherapeutics (sedatives and tranquilizers), opioids, histamine blockers, and L- dopa, which is used for the treatment of Parkinson's disease. Medications used to manage fear and anxiety are capable of inducing postural hypotension. Those drugs most often used in dentistry include nitrous oxide and oxygen-inhalation, diazepam, phenobarbital, midazolam, meperidine and fentanyl.

Addison s disease: Postural hypotension frequently occurs in patients on steroids (with chronic adrenocortical insufficiency) or with Addison's disease. The doctor may manage this condition through the administration of increased dose of corticosteroids to cover the increased stress of a dental appointment. If this is not done, complete vascular collapse may result. Prevention again is the most important crucial aspect. Careful history data is of vital importance. Have they fainted before at the dentist? What medications are you on?

Dental Management

1. With termination of long appointments, gradually upright the patient to help prevent any orthostatic

problem. Slowly upright position when patient recovers.

2. If hypotension persists, assess the basic support of the airway, breathing, and circulation (ABCs).

3. Provide supplemental oxygen.

4. Establish intravenous (IV) line and administer 250 to 500 ml of physiologic solution. This will improve the stroke volume and raise the blood pressure.

5. When this maneuver cannot be accomplished or proves unsuccessful, the patient's heart rate should guide further treatment:

   A. If bradycardia is present (< 60 beats/minute), atropine (0.5 mg every 3 to 5 minutes up to four doses, by IV or submucosal injection) is administered until the rate is within normal limits.

   B. If the rate is greater than 60 beats/minute and pressure remains low, increasing the rate further will do little to improve systolic blood pressure. This merely reduces the time allocated for diastolic filling, and each subsequent stroke volume will decline. Alternatively, attention should be directed to increasing stroke volume, peripheral resistance, or both.

Although several adrenergic drugs may be acceptable, ephedrine is an ideal choice for several reasons. Hypotension encountered during dental practices attributed to either vasovagal episodes or use of sedatives and anesthetics that depress sympathetic outflow to the cardiovascular system. In either case, ephedrine specifically counters these influences indirectly by stimulating norepinephrine release from sympathetic nerve endings (Fig. 3.16).

Also, ephedrine acts directly on α-adrenergic and β-adrenergic receptors, leading to vasoconstriction

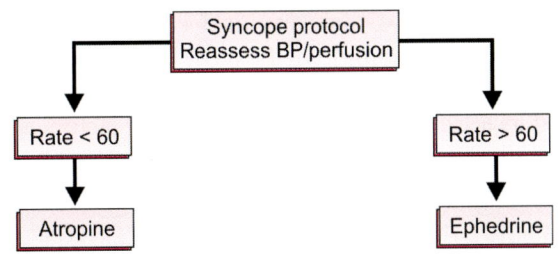

Fig. 3.16: Syncope protocol includes primary assessment (ABC) and oxygen supplementation

and increased cardiac output. Unlike epinephrine and other catecholamines with brief duration of action (5 to 10 minutes), the cardiovascular effects of ephedrine continue for 60 to 90 minutes. Ephedrine should be administered intravenously in 10 mg increments every 3 to 5 minutes or by sublingual injection, 20 to 25 mg. Total dose should not exceed 50 mg (Box 3.2).

Box 3.2: Drugs for hypotension

Action: Anticholinergic, blocks vagal slowing of heart rate.
Preparation: 1 mg/ml, SDV or ampoules.
Dose: IV or sublingual, 0.5 mg every 3 to 5 minutes up to 4 doses.

Ephedrine

Action: Mixed— α/β-receptor agonist, increases systolic/diastolic blood pressures.
Preparation: 50 mg/ml, ampoules or SDV*.
Dose: Sublingual, 25 mg every 3 to 5 minutes up to two doses; IV, 10 mg every 3 to 5 minutes up to five doses.

* SDV, Single-dose vial

HYPERTENSION

- Hypertension is not an independent risk factor, and no benefit is obtained from postponing elective surgery to get better control in patients with stable hypertension and diastolic pressures of 110 mmHg or less.
- Appointments should be in the late morning. Endogenous adrenaline level peaks during morning hours and adverse cardiac events are most likely in the early morning.
- The use of epinephrine in combination with local anesthetics is not contraindicated in the hypertensive patients unless the systolic pressure is over 200 mmHg and the diastolic is over 115 mmHg.
- Concentrations of vasoconstrictors normally used in dental local anesthetic solutions are not contraindicated in patients with cardiovascular disease when administered carefully and with preliminary aspiration "American Dental Association and American Heart Association 1964".
- Avoid anxiety and pain, since endogenous epinephrine released in response to pain or fear may induce dysrhythmias.

Hypertension is generally regarded when either or both systolic or diastolic pressures are persistently raised, and on measurement with systolic pressure over 140 mmHg and diastolic over 90 mmHg. Active treatment is required when the blood pressure at rest exceeds 160/90 mmHg (systolic/diastolic). The ideal is 140/80.

Hypertension is commonly considered to be a chronic (persistently raised) resting blood pressure higher than 140/90. It results from raised peripheral arteriolar resistance. Transient high BP resulting from emotion or exercise is not hypertension. Among other effects, it can weaken the small arteries and cause **aneurysms** (aneurysm = widening). On the other hand, hypotension is chronic low resting BP. It may be a consequence of blood loss, dehydration, anemia, or other factors and is normal in people approaching death.

THE HEMODYNAMIC MECHANISM OF HYPERTENSION

The hemodynamic effects of hypertension primarily involve the left heart. The left ventricle must compensate for the increased load imposed by the elevated peripheral resistance which tends to limit its stroke output. The work of the left heart increases and the increased heart work is nearly proportional to the blood pressure elevation. This high pressure against which the left ventricle must beat causes it to increase in weight to as much as 300 to 400 gm, instead of the usual weight of about 150 gm.

This increase is not accompanied by quite as much increase in coronary blood supply as there is increase in muscle tissue. As the hypertension becomes more and more severe, the left ventricle suffers from relative ischemia or deficient blood supply. In the late stages of hypertension, this can become serious enough that the person develops angina pectoris. Also, very high pressure in the coronary arteries causes rapid development of coronary arteriosclerosis so that the hypertensive patients tend to die of coronary occlusion at much earlier ages than do normal persons.

Factors Transiently Alter the Blood Pressure

1. Increased viscosity of the blood can cause an elevation of blood pressure as a result of an increase in the resistance to flow.

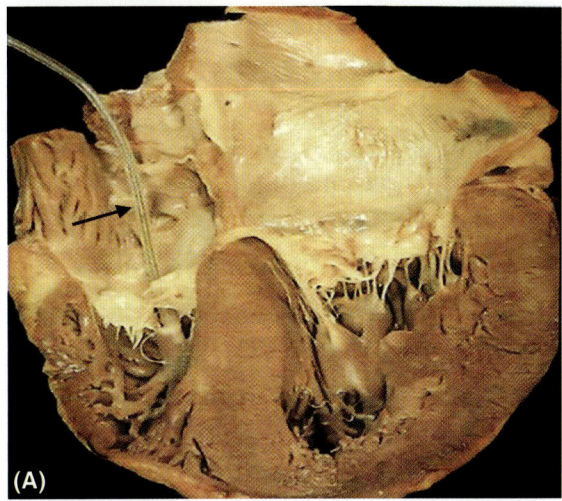 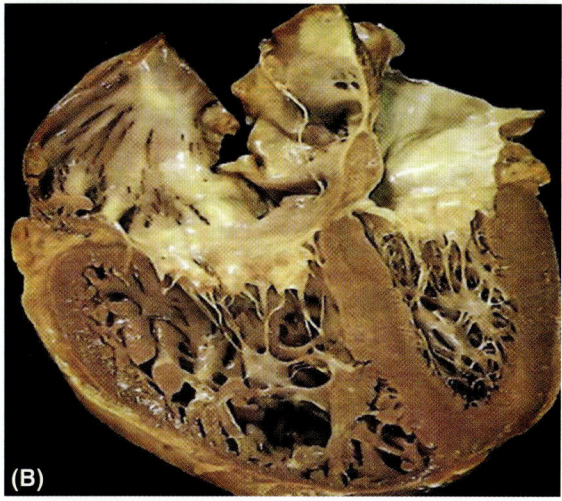

Fig. 3.17: (A) Hypertensive heart disease with thickened left ventricular wall (right side). Arrow indicates incidental pacemaker in the right ventricle. **(B)** Chronic cor pulmonale showing dilated and enlarged right ventricle with thickened wall (left side). *(From Kumae V, Abbas AK, Fausto M: Robbins and Cortan Pathologic Basis of Disease, 7th ed. Philadelphia, WB Saunders, 2005)*

2. Increase in blood volume or tissue fluid volume: A decrease in blood volume or tissue fluid volume will reduce blood pressure, and conversely an increase in blood volume or tissue fluid volume will increase blood pressure.

3. Increased cardiac output associated with exercise and fever increases the blood pressure.

4. *Acute emotions:* About 40% of hypertensive patients have raised levels of the circulating catecholamines, epinephrine or norepinephrine and may, therefore, have abnormal sympathetic activity. Acute emotions, particularly anger, fear, and anxiety play a role in raising the catecholamines level in the blood and ultimately result in hypertension.

5. Hypertension may be secondary to defined causes such as renal disease, endocrine disorders (thyrotoxicosis), pregnancy, or an oral contraceptive but in only 10% of patients.

6. Some drugs can raise the blood pressure as cocaine, amphetamines, immunosuppressives, glucocorticoids, mineralocorticoids, anabolic steroids, and some non-steroidal anti-inflammatory drugs.

7. *Failure in the regulation of vascular resistance:* In sustained hypertension, however, the basic underlying defect is a lack of control of vascular resistance. Control of vascular resistance is multifactorial and abnormalities may exist in one or more areas. Mechanism of control includes neural reflexes and ongoing maintenance of sympathetic vasomotor tone, neurotransmitters such as norepinephrine, extracellular fluid, sodium stores, the rennin-angiotensin-aldosterone pressor system, and locally active hormones such as prostaglandin, kinins, adenosine, and hydrogen ions (H^+). In isolated systolic hypertension, commonly seen in the elderly, the underlying defect is loss of elasticity of the aorta.

8. *Postoperative hypertension:* Common causes of postoperative hypertension are fluid overload, hypercapnia (hypoventilation), pain, and urinary bladder distension. Improvement of these potential causes must be done in conjunction with antihypertensive drugs.

TYPES OF HYPERTENSION

Hypertension is generally divided into benign or essential hypertension and accelerated or malignant hypertension. Any person having an arterial pressure of greater than 140/90 and who have no obvious cause for the hypertension is considered to have essential hypertension. About 90% of all persons who have hypertension have this variety. It is more frequent as age advances, and appears to be related to genetic influences, obesity, and various other factors.

Malignant hypertension usually develops after many years of moderately severe hypertension and seems clearly related to a rise over several months (Table 3.3).

Also hypertension is categorized as **primary** (essential) hypertension and **secondary** hypertension.

Table 3.3: Classification of blood pressure for adults aged 18 years and older*

Category	Systolic (mmHg)	Diastolic (mmHg)
Normal	<130	<85
High normal	130 to 139	85 to 89
Hypertension		
Stage I (mild)	140 to 159	90 to 99
Stage II (moderate)	160 to 179	100 to 109
Stage III (severe)	180 to 209	110 to 119
Stage IV (very severe)	>210	≥ 120

*When systolic and diastolic pressures fall into different categories, the higher category should be selected to classify the individual's blood pressure status.

Primary Hypertension

Primary hypertension is also known as idiopathic hypertension and it involves 90% of patients who have no identifiable cause for their disease, which accounts for 90% of cases, it results from such a complex web of behavioral, hereditary, and other factors that it is difficult to sort out any specific underlying cause. It was once considered such a normal part of the "essence" of aging that it continues to be called by another name, *essential hypertension.* That term suggests a fatalistic resignation to hypertension as a fact of life, but this need not be. Many risk factors have been identified, and most of them are controllable. Hypertension along with several other risk factors, are major determinants of cardiovascular complications. Those risk factors include obesity and dietary factors (hypercholesterolemia), and cigarette smoking.

Obesity: One of the chief risk factors is obesity. Each pound of extra fat requires miles of additional blood vessels to serve it, and all of this added vessel length increases peripheral resistance and blood pressure. Just carrying around extra weight, of course, also increases the workload on the heart. Even a small weight loss can significantly reduce blood pressure.

Sedentary behavior is another risk factor. Aerobic exercise helps to reduce hypertension by controlling weight, reducing emotional tension, and stimulating vasodilation.

Dietary factors: Dietary factors are also significant contributors to hypertension.

Diets high in cholesterol and saturated fat contribute to atherosclerosis. Potassium and magnesium reduce blood pressure; thus, diets deficient in these minerals promote hypertension. The relationship of salt intake to hypertension has been a very controversial subject. The kidneys compensate so effectively for excess salt intake that dietary salt has little effect on the blood pressure of most people. Reduced salt intake may, however, help to control hypertension in older people and in people with reduced renal function.

Nicotine: Nicotine makes a particularly devastating contribution to hypertension because it stimulates the myocardium to beat faster and harder; it also stimulates vasoconstriction and thus increases the afterload against which the myocardium must work. Just when the heart needs extra oxygen, nicotine causes coronary vasoconstriction and promotes myocardial ischemia.

Some risk factors cannot be changed at will—race, heredity, and sex. Hypertension runs in some families. A person whose parents or siblings have hypertension is more likely than average to develop it. The incidence of hypertension is about 30% higher, and the incidence of strokes about twice as high, among blacks as among whites. From ages 18 to 54, hypertension is more common in men, but above age 65, it is more common in women. Even people at risk from these factors, however, can minimize their chances of hypertension by changing risky behaviors.

Secondary Hypertension

Secondary hypertension is a high blood pressure that is secondary to (results from) other identifiable disorders. These include kidney disease (which may cause rennin hypersecretion), atherosclerosis, hyperthyroidism, Cushing's syndrome, and polycythemia. *It* accounts for about 10% of cases. Secondary hypertension is corrected by treating the underlying disease (Box 3.3).

SIGNS AND SYMPTOMS

Hypertension may remain asymptomatic for many years, but when symptoms do occur, they include headache, tinnitus, and dizziness. Late signs and symptoms are related to involvement of various target organs, including kidneys, brain, heart, or eyes (Box 3.4).

COMPLICATIONS OF HYPERTENSION

Hypertension is a "silent killer" that can wreak its destructive effects for 10 to 20 years before its effects are first noticed. Hypertension predisposes to damage to heart, kidneys, brain, and eyes (Fig. 3.18). Hypertension is the major cause of heart failure, stroke, and

Box 3.3: Identifiable causes of hypertension

- Chronic kidney disease.
- Coarctation of the aorta.
- Cushing's syndrome and other glucocorticoid excess states, including chronic long-term steroid therapy.
- Drug-induced or drug-related (e.g. NSAIDs, oral contra-ceptives, decongestants).
- Obstructive uropathy.
- Primary aldosteronism and other mineralocorticoid excess states.
- Renovascular hypertension.
- Sleep apnea.
- Thyroid or parathyroid disease.

Box 3.4: Signs and symptoms of hypertensive disease

Early
- Elevated blood pressure readings
- Narrowing and sclerosis of retinal arterioles
- Headache
- Dizziness

Advanced
- Rupture and hemorrhage of retinal arterioles
- Papilledema
- Left ventricular hypertrophy
- Proteinuria
- Congestive heart failure
- Angina pectoris
- Renal failure
- Dementia
- Encephalopathy

kidney failure. It damages the heart because it increases the afterload, which makes the ventricles work harder to expel blood. The myocardium enlarges up to a point (the *hypertrophic response),* but eventually it becomes excessively stretched and less efficient. Hypertension strains the blood vessels and tears the endothelium, thereby creating lesions that become focal points of atherosclerosis which is a major cause of hemorrhage into the brain from arterial rupture or of thrombosis complicating an atheromatous plaque. Atherosclerosis then worsens the hypertension and establishes an insidious positive feedback cycle.

Another positive feedback cycle involves the kidneys. Their arterioles thicken in response to the stress, their lumens become narrower, and renal blood flow declines. When the kidneys detect the resulting drop in blood pressure, they release renin, which leads to the formation of the vasoconstrictor angiotensin II and the release of aldosterone, a hormone that promotes salt retention. These effects worsen the hypertension that already existed. Persistent hypertension also leads to retinal damage, retinal hemorrhage and optic neuropathy. If diastolic pressure exceeds 120 mmHg, blood vessels of the eye hemorrhage, blindness ensues, the kidneys and heart deteriorate rapidly, and death usually follows within 2 years.

MEDICAL MANAGEMENT OF HYPERTENSION

Specific antihypertensive therapy is urgently indicated where the systolic pressure exceeds 200 mmHg, or the diastolic 110 mmHg and may be indicated at lower levels particularly if there are vascular complications, diabetes, or renal impairment.

For primary hypertension, lifelong treatment is usually necessary as:
1. Lifestyle modifications
2. Medical therapy

1. Lifestyle Modifications

Relaxation, weight loss, salt restriction, restricting alcohol consumption, restricting caffeine intake, stopping smoking and more exercise (Box 3.5).

2. Medical Therapy

Drugs used in hypertensive therapy are:
- *Diuretics* lower blood volume and pressure by promoting urination.
- *Ganglionic blocking agents* reduce autonomic vasoconstriction.
- *Norepinephrine antagonists* block production or compete for receptor sites.
- Smooth muscle relaxants. **Beta adrenergic blocking agents** work at the receptor sites. Beta blockers such

Box 3.5: Lifestyle modifications for the prevention and reduction of high blood pressure

- Weight loss.
- DASH (dietary approaches to stop hypertension) diet:
  - Fruits.
  - Vegetables.
  - Low-fat dairy products.
- Reduce cholesterol.
- Reduce saturated and total fat.
- Reduce sodium to <2.4 g/day.
- Regular aerobic physical activity on most days (30 minutes of brisk walking).
- Limited alcohol intake not more than 1 oz/day (2 drink for men and 1 drink for women).

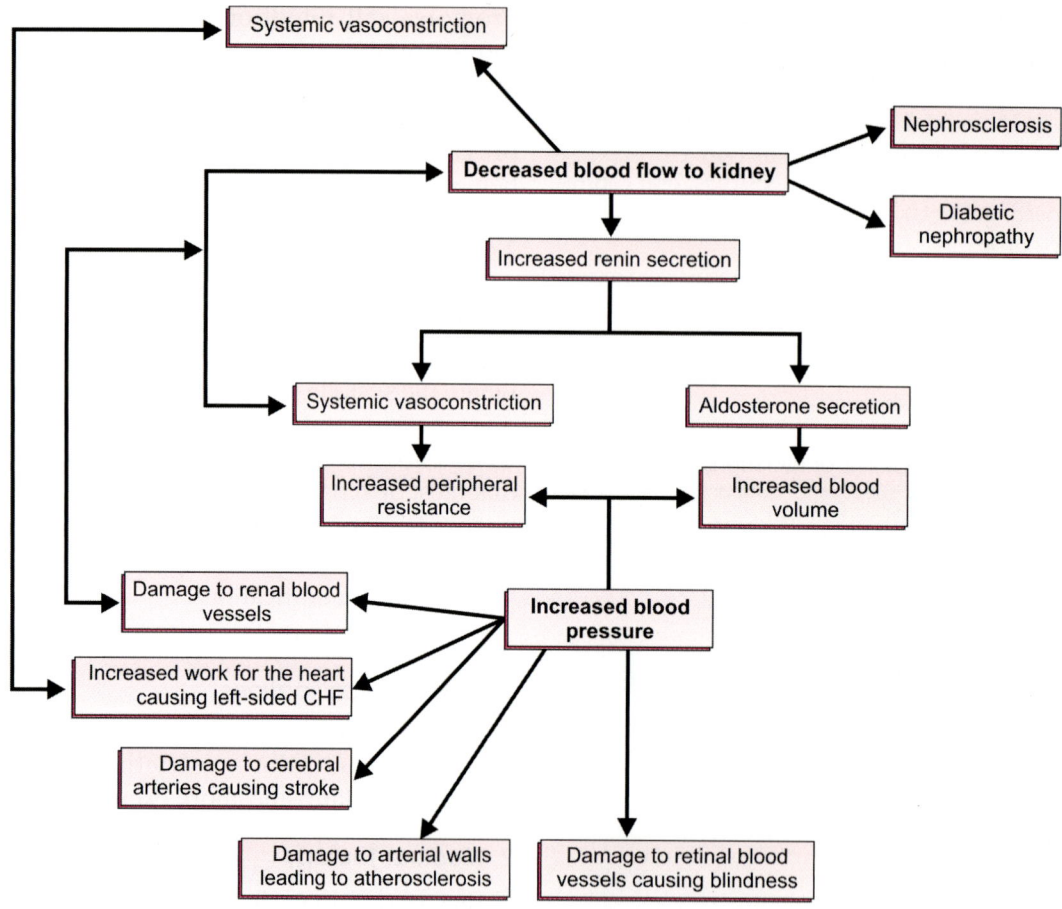

Fig. 3.18: Development and complications of hypertension

as propranolol block the vasoconstrictive action of the sympathetic nervous system.

- *CNS agents* work on spinal or thalamic vasomotor centers.

  Tranquilizers work on the psychogenic component of hypertension. Angiotensin-converting enzyme inhibitors (ACE inhibitors) block the formation of the vasoconstrictor angiotensin.

- *Calcium channel blockers*, the walls of the arteries contain smooth muscle that contracts or relaxes to change their diameter. These changes modify the blood flow and strongly influence blood pressure. Blood pressure rises when the arteries constrict and falls when they relax and dilate. Excessive, widespread vasoconstriction can cause hypertension and vasoconstriction in the coronary blood vessels of the heart can cause pain (angina) due to inadequate blood flow to the cardiac muscle. In order to contract, a smooth muscle cell must open calcium channels in its plasma membrane and allow calcium to enter

from the extracellular fluid. Drugs called *calcium channel blockers* prevent calcium channels from opening. Thus they help to relax the arteries, relieve angina, and lower blood pressure, and promoting vasodilation and reduced cardiac workload.

Antihypertensive medication should be continued as usual preoperatively, including the morning of dental visit, and postoperatively in patients diagnosed and adequately treated.

DENTAL MANAGEMENT (Box 3.6, Table 3.4)

1. At least two or three blood pressure recordings separated by several minutes should be taken on all hypertensive patients during the first dental appointment, and the results averaged. To avoid erroneous results, the measurements should not be taken immediately after entering the office but after the patient has had time to become accustomed to the surroundings. This average figure represents the blood pressure for that

Table 3.4: Dental modification for hypertensive patient. Follow-up and treatment

Normal	<130	<85	Recheck in 2 years	No restrictions
High normal	130 to 139	85 to 89	Recheck in 1 year	No restrictions
Hypertension				
Stage I (mild)	140 to 159	90 to 99	Recheck in 2 months	No restrictions
Stage II (moderate)	160 to 179	100 to 109	Refer to physician within 1 month,	No restrictions
Stage III (severe)	180 to 209	110 to 119	Refer to physician promptly (within 1 week)	Urgent care only: avoid use of vasoconstrictors.
Stage IV (very severe)	≥ 210	≤ 120	Refer to physician immediately	Palliation only; avoid use of vasoconstrictors.

Box 3.6: Dental management recommendation for patients with hypertension

- Stress/anxiety reduction. Short morning appointments.
- Consider premedication with sedative/anxiolytics.
- Consider intraoperative use of nitrous oxide/oxygen.
- Obtain excellent local anesthesia, ok to use epinephrine in modest amounts.
- Cautious use of epinephrine in local anesthesia in patients taking non-selective β-blockers or peripheral adrenergic antagonists.
- Avoid the use of epinephrine-impregnated gingival retraction cord.
- Consider periodic intraoperative BP monitoring for patients with upper level stage 2 hypertension; terminate appointment, if BP rises above 179/109.
- Slow position changes to prevent orthostatic hypotension.

appointment. The blood pressure is recorded for three reasons. First, it serves as a base line from which to make decisions for the emergency management of the patient should an untoward reaction occur during dental treatment. Second, it is used to screen patients (along with a medical history) to identify those who have or may have hypertension and to monitor compliance. Finally, it is a medicolegal necessity.

2. Avoid anxiety and pain, since endogenous epinephrine released in response to pain or fear may induce dysrhythmias. A critical factor in providing "anxiety free" situation is the relationship established among the dentist, office staff, and patient. Anxiety can be reduced by premedication with a benzodiazepine such as diazepam (Valium). An effective approach is to prescribe 2 to 5 mg at bedtime the night before and 2 and 5 mg one hour before the dental appointment.

3. Appointments should be in the late morning. Endogenous adrenaline level peaks during morning hours and adverse cardiac events are most likely in the early morning. Long appointments or stressful appointments are best avoided. If the patient becomes anxious or apprehensive during the appointment, it should be terminated and the patient scheduled for another day.

4. When administering local anesthesia, aspirating dental syringe should be used, since adrenaline in the anesthetic given intravenously may (theoretically) increase hypertension and precipitate dysrhythmias.

5. Adrenaline containing anesthetics should not be given in large doses to patients taking beta-blockers, since interactions between epinephrine and the beta-blocking agent may induce hypertension and cardiovascular complications (Box 3.7). Lidocaine should be used with caution in patients taking beta-blockers.

6. The use of epinephrine in combination with local anesthetics is not contraindicated in the hypertensive patients unless the systolic pressure is over 200 mmHg and the diastolic is over 115 mmHg (Table 3.4). Gingival retraction cords containing epinephrine should be avoided.

Vasoconstrictor Ingredient of the Local Anesthetic Cartridge

One of the most common concerns encountered when planning dental treatment for patients with hypertension and other cardiovascular disorders regards the use of a vasoconstrictor in the local anesthetic.

It is well to recall the purpose for including a vasoconstrictor in the local anesthetic. These are (1) to

Box 3.7

- One, and probably two, carpules of 2% lidocaine with 1:100,000 epinephrine (0.18 to 0.036 mg epinephrine) are of little significance in most patients with hypertension or other cardiovascular disease.
- Try to avoid the use of norepinephrine and levonordefrine in patients with hypertension due to their unopposed σ1 stimulation.
- Relative contraindications to the use of vasoconstrictors include patients with severe and very severe, uncontrolled hypertension, refractory arrhythmias, recent myocardial infarction (≤ 6 months), recent stroke (≤6 months), unstable angina, recent coronary artery bypass graft (≤3 months), uncontrolled congestive heart failure, and uncontrolled hyperthyroidism.

delay systemic absorption of the solution, which increases duration and depth of anesthesia as well as decreasing the chances of toxicity and (2) to provide local hemostasis, which enhances working conditions in the operative field. These properties allow for enhanced quality and duration of pain control and markedly facilitate the technical procedures to be performed. Without these advantages, the local anesthetic is of much shorter duration, of less effectiveness, and is absorbed more quickly, thus enhancing the possibility of toxicity. In addition, the anesthetic solution itself often has mild vasodilatory properties that can result in increased bleeding into the operative field.

A stressed patient can release up to 40 times his or her baseline catecholamine level. We also know that the half-life of epinephrine is only 2 to 5 minutes. It is rapidly inactive by catechol-O-methyltransferase. Many, therefore, feel vasoconstrictors are not contraindicated for treating hypertensive patients, especially for painful procedures where vaso-constrictor-free local anesthetics often fail to produce profound or lasting anesthesia. Dentist should strive to limit the total quantity of circulating epinephrine, which includes that administrated by the dentist in the local anesthesia and that released by the patient's adrenal medulla. Avoiding any "extra" vasoconstrictor, however, seems prudent on all compromised patients. For such patients, the dentist is thus wise to choose a norepinephrine-containing gingival retraction cord.

Caution should be taken to avoid direct intravascular injections and the use of the periodontal ligament syringe with 1:50,000 epinephrine is ill-advised due to potential rapid epinephrine absorption. Also recommended is a giving local anesthetic injection for hypertensive patients' one quadrant at a time, especially those with existing end-organ damage. For long procedures where multiple injections contemplated, the dentist should take BP readings every 10 to 15 minutes throughout the procedures.

Drug Interaction with Epinephrine

The potential danger in administering a local anesthetic containing epinephrine or other vasoconstrictor to a patient with hypertension, or other cardiovascular disease, is untoward increase in the blood pressure or development of an arrhythmia. In most cases, the amount of epinephrine administered is typically in amounts ranging from 0.018 mg to 0.054 mg (one to three cartridges of 2% lidocaine containing 1:100,000 epinephrine). The ability of epinephrine to react with various antihypertensive agents (and other drugs) to potentially yield cardiovascular complications is the subject of much research and debate. A summary of epinephrine and drug interactions follows:

Epinephrine and nonselective beta-blockers: Hypertension and a reflex bradycardia are potential consequences of this drug combination.

Epinephrine and tricyclic antidepressants: This mix also yields acute hypertensive changes, but is more of a problem with the vasoconstrictors levonordefrin and norepinephrine.

Epinephrine and diuretics: Diuretics often produce hypokalemia, which is exacerbated by epinephrine use. Low blood potassium levels increase the risk for dysrhythmias.

Epinephrine and cocaine: Although sometimes difficult to obtain from the patient history, any suspicion of cocaine use should prompt the dentist to use epinephrine with extreme caution. Those drugs together often result in BP spikes and fatal dysrhythmias. Avoiding any dental care for 24 hours following suspected cocaine use is rational.

CARDIAC ARRHYTHMIAS

Cardiac Rhythm

Contraction is called systole and relaxation is diastole. These terms can refer to a specific part of the heart (e.g. atrial systole). Normally, the chambers of the heart (atria and ventricles) contract in a coordinated manner. The contractions are caused by an electrical signal that begins in the sinoatrial node (SA), is conducted through the atria (the upper heart chambers) and stimulates the atria to contract. The electrical signals then passes through the atrioventricular node (AV), on into the bundle of His, and travels through the ventricles (the larger, lower heart chambers), stimulating them to contract. Following excitation and depolarization, the conductive tissue repolarizes to be ready for the next pulse. The normal heart beat triggered by the sinoatrial node (SA node) is called the sinus rhythm. At rest, the adult heart rate is usually around 70 to 80 beats per minute (bpm). Left to itself, the SA node would fire more often than this, but the vagus nerves inhibit it and hold it down to this rate at rest. Stimuli such as hypoxia, electrolyte imbalances, caffeine, nicotine, and other drugs can cause other parts of the conduction system to fire before the SA node does, setting off an extra heartbeat (extrasystole). Any region of spontaneous firing other than the SA node is called an Ectopic* focus. If the SA node is damaged, an ectopic focus may take over the governance of the heart rhythm. The most common ectopic focus is the AV node, which produces a slower heartbeat of 40 to 50 bpm called a nodal rhythm. If neither the SA nor AV node is functioning, other ectopic foci fire at rates of 20 to 40 bpm. The nodal rhythm is sufficient to sustain life, but a rate of 20 to 40 bpm provides too little flow to the brain to be survivable. This condition calls for an artificial pacemaker.

* ec = out of; top = place.

Cardiac Arrhythmias

- Arrhythmias may arise in the atria or ventricles (Fig. 3.19).
- The most common arrhythmias are extrasystoles and atrial fibrillation.
- Arrhythmias may be symptomless but often reduce cardiac efficiency and cardiac output and may cause dyspnea, palpitations and syncope.
- Arrhythmias may also increase the risk of: angina, myocardial infarction, cardiac failure, stroke and transient ischemic attacks, death from sudden cardiac arrest.

a = without; = rhythm; ia = condition.

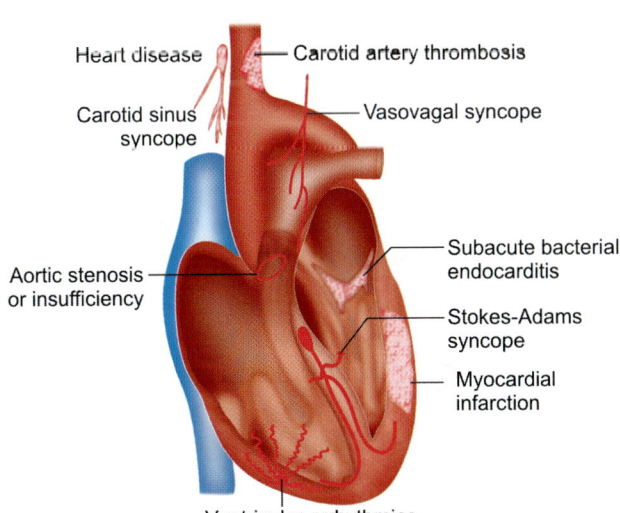

Fig. 3.19: Pathologic processes involving the heart including arrhythmias

A cardiac arrhythmia is any variation in the normal rhythm of the heart beat (abnormal cardiac rhythm). Normal cardiac function depends on cellular automaticity (impulse formation), conductivity, excitability and conductivity form the basis of the vast majority of cardiac arrhythmias. Cardiac arrhythmias may be disturbances of rhythm, rate, or conduction of the heart. They may be found in healthy individuals, patients on various medications, as well as in those with various forms of cardiovascular disease.

One cause of arrhythmia is a **heart block**—the failure of any part of the cardiac conduction system to transmit signals, usually as a result of disease and degeneration of conduction system fibers. A *bundle branch block,* for example, is due to damage to one or both bundle branches. Damage to the AV node causes *total heart block,* in which signals from the atria fail to reach the ventricles and the ventricles beat at their own intrinsic rhythm of 20 to 40 bpm.

SIGNS AND SYMPTOMS OF CARDIAC ARRHYTHMIAS

The arrhythmias may be asymptomatic, symptomatic, or even life-threatening. Although arrhythmias may be asymptomatic, however, it can be detected because of a change in the rate and/or rhythm of the pulse (Boxes 3.8 and 3.9).

Box 3.8: Identification of cardiac arrhythmias

1. *Undetected arrhythmia*
   a. Rapid or slow pulse rate.
   b. Irregular pulse rate.
   c. Associated symptoms:
      1. Palpitations.
      2. Dizziness.
      3. Syncope.
      4. Angina.
      5. Dyspnea.
2. *Susceptible to development of arrhythmia during dental treatment*
   a. History of ischemic heart disease.
   b. History of valvular heart disease.
   c. History of thyroid disease.
   d. History of obstructive pulmonary disease.
3. *Under medical treatment of arrhythmia*

Box 3.9: Signs and symptoms of cardiac arrhythmias

Signs	Symptoms
Slow heart rate (less than 60 beats/minute)	• Fatigue • Dizziness • Syncope
Fast heart rate greater than 100 beats/minute)	• Congestive heart failure • Angina

A slow pulse may indicate a form of bradycardia, and a fast pulse may indicate a tachycardia. Electro-cardiographic monitoring is needed to identify the true nature of many cardiac arrhythmias. Symptoms that may indicate the presence of an arrhythmia include fatigue, dizziness, syncope. The patient may complain of heart palpitation occurring on a regular basis.

Patients with cardiac arrhythmias are presented clinically with atrial fibrillation (flutter), premature ventricular contractions, and ventricular fibrillation.

ATRIAL FIBRILLATION

Atrial fibrillation (AF) affects around 10% of older people. It consists of totally uncoordinated and ineffectual atrial contractions. It occurs when ectopic foci in the atria set off extra contractions and the atria beat 200 to 400 times per minute. Atrial fibrillation is dangerous since it can lead to atrial thrombus formation and release of emboli, for example to the brain, and cause a stroke. Common causes are congestive heart failure, ischemic or rheumatic heart disease, or thyrotoxicosis. Atrial fibrillation causes impaired ventricular filling and an irregular, usually rapid, ventricular rate. Atrial fibrillation can also cause heart failure.

PREMATURE VENTRICULAR CONTRACTIONS (PVCs) AND FIBRILLATION

PVCs occur singly or in bursts as a result of early firing of an ectopic focus. PVCs are often due to irritation of the heart by stimulants, emotional stress, or lack of sleep, but they sometimes indicate more serious pathology.

Ventricular fibrillation is the most serious type of arrhythmias and is the most common cause of death. It is a consequence of myocardial infarction, occasionally of idiopathic fibrosis affecting the conduction system, thyrotoxicosis, halothane anesthesia, or epinephrine, cocaine or digitalis overdosage, causing electrical signals arriving at different regions of the myocardium at widely different times. A fibrillating ventricle exhibits squirming, uncoordinated contractions; it has been described as looking like a "bag of worms." Since a fibrillating heart does not pump blood, there is no coronary perfusion (blood flow) and the myocardium rapidly dies of ischemia. Fibrillation kills quickly, if it is not stopped.

Cardiac arrest is the cessation of all activity in the heart. There is no conduction of impulses, and the ECG shows a flat line. Lack of contractions means that no cardiac output occurs, depriving the brain and heart itself of oxygen. Loss of consciousness takes place immediately, and respiration ceases. There is no pulse at any site, including the apical and carotid sites.

Arrest may occur for many reasons; for example, excessive vagal nerve stimulation may slow be insufficient oxygen to maintain the heart tissue due to severe shock or ventricular fibrillation. In order to resuscitate a person, blood flow to the heart and brain must be maintained.

MEDICAL MANAGEMENT OF CARDIAC ARRHYTHMIA

The management of cardiac arrhythmias involves medication, a pacemaker, surgery, or implantable cardioversion (defibrillators) or external cardiac defibrillators.

Pacemakers are small implanted electronic devices that stimulate the heart to beat and "pace" the heart rate when it is too slow (bradycardia). This battery operated device is implanted in the chest with electrical leads to the heart of a person whose natural pacemaker (the SA node) has become erratic (Fig. 3.20). In a relatively simple operation, electrode leads (catheters) from the pacemaker are passed beneath the skin, through the external jugular vein (or other neck vein), into the superior vena cava, into the right atrium, through the tricuspid valve, and into the myocardium of the right ventricle (see drawing).

The pacing system consists of a generator that will produce an electric impulse that is transmitted by a lead to an electrode that is in contact with endocardial or myocardial tissue. A variety of pacing systems is available. Modern pacemakers are bipolar, implanted transvenously via the subclavian or cephalic vein and typically located in the right ventricle, or on the chest wall either within the pectoral muscle or underneath the skin, or in the abdominal wall (Fig. 3.20).

Defibrillation is an emergency procedure in which the heart is given a strong electrical shock with a pair of electrodes (Fig. 3.21). The purpose is to depolarize the entire myocardium and stop the fibrillation, with

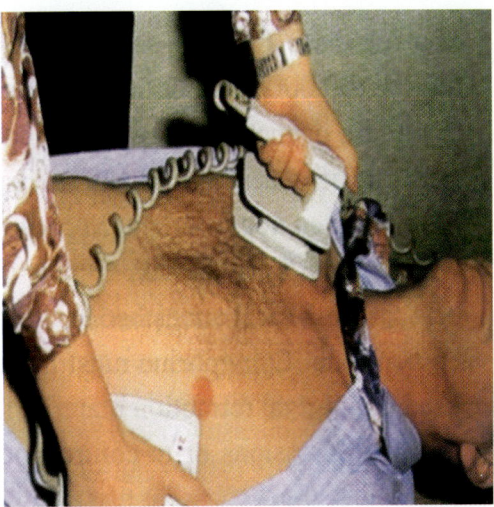

Fig. 3.21: External DC defibrillation should be performed, if the heart has not restarted or the ECG shows ventricular fibrillation, or both. The electrodes must be well separated to avoid a short circuit, electrolyte jelly is necessary for good contact with the skin, and all personnel should stand clear of the patient to avoid receiving an electric shock. Note the placement of cardioversion/defibrillation paddles on the chest *(McKliney and O'houghlin, 2006)*

the hope that the SA node will resume its sinus rhythm. This does not correct the underlying cause of the arrhythmia, but it may sustain a patient's life long enough to allow for other corrective action.

Implantable Cardioverter Defibrillators (ICDs)

ICDs are electronic devices that are the most successful treatment to prevent ventricular fibrillation. They are 99% effective in stopping life-threatening arrhythmias. They continuously monitor the heart rhythm, automatically function as pacemakers for heart rates that are too slow, and deliver life saving shocks, if a dangerous rhythm is detected.

Dental Management of Patient with Cardiac Arrhythmias

Individuals seeking dental treatment may have various forms of cardiac arrhythmias. Some of these arrhythmias are of little concern to the patient or dentist, however, many can produce symptoms, and a few can be life-threatening, including arrhythmias that can occur secondary to anxiety (e.g. those associated with dental treatment).

Patients with significant arrhythmias must be identified prior to undergoing dental treatment. The drugs which may cause cardiac arrhythmias include: Digitalis, morphine, beta blockers, calcium channel

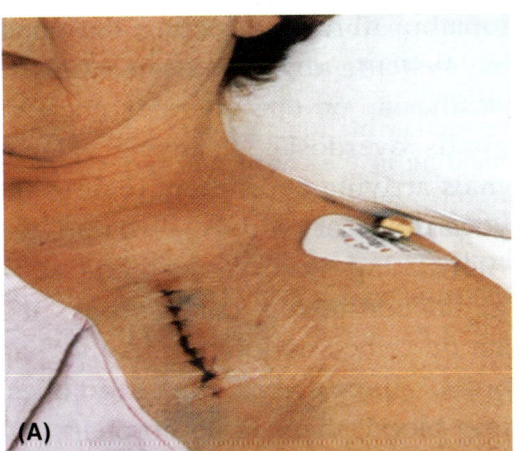

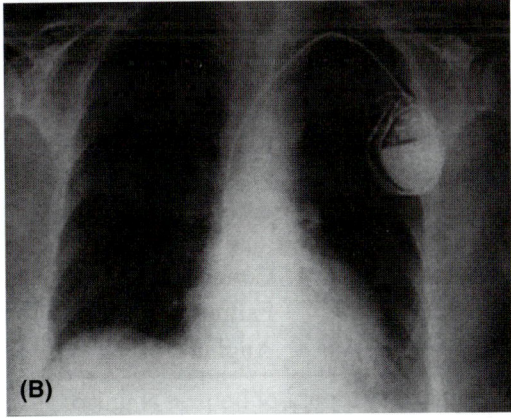

Fig. 3.20: (A) The site of implantation of a pacemaker. The pacemaker is usually implanted in the left pectoral region, but may be placed elsewhere, if necessary. **(B)** Chest X-ray showing an implanted pacing system (same patient as the previous figure). The pacemaker is in the left pectoral region, and the endocardial pacing wire is positioned at the tip of the right **ventricle,** in contact with the endocardium. *(From Chabner DA: The Language of Medicine, 6th ed. Philadelphia, WB Saunders, 2001)*

blockers, atropine, epinephrine, nicotine, caffeine, alcohol, and tricyclic antidepressants.

The following procedures should be followed:

1. *Reduce the patient anxiety:* Any increases in sympathetic tone can precipitate an arrhythmia. Premedication with diazepam (Valium) 5 mg on the night before the appointment may be used. Nitrous oxide inhalation can be initiated. An open honest approach with the patient explaining what will happen is most important.

2. *Minimize stressful situations:* Patients with coronary atherosclerotic heart disease, ischemic heart disease, or congestive heart failure should be managed to prevent or minimize acute exacerbation of these conditions that might trigger significant arrhythmias.

3. *Avoid excessive amounts of vasoconstrictive agents:* At the same time, however, vasoconstrictors in appropriate concentration in the local anesthetic are indicated. The need to achieve profound local anesthesia and hemostasis far outweighs the very slight risk of using these agents in small amounts (e.g. 1:100,000 epinephrine). However, the use of more than two cartridges (1.8 ml) of anesthetic is not advised for any given appointment. In patients with severe arrhythmias, it may be best to use a local anesthetic without epinephrine. Epinephrine must not be used in gingival retraction material for crown impressions or to control local bleeding.

4. *Avoid general anesthesia:* Patient susceptible to developing significant cardiac arrhythmias should

Box 3.10: Sources of electromagnetic interference with pacemaker function

Television set	Diathermy unit
Electrocautery unit	Radio transmitter
Radar transmitter	Boat or automobile motor
Any electric Cavitron	Electric pulp tester
Microwave oven	Arc welder

not be given general anesthesia in the dental office. Be careful when using electrical equipment. During the medical consultation for patients with pacemaker, the risk for electromagnetic interference from electrical equipment used in the dental office should be established. Patients with a new well-shielded generator are at low risk. However, patients with poor shielding may be at high risk for complications in pacing because of *electromagnetic interference.* Pulp testers, motorized dental chairs, belt driven handpieces, and ultrasonic sealers all may be capable of causing pacemaker malfunction in a patient with poor shielding in the pacemaker generator. Electrosurgery units can be of risk to all pacemaker patients, and their use in these patients is contraindicated (Box 3.10).

5. *Minimize prophylactic antibiotics:* Although patients with a pacemaker are potentially susceptible to infective endocarditis, the incidence of this is extremely low; therefore, antibiotic prophylaxis is not generally indicated.

The precautions that must be taken during dental treatment for patients with cardiac arrhythmias is mentioned in Box 3.11.

Box 3.11: Precautions must be taken during dental treatment for patients with cardiac arrhythmias

Stress and anxiety reduction

- Establish good rapport.
- Short schedule, morning appointments.
- Ensure comfortable chair position.
- Provide preoperative sedation (short-acting benzodiazepine night before and/or 1 hour before appointment).
- Administer intraoperative sedation (nitrous oxide/oxygen).
- Obtain pretreatment vital signs.
- Ensure profound local anesthesia.
- Provide adequate postoperative analgesia.

Vasoconstrictors

- Epinephrine-containing local anesthetic can be used with minimal risk, if the dose is limited to 0.036 mg epinephrine (2 carpules containing 1: 100,000 concentrations). Higher doses may be tolerated, but the risk of complications increases with dose. Avoid the use of epinephrine in retraction cord.

Contd...

Contd...

For patients with atrial fibrillation who are taking warfarin (Coumadin)

- Should have current international normalized ratio (INR) (within 24 hours of surgical procedure).
- If INR is within the therapeutic range (INR, 2.0–3.5), dental treatment, including minor oral surgery, can be performed without stopping or altering the coumadin.
- Local measures include gelatin sponge or oxidized cellulose in sockets, suturing, gauze pressure packs, preoperative stents, and tranexamic acid or E-aminocaproic acid mouth rinse and/or to soak gauze.

For patients with pacemakers

- Antibiotic prophylaxis to prevent bacterial endocarditis is not recommended.
- Avoid the use of electrosurgery and ultrasonic sealers.

For patients taking digoxin

- Watch for signs or symptoms of toxicity (e.g. hypersalivation).
- Avoid epinephrine or levonordefrine.

For the high-risk patient who requires urgent care, consider treating in special care clinic or hospital

- Consult with physician
- Provide limited care only for pain control, treatment acute infection, or control of bleeding
  - Intravenous line
  - Sedation
  - Electrocardiogram (ECG) monitoring
  - Pulse oximeter
  - Blood pressure monitoring
  - Avoid or limit epinephrine

ISCHEMIC HEART DISEASES

Myocardial ischemia can be manifested clinically as brief pain (angina pectoris), prolonged pain (myocardial infarction), or sudden death (usually due to arrhythmia). Angina pectoris and consequently myocardial infarction occur when there is a deficit of oxygen for the heart muscle. This can occur when the blood or oxygen supply to the myocardium is impaired.

The Coronary Circulation

If your heart beats an average of 75 times a minute for 80 years, it will beat more than 3 billion times and pump more than 200 million liters of blood. Understandably, it requires an abundant supply of oxygen and nutrients. Even though the heart is only 0.5% of the body's weight, it uses 5% of the circulating blood to meet its own metabolic needs. The cardiac muscle is not nourished to any great extent by the blood flowing through the heart chambers. Instead, it has its own supply of arteries and capillaries that deliver blood to every cell of the myocardium. The blood vessels of the heart wall constitute the coronary circulation. At rest, these vessels supply the myocardium with about 250 ml of blood per minute.

ANGINA PECTORIS (ATHEROSCLEROSIS OF THE CORONARY ARTERIES)

ANATOMY OF CORONARY ARTERIES

Immediately after the aorta leaves the left ventricle, it gives off right and left coronary arteries (Fig. 3.22). Each coronary artery begins at an opening deep in the cup formed by a cusp of the aortic valve, like a hole in the bottom of a pocket. The **left coronary artery** passes under the left auricle and divides into two branches:

1. The **anterior interventricular artery** travels down the anterior interventricular sulcus toward the apex. It issues smaller branches to the interventricular septum and anterior walls of both ventricles. Clinically, this vessel is also called the *left anterior descending (LAD) artery.*

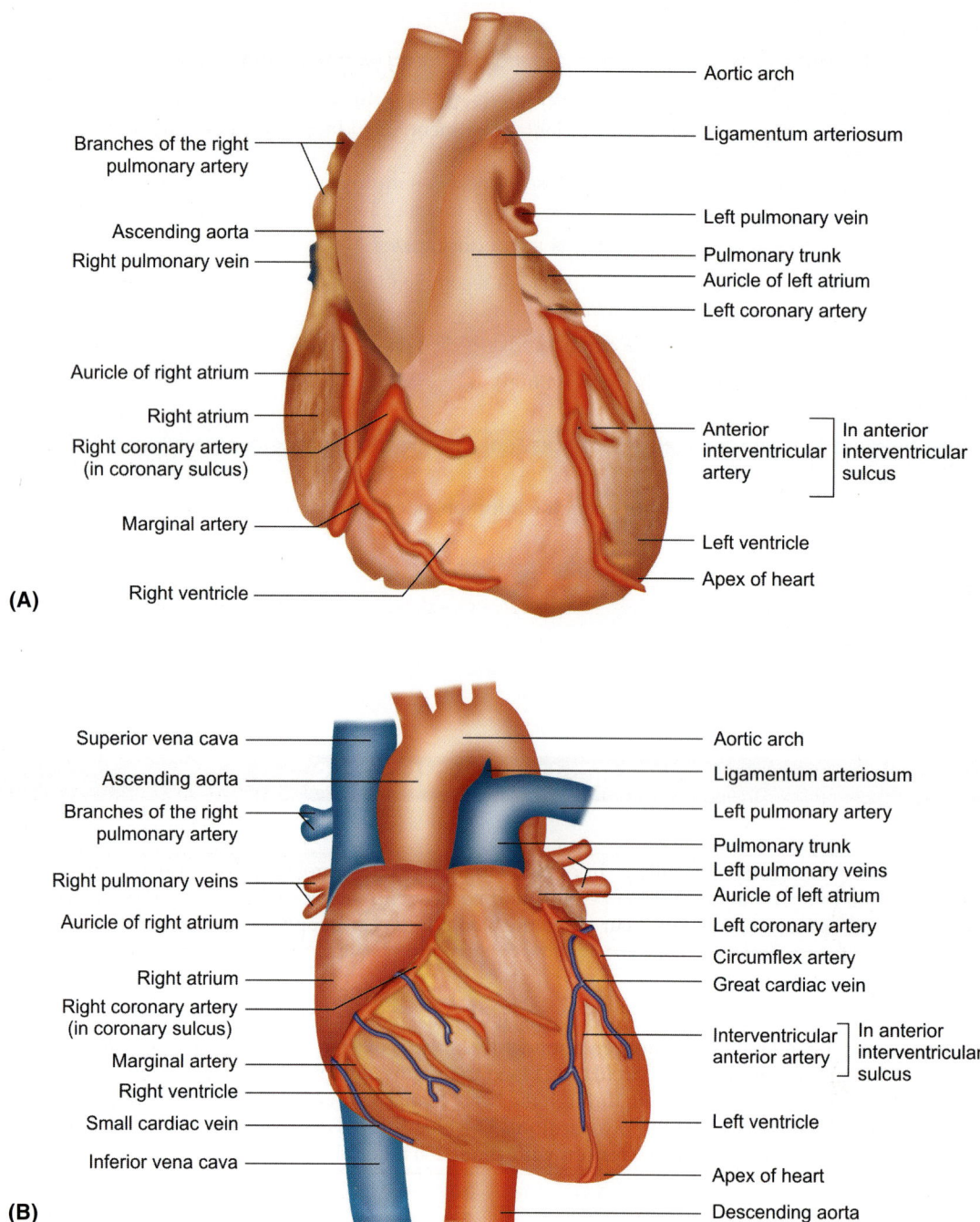

Fig. 3.22: External anatomy and features of the heart. **(A)** A cadaver photo shows the right atrium, right ventricle, and apex of the heart in an anterior view. **(B)** A drawing show the left atrium, left ventricle and base of the heart in a posterior view *(McKliney & O'houghlin, 2006)*

2. The **circumflex artery** continues around the left side of the heart in the coronary sulcus. It supplies blood to the left atrium and posterior wall of the left ventricle.

3. The **right coronary artery** supplies the right atrium, continues along the coronary sulcus under the right auricle, and then gives off two branches:

a. The **marginal artery** supplies the lateral aspect of the right atrium and ventricle.

b. The **posterior interventricular artery** travels down the corresponding sulcus and supplies the posterior walls of both ventricles.

The accumulation of lipid-laden cells in the intima of a blood vessel is the underlying cause for the development of atherosclerosis.

PATHOLOGY

Atherosclerosis is a disorder in which fatty deposits form in an artery, obstruct the lumen, and cause deterioration of the arterial wall (Figs 3.23 and 3.24). It is especially critical when it occurs in the coronary arteries and threatens to cut off the blood supply to the myocardium. Atherosclerosis is also a leading contributor to stroke and kidney failure.

Atherosclerosis is the underlying cause not only of coronary heart disease (heart attack), but also of cerebrovascular disease (stroke), and peripheral arterial disease (intermittent claudication). The atherosclerotic process primarily affects the intima of the artery, causing the intima to thicken, resulting in a narrowed lumen and diminished blood flow and oxygen supply.

The consequent narrowing of the involved coronary artery leads to a decrease in blood flow to a portion of

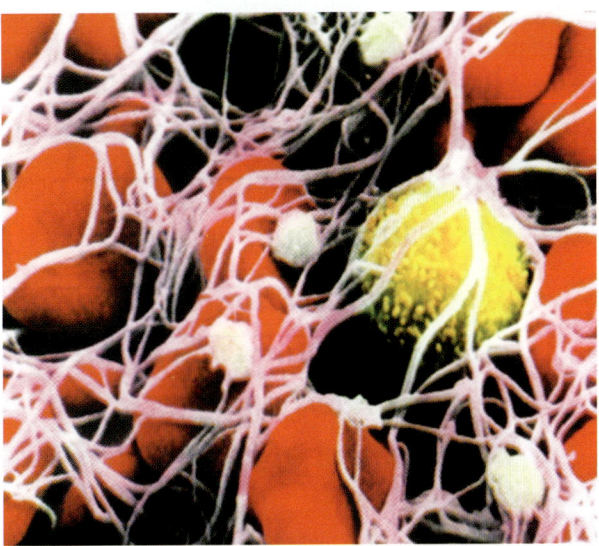

Fig. 3.24: The end product of the coagulation system, which shows a fibrin clot or thrombus. White threads are fibrin, the structure with yellow on the surface is white blood cell, platelets are green, and the red structures are red blood cells *(Little JW, Falace DA, Miller CS, Rhodus, naRhodus NL: Dental Management of the Medically Compromised Patient. Mosby Inc, 2008)*

athero = fat, fatty; Sclerosis = hardening

angio = vessel; plasty = surgical repair

the heart muscle, resulting in myocardial ischemia and affects the efficiency of the heart as a pump. In these instances, the myocardial blood supply cannot be sufficiently increased to meet the increased oxygen requirements of the cardiac muscle.

A discrepancy exists between the myocardial oxygen demands and the ability of the coronary arteries to supply oxygen-carrying blood.

The myocardial oxygen demand can be increased generally by exertion, anxiety, or during digestion of heavy meal, i.e. during physical or emotional stress 'angina of effort' (Fig. 3.25).

As atherosclerosis (atheroma) grows, more and more of the arterial lumen becomes obstructed. Angina pectoris and other symptoms begin to occur when the lumen of a major coronary artery is reduced by at least 75%. When platelets adhere to lesions of the arterial wall, they release clotting factors, so an atheroma can become a focus for thrombosis. A clot can block what remains of the lumen, or it can break free and become an embolus that travels downstream until it lodges in a smaller artery. Part of an atheroma itself can also break loose and travel as a *fatty embolus.*

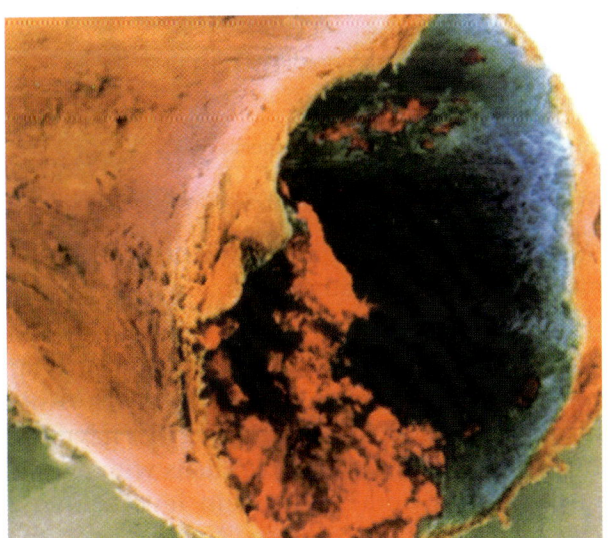

Fig. 3.23: A colored scanning electron micrograph of a blood clot or thrombus inside the coronary artery of a human heart. *(Little JW, Falace DA, Miller CS, Rhodus NL: Dental Management of the Medically Compromised Patient. Mosby Inc, 2008, p 400)*

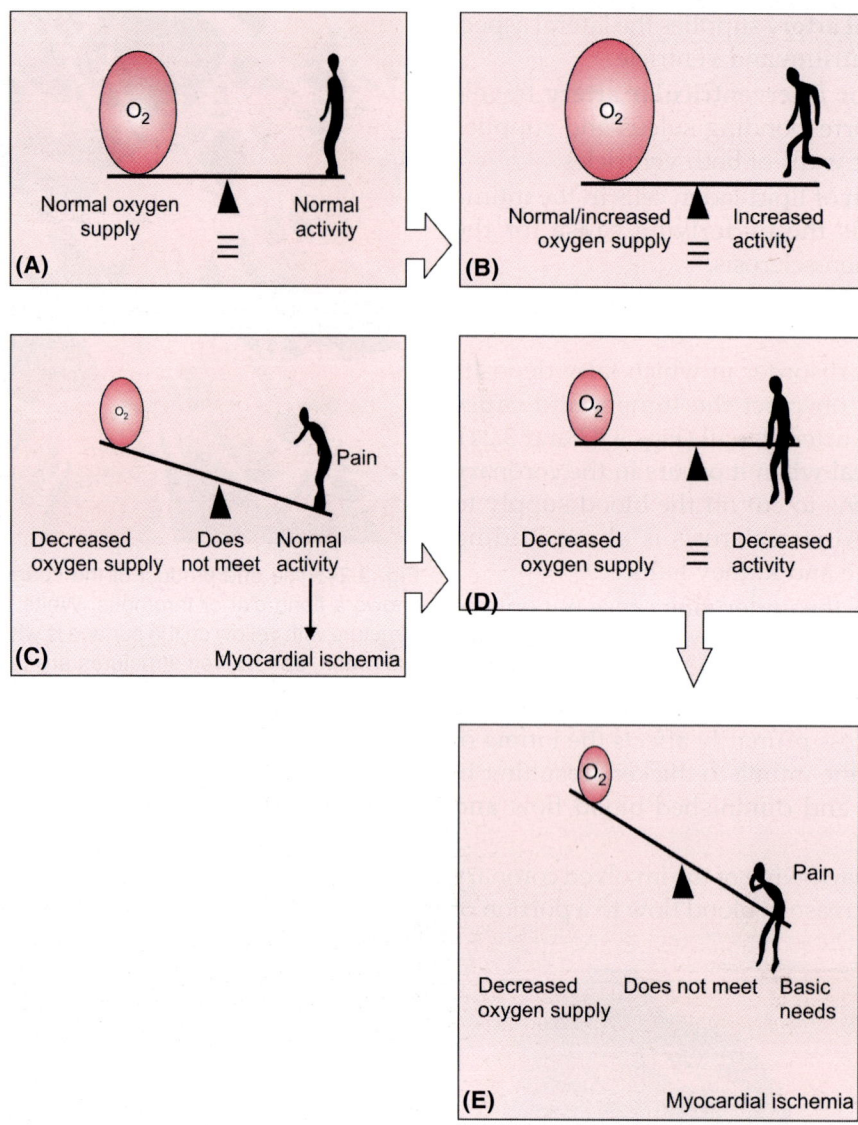

Fig. 3.25: Angina—an imbalance between oxygen supply and demand *(Gould, 2006)*

Atheromas also contribute to coronary artery spasms. Healthy endothelial cells secrete nitric oxide (NO), which causes the arteries to dilate. Vessels damaged by atherosclerosis release less NO, and the coronary arteries exhibit spasms. With much of the lumen already obstructed by the atheroma and perhaps a thrombus, an arterial spasm can temporarily shut off the remaining flow and precipitate an attack of angina (Fig. 3.26).

RISK FACTORS

The cause of coronary atherosclerosis is multifactorial and related to a variety of risk factors. Major risk factors are sex, familial history, hyperlipidemia, cigarette smoking, and diabetes mellitus.

Elevation of serum lipid levels is considered to be a major risk factor for atherosclerosis.

Increased level of low density lipoprotein (LDL) cholesterol carry the greatest risk for coronary atherosclerosis, whereas increased levels of high density lipoprotein (cholesterol, HDL) have been shown to reduce the risk. Individuals with elevated triglyceride or beta-lipoprotein levels have an increased risk for the disease. A diet rich in total calories, saturated fats, cholesterol, sugars, and salts also increases the risk.

Increased blood pressure appears to be one of the most significant unequivocal risk factors in coronary atherosclerotic heart disease. It has been reported that

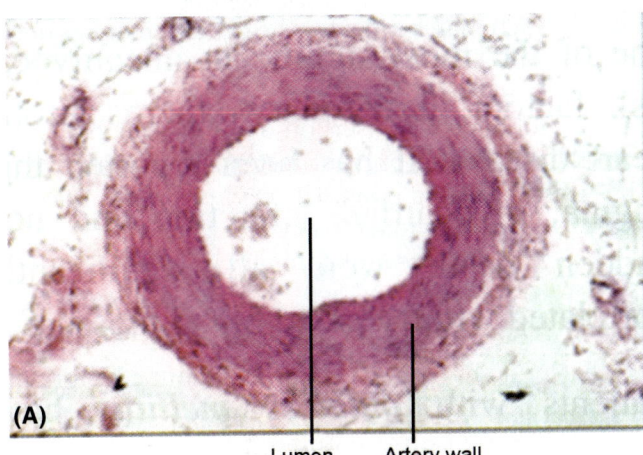

(A)

Lumen   Artery wall

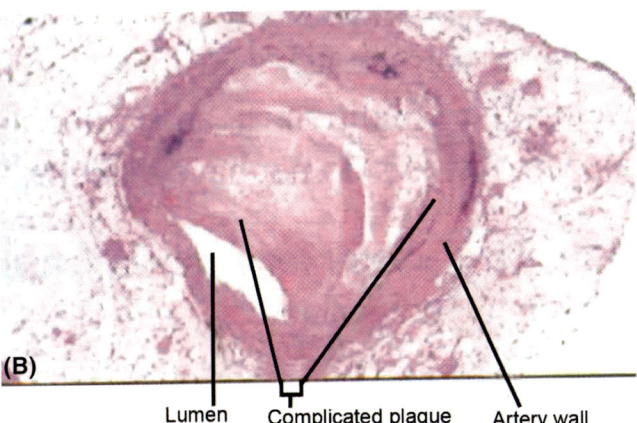

(B)

Lumen   Complicated plaque   Artery wall

Fig. 3.26: Atherosclerosis. (A) Cross-section of a healthy artery. **(B)** Cross-section of an artery with advanced atherosclerosis. The lumen is reduced to a small space that can easily be blocked by thrombosis, embolism, or vasoconstriction. Most of the original lumen is obstructed by a complicated plaque composed of calcified scar tissue *(Saladin: Anatomy and Physiology: The Unity of Form and Function; McGraw-Hill Co. 3rd ed. 2003)*

angina, myocardial infarction and non-sudden death were all significantly correlated with elevated blood pressure.

Patients with *diabetes mellitus* have been found to have a greater incidence of coronary atherosclerotic heart disease, to have more extensive lesions, and to develop the condition at an earlier age than persons who do not have diabetes.

Most risk factors for atherosclerosis, however, are preventable:

- A sedentary lifestyle promotes LDL formation, whereas exercise promotes the formation of *high-density lipoproteins (HDLs)*, which not only contribute to coronary disease but also help to lower blood cholesterol.
- Obesity is a risk factor that can be reduced by exercise.
- Aggressiveness, anxiety, and emotional stress promote hypertension and atherosclerosis.
- The risk for developing coronary atherosclerotic heart disease in *cigarette smokers* is approximately twice that of non-smokers. The incidence of coronary heart disease is proportional to the number of cigarettes smoked per day and the number of years a person has been a smoker. This is reversible; people who quit smoking drop to normal risk levels within 5 years.
- Diet, of course, is an overwhelmingly important factor. Eating animal fat reduces the number of LDL receptors and raises plasma LDL levels. Foods high in soluble fiber (such as beans and apples) lower blood cholesterol by an interesting mechanism. The liver normally converts cholesterol to bile acids, which it secretes into the small intestine to aid fat digestion. The bile acids are reabsorbed farther down the intestine and recycled to the liver for reuse. Soluble fiber, however, binds bile acids and carries them out in the feces. To replace them, the liver must synthesize more, thus using more cholesterol and lowering the blood cholesterol.

In the 1970s, scientists found that the Eskimos of Greenland had unusually low rates of coronary atherosclerosis despite the fact that their diet consisted entirely of meat—averaging a pound of whale meat and a pound of fish per day. Japanese and other groups with large amounts of fish in their diets also show low blood cholesterol levels. It is suspected that this is due to *omega-3 polyunsaturated fatty acids (PUFAs)* in fish oil. PUFAs increase the fluidity of plasma membranes and enable cells to remove more lipid from the blood. However, a daily capsule of fish oil does not hold much promise for controlling cholesterol. Doses of PUFAs high enough to reduce blood cholesterol would be prohibitively expensive and have undesirable side effects, including suppression of the immune system. Studies on the effectiveness of PUFAs remain inconclusive.

TREATMENT OPTIONS

The first pioneering approach to treating atherosclerosis, and still a common standby, is *coronary artery bypass surgery* (Fig. 3.27). Sections of the great saphenous vein of the leg or small arteries

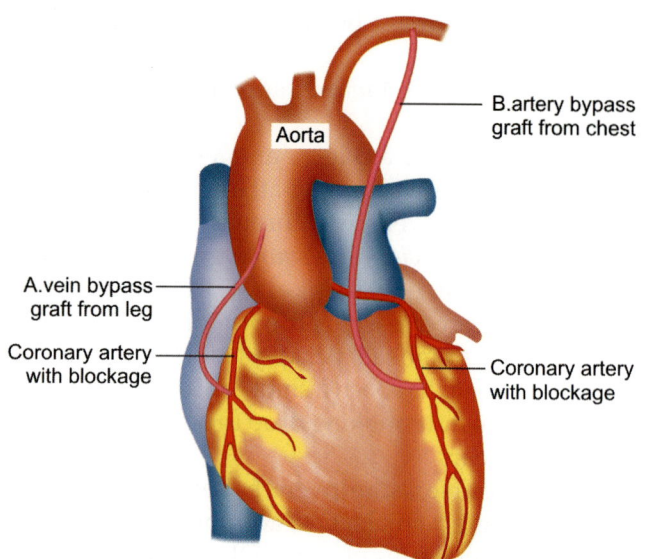

Fig. 3.27: Coronary artery bypass graft (CABG) surgery *(from Chabner DE: The Language of Medicine, 7th ed, Philadelphia, WB Saunders, 2004)*

from the thoracic cavity are used to construct a detour from the aorta to a point on a coronary artery beyond the obstruction.

Balloon angioplasty is a technique in which a thin, flexible catheter is threaded into a coronary artery to the point of obstruction, and then a balloon at its tip is inflated to press the atheroma against the arterial wall, opening up the lumen. Its usefulness is limited to well-localized atheromas.

In another method, *laser angioplasty*, an illuminated catheter enables the surgeon to see inside a diseased artery on a monitor and to use a laser to vaporize atheromas and reopen the artery. These methods are cheaper and less risky than bypass surgery. However, there is some concern that these procedures may cause new injuries to the arterial

walls, which may be foci for the development of new atheromas. Also, angioplasty is often followed by *restenosis*— atheromas grow back and reobstruct the artery months later. Insertion of a tube called a *stent* into the artery can prevent restenosis, ensuring that the vessel remains open. Clearly, prevention is the least expensive, least risky, and most effective approach to the threat of coronary artery disease.

DENTAL MANAGEMENT

Patients who have stable angina without a history of infarction generally have a much lower risk of complications occurring in the dental office than do patients who have unstable angina or a history of a recent myocardial infarction.

1. Careful history taking of the case. The patient should be questioned about the events that precipitate the angina, the frequency, duration, and severity of angina, and the response to medication. Since the treatment includes the use of vasodilators when pain is experienced, details of the frequency of need for these tablets will give an indication of the severity of the disease.

2. Consultation with the patient's physician. Where use of the drug is frequent, or increasing in frequency, advice should be thought from the patient's physician.

3. The patients should be given short morning appointments.

4. The dental management of the dental patient with a history of ischemic heart disease who develops chest pain, "patient with stable angina pectoris or history of myocardial infarction" is mentioned in Box 3.12. Refer to Chapter 15, Page 704 "H" Angina Pectoris.

Box 3.12: Management of dental patient with a history of ischemic heart disease who develops chest pain, "patient with stable angina pectoris or history of myocardial infarction"

1. Pretreatment home
   - Benzodiazepine (5 mg diazepam) night before and one hour before appointment.
   - Application of long acting dermal nitroglycerine.
   - Pretreatment vital signs.
   - Patients receiving daily aspirin therapy may have increased bleeding, but is usually not clinically significant.
   - If patient is taking warfarin sodium (coumadin) for anticoagulation, pretreatment prothrombin time should be less than 2 times (normal international normalized ratio (INR) <3.0).
2. Avoid elective dental care.
3. Short appointments (AM appointment probably preferable).
4. Semisupine chair position for comfort.
5. Patient should bring own supply of nitroglycerine for use, if necessary.

Contd....

Contd....

6. Ensure good pain control: Use local anesthetic with vasoconstrictor (epinephrine, maximum dose 0.036 mg; levonordefrine 0.20 mg).
7. Avoid use of epinephrine in retraction cord.
8. Avoid anticholenergic drugs (scopolamine or atropine).
9. If patient becomes fatigued or has a change in pulse rate or rhythm,
   - Stop dental procedure.
   - Give patient nitroglycerine tablet under tongue.
   - Administer O_2
   - Periodic or continuous monitoring of vital signs:
     a. If pain is relieved within 5 minutes, let patient rest and continue with appointment or terminate appointment and reschedule for another day.
     b. If pain is not relieved within 5 minutes:
       i. Take patient's blood pressure and pulse
       ii. If patient's condition is stable, give second nitroglycerine tablet, if pain is relieved within 5 minutes manage simple dental procedure, e.g. temporary filling.
       iii. If patient's condition remains stable but pain continues, give third nitroglycerine tablet, if pain is relieved within 5 minutes, manage as in the above.
       iv. If pain is not relieved following three nitroglycerine tablets given within 15 minute period, or if patient becomes unstable at any time, call for immediate transport to emergency unit.

* Trinitroglycerine. Inpatients with frequent attacks of angina, especially those whose attacks are triggered by situational anxiety, it may be useful to administer sublingual nitroglycerine just before injection of the local anesthetic agent. Such injections frequently are the most stressful point of an outpatient oral surgery visit.

MYOCARDIAL INFARCTION

The cardiac tissue is supplied by a system of coronary blood vessels. Blockage of any major coronary artery can cause myocardial infarction, death of cardiac muscle due to lack of oxygen.

PHYSIOLOGY

The **myocardium** (Fig. 3.28), by far the thickest layer, is composed of cardiac muscle and performs the work of the heart.

Its muscle cells spiral around the heart and are bound together by a meshwork of collagenous and elastic fibers that make up the **fibrous skeleton.** The fibrous skeleton has at least three functions: to provide structural support for the heart, especially around the valves and the openings of the great vessels; to give the muscle something to pull against; and, as a nonconductor of electricity, to limit the routes by which electrical excitation travels through the heart. This insulation prevents the atria from stimulating the ventricles directly and is important in the timing and coordination of electrical and contractile activity. Elastic recoil of the fibrous skeleton may also aid in refilling the heart with blood after each beat, but physiologists are not in complete agreement about this. The **endocardium** consists of a simple squamous endothelium overlying a thin areolar tissue layer. It forms the smooth inner lining of the chambers and valves and is continuous with the endothelium of the blood vessels.

PATHOLOGY

Myocardial infarction is necrosis of the myocardium supplied by a coronary artery that becomes narrowed or completely occluded and does not spontaneously reopen within a few minutes (Figs 3.29 and 3.30).

If the degree of ischemia resulting from coronary atherosclerosis is significant, the area of myocardium supplied by that vessel can undergo necrosis. The infarction may be subendocardial or transmural, the latter involving the entire thickness of the myocardium.

Signs and Symptoms

Acute myocardial infarction may be silent (i.e. without anginal symptoms) without untoward events or silent with development of arrhythmias, heart block, bundle branch block, or heart failure.

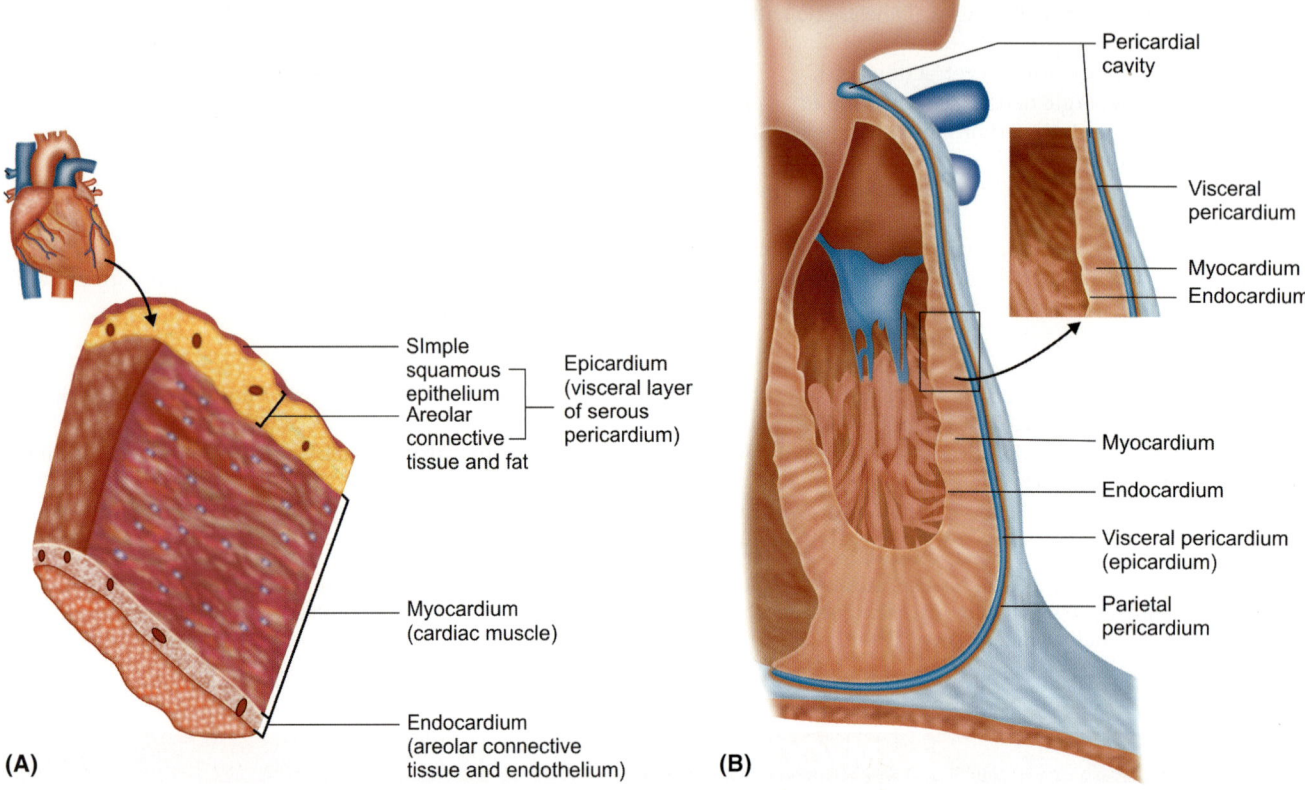

Fig. 3.28: **(A)** The layers of the heart wall (peri-, endo-, and myocardium). **(B)** Organization of the heart wall. The heart wall contains an outer epicardium (visceral layer of serous pericardium), a middle myocardium (composed of cardiac muscle), and an inner endocardium (composed of areolar connective tissue and an endothelium) *(McKliney & O'houghlin,2006)*

The signs and symptoms disappear once the myocardial work requirements are lowered or the oxygen supply to the heart is increased. Heart failure occurs when 30% of the left ventricle is infarcted, and cardiogenic shock when 40% is infracted.

When signs and symptoms develop, the following are common:

1. The feeling of heavy pressure, squeezing sensation or severe pain of short duration in the substernal region. When the chest pain lasts over 30 minutes and not relieved by nitroglycerine it has to be considered infarction unless not confirmed by ECG and cardiac enzyme studies, or myocardial scanning with technetium –99, if the ECG and enzymes are not definitive.

2. Radiation of the sternal pain to the left shoulder, arm, and the submandibular region.

3. As a result of stimulation of the vagus nerve activity, which generally follows, there is nausea, sweating, and bradycardia.

Complications

Complications of myocardial infarction include weakened heart muscle resulting in acute congestive heart failure, post-infarction angina, infarct extension, cardiogenic shock, pericarditis, and arrhythmias. As a general rule, elective surgery should not be done 6 months of a myocardial infarction and 3 months of coronary bypass surgery. The risk of reinfarction is 20 to 30% within the first 3 months, 10 to 15% after 4 to 6 months, and 5% after 6 months. Three months is a safe estimate after bypass surgery.

Management (Box 3.13)

1. Patients should be asked to bring their nitroglycerine with them to each appointment and keep it handy should they experience angina during the dental appointment. Some dentists advice premedication with glyceryl trinitrate tablets or sublingual spray. The vasodilator effect lasts about half an hour.

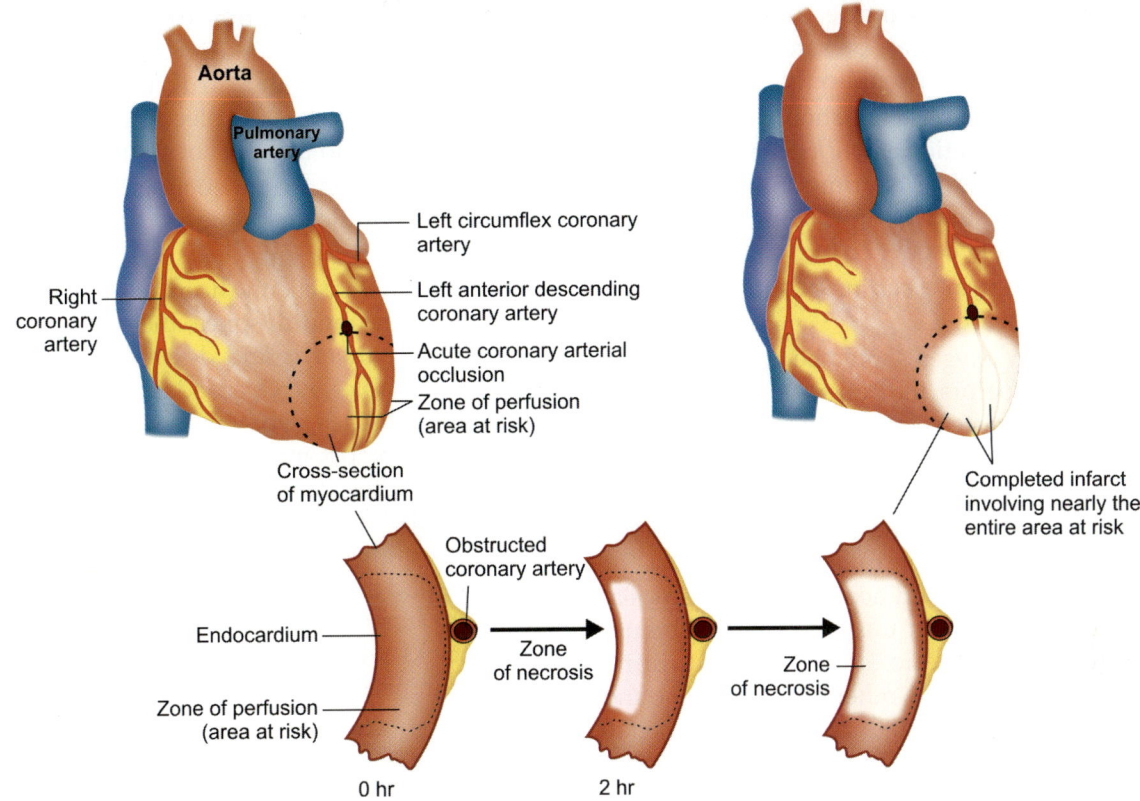

Fig. 3.29: Progression of myocardial necrosis after coronary artery occlusion *(Schoen FJ. The heart. In Kumar V, Abbas AK, Fusto N [eds]. Robbins and Cotran Pathologic Basis of Disease, 7th ed. Philadelphia, Saunders, 2005)*

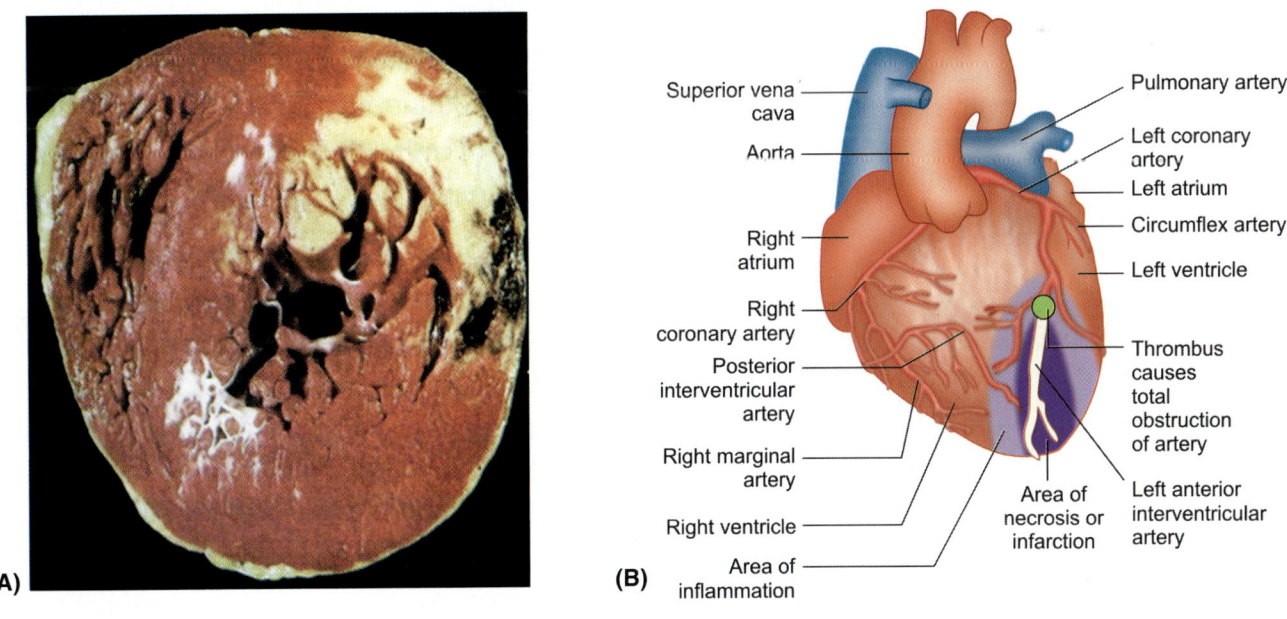

Fig. 3.30: (A) Damage caused by myocardial infarction. **(B)** Acute myocardial infarct of the posterolateral left ventricle, shown by lack of stain in the necrotic area. Note the dark area on the right indicating hemorrhage and ventricular rupture. The white area on the lower left indicates an old infarct *(From Kumar V, Abbas AK, Fausto M: Robbins and Cotran Pathologic Basis of Disease, 7th ed. Philadelphia, WB Saunders, 2005)*

2. Once the decision is made that ambulatory elective oral surgery can be safely proceed, the vital signs should be periodically monitored.

3. Anxiety reduction protocol should be followed. Anxiolytic medication such as diazepam, 2 to 5 mg, can be given at bedtime the night before the appointment and again one hour before the appointment, if needed.

4. Keep the patient in a supine position to reduce strain on the heart.

5. Supplementary oxygen should be available. When anginal attack occurs, the patient is laid down and oxygen is administered at 6 liters/minute.

6. Profound local anesthetic is the best means of limiting patient's anxiety. Although some controversy exists over the use of local anesthetics containing epinephrine in angina patients, the benefits (prolonged and accentuated anesthesia) outweight the risks. In unstable angina, the use of a local anesthetic solution containing octapressin is indicated, otherwise lignocaine and adrenaline may be used. Care should be taken to avoid excessive epinephrine administration by using proper injection techniques. Some clinicians also advise giving no more than 4 ml of a local anesthetic containing 1:100,000 concentration of epinephrine or a total adult dose of 0.04 mg in any thirty-minute period. Generally, the amount of epinephrine should be limited to 0.036 mg and of levonordefrine to 0.20 mg. Gingival retraction cord impregnated with epinephrine should not be used.

7. Regular verbal contact with the patient should be maintained.

8. Patients with angina or post-myocardial infarction may be taking daily aspirin as an antiplatelet aggregation drug. In this case, one can expect some increase in bleeding, but it is locally controllable and usually not clinically significant.

9. Anticholinergic drugs such as scopolamine or atropine should be avoided due to a resulting tachycardia.

If a patient with ischemic heart disease experiences chest pain, sweat, and dyspnea, the dental procedure is halted, the patient is laid down and a sublingual nitroglycerine tablet and O_2 are administered (Box 3.13). If the pain subsides, work may be resumed or the patient may be reappointed. If the pain does not subside within 5 minutes, another nitroglycerine tablet is administered. After 5 minutes, if pain persists, a third tablet can be given. If after three tablets within 15 minutes period the pain persists, the patient should be referred to hospital and not sent directly home. In severe attacks where pain persists, morphine sulfate 20 mg is administered subcutaneously to cease the pain.

Box 3.13: Value of oxygen

In many cardiac patients, oxygen administered by nasal prongs is recommended for various reasons:
1. Breathing air with elevated proportions of oxygen is known to produce a mild euphoria independent of its other physiologic effects.
2. Increasing the oxygen content of inspired air provides better tissue perfusion with no increase in cardiac output, heart rate, or work of the heart.
3. When myocardial oxygenation is improved, ischemic events are less likely, as are arrhythmias.
4. Should cardiopulmonary resuscitation become necessary, an initially well-oxygenated patient is at an advantage from the standpoint of both cerebral ischemia and metabolic acidosis.

ENDOCARDITIS

As mentioned before, the **endocardium** consists of a simple squamous endothelium overlying a thin areolar tissue layer. It forms the smooth inner lining of the chambers and valves and is continuous with the endothelium of the blood vessels.

Physiology of the Valves

To pump blood effectively, the heart needs valves that ensure a predominantly one-way flow. There is a valve between each atrium and its ventricle and at the exit from each ventricle into its great artery (Fig. 3.31). The four heart valves allow blood to flow through the hear in only one direction, thus preventing the backflow of blood. The two atrioventricular valves allow blood to flow from the atria to the ventricles, and the two semilunar valves allow blood to flow from the right ventricle to the pulmonary artery (on the way to the lungs) and from the left ventricle to the aorta (on the way to the rest of the body).

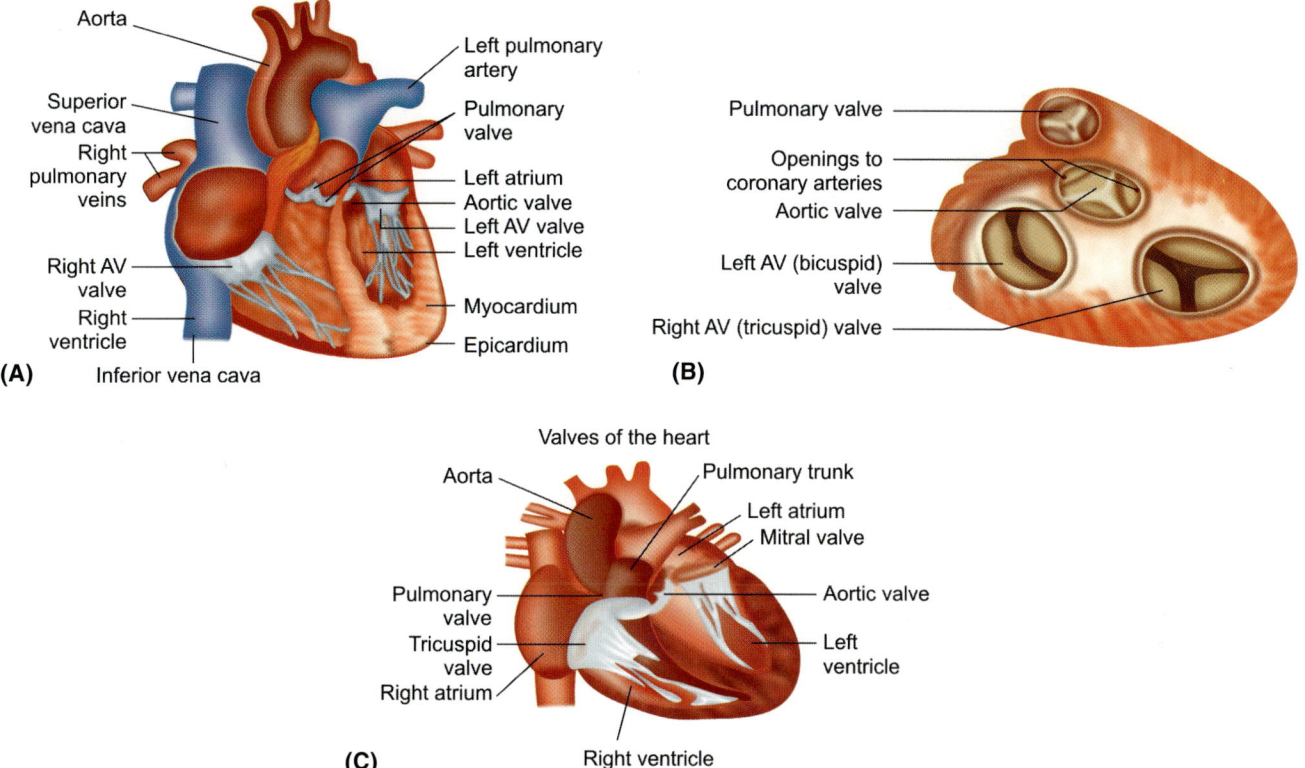

Fig. 3.31: (A) Internal anatomy of the heart. **(B)** Heart valves. **(C)** Superior view of the heart with the atria removed

Each valve consists of two or three fibrous flaps of tissue called **cusps**, covered with endothelium. The **atrioventricular (AV) valves** regulate the openings between the atria and ventricles. The **right AV (tricuspid) valve** has three cusps and the **left** AV **(bicuspid) valve** has two. The left AV valve is also known as the **mitral valve** after its resemblance to a miter the headdress of the catholic bishop.

The **semilunar valves** (pulmonary and aortic valves) regulate the openings between the ventricles and the great arteries. The **pulmonary valve** controls the opening from the right ventricle into the pulmonary trunk, and the **aortic valve** controls the opening from the left ventricle into the aorta. Each has three cusps shaped somewhat like shirt pockets.

The opening and closing of heart valves is the result of pressure gradients between the "upstream" and "downstream" sides of the valve (Fig. 3.32). When the ventricles are relaxed, the AV valve cusps hang down limply, both AV valves are open, and blood flows freely from the atria into the ventricles. When the ventricles have filled with blood and begin to contract, their internal pressure rises and blood surges against

the AV valves. This pushes their cusps together, seals the openings, and prevents blood from flowing back into the atria. The papillary muscles contract with the rest of the ventricular myocardium and tug on the chordae tendineae, which prevents the valves from bulging excessively (prolapsing) into the atria or turning inside out like windblown umbrellas. When rising "upstream" pressure in the ventricles exceeds the "downstream" blood pressure in the great arteries, the ventricular blood forces the semilunar valves open and blood is ejected from the heart. Then as the ventricles relax again and their pressure falls below that in the arteries, arterial blood briefly flows backward and fills the pocket like cusps of the semilunar valves. The three cusps meet in the middle of the orifice and seal it, thereby preventing blood from reentering the heart.

HEART VALVE DISEASES

I. Valvular Insufficiency (Incompetence)

Refers to any failure of a valve to prevent *reflux (regurgitation)—the* backward flow of blood (Fig. 3.33). **Valvular stenosis** *(steno* = narrow) is a form of

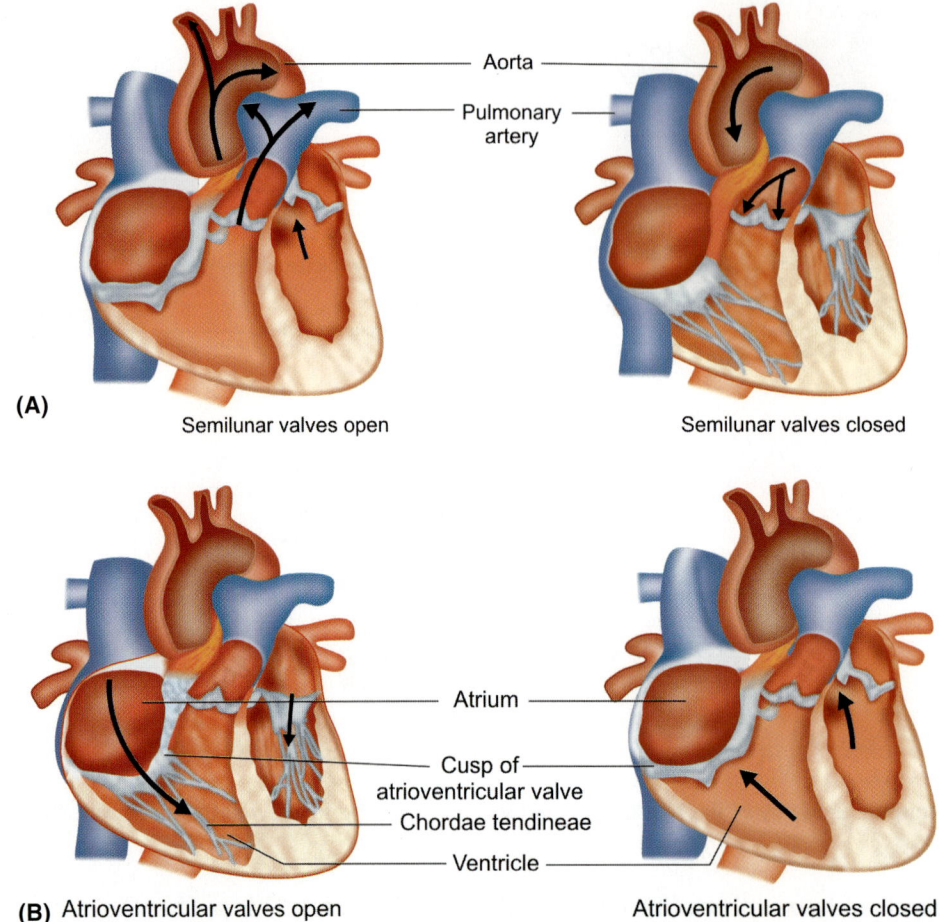

Fig. 3.32: Operation of the heart valves. **(A)** The semilunar valves. When the pressure of the ventricle is greater than the pressure in the artery, the valve is forced open and blood is ejected. When the ventricular pressure is lower than the arterial pressure, arterial blood holds the valve closed. **(B)** The atrioventricular valves. When atrial pressure is greater than ventricular pressure, the valve opens and blood flows through. When ventricular pressure rises above atrial pressure, the blood in the ventricle pushes the valve cusps closed

insufficiency in which the cusps are stiffened and the opening is constricted by scar tissue. It frequently results from rheumatic fever, an autoimmune disease in which antibodies produced to fight a bacterial infection also attack the mitral and aortic valves. As the valves become scarred and constricted, the heart is overworked by the effort to force blood through the openings and may become enlarged. Regurgitation of blood through the incompetent valves creates turbulence that can be heard as a *heart murmur*.

II. Mitral Valve Prolapse (MVP)

It is an insufficiency in which one or both mitral valve cusps bulge into the atrium during ventricular contraction. It is often hereditary and affects about 1 out of 40 people, especially young women. In many cases, it causes no serious dysfunction, but in some people it causes chest pain, fatigue, and shortness of breath. An incompetent valve can eventually lead to heart failure. A defective valve can be replaced with an artificial valve or a valve transplanted from a pig heart.

III. Endocarditis

It is a life-threatening infection of the heart valves, associated with either congenital or disease-induced anomalies of native or prosthetic valves.

The pathologic process of endocarditis involves the indolent form (formerly known as subacute bacterial endocarditis), to the acutely progressive type (formerly known as acute bacterial endocarditis).

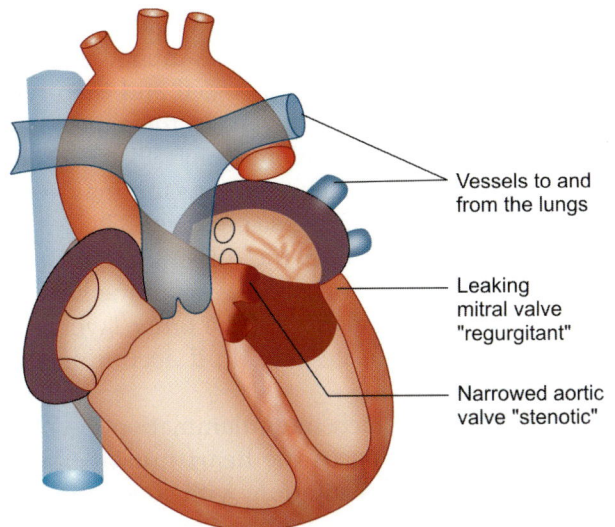

Fig. 3.33: Mitral valve stenosis

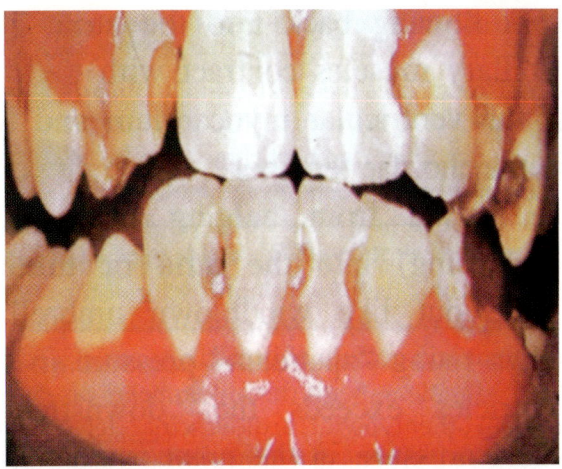

Fig. 3.34: Severe dental caries and gingivitis predisposes patients to episodes of bacteremia, and thus to infective endocarditis in the presence of a congenital or acquired cardiac abnormality. Full treatment of caries or appropriate dental extraction should be carried out with antibiotic prophylaxis all such patients

These differences reflect the relative contributions of immunological activation, systemic sepsis and valvular damage, and in part depend upon the nature of the infecting organism.

Infective endocarditis results from two main predisposing factors bacteremia and a cardiac lesion where there is turbulent blood flow (Figs 3.34 and 3.35).

Although an enormous variety of organisms have been reported as causing endocarditis, the main causative microorganisms are *Streptococcus viridans* (present in enormous numbers in the mouth and the gastrointestinal tract), *Streptococcus mutans* and

Streptococcus sanguis. Streptococcus viridans proliferates where oral hygiene is lacking and proliferate into the bloodstream in large numbers particularly during tooth extraction, during chewing and home oral hygiene procedures. Oral bacteremia after tooth extraction is generally transient and lasts for less than 15 minutes, but occasionally last for up to one hour.

Any dental procedure that causes injury to the soft tissue or bone, resulting in bleeding, can produce a transient bacteremia and in susceptible patient, can result in endocarditis. Even minor dental manipulation, such as the cleaning of teeth or the placement

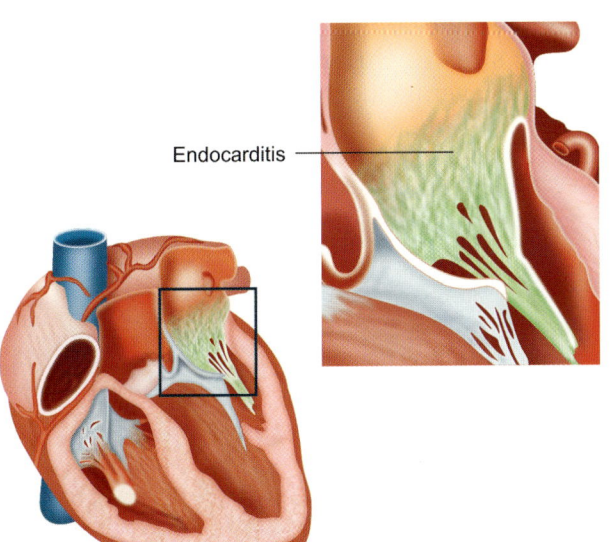

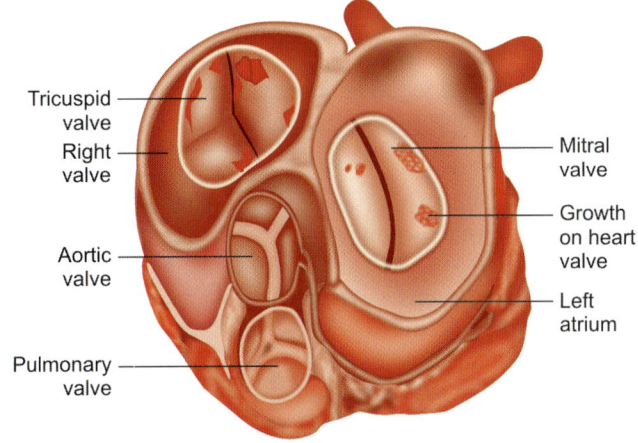

Fig. 3.35: Infective endocarditis is an infection of the heart chambers or valves. The figures show germination of microorganisms over the mitral valve

of a matrix band, can result in a transient bacteremia (Table 3.5). In normal patients, the body's defensive mechanism handles these bacteremias, and usually no serious problem develops. However, in the patient with a heart defect, such as rheumatic heart disease, the anatomy and function of the affected valve are altered because of the scarring following the acute rheumatic fever attack. When bacteremias occur, the altered valvular tissue with non-bacterial thrombotic endocarditis (NBTE) provides an ideal location for attachment and growth of bacteria.

Thus in patients with rheumatic heart disease, or those with other types of cardiovascular defects, there is a very real threat of endocarditis during every period of bacteremia. Platelets and fibrin deposits accumulate at sites where there is turbulent blood flow over damaged valves (non-bacterial thromboembolic endocarditis). These sterile vegetations can thereafter readily be infected during bacteremias resulting in infective endocarditis. Cardiac valves already damaged by infective endocarditis, or prosthetic cardiac valves, can particularly become infected (prosthetic valve endocarditis).

IV. Rheumatic Heart Disease

Rheumatic fever is a disease which sometimes follows a sore throat caused by certain strains of beta-hemo-lytic streptococci. Children between 5 and 15 years are predominantly affected. Rheumatic fever may occasionally be followed by chronic rheumatic carditis with permanent cardiac valvular damage.

The infection commonly appears as an upper respiratory infection, tonsillitis, pharyngitis, or strep throat (awareness of the risk of rheumatic fever has led to increased use of throat cultures to quickly identify and treat a *Streptococcus* infection). Antibodies to the *Streptococcus* organism form as usual and then react with connective tissue (collagen) in the skin, joints, brain, and heart, causing inflammation (Fig. 3.36). The heart is the only site where scar tissue may form, leading to rheumatic heart disease (Fig. 3.37).

During the acute stage, the inflammation in the heart may involve one or more layers of the heart:

• Pericarditis, inflammation of the outer layer, may include effusion (excessive fluid accumulation), which impairs filling.

• Myocarditis, in which the inflammation develops as localized lesions in the heart muscle, called Aschoff bodies, may interfere with conduction.

• Endocarditis, the most common problem, affects the valves, which become edematous. And verrucae form. Verrucae are rows of small, wart-like vegetations along the outer edge of the valve cusps. The mitral valve is affected most frequently. The inflammation disrupts the flow of blood and the effectiveness of the left ventricle. Eventually, the valve may be scarred, leading to stenosis, if the cusps fuse together or to incompetence, if fibrous tissue shrinks, or to a combination of these, ending in rheumatic heart disease (Fig. 3.37B). In some cases the chordate tendinae are involved in the inflammatory reaction, and fibrosis ensues, leading to shortened chordate and malfunctioning valve. Recurrent inflammation is likely to cause more damage to the valves, which are also at risk for infective endocarditis.

Other sites of inflammation in patients with rheumatic fever include:

Table 3.5: Reported frequency of bacteremia associated with various dental procedures and oral manipulation

Dental procedure/oral manipulation	Reported frequency of bacteremia
Tooth extraction	10–100%
Periodontal surgery	36–88%
Scaling and root planning	8–80%
Teeth cleaning	<40%
Rubber dam matrix/wedge placement	9–32%
Endodontic procedures	≤20%
Tooth brushing and flossing	20–68%
Use of wooden toothpicks	20–40%
Use of water irrigation devices	7–50%
Chewing food	7–51%

Data compiled from Wilson W, Taubert KA, Gewitz M, Lockhart PB, Baddour LM, Levison M, et al. Prevention of Infective Endocarditis: Guidelines from the American Heart Association. Circulation 2007;115:1–17

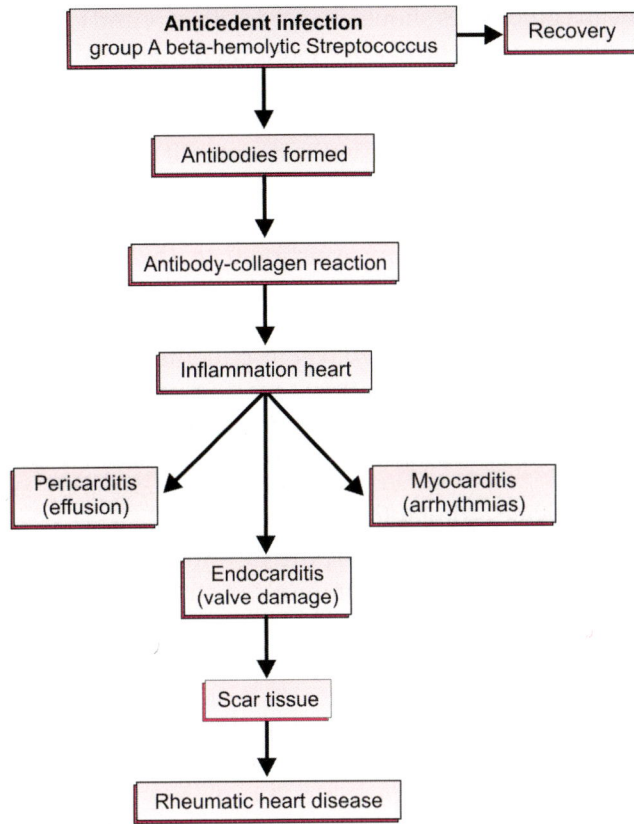

Fig. 3.36: Development of rheumatic fever and rheumatic heart disease *(Gould, 2006)*

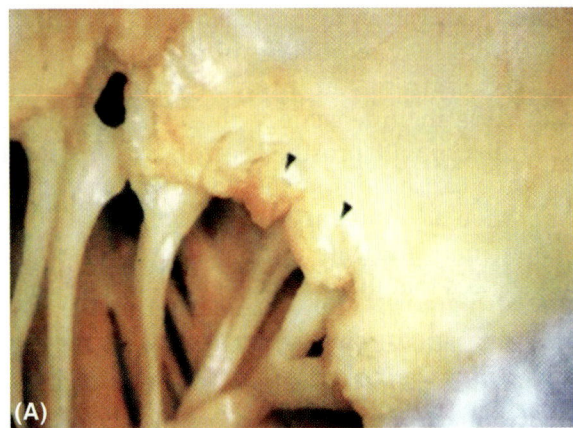

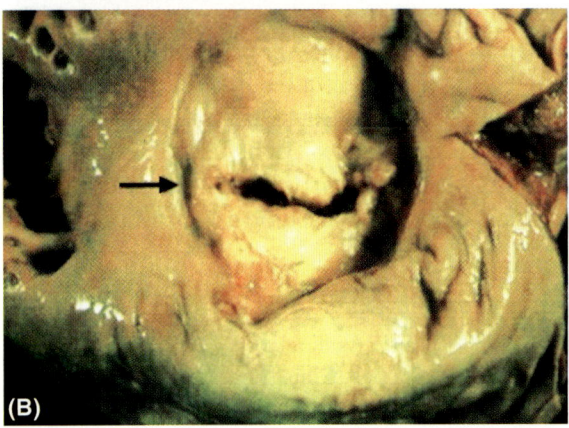

Fig. 3.37: Rheumatic heart disease: **(A)** Acute rheumatic: mitral valvulitis superimposed on rheumatic heart disease (note thick cords). Verrucae (arrows) are visible along the edge of mitral valve leaflet. **(B)** Mitral stenosis with fibrous thickening and distortion of valve leaflets. Arrow marks commissural fusion. *(From Kumar V, Abbas AK, Fausto M: Robbins and Cortan Pathologic Basis of Disease, 7th ed. Philadelphia, WB Saunders, 2005)*

- The large joints, particularly in the legs, which may be involved with synovitis in a migratory polyarthritis (often multiple joints affected).

- The skin, which may show a nonprutitic rash known as erythema marginatum (red macules or papules that enlarge and have white centers).

- The wrists, elbows, knees, or ankles, where small, non-tender subcutaneous nodules usually form on the extensor surfaces.

- The basal nuclei in the brain (more frequently in girls) causing involuntary jerky movements of the face, arms, and legs (Sydenham's chorea or Saint Vitus dance).

Rheumatic heart disease develops years later in some individuals, when scarred valves or arrhythmias compromise heart function. Congestive heart failure may occur in either the acute or chronic stage.

Patients suspected of having rheumatic heart disease should receive proper antibiotic coverage, the standard amoxicillin regimen or a parenteral regimen. The oral route of administration for antibiotics is preferred because of the lower incidence of allergic sensitivity. The dentist should plan to do as much treatment as possible during each coverage period (period of time patient is taking antibiotics) so the patient's dental treatment will not be spread over too long time, and thus the number of necessary coverage periods can be kept to a minimum. One to two weeks or more should elapse between coverage periods.

At least two blood cultures from different sites and at different times are required: the first two results are positive in 95% of cases of culture-positive endocarditis. Blood culture bottles should be filled according to the instructions. It is important to use the correct blood volume for the culture system being used.

It is obligatory to try to prevent the onset of infective endocarditis in view of the high morbidity and mortality. Patients at high risk for infective endocarditis include mainly those with previous endocarditis, or with prosthetic cardiac valves. Dental procedures carried out in these patients necessitate preoperative administration of antibiotics. Clinical judgment may indicate antibiotic use in selected circumstances that may create significant bleeding.

DENTAL PROCEDURES AND ENDOCARDITIS PROPHYLAXIS

Infective endocarditis is often exceedingly insidious in origin and can develop 2 or more months after the operation that might have precipitated it. There is no need for antibiotic prophylaxis for procedures that do not include bleeding (Box 3.14 A and B).

Antibiotic prophylaxis is recommended in procedures likely to create transient bacteremia in patients at risk (Box 3.15). The evidence for prophylaxis in endocarditis is circumstantial and recommendations are based on a body of opinion. This

Box 3.14A: Endocarditis prophylaxis not recommended

1. Restorative dentistry (operative and prosthodontics) with or without retraction cord.
2. Local anesthetic injections (non-intraligamentary).
3. Intracanal endodontic treatment and post-placement and build up.
4. Placement of rubber dams.
5. Postoperative suture removal.
6. Placement of removable prosthodontic or orthodontic appliances.
7. Taking of oral impressions.
8. Fluoride treatments.
9. Taking of oral radiographs.
10. Orthodontic appliance adjustment.
11. Shedding of primary teeth.

Box 3.14B: Endocarditis prophylaxis recommended

- Dental extractions, periodontal procedures, including surgery, scaling and root planning, probing, and recall maintenance.
- Dental implant placement and reimplantation of avulsed teeth
- Endodontic (root canal) instrumentation or surgery beyond the apex
- Subgingival placement of antibiotic fibers or strips
- Initial placement of orthodontic bands but not brackets
- Intraligamentary local anesthetic injections
- Prophylactic cleaning of teeth or implants where bleeding is anticipated.

means guidelines should be used with care and clinical judgement should be exercised. The aim of prophylaxis is to reduce the risk of transient bacteremia in patients who are at risk of endocarditis because of underlying valve disease. It is important to identify *'patients at risk'* to ensure antibiotics are recommended only for appropriate patients. In general, the risk is proportional to the degree of hemodynamic turbulence associated with a structural defect that may eventually allow vegetation formation. As a prophylaxis in patients at risk who will carry out extraction, scaling, and surgery involving the periodontal tissues, it is recommended to carry out the following steps.

1. Antibiotic Administration

It is particularly important in endocarditis that antibiotics should be administered strictly according to the scheduled dosages.

The risk of endocarditis is almost always greater than the risk of antibiotic toxic effects. The next 1 to 2 hours of the coverage period (period of time patient is taking antibiotics) should be used to do as much dental treatment as possible. It is during this period that the patient is best protected. If additional coverage periods are needed, at least one week should elapse before another coverage period is initiated.

This will allow the oral flora to return to normal. However, the last recommendation of the American Heart Association (2007) concerning the prophylactic regimens for the prevention of endocarditis in patients undergoing dental procedures is shown in Tables 3.6 to 3.9. Prophylactic indications of antibiotic is discussed in Chapter 15, "A": Antibitotics, page 435 and "B": Bacterial Endocarditis, page 437.

The principles for effective prophylaxis include:
1. The specific organism involved should be known, and an antibiotic effective against that organism should be selected.
2. High doses of antibiotic at the time of bacteremia should be provided and continued for an adequate length of time, i.e. continued as long as bacteria can be released, which is usually for a short duration.

There are several problems with the current use of antibiotic prophylaxis against endocarditis. The risk of developing the disease in susceptible patients is not known. A number of different microorganisms are found to cause endocarditis;

Table 3.6: American Heart Association recommended standard prophylactic regimen for dental procedures 2007*

Adults	Amoxicillin 2 g, orally, 1 hour before procedure, then 1.5 g 6 hours after initial dose.
Children	Amoxicillin 50 mg/kg, orally, 1 hour before procedure, then half initial dose 6 hours later.
	Children less than 15 kg: initial dose 750 mg amoxicillin.
	Children 15 to 30 kg: initial dose, 1500 mg amoxicillin.
	Children over 30 kg: initial dose, 300 mg amoxicillin.
	Children 1 hour before procedure followed 6 hours later with half initial dose.

Used in all-risk patients, including those with prosthetic heart valves. Children's doses should not exceed adult dose.

Table 3.7: Recommended standard prophylactic regimen for dental therapy for rheumatic fever prevention. Patients unable to take oral medications. American Heart Association (2007)

Ampicillin	
Adults	2.0 g intramuscular or intravenous 30 min before the procedure.
Children	50 mg/kg intramuscular or intravenous 30 minutes before the procedure.

Table 3.8: Recommended standard prophylactic regimen for dental therapy for rheumatic fever prevention. Procedures in patients allergic to amoxicillin/penicillin or who are on long-term penicillin (AHA 2007)

Clindamycin (cleocin)	
Adults	600 mg PO (oral), 1 h. before the procedure
Children	20 mg/ kg PO 1 h. before the procedure
Cephaloxin (keflex)**	
Adults	2.0 g oral 1 h. before the procedure
Children	50 mg/ kg oral 1 h. before the procedure.
Azithromycin or clarithromycin	
Adults	500 mg oral 1 h. before the procedure
Children	15 mg/kg oral 1 h. before the procdure

Table 3.9: Recommended standard prophylactic regimen for dental therapy for rheumatic fever prevention. Penicillin-allergic patients unable to take oral medications (AHA 2007)

Cefazolin (ancef) or ceftriaxone (rocephin)**	
Adults	1.0 g IV or IM 30 min. before the procedure
Children	50 mg/kg IM or IV 30 min. before the procedure
Systemic clindamycin	
Adults	600 mg/kg IV or IM before the procedure
Children	20 mg/kg IV 30 min. before the procedure

* Children doses should not exceed adult doses.
** Avoid cephalosporins in patients with immediate-type hypersensitivity/acute anaphylaxis reaction to penicillin.

therefore, no one antibiotic is effective in preventing the disease. The duration of coverage is not known for oral wounds healing by secondary intension. Bacterial resistance during the coverage period is becoming a problem, as is the presence of resistant strains in the oral flora before antibiotic prophylaxis is initiated. If the antibiotic regimen is too complicated and expensive, the patient may be discouraged from seeking needed dental treatment.

2. Mouthwash

To reduce the severity of the resulting bacteremia, chlorhexidine 0.2% mouth rinses and application of an antiseptic such as 10% povidene iodine or 0.5% chlorhexidine gel to the gingival crevice should be performed before any surgical procedure.

3. Effective Preventive Dental Procedures

The primary goal of dentist while dealing with patients susceptible to endocarditis is to encourage excellent dental repair and effective preventive dental procedures including regular dental checkup, fluoridation, diet modification to reduce the risk of caries and periodontal disease, arid daily oral hygiene (with effective brushing and flossing of the teeth).

CONGESTIVE HEART FAILURE

Congestive heart failure (CHF) is a syndrome resulting from diseases or structural defects that make the heart an ineffective pump. Heart failure is due to the inability of the heart to function as a pump.

PATHOLOGY

Congestive heart failure results from the failure of either ventricle to eject blood effectively. It is usually due to a heart weakened by myocardial infarction, chronic hypertension, valvular insufficiency, or congenital defects in cardiac structure. If the left ventricle fails, it results in an inadequate emptying of the ventricles during systole, blood backs up into the lungs and causes pulmonary edema (fluid in the lungs), shortness of breath, and a sense of suffocation.

If the right ventricle fails, it results in an incomplete filling of the ventricles during diastole, blood backs up into the venae cavae and causes systemic, or generalized, edema. Systemic edema is marked by enlargement of the liver, ascites (the pooling of fluid in the abdominal cavity), distension of the jugular veins, and swelling of the fingers, ankles, and feet. Failure of one ventricle eventually increases the workload on the other ventricle, which stresses it and leads to its eventual failure as well. Thus heart failure may be defined as a state in which cardiac dysfunction results in a diminished functional capacity and an impaired quality of life. Conditions that can result in congestive heart failure, when they are severe enough, include the following:

1. Myocardial infarction when 30% of the left ventricle is infracted. When more than 40% is lost, cardiogenic shock ensues, carrying a 75% mortality. Infarction of the right ventricle rarely results in failure.
2. Cardiomyopathy when cardiac muscle's contractile ability is severely diminished owing to toxic substances (e.g. alcohol, cobalt) or idiopathic (possibly viral) causes.
3. Structural changes that cause inefficient pumping and overloading of heart chambers, such as stenosis and regurgitation of valves and ventricular septal defects.
4. Persistent severe hypertension, either pulmonary or systemic, which can lead to a contractile deficit in the ventricles.

The left ventricular heart failure is brought on by either increased workload or disease of the heart muscle. The increased workload may result from a variety of entities, including aortic valve disease, and arterial hypertension. The outstanding symptoms of left ventricular failure is dyspnea, which results from blood accumulation in the pulmonary vessels. Acute pulmonary edema often is associated with left ventricular failure. Left sided heart failure leads to pulmonary hypertension which increases the work of the right ventricle, pumping against the increased pressure, and often leads to right sided heart failure as well. An important feature of left ventricular failure is the retention of sodium and water and the insufficient emptying of the left ventricle during systole.

The New York Heart Association (NYHA) has devised a functional classification of heart disease that grades the severity of chronic heart failure. It is useful in following the course of the disease and assessing the effects of therapy. It also can be used to aid in the dental management of patients.

Class I: No limitation of physical activity. No dyspnea, fatigue, or palpitation with ordinary physical activity.

Class II: Slight limitation of physical activity. These patients have fatigue, palpitations and dyspnea with ordinary physical activity but are comfortable at rest.

Class III: Marked limitation of activity. Less than ordinary physical activity results in symptoms but patients are comfortable at rest.

Class IV: Symptoms are present at rest, and any physical exertion exacerbates the symptoms.

Signs and Symptoms

The heart generally calls little attention to itself in failure. Pain is rare unless an episode of myocardial infarction occurs in conjunction, palpitation is uncommon unless the patient has been given digitalis and develops arrhythmias because of it.

If one listens to the chest of a person in heart failure, he may hear three silent sounds instead of two. The third sound of the heart beat is the 'gallop' rhythm which is very characteristic and striking.

Another sign is *pulsus alternans.* The pulse has a regular alternation of one strong beat and a weak beat.

The signs of congestive heart failure usually include rapid shallow breathing, hyperventilation alternating with apnea (Cheyne-Stokes respiration), inspiratory rates, increased venous pressure (Fig. 3.40), cardiac enlargement on chest radiograph, distended neck veins, large and tender liver, jaundice, pitting dependent peripheral edema (Fig. 3.38), ascites, cyanosis, and clubbing of fingers (Fig. 3.39). The symptoms of congestive heart failure include fatigue and weakness, dyspnea (breathlessness), orthopnea (dyspnea brought on by lying down, paroxysmal nocturnal dyspnea (dyspnea awakening patient from sleep), hyperventilation followed by apnea, low grade fever, anorexia, nausea, vomiting and constipation, liver pain, cough, and expectoration often severe enough to interfere with sleep; rusty sputum, insomnia, history of sweating, dizziness and confusion.

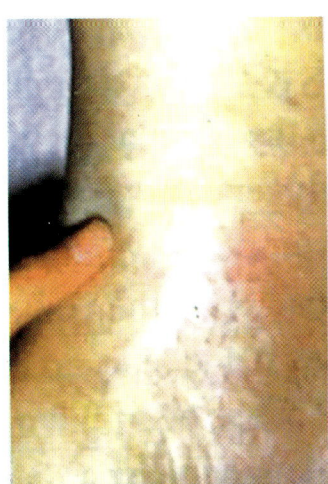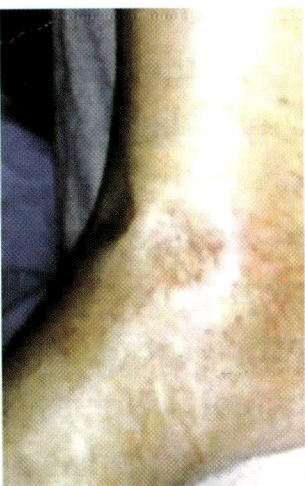

Fig. 3.38: Pitting edema in a patient with heart failure. A depression "pit" remains in the edematous tissue for some minutes after firm fingertip pressure is applied *(Forbes CD, Jakson WE. Color Atlas and Text of Clinical Medicine. Edinburgh, Mosby, 2004)*

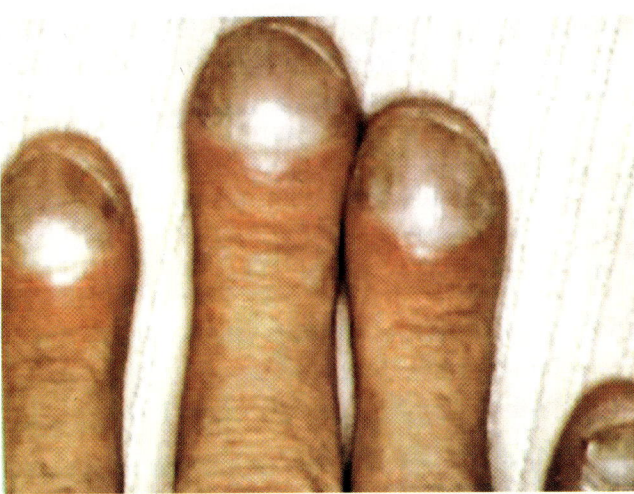

Fig. 3.39: Clubbing of the fingers in a patient with congestive heart failure. *(Little JW, Falace DA, Miller CS, Rhodus, NL: Dental Management of the Medically Compromised Patient. Mosby Inc, 2008)*

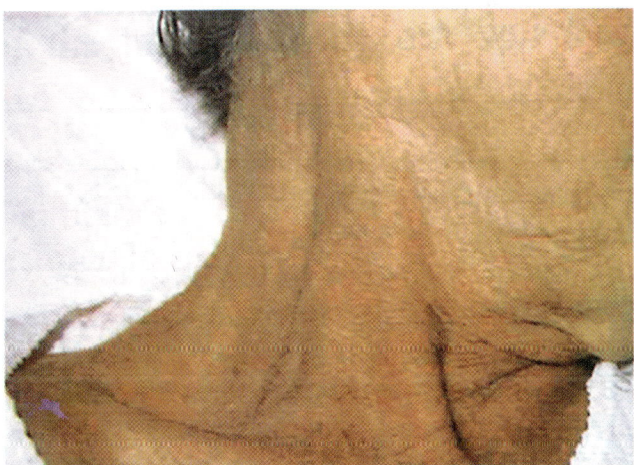

Fig. 3.40: Elevated external jugular vein pressure. The pressure in the internal and external jugular veins is elevated in right heart failure

DENTAL MANAGEMENT (Box 3.15)

Any history of exertional dyspnea, orthopnias, or paroxysmal nocturnal dyspnea provides a useful indicator of this and should alert the dental practitioner.

1. Patients who are under good control, with no complications, can receive routine dental care.
2. Short stress free appointments are advised. Local anesthetics with epinephrine may be used, although any intravascular injection resulting in tachycardia may cause decompensation and acute pulmonary edema with sudden onset of shortness of breath.

3. Under local anesthesia, the most desirable position for operating may be unsatisfactory for the patient comfort. Patients with poorly compensated heart failure may not tolerate a supine chair position due to pulmonary edema and will need a semisupine or upright chair position (cardiac position). This promotes venous return from the extremities, relieves neck vein engorgement, and eases respiration.

4. Patients taking digitalis glycoside (digoxin) should be given epinephrine or levonordefrine cautiously as the combination can potentially precipitate arrhythmias. A maximum of 0.036 mg epinephrine (two carpules of 2% lidocaine with 1:100,000 epinephrine) is recommended.

5. In patients who are NYHA class III or IV, vasoconstrictors should be avoided. Nitrous oxide–oxygen sedation can be used to provide adequate O_2 flow (at least 30%) is maintained. Refer to Chapter 15, Page 706 "Heart Failure".

CARDIAC ARREST

Cardiac arrest, is a clinical term used to describe the absence of pulse. In dental practice, cardiac arrest is most likely to follow prolonged hypoxia, hypotension, or acute ischemic event.

In circulatory arrest, all blood flow abruptly stops, due either to cardiac arrest or ventricular fibrillation. The real problem in circulatory arrest is to prevent detrimental effects in the brain.

Four or five minutes of circulatory arrest causes permanent brain damage in over 50% of patients. Ventricular fibrillation, ventricular asystole, and agonal rhythm are the three types of arrhythmias associated with cardiac arrest. They are all lethal arrhythmias that require immediate therapy for survival.

Ventricular fibrillation: Ventricular fibrillation is represented as chaotic activity on the ECG, with the ventricles contracting very rapidly but ineffectively. This usually is a terminal arrhythmia unless therapy is administered rapidly. Coronary atherosclerosis is the most common form of heart disease predisposing to ventricular fibrillation. Other causes of this arrhythmia include rheumatic heart disease, anaphylaxis, blunt cardiac trauma, mitral valve prolapse, cardiac surgery, digitalis intoxication, and cardiac catheterization.

Ventricular asystole: In ventricular asystole, cardiac standstill occurs when no impulses are being conducted to the ventricles (ECG is a flat line) and no muscular activity is taking place. The condition

Box 3.15: Dental management of the patient with heart failure

1. Evaluate patient for history, signs, or symptoms of heart failure (HF).
2. For patients with symptoms of untreated or uncontrolled HF, defer elective dental care and refer to physician.
3. For patients diagnosed and treated for HF:
   – Confirm status with patient or physician.
   – New York Heart Association (NYHA) class 1 patients (asymptomatic)—provide routine care.
   – NYHA class II (and some class III) patients obtain consultation with physician for medical clearance and provide routine care.
   – NYHA (some class III and class IV) patients obtain consultation with physician; consider treatment in a special care or hospital setting.
   – Identify underlying cardiovascular disease (i.e. coronary artery disease, hypertension, cardiomyopathy, valvular disease), and manage appropriately.
4. Drug considerations:
   – For patients taking digitalis, avoid epinephrine; if considered essential, use cautiously (maximum 0.036 mg epinephrine or 0.20 mg levonordefrine); avoid gag reflex; avoid erythromycin, which may increase the absorption of digitalis and lead to toxicity (signs of digitalis toxicity are tachycardia, hypersalivation, visual disturbances, etc.).
   – For patients with NYHA class III and IV congestive heart failure, avoid use of vasoconstrictors; if use is considered essential, discuss with physician.
   – Avoid epinephrine-impregnated retraction cord.
5. Schedule short, stress-free appointments.
6. Use semisupine or upright chair position.
7. Watch for orthostatic hypotension, make position or chair changes slowly and assist patient into and out of chair.
8. Avoid the use of nonsteroidal anti-inflammatory drugs (NSAIDs).
9. Nitrous oxide/oxygen sedation may be used with a minimum of 30% oxygen.

causing ventricular fibrillation also can lead to ventricular asystole.

Agonal rhythm: Again, in agonal rhythm, effective ventricular contraction ceases. Although impulse conduction is taking place, the ECG shows wide distorted complexes, with no mechanical activity in the ventricles.

Closed chest cardiac massage will circulate blood regardless of whether the heart is in arrest or in fibrillation. Inflation of the lungs with oxygen will help to restore adequate amount of oxygen to the brain and to the coronary arteries. Ventilations should be performed using a positive pressure device with 100% oxygen source.

Because early cardiac arrest is caused by ventricular tachycardia or fibrillation, definitive treatment requires electrical defibrillation as soon as it is available. The beneficial role of cardiopulmonary resuscitation (CPR) likely rests in its modest influence on coronary perfusion, which may sustain electrical activity until defibrillation is available. This concept is supported by data illustrating greatest success when cardiopulmonary resuscitation is initiated immediately and is followed by advanced cardiac life support (ACLS) within 8 to 10 minutes of cardiac arrest. Coronary perfusion is essential to sustain myocardial viability, and the protocol for cardiac arrest includes attempts to improve peripheral resistance to facilitate this effort. For this reason, epinephrine is indicated in all cases of cardiac arrest, and this actually precludes an absolute requirement for ECG standards recommend a 1 mg dose repeated every 5 minutes as necessary during cardiopulmonary resuscitation. This can be accomplished by injecting either 10 ml of a 1:10,000 solution into antecubetal vein. An alternative is to inject 1 or 2 ml of a 1:1000 solution sublingually. If the cardiac muscle is not well oxygenated, it is very difficult to restore its normal cycle.

4

Respiratory System

- Anatomy
  - Pulmonary Circulation
- Physiology of Respiration
  - Gas Exchange and Transport
  - Concentration Gradients of the Gases
  - Control of Respiration
  - Clinical Terminology of Ventilation
- Chronic Obstructive Pulmonary Diseases
- Bronchial Asthma
  - Dental Management
  - Drugs for Asthmatic and Allergic
- Emphysema
  - Tuberculosis
- Aspiration

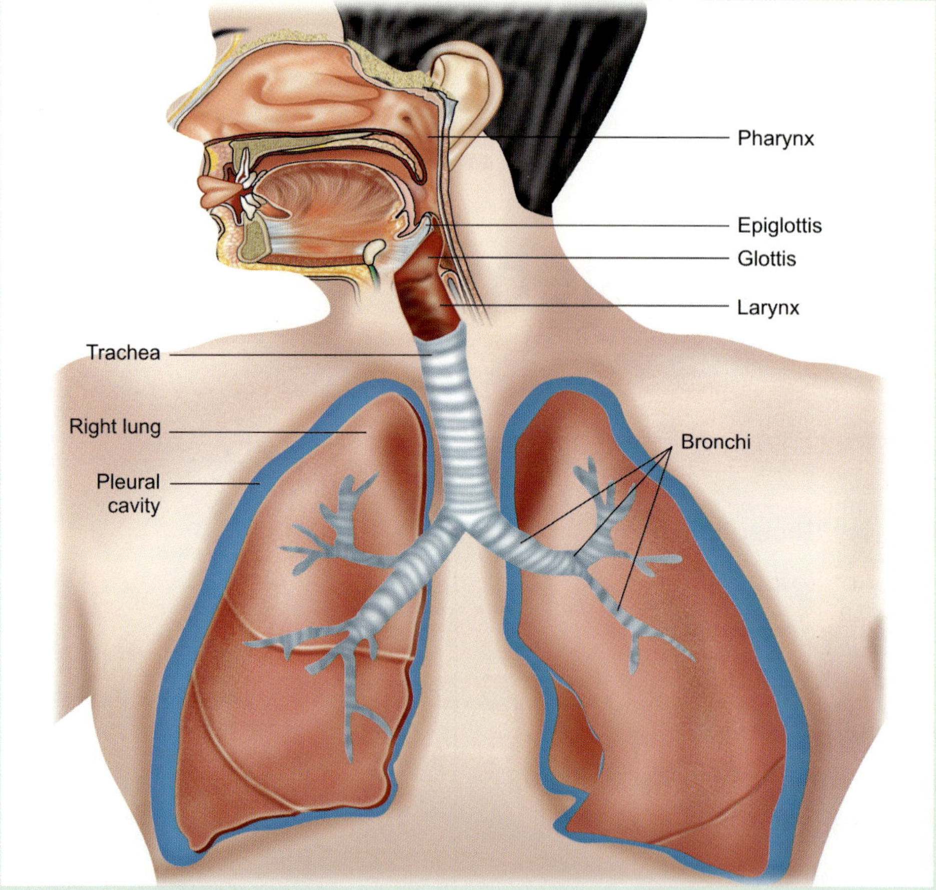

(A) Gross anatomy of the respiratory system

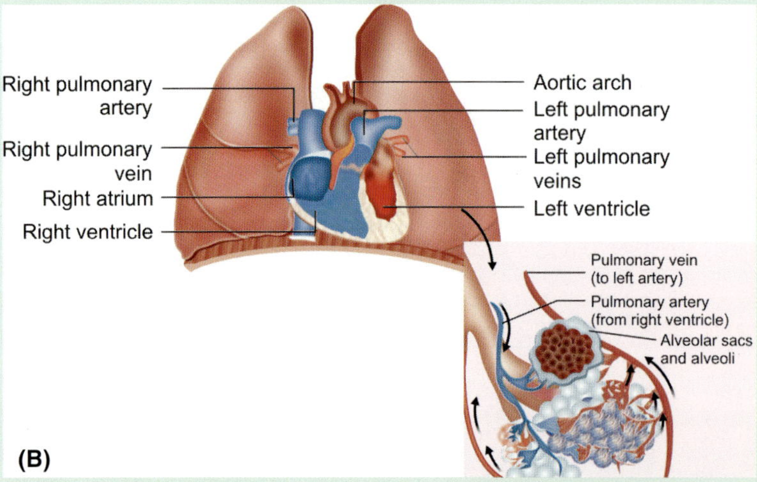

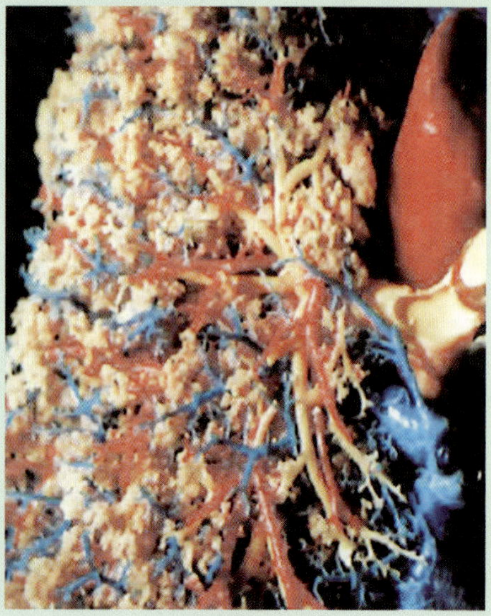

Plate II **(A)** Gross anatomy of the respiratory system. **(B)** The pulmonary circulation. Microscopic anatomy of the blood vessels that supply the pulmonary alveoli. **(C)** A resin cast of the lung, with arteries in blue, veins in red, and the bronchial tree and alveoli in yellow *(Saladin: Anatomy and Physiology: The Unit of Form and Function. McGraw-Hill Co. 3 ed. 2003)*

ANATOMY

The term respiration has three meanings: (1) ventilation of the lungs (breathing), (2) the exchange of gases between air and blood and between blood and tissue fluid, and (3) The use of oxygen in cellular metabolism. The principal organs of the respiratory system are the nose, pharynx, larynx, trachea, bronchi, and lungs (Plate II). These organs serve to receive fresh air, exchange gases with the blood, and expel the modified air. Within the lungs, air flows along a dead-end pathway consisting essentially of bronchi, bronchiole and alveoli. Incoming air stops in the alveoli (millions of thin-walled, microscopic air sacs in the lungs), exchanges gases with the bloodstream across the alveolar wall, and then flows back out. An alveolus (Figs 4.1 and 4.2) is a pouch about 0.2 to 0.5 mm in diameter. Its wall consists predominantly of squamous thin alveolar cells—cells that allow for rapid gas diffusion between the alveolus and bloodstream.

The conducting division of the respiratory system consists of those passages that serve only for airflow, essentially from the nostrils through the bronchioles. The respiratory division consists of the alveoli and other distal gas-exchange regions.

The airway from the nose through the larynx is often called the upper respiratory tract (i.e. the respiratory organs in the head and neck), and the regions from the trachea through the lungs compose the lower respiratory tract (the respiratory organs of the thorax).

A resting adult breathes 10 to 15 times per minute, inhaling about 500 mL of air during inspiration and exhaling it again during expiration. A resting adult breathes 10 to 15 times per minute, inhaling about 500 mL of air during inspiration and exhaling it again during expiration.

Pulmonary Circulation

The pulmonary circulation is composed of the pulmonary arteries, which brings venous blood (dark blue in color) from the right side of the heart to be oxygenated; the pulmonary capillaries, in which diffusion or gas exchange occurs; and the pulmonary veins, which returns the oxygenated blood (bright red) to the left side of the heart, which then pumps it out into the systemic circulation.

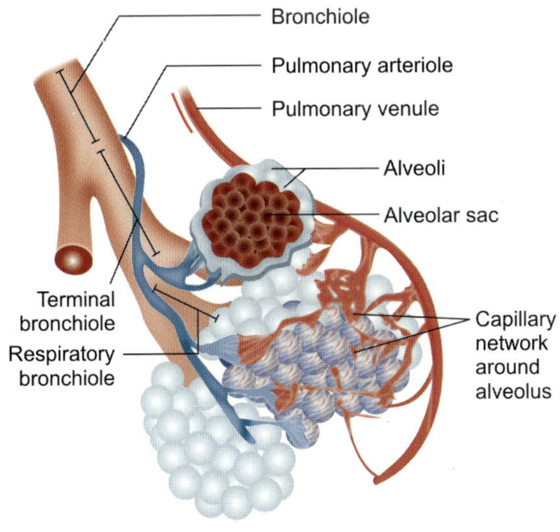

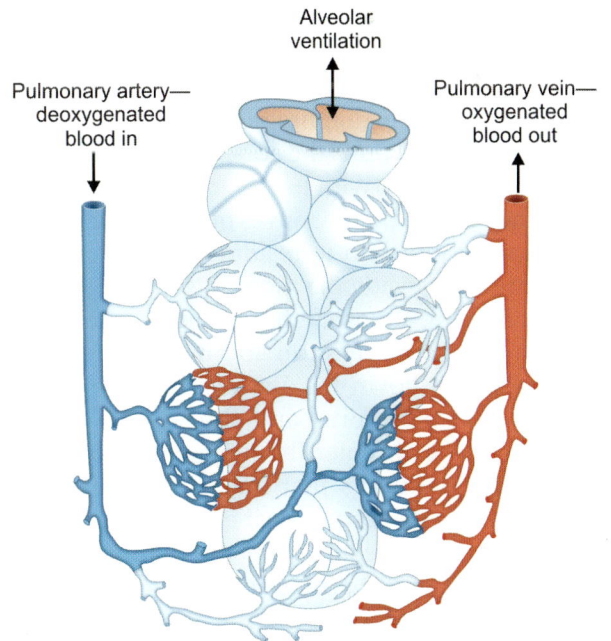

Fig. 4.1: Pulmonary alveoli. Clusters of alveoli and their blood supply. *(Saladin: Anatomy and Physiologyi. The Unity of Form and Function. Mc-Graw-Hill Co. 3 ed. 2003)*

Fig. 4.2: The acinus—the basic gas exchange unit of the lung *(Haslett C, Chilvers ER, Boon NA and Colledge NR: Davidson's Principles and Practice of Medicine. 19 ed. Livingstone C 2002)*

PHYSIOLOGY OF RESPIRATION

"The process of inspiration and expiration"

Airflow during inspiration and expiration depends on a passive gradient, with air always moving from a high pressure area to a low pressure area (flow in one way only). If atmospheric pressure is higher than air pressure inside the lungs, air will move from the atmosphere into the lungs (inspiration).

For expiration to occur, pressure must be higher in the lungs than in the atmosphere. These pressure changes in the lungs result from alternations in the size of the thoracic cavity. As the size of the thoracic cavity decreases, the pressure inside the cavity increases.

A sequence of events is responsible for the change in size of the thorax and the changes in airflow with inspiration and expiration:

1. Normal quiet inspiration begins with contraction of the diaphragm and the external intercostal muscles.
2. The diaphragm flattens and descends, increasing the length of the thoracic cavity.
3. The external intercostal muscles raise the ribs and sternum up and outwards, increasing the transverse and anteroposterior diameters of the thorax.
4. The increased size of the thoracic cavity results in decreased pressure in the pleural cavity and in the alveoli and airways.
5. As the ribs and diaphragm move, the attached parietal pleura pulls the adhering visceral pleura and lungs along with it.
6. As the visceral pleura moves outwards, the elastic lungs expand with it, resulting in a decrease in air pressure inside the lungs.
7. At this point, atmospheric pressure is greater than intra-alveolar pressure, so air flows from the atmosphere down the airways into the alveoli; Note that the thorax and lungs must expand before more air enter the lungs; it is not the air entering the lungs that makes them expands. Breathing requires physical effort and energy.
8. During normal expiration, the diaphragm and external intercostal muscles relax, leading to a decrease in thoracic size.
9. This decrease, combined with the natural elastic recoil of the alveoli, results in increased intra-alveolar pressure (greater than atmospheric pressure).
10. Therefore, air flows out of the alveoli into atmosphere.

Gas Exchange and Transport

Air is a mixture of gases (nitrogen, oxygen, carbon dioxide), each of which contributes a share, called its **partial pressure,** to the total atmospheric pressure. Partial pressure is abbreviated P followed by the formula of the gas. The partial pressure of nitrogen is PN_2, for example. Nitrogen constitutes about 78.6% of the atmosphere; thus at 1 atm of pressure, $PN_2 = 78.6\% \times 760$ mmHg = 597 mmHg.

Dalton's law states that the total pressure of a gas mixture is the sum of the partial pressures of the individual gases. That is, $PN_2 + PO_2 + PH_2O + PCO_2 = 597.0 + 159.0 + 3.7 + 0.3 = 760.0$ mmHg. These partial pressures are important because they determine the rate of diffusion of a gas and, therefore, strongly affect the rate of gas exchange between the blood and alveolar air.

Concentration Gradients of the Gases

The PO_2 is about 104 mmHg in the alveolar air and 40 mmHg in the blood arriving at an alveolus. Oxygen, therefore, diffuses from the air into the blood, where it reaches a PO_2 of 104 mmHg. Before the blood leaves the lung, however, this drops to about 95 mmHg because blood in the pulmonary veins receives some oxygen-poor blood from the bronchial veins by way of anastomoses.

The PCO_2 is about 46 mmHg in the blood arriving at the alveolus and 40 mmHg in the alveolar air. Carbon dioxide, therefore, diffuses from the blood to the alveoli (Fig. 4.3). These changes are summarized here.

Blood entering lung	Blood leaving
PO_2 40 mmHg	PO_2 95 mmHg
PCO_2 46 mmHg	PCO_2 40 mmHg

These gradients differ under special circumstances such as high altitude and *hyperbaric oxygen therapy* (treatment with oxygen at greater than 1 atm of pressure). At high altitudes, the partial pressures of all atmospheric gases are lower. Atmospheric PO_2, for example, is 159 mmHg at sea level and 110 mmHg at 3,000 m (10,000 ft).

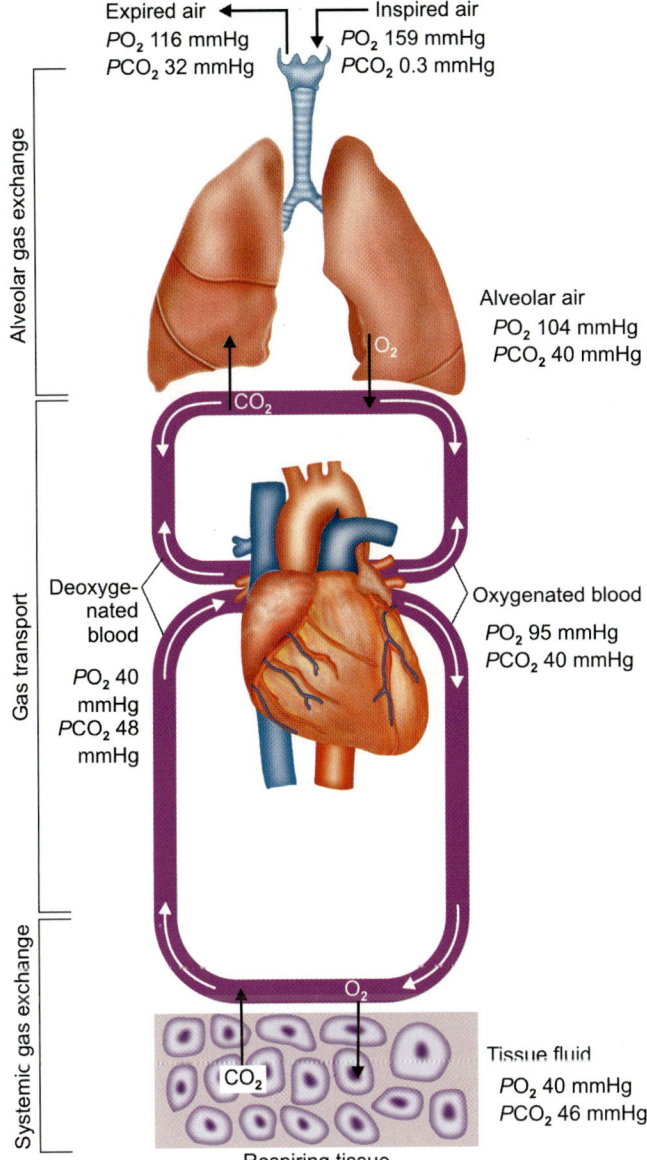

Expired air
PO_2 116 mmHg
PCO_2 32 mmHg

Inspired air
PO_2 159 mmHg
PCO_2 0.3 mmHg

Alveolar air
PO_2 104 mmHg
PCO_2 40 mmHg

O_2

CO_2

Deoxyge-
nated
blood

PO_2 40
mmHg
PCO_2 48
mmHg

Oxygenated blood
PO_2 95 mmHg
PCO_2 40 mmHg

O_2

CO_2

Tissue fluid
PO_2 40 mmHg
PCO_2 46 mmHg

Respiring tissue

Alveolar gas exchange

Gas transport

Systemic gas exchange

Fig. 4.3: Changes to PO_2 and PCO_2 along the circulatory route. Trace the partial pressure of oxygen from inspired air to expired air and explain each change in PO_2 along the way. Do the same for PCO_2

The O_2 gradient from air to blood is proportionately less, less O_2 diffuses into the blood. In a hyperbaric oxygen chamber, by contrast, a patient is exposed to 3 to 4 atm of oxygen to treat such conditions as gangrene (to kill anaerobic bacteria) and carbon monoxide poisoning (to displace the carbon monoxide from hemoglobin). The PO_2 ranges between 2,300 and 3,000 mmHg. Thus, there is a very steep gradient of PO_2 from alveolus to blood and diffusion into the blood is accelerated.

Control of Respiration

The control centers for breathing are located in the medulla and the pons. The medulla has two respiratory nuclei. One of them, called the inspiratory center, is composed primarily of neurons, which fire during inspiration, and stimulate the muscles of inspiration. The more frequently they fire, the more motor units are recruited and the more deeply you inhale. If they fire longer than usual, each breath is prolonged and the respiratory rate is slower. When they stop firing, elastic recoil of the lungs and thoracic cage produces passive expiration.

The inspiratory center in the medulla controls the basic rhythm by stimulating the phrenic nerves to the diaphragm and the intercostal nerves to the external intercostal muscles. These stimuli occur spontaneously in a rhythmic fashion, each lasting about two seconds.

The other nucleus is the expiratory center, which fire during forced expiration. The expiratory center inhibits the inspiratory center when deeper expiration is needed. Conversely, the inspiratory center inhibits the expiratory center when an unusually deep inspiration is needed. Fibers from these neurons travel down the spinal cord and synapse with lower motor neurons in the cervical to thoracic regions. From here, nerve fibers travel in the phrenic nerves to the diaphragm and intercostal nerves to the intercostal muscles. Additional centers in the pons play a role in coordinating inspiration, expiration, and intervals of each.

Any depression of the central nervous system activity, for example, by drugs, can lead to slow, shallow breathing. Other factors include activity of the hypothalamus, perhaps in response to emotions; or stretch receptors in the lungs or the Hering-Breuer reflex, which prevents excessive lung expansion; or voluntary control, as required when singing. However, voluntary control is limited by the level of carbon dioxide in the blood. When the concentration or partial pressure of carbon dioxide (PCO_2) in the blood rises, breathing resumes automatically. For this reason, a child who intensionally holds to stop her breath will eventually have to breathe spontaneously.

Other factors are most important in respiratory control.

Chemoreceptors (Fig. 4.4) sense changes in the levels of carbon dioxide, hydrogen ions, and oxygen in the blood or CSF.

• *The central chemoreceptors* are paired areas close to the surface of the medulla oblongata, ventral to the

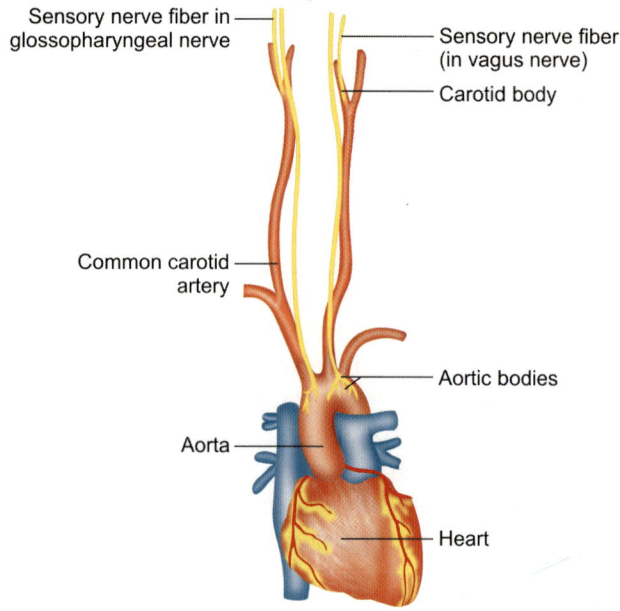

Sensory nerve fiber in glossopharyngeal nerve

Sensory nerve fiber (in vagus nerve)

Carotid body

Common carotid artery

Aortic bodies

Aorta

Heart

Fig. 4.4: Nervous pathways from the peripheral chemoreceptors to the respiratory centers of the medulla oblongata

The central chemoreceptors in the medulla respond quickly to slight elevation in PCO_2 (from a normal 40 to 43 mmHg) or to a decrease in pH (increased H^+) of the cerebrospinal fluid.

- *The peripheral chemoreceptors*, located in the carotid bodies at the bifurcation of the common carotid arteries and in the aortic body in the aortic arch, are sensitive to decreased oxygen levels in arterial blood as well as low pH.

Normal oxygen levels provide a substantial reserve of oxygen in the venous blood. A marked decrease in oxygen (from approximately 105 to 60 mm Hg) is necessary before the chemoreceptors respond to hypoxia. The control mechanism can be important when individuals with chronic lung disease adapt to a sustained elevation in PCO_2 and move to a hypoxia drive. Such individuals are dependent on low oxygen levels rather than the normal slight elevation in carbon dioxide to stimulate inspiration. Therefore, it is important for these patients always to remain slightly hypoxic and not be given excessive amounts of oxygen at any time.

When carbon dioxide levels in the blood increase (hypercapnia), the gas easily diffuses into the CNF,

inspiratory center. They primarily monitor the pH of the cerebrospinal fluid (CSF) and the tissue fluid of the brain.

Pulmonary ventilation is adjusted to maintain the pH of the brain. Hydrogen ions cannot freely cross the blood–CSF barrier, but CO_2 does. In the CSF, CO_2 reacts with water and releases H^+. H^+ then strongly stimulates the central chemoreceptors, which transmit signals to the inspiratory center.

Normally, the blood has a pH of 7.40± 0.05. Deviation from this range is called acidosis when the pH falls below 7.35 and alkalosis when it rises above 7.45. The most common cause of acidosis is hypercapnia, a $PCO_2 > 43$ mmHg. The most common cause of alkalosis is hypocapnia, a $PCO_2 < 37$ mmHg. Whenever there is a CO_2 imbalance in the blood, CO_2 diffusion across the blood–CSF barrier creates a parallel shift in the pH of the CSF.

Clinical Terminology of Ventilation

Apnea: Temporary cessation of breathing (one or more skipped breaths).

Dyspnea: Labored, gasping breathing; shortness of breath.

Eupnea: Normal, relaxed, quiet breathing; typically 500 mL/breath, 12 to 15 breaths/min.

Hyperpnea: Increased rate and depth of breathing in response to exercise, pain, or other conditions.

Hyperventilation: Increased pulmonary ventilation in excess of metabolic demand, frequently associated with anxiety; expels CO_2 faster than it is produced, thus lowering the blood CO_2 concentration and raising the pH.

Hypoventilation: Reduced pulmonary ventilation; leads to an increase in blood CO_2 concentration, if ventilation is insufficient to expel CO_2 as fast as it is produced.

Orthopnea: Dyspnea that occurs when a person is lying down.

Respiratory arrest: Permanent cessation of breathing (unless there is medical intervention).

Tachypnea: Accelerated respiration.

Smoking is one of the most important modifiable factors contributing to disease and premature death. It significantly increases the risk and severity of atherosclerosis, and is directly related to the development of cancers of the lung, esophagus, stomach, and urinary bladder. Current studies also indicate an association between second-hand smoke exposure and an increased risk of bronchitis, ear infections, and asthma in children. The most common smoking-related diseases are emphysema and several types of cancers (Plate III).

lowering the pH and stimulating the respiratory center, resulting in an increased rate and depth of respirations (hyperventilation). Hypercapnia causes respiratory acidosis, and acidosis depresses the nervous system. Hypocapnia, or low PCO_2, may be caused by hyperventilation after excessive amounts of carbon dioxide have been expired. Hypocapnia causes respiratory alkalosis.

CHRONIC OBSTRUCTIVE PULMONARY DISEASES

Chronic obstructive pulmonary disease (COPD) refers to any disorder in which there is a long-term obstruction of airflow and a substantial reduction in pulmonary ventilation. The major COPDs are *asthma, chronic bronchitis* and *emphysema.*

Chronic Bronchitis

Beginning smokers exhibit inflammation and hyperplasia of the bronchial mucosa. In **chronic bronchitis,** the cilia are immobilized and reduced in number, while goblet cells enlarge and produce excess mucus. With extra mucus and fewer cilia to dislodge it, smokers develop a chronic cough that brings up **sputum,** a mixture of mucus and cellular debris. Thick, stagnant mucus in the respiratory tract provides a growth medium for bacteria, while cigarette smoke incapacitates the alveolar macrophages and reduces defense mechanisms against respiratory infections. Smokers, therefore, develop chronic infection and bronchial inflammation, with symptoms that include dyspnea, hypoxia, cyanosis, and attacks of coughing.

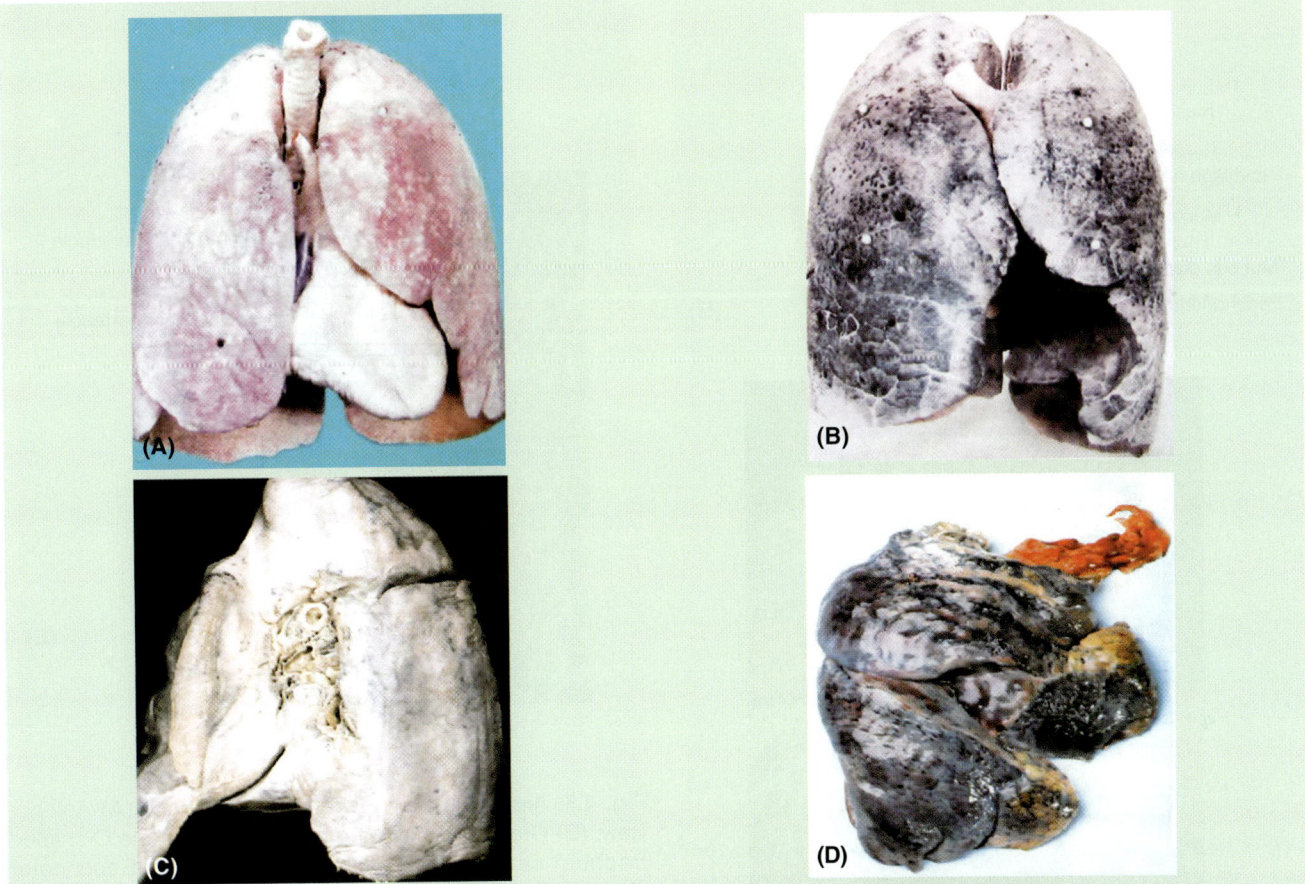

Plate (III) (A) Non-smoker's lung. **(B)** Smoker's lung *(McKliney and O'houghlin, 2006),* Effect of smoking. **(C)** A healthy adult lung. **(D)** A smoker's lung with carcinoma

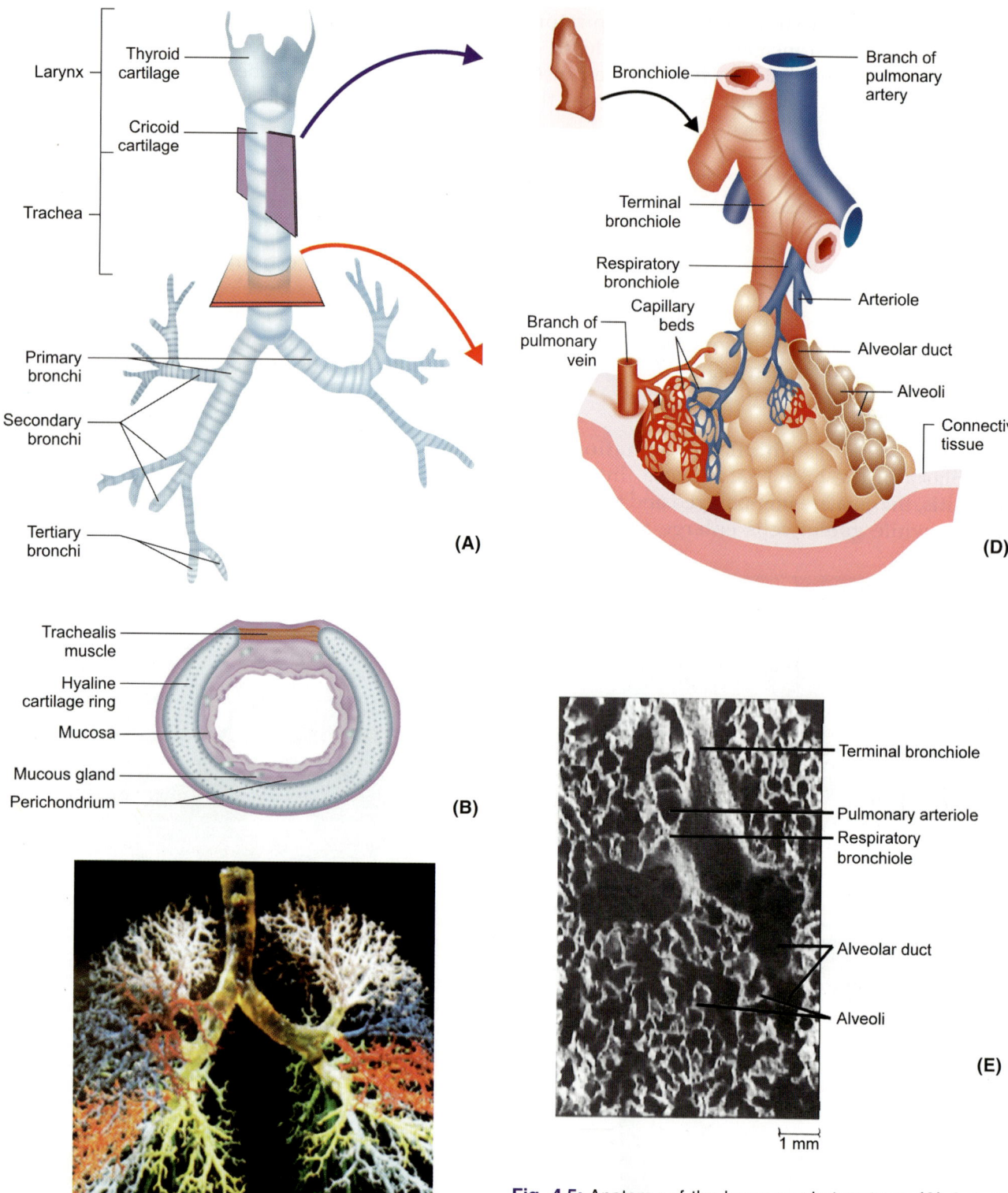

Fig. 4.5: Anatomy of the lower respiratory tract. **(A)** Anterior view. **(B)** Cross-section of the trachea showing the C-shaped tracheal cartilage. **(C)** The bronchial tree. Each color identify a bronchopulmonary segment by a tertiary bronchus. **(D)** Terminal bronchioles, **(E)** Pulmonary alveoli *(McKliney and O'houghlin,2006)*

Branch into respiratory bronchioles, which then branch into alveolar ducts and alveoli. The pulmonary vessels travel with the bronchioles, and the proximal capillaries wrap around the alveoli for gas exchange (Fig. 4.5).

Asthma

In asthma, an allergen triggers the release of histamine and other inflammatory chemicals that cause intense bronchoconstriction and sometimes suffocation. The other COPDs are almost always caused by cigarette smoking but occasionally result from air pollution or occupational exposure to airborne irritants. Beginning smokers exhibit inflammation and hyperplasia of the bronchial mucosa.

Emphysema

In **emphysema,** alveolar walls breakdown and the lung exhibits larger but fewer alveoli (Figs 4.6 and 4.7). Thus, there is much less respiratory membrane available for gas exchange. The lungs become fibrotic and less elastic. The air passages open adequately during inspiration, but they tend to collapse and obstruct the outflow of air.

Air, therefore, becomes trapped in the lungs, and over a period of time, a person becomes barrel-chested. The overly stretched thoracic muscles contract weakly, which further contributes to the difficulty of expiration. People with emphysema become exhausted because they expend three to four times the normal amount of energy just to breathe. Even slight physical exertion, such as walking across a room, can cause severe shortness of breath.

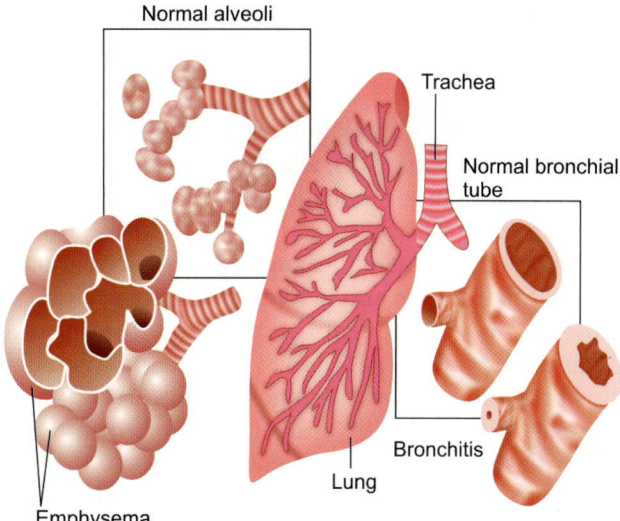

Emphysema
With emphysema, the walls of alveoli are damaged by inflammation. Alveoli can lose their natural elasticity become overstretched and rupture forming 1 large space instead of small ones.

Chronic brochitis is a chronic inflammation and thickening of the walls of your bronchial tubes which narrows them. It often induces coughing spells.

Fig. 4.6

All of the COPDs tend to reduce pulmonary compliance and vital capacity and cause hypoxemia, hypercapnia, and respiratory acidosis. Hypoxemia stimulates the kidneys to secrete erythropoietin, which leads to accelerated erythrocyte production and polycythemia, COPD also leads to **cor pulmonale**—hypertrophy and potential failure of the right heart due to obstruction of the pulmonary circulation. Asthma and emphysema will be discussed in detail.

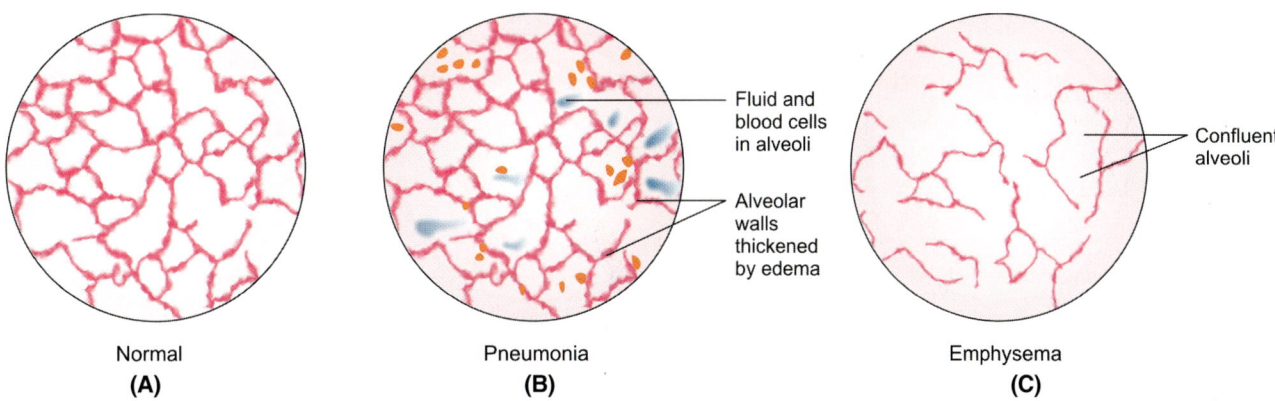

Normal
(A)

Fluid and blood cells in alveoli

Alveolar walls thickened by edema

Pneumonia
(B)

Confluent alveoli

Emphysema
(C)

Fig. 4.7: Pulmonary alveoli in health and disease. **(A)** In a healthy lung, the alveoli are small and have thin respiratory membranes. **(B)** In pneumonia, the respiratory membranes (alveolar walls) and thick with edema, and the alveoli contain fluid and blood cells. **(C)** In emphysema, alveolar membranes breakdown and neighboring alveoli join to form larger, fewer alveoli with less total surface area

BRONCHIAL ASTHMA

Asthma is a complex inflammatory condition involving many inflammatory cells, which release a wide variety of mediators. These mediators act on cells of the airway leading to smooth muscle contraction, mucus hypersecretion, plasma leakage, edema, activation of cholinergic reflexes and activation of sensory nerves, which can lead to amplification of the ongoing inflammatory response (Fig. 4.8). Chronic inflammation also leads to structural changes, such as subepithelial fibrosis and smooth muscle hypertrophy and hyperplasia, which are less easy to reserve than the acute processes. Inadequately treated chronic asthma is thus associated with structural changes in the lungs.

In asthma, the tracheobronchial tree is hyperirritable and overly responds to a variety of stimuli. The principle features of an acute asthmatic attack are mucous secretion and acute bronchospasm. Patients with chronic forms of respiratory disease (e.g. chronic obstructive pulmonary disease) are also a risk for bronchospasm (Fig. 4.9). Dyspnea and wheezing herald the onset of an acute asthmatic attack and demand immediate intervention.

Asthma runs in families and seems to result from a combination of hereditary factors and environmental irritants. Generally, asthma is most common, paradoxically, in two groups: (1) Inner-city children who are exposed to crowding, poor sanitation and

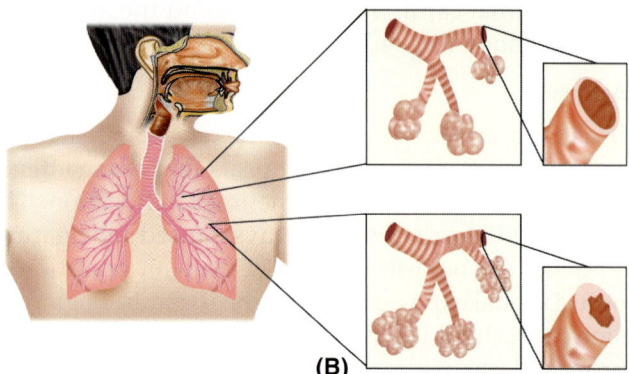

Fig. 4.9: (A) In normal bronchioles, the airway is open and unobstructed. **(B)** During an attack, the bronchioles of an asthma sufferer are constricted by bands of muscle around them. They may be further obstructed by increased mucus production and tissue inflammation

ventilation, and who do not go outside very much or get enough exercise; and (2) Children from extremely clean homes, perhaps because they have too little opportunity to develop normal immunities. Asthma is also more common in countries where vaccines and antibiotics are widely used. It is less common in developing countries.

Basic pathology is hyperactive airways with bronchospasm and increased mucous secretion.

The precipitant factors are (Figs 4.10 and 4.11):

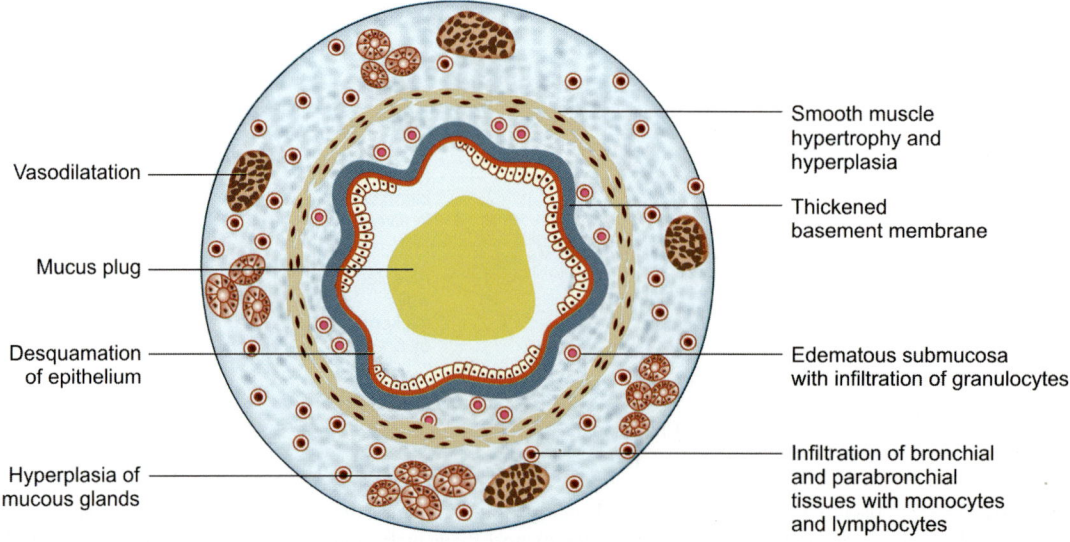

Vasodilatation

Mucus plug

Desquamation of epithelium

Hyperplasia of mucous glands

Smooth muscle hypertrophy and hyperplasia

Thickened basement membrane

Edematous submucosa with infiltration of granulocytes

Infiltration of bronchial and parabronchial tissues with monocytes and lymphocytes

Fig. 4.8: Pathological changes seen in the bronchus of an asthmatic. Notice the inflammatory cells in the bronchial tissues, and the presence of mucus plug expectorated by the patient *(Haslett et al, 2002)*

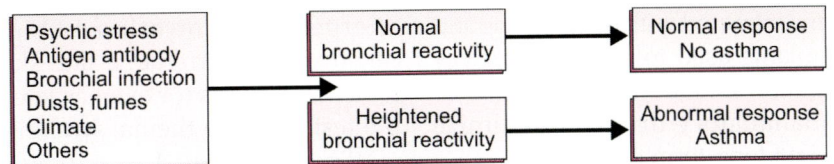

Fig. 4.10: Precipitating factors of bronchial asthma

1. Foods cow's milk, eggs, fish, chocolate, shellfish, tomatoes.
2. Drugs penicillin, vaccines, aspirin, nonsteroidal anti-inflammatory drugs (NSAIDs), cholinergic drugs, and beta-adrenergic blocking drugs.
3. Exercise or stress.
4. Viral respiratory tract infections.
5. Environmental allergies.
6. Cold air.
7. Smoke.
8. Chemicals and highly emotional states such as anxiety, stress and nervousness.

Metabisulfite preservatives of food and drugs (local anesthetics containing epinephrine) may cause wheezing, when low levels of the enzyme sulfite oxidase are present. Sulfur oxide is produced in the absence of sulfite oxidase. The buildup of sulfur dioxide in the bronchial tree precipitates an acute asthma attack.

Exercise-induced asthma is a form of asthma that is stimulated by exertional activity. It is believed that thermal changes during inhalation of cold air provoke mucosal irritation and airway hyperactivity. Children and young adults are more severely affected owing to their high level of physical activity.

Patients with infectious asthma develop bronchial constriction and increased airway resistance due to the inflammatory response of the bronchi to infection. Causative agents often are viruses, bacteria and fungi. Treatment of infection usually improves control of the pulmonary constriction.

The respiratory crisis is triggered by allergies in pollen, mold, animal dander, food, dust mites (Fig. 4.11), or cockroaches. The allergens stimulate plasma cells to secrete IgE, which binds to mast cells of the respiratory mucosa. Re-exposure to the allergen causes the mast cells to release a complex mixture of histamine, interleukins, and several other inflammatory chemicals, which trigger intense airway inflammation.

Within minutes, the bronchioles constrict spasmodically *(bronchospasm),* and a person exhibits

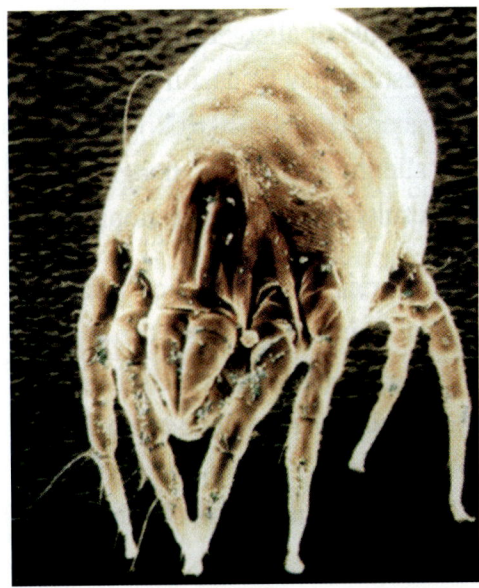

Fig. 4.11: The housedust mite. The fecal particles of this and related mite species are the most common cause of allergic asthma worldwide. The fecal particles are small enough to be inhaled into the peripheral airways in the lung. Dust mites are most common in moist, temperate environments. They feed on shed scales of human and animal skin, and commonly infest mattresses, pillows, carpets and soft furnishings. Their growth is encouraged by the low rate of air turnover in modern insulated houses. They are about 0.5 mm in length and invisible to the naked eye. Dust-mite allergy also plays a major role in peripheral rhinitis and possibly eczema *(Forbes and Jackson, 2003)*

severe coughing, wheezing, and sometimes fatal suffocation. A second respiratory crisis often occurs 6 to 8 hours later. Interleukins attract eosinophils to the bronchial tissue, where they secrete proteins that paralyze the respiratory cilia, severely damage the epithelium, and lead to scarring and extensive long-term damage to the lungs. The bronchioles also become edematous and plugged with thick, sticky mucous.

People who die of asthmatic suffocation typically show airways so plugged with gelatinous mucus that they could not exhale. The lungs remain hyperinflated even at autopsy. Asthma is treated with epinephrine and other adrenergic stimulants used to dilate the airway and restore breathing, and inhaled corticosteroids or nonsteroidal anti-inflammatory drugs to minimize airway inflammation and long-term damage.

Skin Test

Skin-prick testing may be useful in establishing the patient's immediate (type I) sensitivity to common allergens, thus confirming the patient's atopic state, and providing useful information about the possible role of allergens in disease. Skin-prick testing may be useful in asthma, rhinitis, allergic conjunctivitis, urticaria and other allergic conditions, though false positive results are common in atopic eczema.

In skin-prick testing, a tiny quantity of allergen is introduced into the superficial layers of the stratum corneum (Fig. 4.12). A true positive skin-prick test reaction (Fig. 4.13) indicates that specific IgE is fixed to mast cells in the skin and has led to a vasoactive response caused by release of histamine. When the allergen concentration is high, or the patient's sensitivity is extreme, a late skin reaction may also follow 4–6 hours (or even as late as 24–48 hours) after the test, with erythema, swelling and induration.

When performed in patients with asthma, with appropriate positive (histamine) and negative (diluent) controls, skin test results correlate well with the results of bronchial challenge testing with the allergens (which is performed routinely), and thus give useful information on the allergen involved; however, the results must always be correlated with clinical history. Skin testing is relatively unreliable for ingested allergens including food, partly because of the nature of the available allergen preparation and partly because reactions to ingested substances are not always mediated by IgE.

Medical Therapy

Drugs for asthmatic and allergic patients are described in Box 4.1.

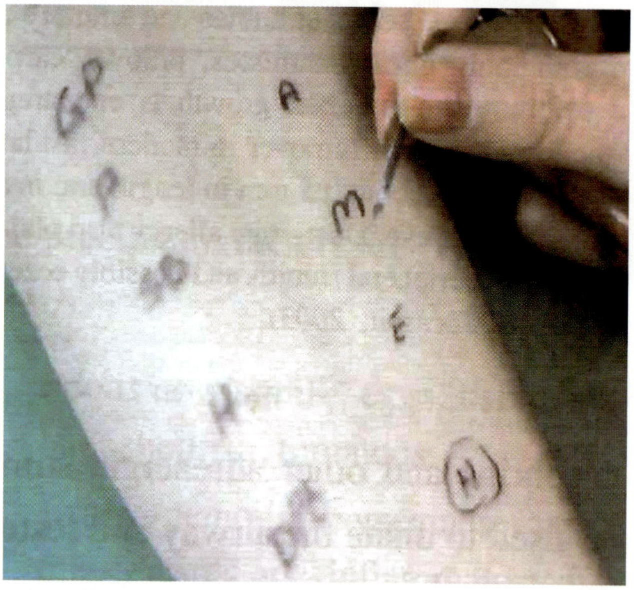

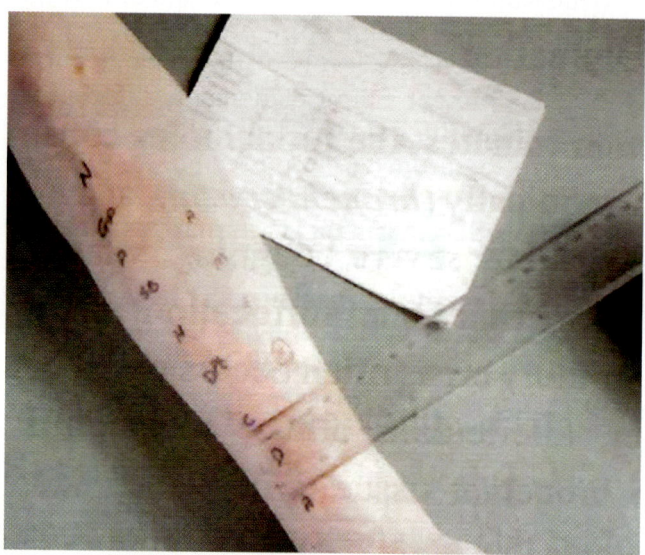

Fig. 4.12: Skin-prick testing. The volar surface of the forearm is cleaned, prick sites are marked, and drops of allergen extract in appropriate concentration are placed on the skin. The test should always include a negative control of 0.5% phenol saline, the suspending solution for the allergens, and histamine 1% as a positive control. A lance or standard needle is introduced through each drop at 45° to the skin surface to a depth of about 1 mm, the skin is lifted slightly, and the lance withdrawn. The procedure is painless, and the puncture sites should not bleed. The skin is blotted dry, and the resultant reaction is assessed at 15–20 minutes

Fig. 4.13: Reading the skin-prick test results. The maximum reaction is usually seen after 15–20 minutes. The saline control (N) should be negative. The histamine control (H) should be positive; recent antihistamine administration may cause a negative result, and this invalidates other negative reactions. The presence of a positive skin response indicates the presence of specific IgE antibody in the blood, and there is a reasonable correlation between the size of the wheal and the significance of different inhaled allergens in a single patient. Positive results are best recorded by measuring the diameter of the wheal in millimeters, using a transport gauge or a ruler. Here the strongest reaction is to grass pollen (GP), and significant positive reactions are also seen to cat © and the housedust mite *(Forbes and Jackson, 2003)*

Box 4.1: Drugs for asthmatic and allergic patients

Albuterol (ventolin, proventil)	
Action:	Selective β2-receptor agonist; relaxes bronchial smooth muscle
Preparation:	Metered dose inhaler
Dose:	1 or 2 inhalations every 3 minutes
Diphenhydramine (benadryl)	
Action:	Selectively blocks histamine receptors; counteracts cutaneous reactions, including pruritis, rash, and urticaria.
Preparation:	50 mg/ml, SDV, ampoules, prefilled syringes
Dose:	IV, 25 mg every 5 minutes up to two doses; *IM,* 50 mg.
Epinephrine	
Action:	α/β receptor agonist; increases cardiac output, bronchodilators and decongests edematous mucosa.
Preparation:	1 mg/ml, ampoules and prefilled syringes
Dose:	*Subcutaneous* 0.3 to 0.5 mg every 5 minutes up to two does.
	0.1 mg every 3 minutes up to five doses.

SVD, Single-vial dose; IV, intravenous; IM, intramuscular

Dental Management (Box 4.2)

1. Stop procedure.
2. Positional changes—usually upright with slight forward tilt.
3. Oxygen supplementation.
4. Administer bronchodilator—ventolin via nebulizer (Figs 4.14 and 4.15).
5. If continues—epinephrine IM 1:1,000 0.3–0.5 mg. (adult).
6. Start aminophylline 5–7 mg/kg and give slowly, if attack continues after epinephrine has been given.
7. Call for medical help.

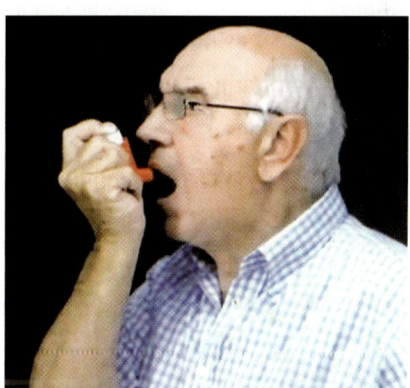

Fig. 4.14: Use of an inhaler by a patient

Drug Considerations in the Dental Management of Asthmatic Patient

1. Avoid aspirin-containing medications (use acetaminophen).
2. Avoid nonsteroidal anti-inflammatory drugs.
3. Avoid barbiturates and narcotics.
4. Avoid erythromycin and macrolide antibiotics in patients taking theophylline
5. Avoid local anaesthetics containing epinephrine or levonordephrine because of sulfite preservative.
6. Patients taking corticosteroid medications may require supplementation.
7. Provision of stress-free environment through establishment of rapport and openness.
8. If sedation is required, use nitrous oxide-oxygen inhalation and/or small doses of oral diazepam.

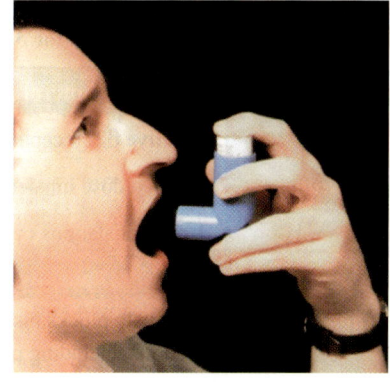

Fig. 4.15: A pressurized metered-dose inhaler (pMDI). All commonly used inhaled therapy for asthma is available in this form. Although convenient and portable, the pMDI requires good coordination between actuation and inhalation by the patient. The drug delivery characteristics of many pMDIs have changed recently, as new propellant gases (HFAs) have replaced CFC gases for environmental reasons

Box 4.2: Dental management of patient with asthma

1. *Identify and assess by history*
   a. Type of asthma (mild, moderate, or severe).
   b. Precipitating factors (and plan for allergen avoidance).
   c. Age at onset.
   d. Level of control (frequency, time of day, and severity of attacks):
      • How usually managed.
      • Medications being taken (how often quick-relief medication is used) and taken correctly on the day of the appointment.
      • Necessity of emergency care (life-threatening attacks, hospitalizations, emergency department visits).
      • Baseline forced expiratory volume (FEV) in 1 second, stable (not decreasing).
2. *Avoid known precipitating factors.*
3. *Obtain medical consultation for patient with severe persistent asthma.*
4. *Ask patient to bring current medication inhaler to every appointment and to keep it available,* (used prophylactically in persons with moderate to severe persistent disease) (Figs 4.14 and 4.15)
5. *Drug considerations:*
   a. Avoid aspirin-containing medications (use acetaminophen).
   b. Avoid nonsteroidal anti-inflammatory drugs (NSAIDs).
   c. Avoid barbiturates and narcotics (histamine lasing drugs).
   d. Avoid erythromycin and macrolide antibiotics in patients taking theophylline.
   e. Discontinue cimetidine 24 hr before intravenous sedation in patients taking theophylline.
6. *Local anesthetic considerations* (may elect to avoid solutions containing epinephrine or levonordefrine because of sulfite preservative).
7. *Patients taking chronic corticosteroid medications over the long term may require supplementation.*
8. *Provide stress-free environment through establishment of rapport and openness.*
9. *If sedation is required, nitrous oxide/oxygen inhalation sedation and/or small doses of oral diazepam recommended.*
10. *Recognize signs and symptoms of a severe or worsening asthma attack:*
    a. Inability to finish sentences with one breath.
    b. Ineffectiveness of bronchodilators to relieve dyspnea.
    c. Tachypnea equal to or greater than 25 breaths per minute.
    d. Tachycardia equal to or greater than 110 beats per minute.
    e. Diaphoresis.
    f. Accessory muscle usage.
    g. Paradoxical pulse.
11. *Administer fast-acting bronchodilator* (Note: Corticosteroids have delayed onset of action), oxygen, and, if needed, subcutaneous 0.3–0.5 ml of epinephrine (1:1000).
12. *Activate emergency medical system (EMS).*
13. *Repeat administration of fast-acting bronchodilator every 5 minutes until EMS arrives.*

EMPHYSEMA
(Emphys = Inflamed)

In emphysema, alveolar walls breakdown and the lung exhibits larger but fewer alveoli. Thus, there is much less respiratory membrane available for gas exchange.

Pulmonary emphysema is a condition characterized by abnormal dilation of the terminal alveoli and of other respiratory structures (Fig. 4.16). Chronic emphysema is one of the most common forms of pulmonary disease. The state of the disease may range from mild form to a severe debilitating state.

PATHOLOGY

In emphysema, alveolar walls breakdown and the lung exhibits larger but fewer alveoli (Fig. 4.7). Thus, there is much less respiratory membrane available for gas exchange. The lungs become fibrotic and less

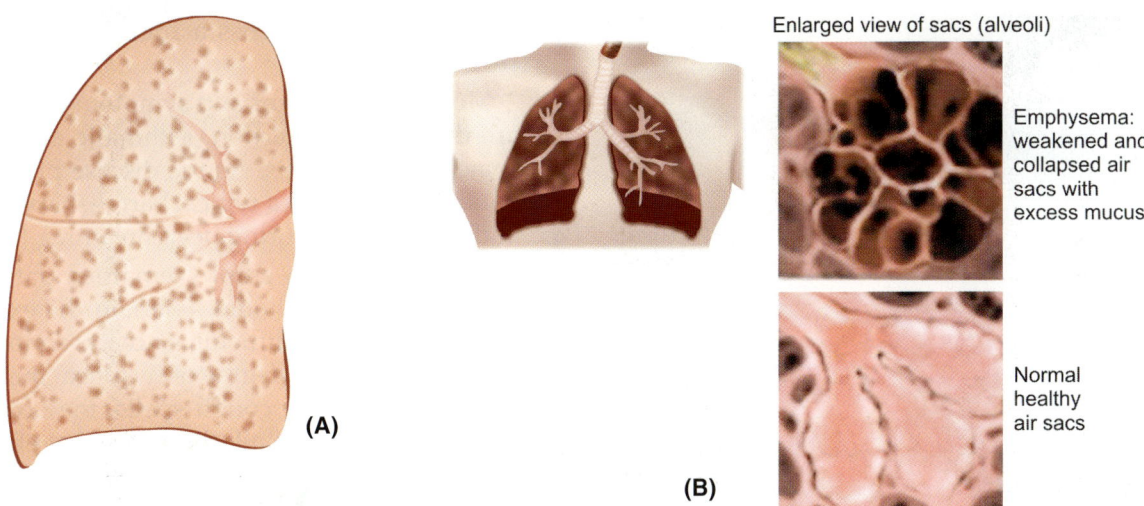

Enlarged view of sacs (alveoli)

Emphysema: weakened and collapsed air sacs with excess mucus

Normal healthy air sacs

(A)

(B)

Figs 4.16A and B: (A) The figure shows the gross and microscopic appearance of a lung involved with emphysema. Note the dilated air spaces and rupture of the alveolar walls in the upper part of the lung. **(B)** Dilation of the alveoli

elastic. The air passages open adequately during inspiration, but they tend to collapse and obstruct the outflow of air (Fig. 4.17).

The overly stretched thoracic muscles contract weakly, which further contributes to the difficulty of expiration (Fig. 4.18). Air, therefore, becomes trapped in the lungs, and over a period of time, a person becomes barrel-chested (Figs 4.19 and 4.20).

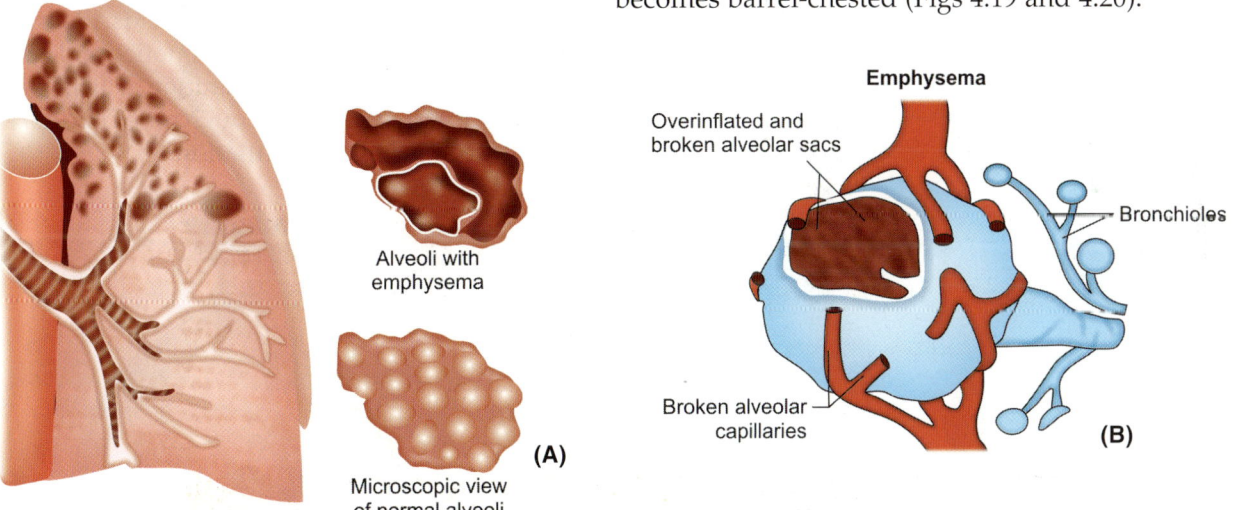

Alveoli with emphysema

Microscopic view of normal alveoli

(A)

Emphysema

Overinflated and broken alveolar sacs

Bronchioles

Broken alveolar capillaries

(B)

Figs 4.17A and B: Breakage of the alveolar sacs. Air trapped in the lungs

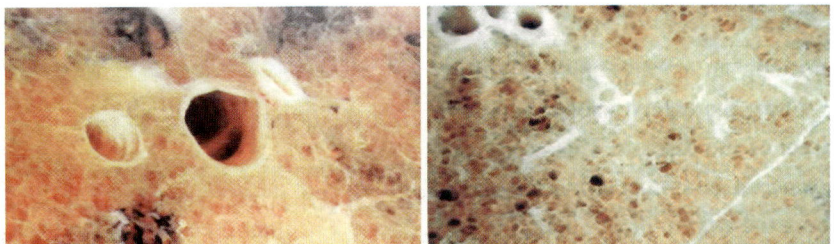

Figs 4.18A and B: The pathology of emphysema. **(A)** Normal lung. **(B)** Emphysematous lung showing gross loss of the normal surface area available for gas exchange *(Haslett et al, 2002)*

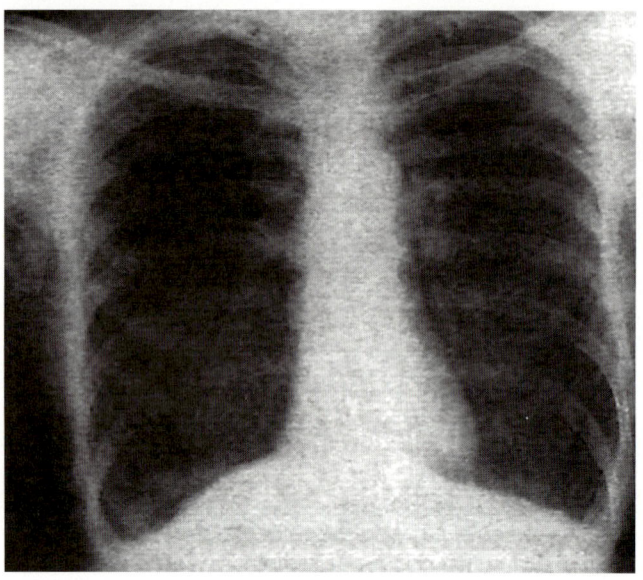

Fig. 4.19: Emphysema. The PA chest X-ray shows hyperinflation of both lung fields, producing depression of both diaphragms and a characteristic long, thin mediastinum. There are also calcified lesions and some scarring at both apices and both hila as a result of old, healed tuberculosis *(Forbes and Jackson, 2003)*

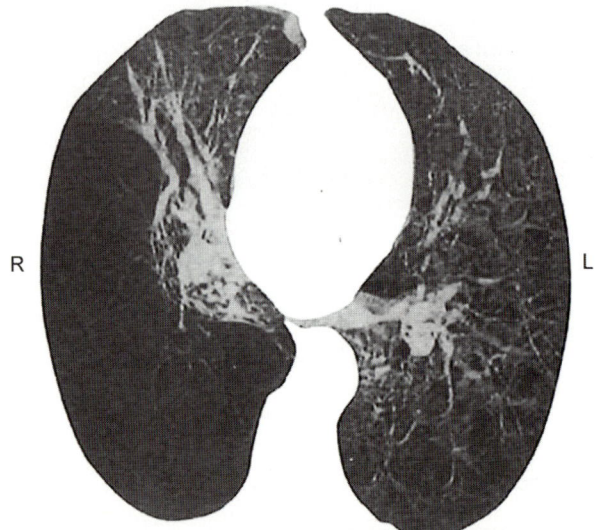

Fig. 4.20: Gross emphysema. High resolution CT showing emphysema most evident in the right lower lobe *(Haslett C, Chilvers E R, Boon N A, and Colledge N R: Davidson's Principles and Practice of Medicine. 19 ed. Livingstone C 2002)*

Signs and Symptoms

People with emphysema become exhausted because they expend three to four times the normal amount of energy just to breathe. Even slight physical exertion, such as walking across a room, can cause severe shortness of breath.

Most common signs and symptoms of emphysema are dyspnea on exertion, asthmatic attacks, and in some cases, cyanosis. As the disease progresses, the patient may exhibit a typical barrel-shaped chest and audible wheezes during deep breathing (Fig. 4.21).

When seeing an emphysematous patient in the office, the dentist should ascertain the extent of the disease. This is not difficult, since it is simply a matter of determining the degree of dyspnea, the frequency and severity of the cough spells, the occurrence of cyanosis, and above all, the restricting effects of the disease on the patient's daily activities.

Like the patient with bronchitis and bronchiectasis, the patient who has emphysema should be asked to clear the tracheobronchial tree as much as possible by deep breathing and coughing just before the appointment. Bronchodilator sprays and expectorants also may be helpful. As a rule, early morning is not a good time for appointments; they should be scheduled later in the day after the patient has had a chance to loosen and clear the lung fields. Preoperative medications such as sedatives, hypnotics, and narcotics should be used with extreme caution, if at all, because they may interfere with the cough reflex or depress an already compromised ventilation.

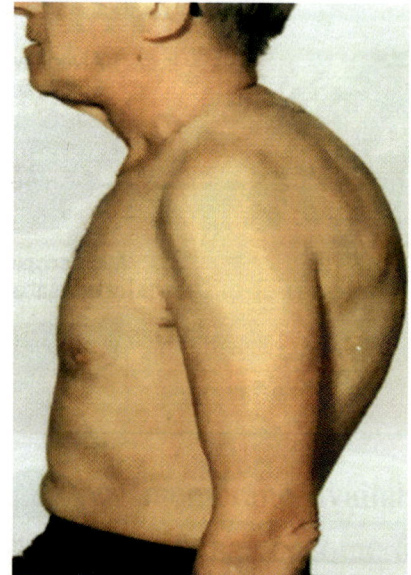

Fig. 4.21: Emphysema. The hyperinflation of the chest and associated kyphosis are typical but not diagnostic. A similar appearance may be seen in any chronic respiratory disorder *(Forbes and Jackson, 2003)*

Diseases of the lung attain significance for local anesthesia when the patient suffers from allergic asthma or present chronic obstruction pulmonary diseases which result in pulmonary insufficiency. Episodes of allergic asthma have been induced by the antioxidant sodium sulfite, which is essential for the stability of the catecholamine. High-risk respiratory patients can be additionally endangered by the methemoglobin of prilocaine. The disorders where the application of local anesthetic is contraindicated as it leads to the production of methemoglobin are shown in Box 4.4.

Tuberculosis is a systemic infectious disease, granulomatous in nature caused by acid-fast bacilli *Mycobacterium tuberculosis* or rarely, *Mycobacterium bovis*. It is of worldwide prevalence (Table 4.1) and have varying clinical manifestations.

Table 4.1 presents data about tuberculosis (TB) in various regions of the world (WHO 1991). Most persons who suffer from TB are found in Africa, Southeast Asia and in the Western Pacific regions. The WHO estimates that 1.7 billion people are infected worldwide. Of critical importance is the increase in TB cases that are resistant to therapy.

Box 4.3: Dental management of chronic obstructive pulmonary disease

Dental management of the patient with COPD

1. Review history for evidence of concurrent heart disease; take appropriate precautions, if heart disease is present.
2. Avoid treating, if upper respiratory infection is present.
3. Treat in upright chair position.
4. Use local anesthetic as usual.
5. Avoid use of rubber dam in severe disease.
6. Use pulse oximetry to monitor oxygen saturation. Use low-flow (2 to 3 L/min) supplemental oxygen when oxygen saturation drops below 95%; it may become necessary when oxygen saturation drops below 91%.
7. Avoid nitrous oxide/oxygen inhalation sedation with severe COPD and emphysema.
8. Consider low dose oral diazepam or other benzodiazepine; these may cause oral dryness.
9. Avoid use of barbiturates, narcotics, antihistamines, and anticholinergics.
10. Supplemental steroids may be needed, if patient is taking steroids and an invasive procedure is planned.
11. Avoid erythromycin, macrolide antibiotics, and ciprofloxacin for patients taking theophylline.
12. Do not use outpatient general anesthesia.

Box 4.4 Disorders which lead to the production of methemoglobin (application of local anesthetics is contraindicated)

1. Anemia.
2. Glucose-6-phosphate-dehydrogenase deficiency.
3. Idiopathic methemoglobinemia.
4. Manifest cardiac insufficiency.
5. Respiratory insufficiency.

Table 4.1: Tuberculosis in various regions of world

Region	Infected population		Fatal cases
	(in millions)	New case	
Africa	171	1400000	660000
America*	117	560000	220000
Eastern Mediterranean Area	52	594000	160000
Southeast Asia[1]	426	2480000	940000
Western Pacific	574	2560000	890000
Europe and other industrialized countries[2]	382	410000	40000
Total	1722	8004000	2910000

*Except United States and Canada; [1]Except Japan, Australia and New Zealand; [2]United States, Japan, Australia, New Zealand

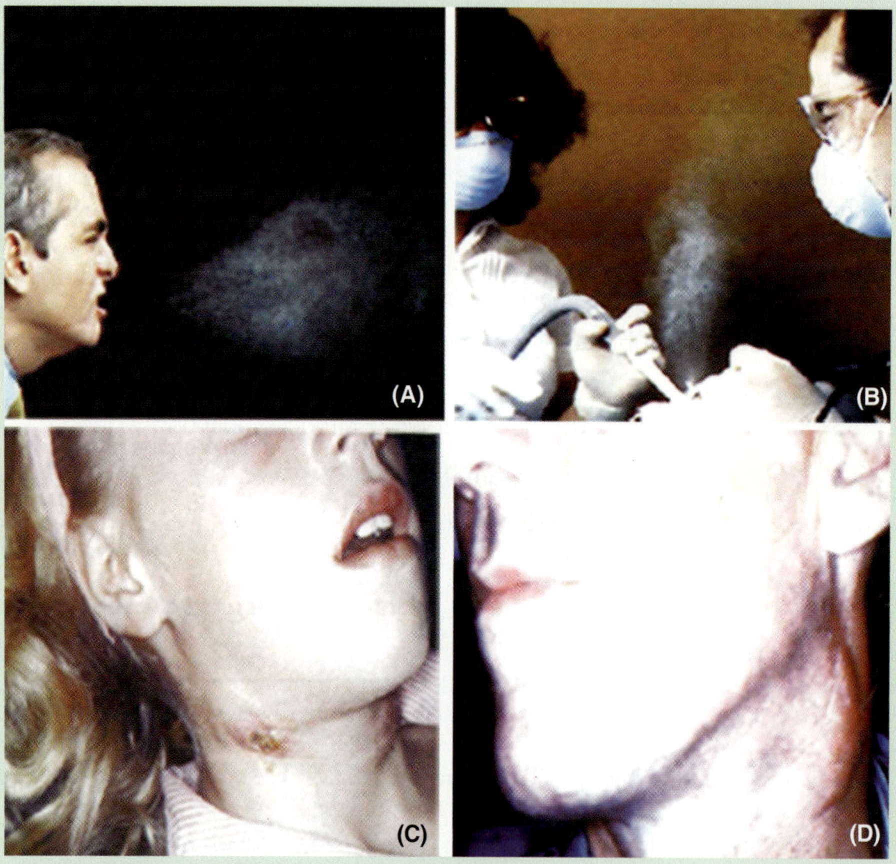

Plate (IV) **(A)** Mycobacterial tuberculosis (MBT) is carried in airborne particles called droplet nuclei that are generated when person with infectious TB disease coughs, sneezes, shouts, signs or talk *(Proteous and Terezhalmy, 2008)*. **(B)** While high-speed and ultrasonic dental instrumentation clearly generate droplet nuclei. There is a paucity of data linking dental instrumentation to the generation of droplet nuclei containing MBT *(Nuala et al, 2008)*. **(C)** Submandibular fistula secondary to tuberculous cervical lymph nodes *(Neville, 2009)*. **(D)** Tuberculosis of the cervical lymph nodes

Types of Oral Tuberculosis

Two main types of oral tuberculosis infection occur, one is primary and other is secondary.

Primary lesion: Develops when bacteria are directly inoculated in the oral tissue of a person who has not acquired immunity to the disease. It involves gingival, tooth extraction socket and buccal fold.

Secondary lesion: Infection is carried in by hematogenous route or through break in the tissue surface, is deposited in the submucosal, subsequently proliferates and ulcerates the overlying mucosa. It occurs more frequently in cases of extrapulmonary tuberculosis.

- *Pulmonary tuberculosis:* A persistence cough, hemoptysis and abundant sputum are usual features of pulmonary tuberculosis. There is also evening rise in temperature of 0.5° to 2°F and night sweats.
- *Miliary tuberculosis:* It spreads through bloodstream and there is wide involvement of many organs like kidney, liver and is called miliary tuberculosis.
- *Pott's disease:* If tubercular involvement of spine occurs in children, then it is called Pott's disease.

Transmission and Prevalence

Prevalence is more in the low income group with low socioeconomic and unhygienic condition. The common cause of entry of the bacillus in body is by inhalation. Infants and young children are at risk in acquiring this disease. Mycobacterial tuberculosis (MBT) is carried in airborne particles called droplet nuclei that are generated when persons with infectious TB disease cough, sneeze, shout, sing, or talk (Plate IV-A).

These droplet nuclei are between 1–5 microns in size, which can remain suspended in air for hours and can be carried in normal air currents throughout a room or building. The probability of a person exposed to MBT becoming infected depends on the concentration of infectious droplet nuclei in the air and the duration of the exposure to a person with infectious TB disease. Enviromental factors such as exposure in confined spaces, inadequate ventilation, and recirculation of air containing infectious droplet nuclei further increase the likelihood of transmission. The persons at highest risk for exposure to an infection with MBT are close contacts of persons who share air space in a household or other enclosed environment with person with pulmonary tuberculosis.

The lung is the most common site for TB disease. Classic symptoms include chronic ill health, coughing with hemoptysis, low-grade fever, weight loss, and night sweats. About 15% of patients with TB disease present with an extrapulmonary site of infection. This is especially common in patients who have both TB and an HIV infection. Expectoration of the infected sputum may cause tuberculous tracheitis, laryngitis (hoarseness, coughing, and pain), and tuberculous ulcers on the tonsils (dysphagia) and nasal cavity (obstruction, perforation, nasal discharge).

The systemic presentation of extrapulmonary tuberculosis is illustrated in Fig. 4.22. Tuberculous lesions of the upper aerodigestive tract have become rare. Tuberculosis may also be presented around the upper aerodigestive tract as parotitis, intraosseous lesions, preauricular swelling and trismus, tracheitis and laryngitis. Infection can occur through ingestion of unpasteurized infected cow milk.

Microorganisms may become disseminated by either bloodstream or lymphatic spread. It can rarely be transmitted through the placenta from the diseased mother to fetus. It is postulated an MBT infection *in utero* is either the result of: (1) hematogenous infection through the umbilical vein or (2) prenatal aspiration of infected amniotic fluid (Cantwell et al, 1994; Li CK et al, 1989; Popli et al, 1998). Congenital TB is rare but fatal, if untreated and it is difficult to diagnose in time to treat successfully without knowledge of a maternal history of TB.

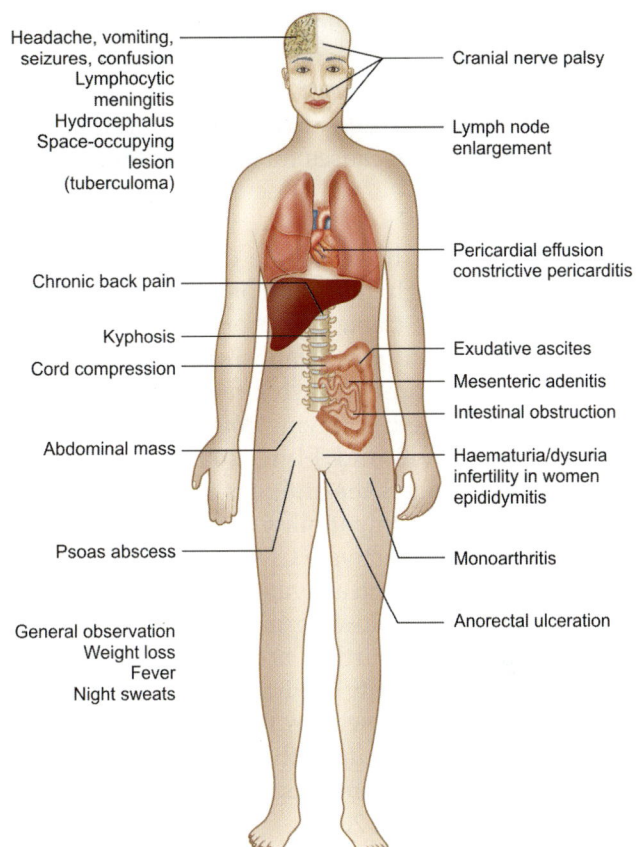

Fig. 4.22: Systemic presentation of extrapulmonary tuberculosis

Etiology

The causative organism first member identified as is *Tuberculous bacillus* and the disease is designated as *Mycobacterium tuberculosis*. The organism is anaerobic, non-motile, non-sporing, rod-shaped and is stained with special Ziehl-Neelson stain. Constitutional factors include: low income group, low and unhygienic living conditions and malnutrition and over-crowding.

Pathogenesis

Initial tuberculosis usually occurs in lungs but occasionally occurs in tonsil or alimentary tract. In most of the patients, primary infection and the associated lymph node lesions heal and calcify. In some cases, caseous tuberculosis focus ruptures into vein and produces acute dissemination throughout the body, a condition called as acute miliary tuberculosis. Meningitis often complicates this condition.

Progressive pulmonary tuberculosis may develop directly from a primary lesion or may occur following reaction of an incompletely healed primary focus. Post-primary pulmonary tuberculosis is a condition in which liquefied center of tuberculosis pulmonary infection is discharged into sinus. Extension of infection into pleura causes tuberculosis pleurisy.

Immunologic Aspect

When susceptible hosts inhale droplet nuclei, the bacilli travel through the mouth or nasal passages, the upper respiratory tract, and bronchi to the alveoli where a local infection is established (Nardell, 1993). The immune response to such infections is predominantly cell-mediated, involving both CD4+ and CD8+ T cells (Lazarevic and Flyn, 2002). Pulmonary macrophages process the antigens and present them to both major histocompatibility complex (MHC) class II molecules, which activate CD4+ cells; and to MHC class I molecules, which activate CD8+ T cells. Within two to ten weeks following exposure, the immune response will limit further multiplication of MET. However, if the quantity or virulence of the TB bacilli is such that they overwhelm the immune response, the bacilli may disseminate throughout the body by lymphatic and hematogenous spread (Glickman MS, Jacobs, 2001; Milburn, 2001).

Latent TB Infection (LTBI)

The immune response to MBT culminates in the formation of tuberculous granulomas at foci of infection. Consequently, not all bacilli are eliminated from the body and those incarcerated in granulomas can remain viable for many years.

At this stage, the person infected is said to have LTBI. Although immunological test results for MBT are positive, these patients have no symptoms, no radiographic abnormalities compatible with tuberculosis, and all bacteriologic studies are negative. Patients with LTBI are not contagious (Saunders and Cooper, 2000).

Oral Manifestations

Tuberculous lesions of the mouth may be either primary or secondary to pulmonary tuberculosis, with secondary lesions being more common. Majority of oral lesions are secondary to infection in some other parts of body. The oral lesions of the disease, although not common, occur in various forms. Orofacial presentation of tuberculous disease includes swelling, pain, loosening of teeth and even the displacement of tooth buds. Other manifestations may include an ulcer, granulomas, involvement of the salivary glands and temporomandibular joints, and tuberculous lymphadenitis.

Lymph Node Involvement

If the microorganisms spreads by lymphatics to lymph nodes, it leads to marked enlargement of the cervical lymph nodes. This glandular form of the disease is called **"scrofula"**. When the cervical lymph nodes are involved:

- They may remain as granulomatous lesion.
- Caseate forming tuberculous abscesses with frequent breakdown of the gland. The chronicity of the infection and the lack of marked pain or acute inflammatory symptoms have resulted in the term **'cold abscess'**.
- In some instances, the involved lymph node undergo fibrosis and calcification.

In any case, swelling of neck is present which is tender, painful and often show inflammation of the overlying skin. When abscess forms, it perforates and discharges pus (Figs 4.23 to 4.28).

Generally, the patient may suffer of episodes of fever and chills, easy fatigability and malaise. There may be gradual loss of weight accompanied by persistent cough with or without hemoptysis. Local symptoms depend upon the tissue or organs involved.

Tuberculous Ulcer

The lesion may be preceded by an opalescent vesicle or nodule, as a result of caseation necrosis, it breaks down into an ulcer. The typical oral lesions consist of a stellate ulcer, most commonly seen on the tongue (Figs 4.29 and 4.30) followed by palate (Fig. 4.31), lips, buccal mucosa (Figs 4.32 and 4.33) and gingiva. The ulcer is usually superficial or deep and painful. It tends to increase slowly in size. In area of trauma may be mistaken as traumatic ulcer or carcinoma. Ulcers are non-specific in their clinical presentation and for this reason they are overlooked by the clinician. The typical tuberculosis ulcer has a shallow irregular granulating floor with ragged undermined edges, minimum induration and often with yellowish granular base.

The mucosa surrounding the ulcer is inflamed and edematous. Crusting and oozing is seen when the lesion involves adjacent cutaneous surface. The differential diagnosis of a tuberculous ulcer of the oral cavity includes aphthous ulcers, traumatic ulcers, syphilitic ulcers and malignancy including squamous cell carcinoma, lymphomas and metastases.

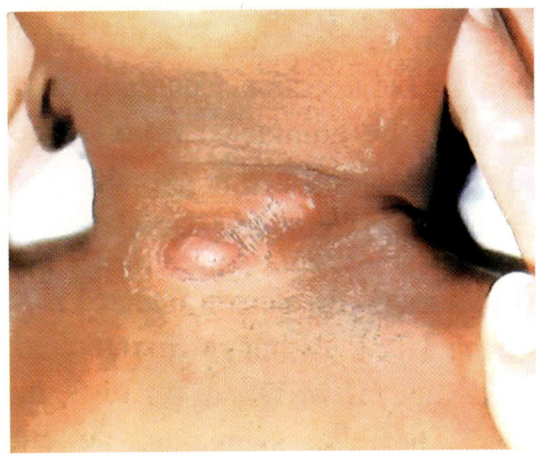

Fig. 4.23: Tuberculous cervical lymphadenopathy *(Scully et al, 2004)*

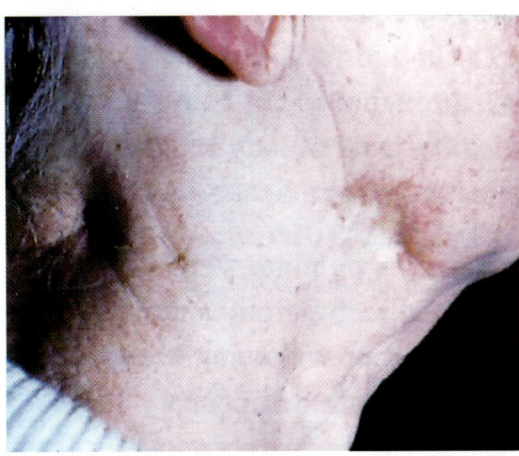

Fig. 4.24: Tuberculous lymphadenitis caseates and discharges through multiple fistulae (scrofula) with scars on healing *(Scully et al, 2004)*

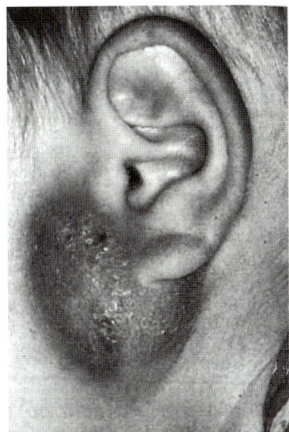

Fig. 4.25: Left sided preauricular swelling due to tuberculous involvement of the superficial lobe of the left parotid gland *(Holmes et al, 2000)*

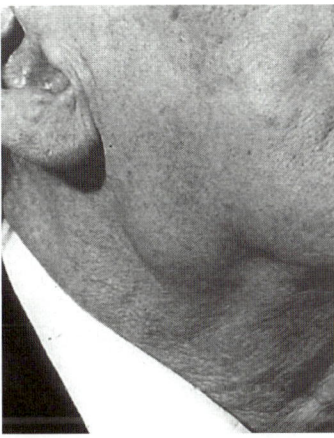

Fig. 4.26: Swelling in tail of right parotid gland infected by tuberculosis *(Holmes et al, 2000)*

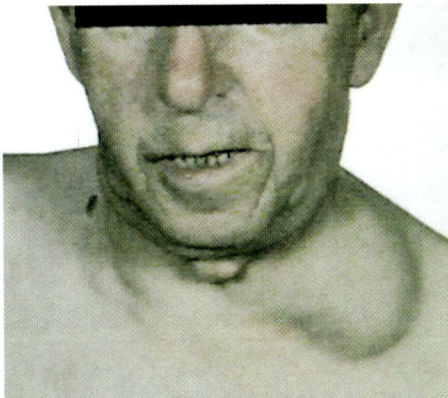

Fig. 4.27: Gross enlargement of supraclavicular and cervical lymph nodes. This is disseminated malignant disease. Biopsy is usually necessary for definitive diagnosis *(Haslett et al, 2002)*

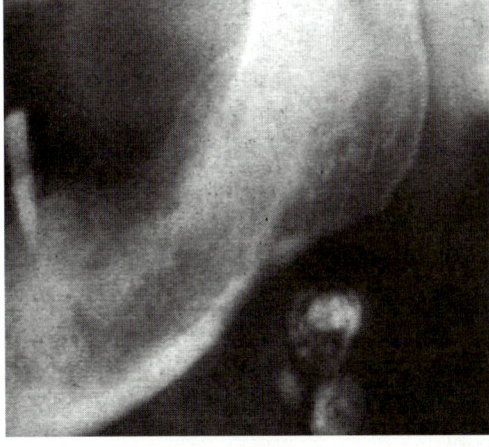

Fig. 4.28: Tuberculosis; multiple calcified cervical lymph nodes *(Neville et al, 2009)*

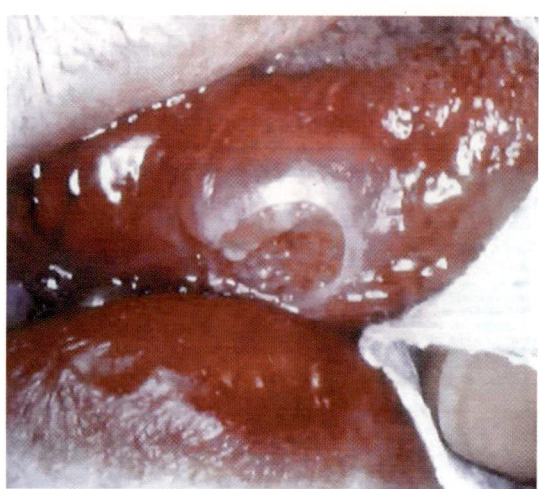

Fig. 4.29: Tuberculosis. Chronic mucosal ulceration of the ventral surface of the tongue on the right side *(Neville et al, 2009)*

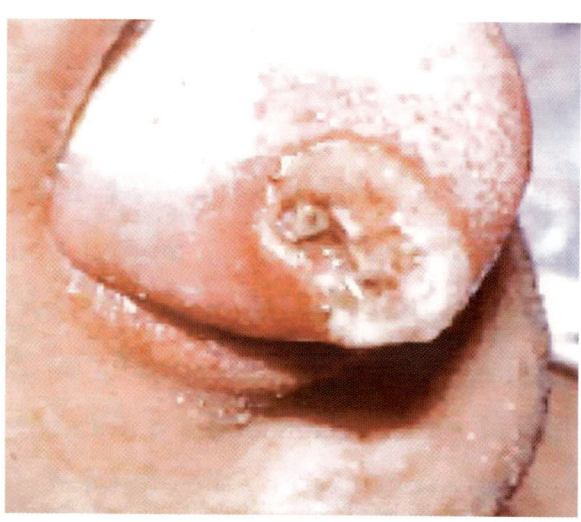

Fig. 4.30: Oral tuberculous lesion of the dorsum of the tongue in a patient with both TB disease and HIV infection *(Porteous and Terezhalmy, 2008)*

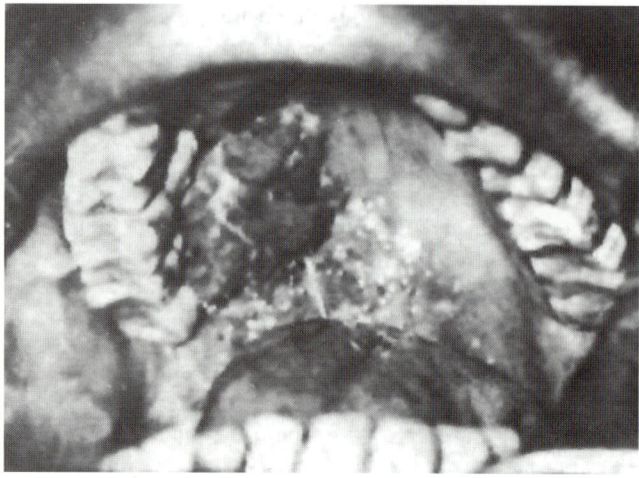

Fig. 4.31: Intraoral photograph showing extensive proliferative lesion of palate and gingivae *(Bryant and Pepys, 1976)*

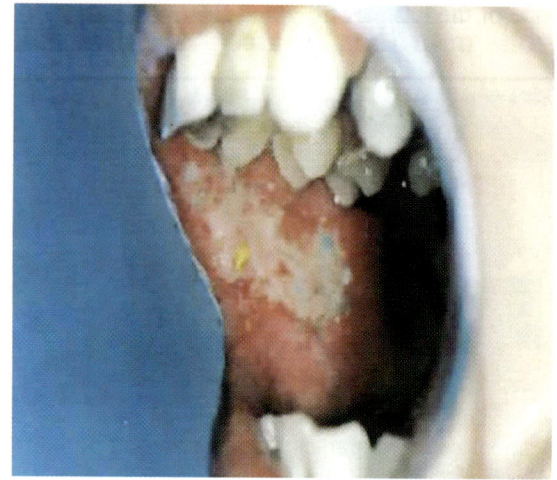

Fig. 4.32: 13 x 1 cm^2 ulcer of the right buccal mucosa *(Von Arex and Husain, 2001)*

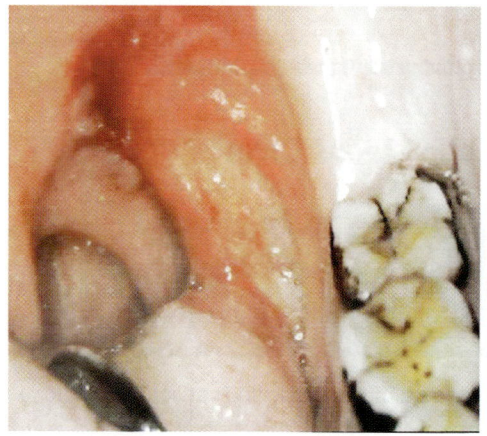

Fig. 4.33: A large crater-like ulceration surrounded by erythema is obvious on the left anterior tonsillar pillar in an AIDS patient. The differential diagnosis should include atypical ulceration, e.g. a major aphtha

Tuberculous Gingivitis

Tubercle involvement of the periapical tissue and tooth socket has been reported. The socket may be filled with so-called tuberculosis granulation tissue, consisting of many small, pink and red elevations. Tuberculosis gingivitis is an unusual form which may appear as diffuse, hyperemic or nodular papillary proliferation (Figs 4.34 to 4.36).

Jaw Bone Involvement

The jaw bones are involved by tuberculosis as a primary or secondary lesion.

1. *As a primary lesion*, the infection may extend to the jaw bone by: Direct transfer from infected sputum or infected raw cow's milk via: (a) Open pulp in a carious tooth, (b) Extraction wound. After trauma, bacilli are possibly transferred from the primary focus in another part of the body and localize in the jaw (Ebenezer et al, 2006; Gupta et al, 2005) or (c) Gingival margin or (d) Perforation of an erupting tooth.

   In the literature reviewed, there have been cases of primary TB of the mandible reported in adults also. As there is no primary focus in the lung, it is probable that either spread from the oral cavity had occurred after dental extraction (Fukuda et al, 1992) or a trivial trauma could have made an occult tubercular focus in the mandible (Gupta et al, 2005).

2. *As a secondary lesion*, extension of tubercular granuloma at the apex of tooth may occur due to hematological spread from a primary lesion developed anywhere in the body and primarily from the lungs.

Mandibular involvement is more frequent than maxillary, with the alveolar and angle regions showing greater affinity (Fukuda et al, 1992; Ebenezer

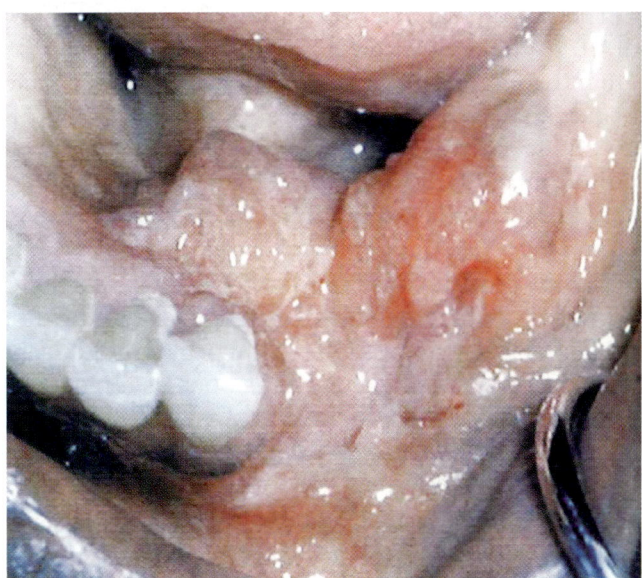

Fig. 4.35: Tuberculosis. Area of granularity and ulceration of the lower alveolar ridge and floor of the mouth *(Neville et al. 2009)*

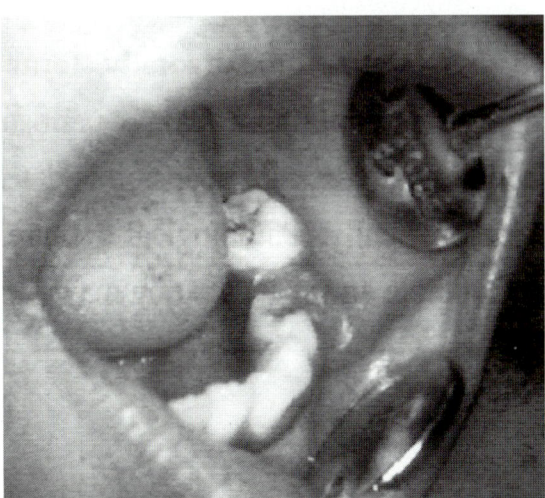

Fig. 4.34: Intraoral photograph showing obliteration of the lower left buccal vestibule extending from the deciduous mandibular left first molar to the mandibular left permanent first molar *(Dinkar and Prabhudessai, 2008)*

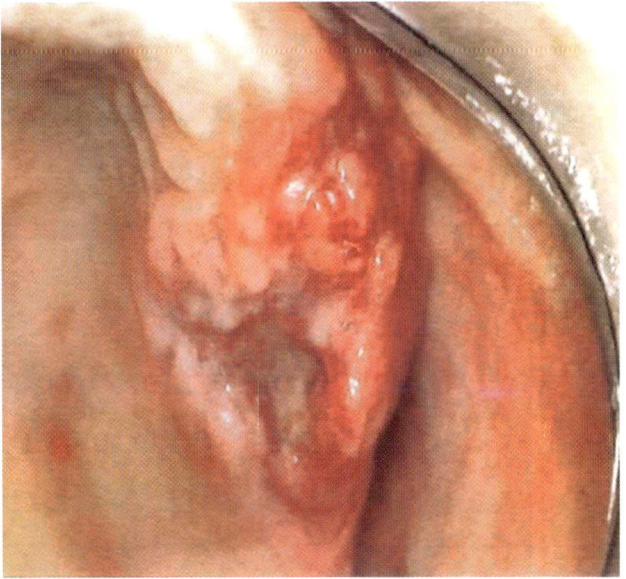

Fig. 4.36: Tuberculosis of the maxillary alveolar ridge *(Regezi et al, 2008)*

et al, 2006; Eramus et al, 1998). Approximately 66% of all cases of TB of the jaw occur in children below the age of 16.

Tubercular involvement of jaw bone causes swelling and the symptoms include difficulty in eating, trismus, paresthesia of the lower lip and enlargement of the regional lymph nodes. Fistulae drain either intraorally or extraorally often with blue margins. In some case, destructive involvement may reach to the TMJ area.

There is no characteristic radiographic appearance of TB of the jaws or alveolar bone and most lesions are indistinguishable from those caused by pyogenic organisms. The radiographic appearance of TB involving the jaw bone varies from apical osteitis and periodontitis with horizontal bone loss to a widespread destructive osteolytic lesion, and the latter may often be mistaken for a dental abscess.

Radiologically, tubercular osteomyelitis resembles non-specific osteomyelitis (Figs 4.37 to 4.40). The first demonstrable change is a small unilocular radiolucent area due to decalcification in the bone as a response to tuberculous infection. Involvement of the zygoma bone of the maxilla (Fig. 4.41) and the femur (Fig. 4.42) bone has been reported.

The lesion is clinically undetectable at this stage. As the disease progresses, the bone is destroyed with an increase in the size of the decalcified area (blurring of trabecular details) and a subperiosteal abscess then

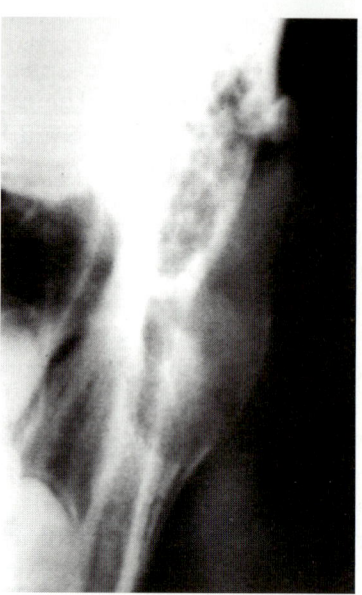

Fig. 4.37: Tuberculous osteomyelitis. PA view shows radiolucency and buccal expansion of right cortical plate of ramus

forms, presenting as a painless, soft swelling. Caseation appears, followed by softening and liquefaction. This cold abscess may burst intra- or extraorally, forming single or multiple sinus(es). A periosteal reaction with cortical expansion is detected radiologically. Pathological fracture of the mandible and sequestration may occur.

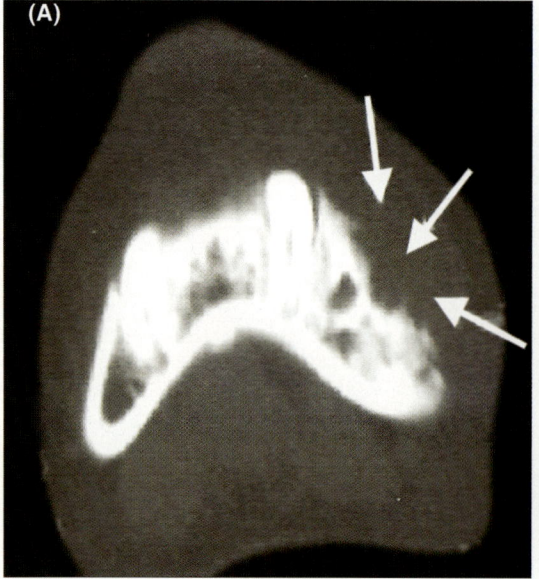
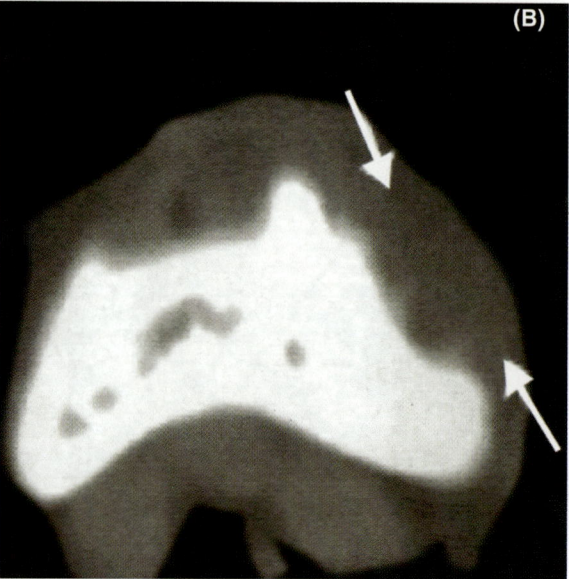

Fig. 4.38: (A) Plain CT scan of the mandible (arrows) showing an osteolytic lesion in the body of the mandible on the left side. **(B)** Plain CT scan of mandible (arrows) showing soft tissue mass in the submandibular region *(Dinkar and Prabhudessai, 2008)*

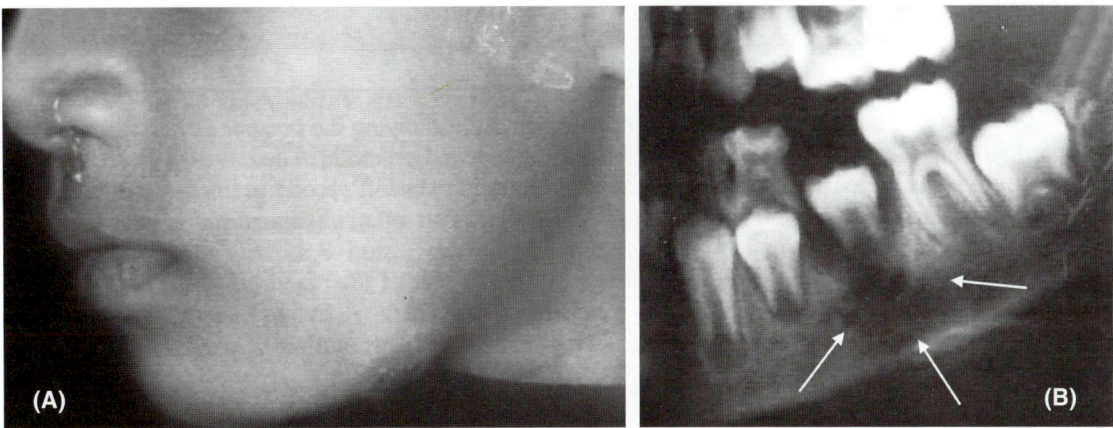

Figs 4.39A and B: (A) Extraoral radiograph showing left unilateral diffuse solitary swelling over the left body of the mandible with a fistula. **(B)** Part of an enhanced panoramic radiograph of the left side showing an ill-defined radiolucent osteolytic lesions (arrows) and destruction of the crypt of the second premolar *(Dinkar and Prabhudessai, 2008)*

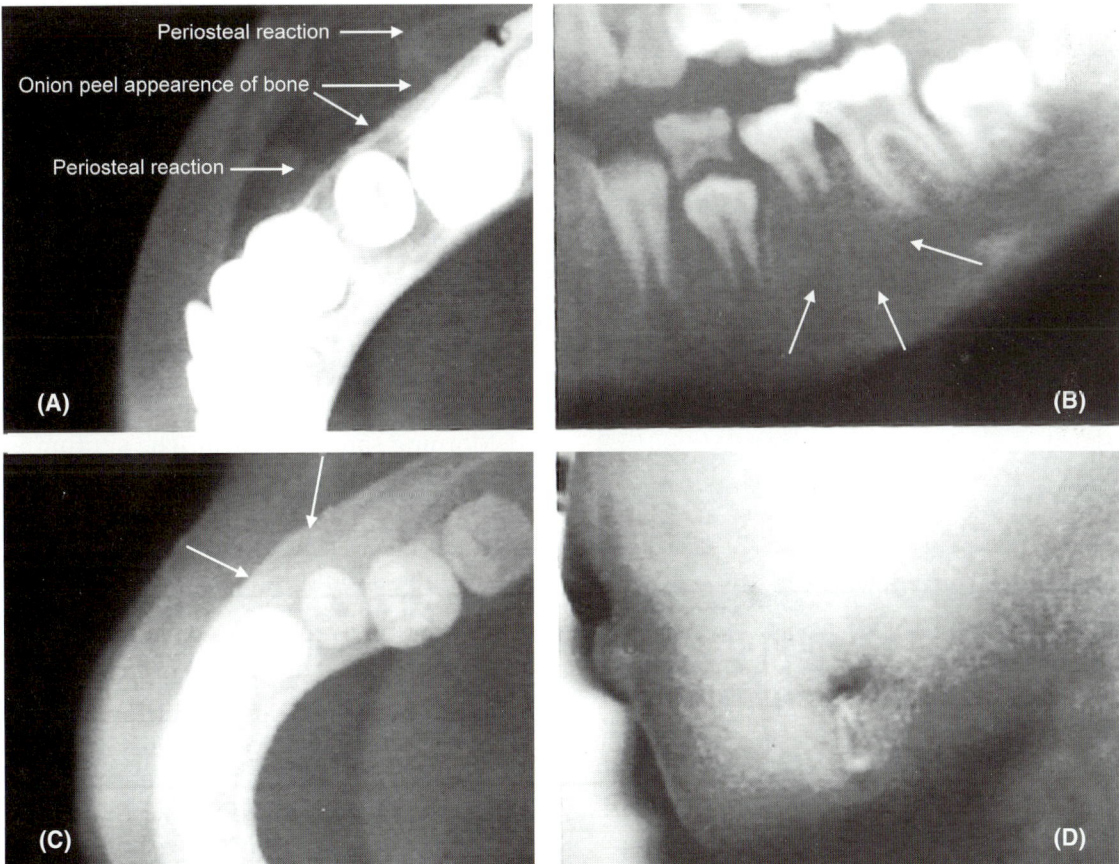

Figs 4.40A to D: (A) Occlusal view of the left side of the mandible showing the presence of an ill-defined osteolytic lesion involving the crypt of the developing lower left second premolar. There was periosteal bone reaction with an onion peel appearance (arrows) in relation to the lower left second premolar and the permanent first and second molars *(Dinkar and Prabhudessai, 2008)*. **(B)** Part of an enhanced panoramic radiograph of the left side of the mandible showing complete healing of the bony lesion 8 months after initiation of antituberculous chemotherapy (arrows). **(C)** Occlusal view of the left side of the mandible showing complete healing of the bone 8 months after initiation of antituberculous chemotherapy (arrows). **(D)** Extraoral photograph showing the residual scar on the left side of the face after complete resolution of the swelling *(Dinkar and Prabhudessai, 2008)*

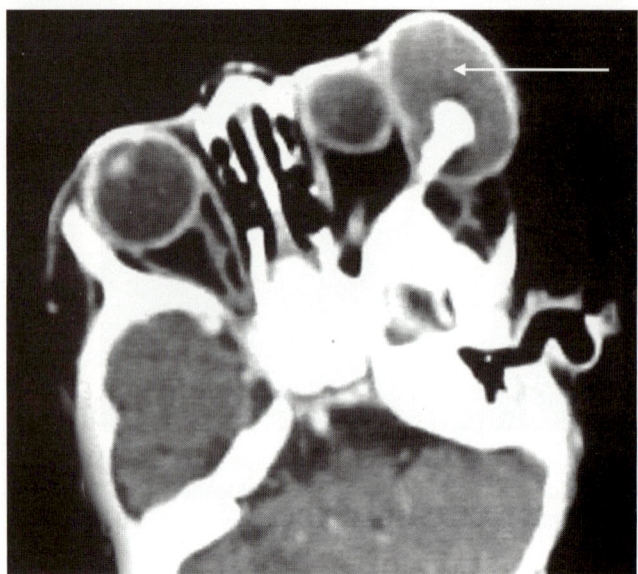

Fig. 4.41: CT scan: Axial cuts showing soft tissue abscess with sclerosis of zygoma (white arrow) *(Sethi et al, 2005)*

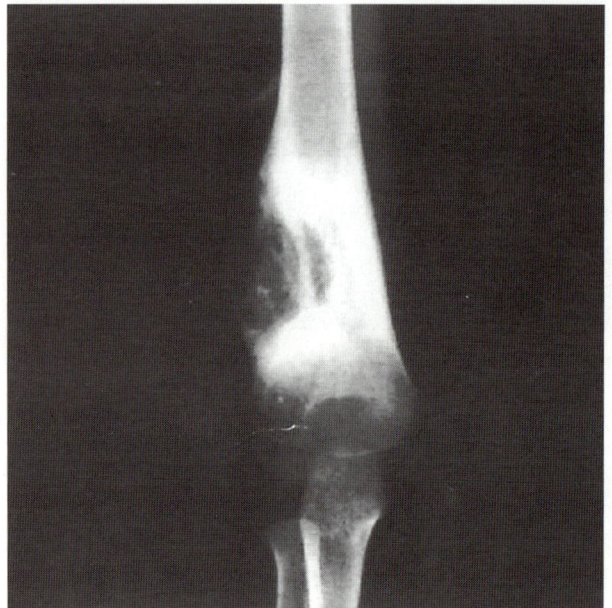

Fig. 4.42: Tuberculous osteomyelitis was also present in the femur of the same patient

Histopathological Features

Foci of caseous necrosis surrounded by epithelioid cells, lymphocytes and multinucleated giant cells, called Langhan's giant cells having horseshoe-shaped nuclear arrangement are seen. Areas of infection demonstrate the formation of granuloma, which are circumscribed collection. This granuloma is called as tubercular granuloma (Fig. 4.43).

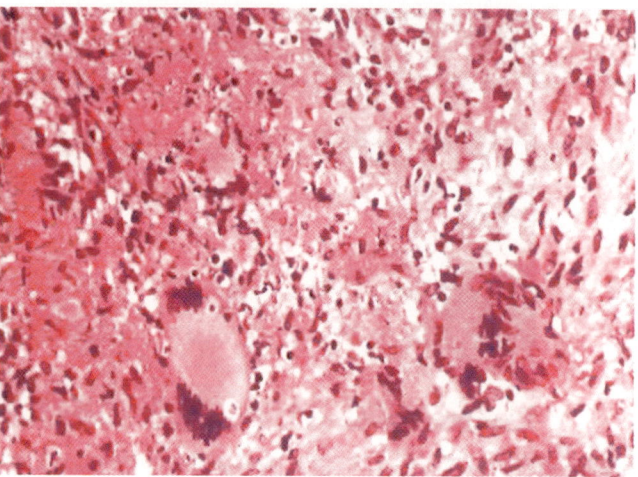

Fig. 4.43: Tuberculosis. Sheets of histiocytes are intermixed with multinucleated giant cells and are as of necrosis *(Neville et al, 2009)*

Diagnosis

Traditionally, the diagnosis of TB is made based on:

1. *Clinical findings*
2. *Imaging:* Chest X-ray (Fig. 4.44), and CT scan, if necessary and radiographic evidence of osteolysis.
3. *Sputum staining and culture:* Since oral tuberculosis is almost always secondary to pulmonary tuberculosis, sputum culture must always be carried out. A pulmonary TB suspect should submit 3 sputum samples for microscopy. Morning sample is ideal. The sputum is stained with Zeihl-Nielsen stain for acid- and alcohol-fast bacilli.
4. *Fine needle aspiration cytology:* FNAC of the swelling should be carried out. Tuberculosis is only considered when the histological specimen reveals a granulomatous lesion. The diagnosis of tuberculosis is confirmed by the presence of acid-fast bacilli in the specimen or more likely by culture of tuberculous bacilli. Ziehl-Neelsen is used for staining Mycobacterium. Usually, a typical caseous material with a white cheesy appearance is aspirated. On microscopic examination, this material demonstrates necrotic material, a large number of neutrophils, few lymphocytes and a few clusters of epithelioid cells. The fine needle aspiration cytology helped to rule out Ewing's sarcoma, which shows small round cells with well-delineated nuclear outlines and ill-defined borders.

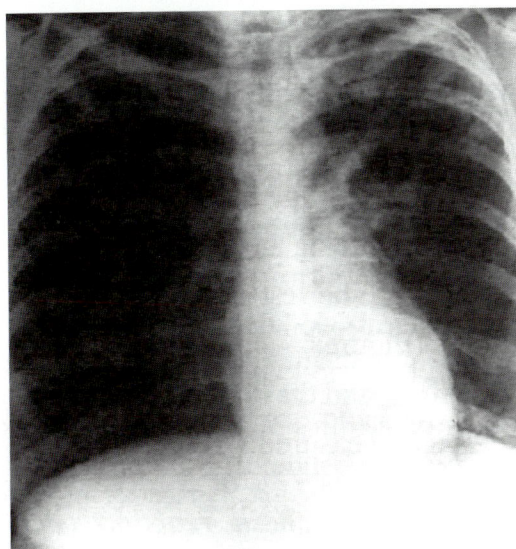

Fig. 4.44: Posteroanterior chest radiograph showing bilateral upper lobe consolidation and cavitation, consistent with pulmonary tuberculosis *(Von Arx and Husain, 2001)*

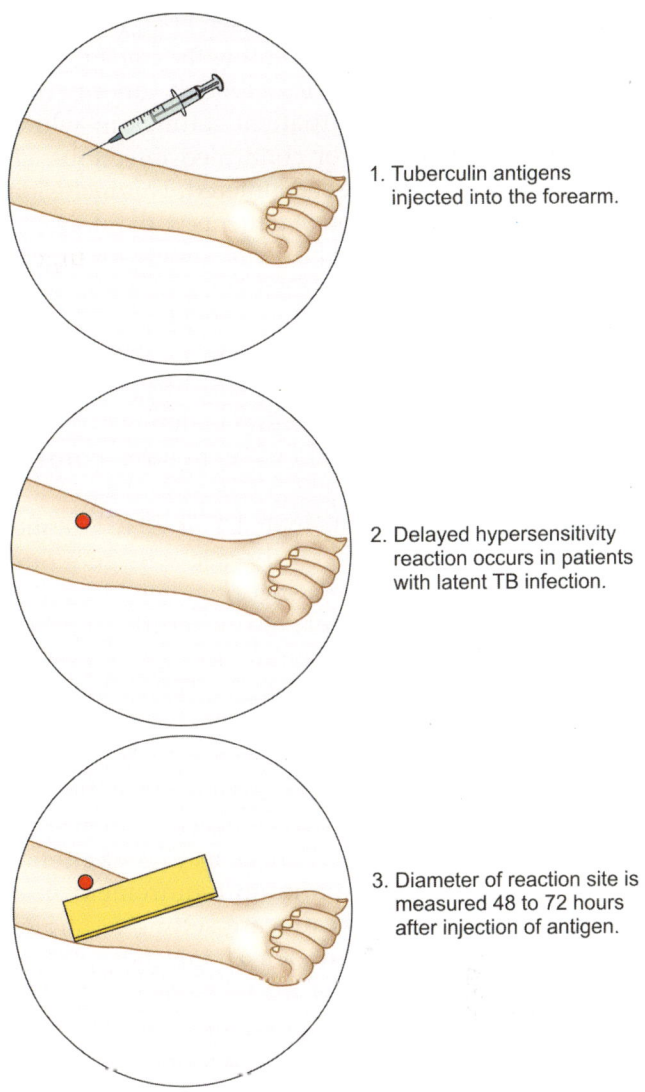

1. Tuberculin antigens injected into the forearm.

2. Delayed hypersensitivity reaction occurs in patients with latent TB infection.

3. Diameter of reaction site is measured 48 to 72 hours after injection of antigen.

Fig. 4.45: Tuberculin skin test

5. *Tuberculosis skin test:* The Mantoux test is the preferred skin test for detecting tuberculosis. It involves the injection of 5 Tuberculin unit of purified protein derivatives (the antigen), usually 0.1 ml intradermal into either the volar or dorsal surface of the forearm. The skin test is read on the basis of millimeters of induration by purified protein derivative (PPD). 10–15 mm induration is required for the test to be positive. The TST evokes a delayed hypersensitivity reaction to the tuberculin mediated by T lymphocytes producing an area of redness and swelling. The test is read at 48 to 72 hours (Fig. 4.45). Erythema is disregarded, and the diameter of the induration is measured.

6. *Polymerase chain reaction (PCR):* This technique amplifies even very small proteins of predetermined target region of *Mycobacterium tuberculosis* complex DNA.

Medical Therapy

Short-term chemotherapy, isoniazid (5 mg/kg with maximum of 300 mg daily or 15 mg/kg two to three times weekly) and rifampicin (10 gm/kg), ethambutol (25 gm/kg daily for no more than 2 months).

Dental Management

For those with pulmonary tuberculosis, close contact are those sharing a house and are most at risk.

Occasionally, a contact at work is close enough to be equivalent to a household contact (Plate IV-B). Casual contacts are most occupational contacts and need only to be examined, if they are unusually susceptible to infection, such as immunocompromized adults.

All staff in regular contact with patients are at potential risk of contracting TB. All health workers at risk should be protected by BCC vaccination. It has been reported by Smith et al (1982) that a dentist who has pulmonary tuberculosis was the source of infection to the patients treated by him at two different clinics.

In 2005, the Centers for Disease Control and Prevention (CDC) published new guidelines for preventing the transmission of *Mycobacterium tuberculosis*

(MET) in healthcare facilities (Jensen et al, 2005). The 2005 CDC guidelines for preventing the transmission of MBT in healthcare facilities explicitly identify oral healthcare settings as outpatient settings in which patients with suspected or confirmed infectious TB disease are expected to be encountered. This inclusion is based on the assumption of patients with infectious TB disease may present in the dental setting for urgent or routine dental care and OHCWs might share air space with persons with infectious TB disease or might come in contact with clinical specimens that contain MET. Consequently, every oral healthcare facility should have a TB infection-control plan that is part of its written infection control/exposure control protocol.

However, it can be anticipated that OHCWs and patients with infectious TB disease will generate droplet nuclei by coughing, sneezing, laughing, and talking; therapeutic intervention could further stimulate coughing and promote the generation of infectious particles. Since patients and OHCWs share the same air space, the potential for the transmission of MET cannot be discounted. The probable transmission of MDR TB disease from patients to two OHCWs has been documented, and there is evidence of TB disease transmission from an oral surgeon to 15 patients following extractions. Minimum requirement in a community-based oral healthcare setting is implementation and enforcement of a TB infection-control protocol which provides for the following:

1. Prompt identification of patients with suspected or confirmed infectious TB disease.
2. Separation of patients with suspected and confirmed TB disease from other OHCWs and patients. Routine dental care should be postponed until a physician confirms that the patient does not have infectious TB disease or until confirmation the patient is no longer infectious.
3. Referral of patients with suspected and confirmed TB disease for a medical evaluation and/or required oral healthcare procedures to a facility with appropriate enviromental controls and respiratory-protection controls.

Consequently, patients with suspected or confirmed TB disease requiring urgent dental care must be promptly referred to an oral healthcare facility that meets the requirements for an airborne infection isolation (AII) room (enviromental controls); while performing procedures on such patients, OHCWs should follow the respiratory-protection rules. The enviromental controls are physical or mechanical measures intended to prevent the spread and reduce the concentration of infectious droplet nuclei 1–5 μm in diameter in ambient air.

a. Patients with suspected or confirmed TB disease requiring urgent dental care must be treated in a room, which meats requirements for an airborne infection isolation (AII) room.
b. AII rooms provide positive pressure in the room (air flows under the door gap out of the room).
c. AII rooms should have a direct exhaust of air from the room to the outside of the building or recirculation of air through a high efficiency particulate air (HEPA) filter.
d. OHCWs performing urgent dental care on a patient with suspected or confirmed TB disease must wear at least N95 disposable respirators.
e. Non-powered disposable respirators with air purifying, particulate-filter respirators.
f. These disposable respirators have filtration efficiency or 95% when challenged with 0.3 μm particles.

ASPIRATION*

Aspiration involves the passage of food or fluid, vomitus, drugs or other foreign materials into the trachea and lungs. The right lower lung is often the destination of aspirated materials because anatomically the right branching bronchus tends to continue almost straight down, whereas the bronchus in the left lung branches at a sharper angle. Normally, a cough removes such material from the upper tract and the vocal cords and epiglottis prevent entry into the lower tract. The characteristics of the aspirate determine the

* Cited from Gould, BA (2006)

specific effects on respiratory function. For example, vomitus may contain solid objects as well as highly acidic gastric secretions, lipids, or alcohol. The common result is a solid object causing obstruction directly or an irritating liquid causing inflammation and swelling. In addition, inflammation may interfere with gas exchange and predispose to pneumonia.

Some examples of the effects of aspirated solid objects are as follows:

- Solid objects lodge in a passageway and totally obstruct airflow at that point. The physical size of the object is one factor, which may be augmented by inflammation and swelling in the area. A small obstruction may be asymptomatic.

- A large object may occlude the trachea and block all airflow, a life-threatening situation. In such cases, no sound can be made to alert others to the problem, and consciousness is lost very quickly as oxygen supplies are depleted.

- Solid objects lodging in a bronchus lead to non-aeration and collapse of the area distal to the obstacle.

- Sometimes solid objects create a ball valve effect, in which air is able to pass the passageway totally closes on expiration, leading to a buildup of air distal to the obstruction.

- Foods such as dried beans may swell after aspiration and become more firmly lodged.

- Sharp pointed objects, such as remaining root of a tooth, or a tooth, bone fragments also lodge in a passageway (Fig. 4.46). Although it does not totally occlude the airway by itself, such an object traumatizes the mucosa, causing an acute inflammatory response that adds to the barrier. The inflammatory response may stimulate bronchoconstriction. Also an object that straddles the airway will collect any other material entering the area increasing the obstruction and fatty or irritating solids such as peanuts also cause inflammation around the area, creating edema and further impeding airflow. If not removed, a granuloma or fibrous tissue develops around such material.

When liquids are aspirated, the effects are somewhat different. Irritating liquids, particularly acids (vomitus), alcohol, or oils (milk), tend to disperse into several bronchi. These materials cause severe inflammation, leading to narrow airways and increased secretions, which make the lungs more difficult to expand. In some cases, the alveoli are involved in the inflammation, and gas diffusion is

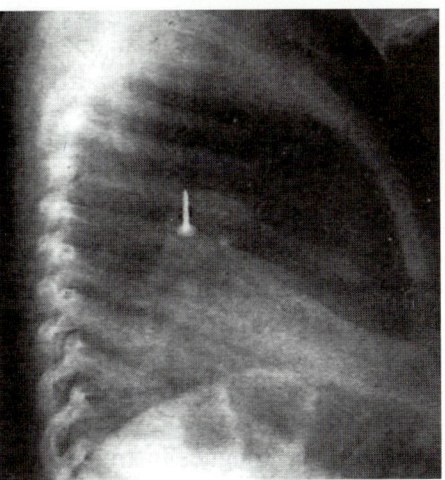

Fig. 4.46: An inhaled foreign body — a nail — impacted in the right lower lobe bronchus. This young patient presented with a persistent cough and wheeze, but did not realize that he had inhaled a nail. Foreign bodies should always be borne in mina as a differential diagnosis of wheezing, especially in children.

impaired. This type of inflammation may be called chemical or aspiration pneumonia; it predisposes to the development of infection later.

Etiology

Aspiration is a common problem in young children. When children are very young, they put most objects in their mouths. Children also tend to move about with objects in their mouths, thus increasing the risk of aspiration. Smooth, round objects are most dangerous. Common examples are chunks of hot dogs, candy, nuts, grapes, and raw carrots. Buttons or coins and balloons are frequent nonfood examples. Children may accidentally aspirate toxic fluids such as cleaning materials or lighter fluid. Some fluids, such as those containing hydrocarbons, for example turpentine, have a low viscosity and a low surface tension and, therefore, tend to spread in a very thin film over a large area of the lung, causing extensive irritation and damage. Inhalation of substances such as baby powder can also cause inflammation in the delicate lung tissue.

Children with congenital anomalies such as a cleft palate or tracheoesophageal fistula are especially at risk for aspiration until repair takes place.

Aspiration can occur under many different circumstances. It is often a complication in individuals of any age when the swallowing or gag reflex is depressed for any reason, for example, following anesthesia or stroke, or in patients with coma or neurologic damage.

Vomitus may be aspirated postoperatively from the effects of anesthetics or drugs. Usually, a patient is not allowed to eat or drink preoperatively to reduce the risk of aspiration but emergency situations do not allow for this precaution.

Individuals who eat or drink or perhaps take medications when lying down also risk aspiration because the gravitational force is of no value in moving food quickly and completely down the esophagus. Residual liquid often remains in the mouth and oropharynx, to drip at a later time into the trachea.

Adults frequently aspirate food or fluid, especially when combining eating with talking at social events (sometimes called a cafe coronary). A chunk of meat is the common culprit, particularly if the food is not well chewed and alcohol intake has depressed protective reflexes. Because such food causes total obstruction, the person cannot speak, but may have time to gesture to the chest or neck before falling unconscious, and this could be interpreted as a heart attack or coronary. In these cases, a life could be saved, if the situation were treated as aspiration rather than as a heart attack.

Common Manifestations

- Coughing and choking with marked dyspnea are common.
- Stridor and hoarseness are characteristic of upper airway obstruction.
- Wheezing occurs with aspiration of liquids into the lungs.
- Tachycardia and tachypnea are responses to respiratory distress.
- Nasal flaring chest retractions, and marked hypoxia occur in individuals with severe respiratory distress and as mentioned earlier, total obstruction at the larynx or trachea prevents any sounds or cough from being produced. A person may reach for the chest or neck area. Cardiac or respiratory arrest quickly ensues.

Other Potential Complications

- Respiratory distress syndrome may develop, if inflammation is widespread.
- Pulmonary abscess may develop, if microbes are in the aspirate and certain materials such as solvents, if aspirated in large amounts, may be absorbed into the blood and cause systemic effects.

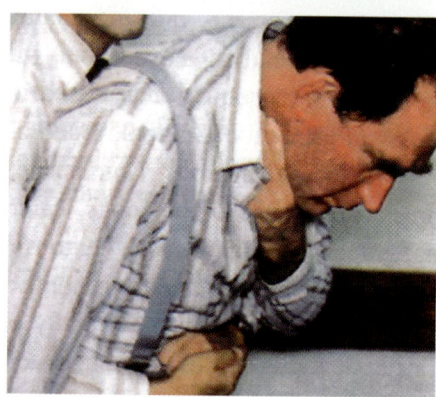

Fig. 4.47: The Heimlich abdominal thrust maneuver can be used in an attempt to dislodge an inhaled foreign body in a conscious patient. One fist is clenched and positioned in the epigastrium and the other hand is placed on top. The patient is squeezed suddenly so that the fist moves backwards and upwards, causing a violent expulsion of air from the lungs *(Forbes & Jackson, 2003)*

Treatment

Aspiration is easier to prevent than to treat. Avoiding talking or moving when chewing and swallowing reduces the risk. Small objects or fluid can frequently be coughed up.

Emergency Treatment for Aspiration

1. The Heimlich maneuver (Fig. 4.47) to dislodge the solid object is recommended (stand behind the victim with encircling arms, position a fist, thumb side against the other hand over the first and thrus forcefully inward and upward).
2. A foreign object may be ejected from an infant by back blows administered between the infant's shoulder blades, while the infant's body is supported over an arm or leg, head lower than the trunk.

Sometime an individual can use finger probe successfully to access an object at the back of the tongue. Instrumentation may be necessary in some cases to remove the offending object. In case of total obstruction, an emergency tracheotomy is necessary. Patients with widespread inflammation should be monitored for adult respiratory distress syndrome (ARDS) or pneumonia. Oxygen and supportive therapy may be required as well as prophylactic antibiotics.

5

Liver

- **Anatomy**
  - **Normal Hepatic Physiology**
    - **Liver Function Testing**
- **Hepatitis**
- **Viral Hepatitis**
- **Dental Management**
- **Cross-infection**
- **Infection Control Checklist**
- **Prophylaxis of Viral Hepatitis**
- **Practice Infection Control Policy**

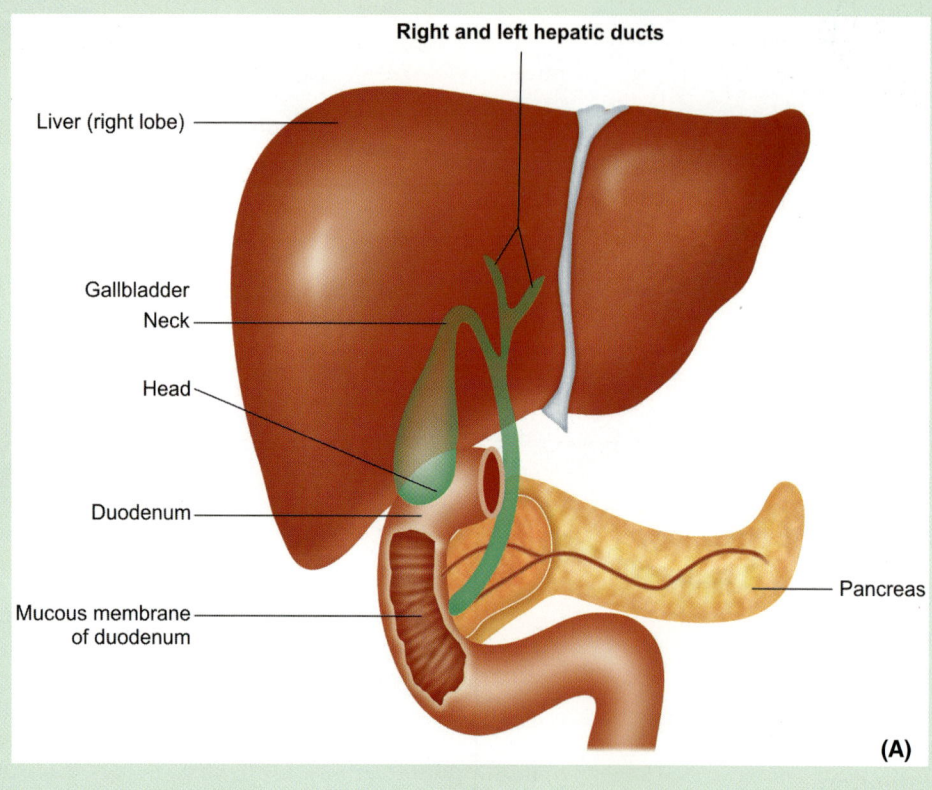

Right and left hepatic ducts

Liver (right lobe)

Gallbladder
Neck

Head

Duodenum

Mucous membrane
of duodenum

Pancreas

(A)

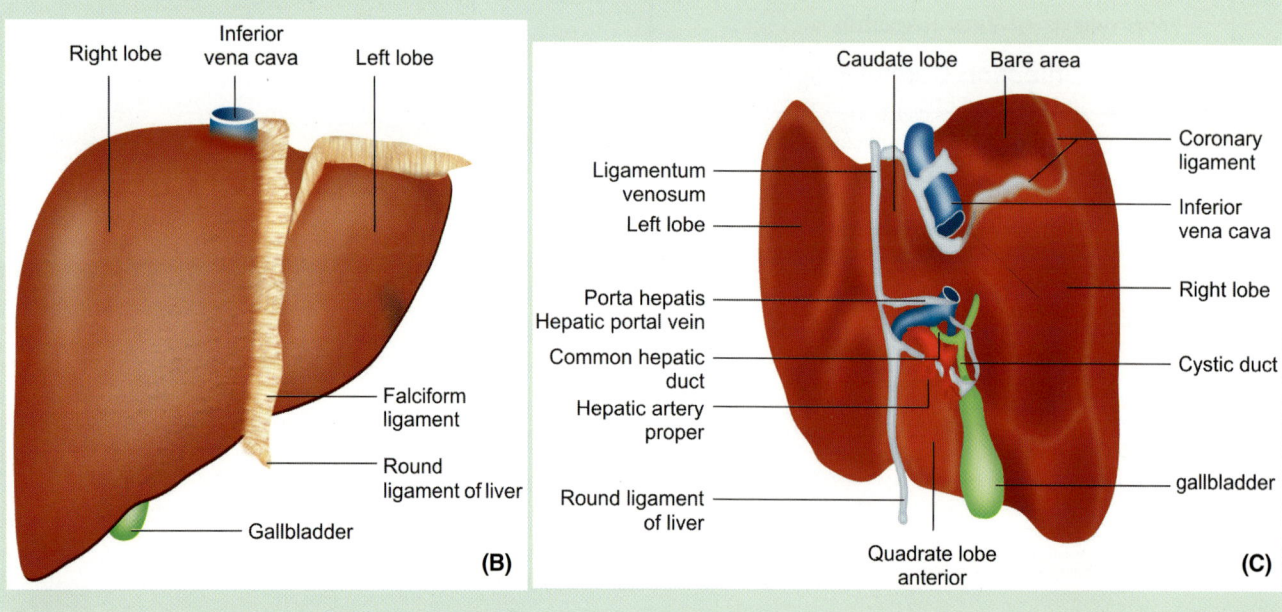

Right lobe — Inferior vena cava — Left lobe

Falciform
ligament

Round
ligament of liver

Gallbladder

(B)

Caudate lobe — Bare area

Ligamentum
venosum

Left lobe

Porta hepatis
Hepatic portal vein

Common hepatic
duct
Hepatic artery
proper

Round ligament
of liver

Quadrate lobe
anterior

Coronary
ligament

Inferior
vena cava

Right lobe

Cystic duct

gallbladder

(C)

Plate V: Gross Anatomy of the liver. **(A)** Relation of liver to the surrouding organs, the liver is in the upper right quadrant of the abdomen. **(B)** Anterior and **(C)** Posteroinferior views show the four lobes of the liver as well as gallbladder and the porta hepatis

Introduction

The liver is the body's 'factory' carrying out hundreds of jobs that are vital to life. It is very tough and able to continue to function when most of it is damaged. It can also repair itself—even renewing large section.

The liver has around 500 different functions, importantly it:
- Fights infections and disease.
- Destroys and deals with poisons and drugs.
- Filters and cleans the blood.
- Controls the amount of cholesterol.
- Produces and maintains the balance of hormones.
- Produces chemicals, enzymes and other proteins—responsible for most of the chemical reactions in the body, for example, blood clotting and repairing tissue.
- Processes food once it has been digested.
- Produces bile to help breakdown food in the gut.
- Stores energy that can be used rapidly when the body need it most.
- Stores sugar, vitamins and minerals, including iron.
- Repairs damage and renews itself.

Liver damage develops over time. Any inflammation of the liver is known as hepatitis, where its cause is viral or not. A sudden inflammation of the liver is known as acute hepatitis. Where inflammation of the liver lasts longer than six months the condition is known as chronic hepatitis.

Fibrosis is where scar tissue is formed in the inflamed liver. Fibrosis can take a variable time to develop. Although scar tissue is present, the liver keeps on functioning quite well. Treating the cause of inflammation may prevent the formation of further liver damage and may reverse some or all of the scarring. Cirrhosis is where inflammation and fibrosis has spread throughout the liver and disrupts the shape and function of the liver. With cirrhosis, the scarring is more widespread and can show up on an ultrasound scan. Even at this stage, people can have no signs or symptoms of liver disease. Where the working capacity of liver cells has been badly impaired and they are unable to repair or renew the liver, permanent damage occurs.

This permanent cell damage can lead to liver failure or liver cancer. All the chemicals and waste products that the liver has to deal with build up in the body. The liver is now so damaged that the whole body becomes poisoned by the waste products and this stage is known as end-stage liver disease. In the final stages of liver disease, the building up of waste products affects many organs. This is known as multiple organ failure. Where many organs are affected, death is likely to follow.

ANATOMY

The liver is a reddish brown gland located in the right upper abdominal quadrant beneath the diaphragm and is normally protected by the ribs and costal margin (Fig. 5.1). It fills most of the right hypochondriac and epigastric regions. It is the body's largest gland, weighing about 1.4 kg (3 lb). The liver has a tremendous variety of functions, but only one of them, the secretion of bile, contributes to digestion.

GROSS ANATOMY

The liver has four lobes called the right, left, quadrate, and caudate lobes. From an anterior view, we see only a large *right lobe* and smaller *left lobe* (Plate V).

They are separated from each other by *the falciform ligament,* a sheet of mesentery that suspends the liver from the diaphragm and anterior abdominal wall. The *round ligament (ligamentum teres),* also visible anteriorly, is a fibrous remnant of the umbilical vein, which carries blood from the umbilical cord to the liver of a fetus.

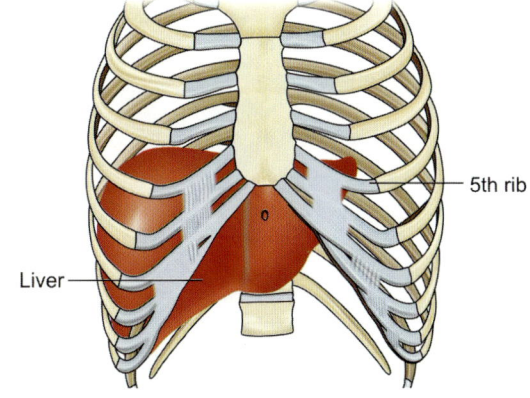

5th rib

Liver

Fig. 5.1: The liver is protected by the ribs and costal margin

From the inferior view, we also see a squarish **quadrate lobe** next to the gallbladder and a tail-like **caudate lobe** posterior to that. An irregular opening between these lobes, the **porta hepatis,** is a point of entry for the hepatic portal vein and proper hepatic artery and a point of exit for the bile passages, all of which travel in the lesser omentum.

The gallbladder adheres to a depression on the inferior surface of the liver between the right and quadrate lobes. The posterior aspect of the liver has a deep groove (sulcus) that accommodates the inferior vena cava. The superior surface has a *bare area* where it is attached to the diaphragm. The rest of the liver is covered by a serosa.

MICROSCOPIC ANATOMY

The interior of the liver is filled with innumerable tiny cylinders called hepatic lobules, about 2 mm long by 1 mm in diameter. A lobule consists of a central vein passing down its core, surrounded by radiating sheets of cuboidal cells called hepatocytes (Fig. 5.2).

Imagine spreading a book wide open until its front and back covers touch. The pages of the book would fan out around the spine somewhat like the plates of hepatocytes fan out from the central vein of a liver lobule. Each plate of hepatocytes is an epithelium one or two cell thick. The spaces between the plates are blood-filled channels called hepatic sinusoids.

There are two main hepatic blood supplies the hepatic artery and the portal vein. The common hepatic artery, a branch of the celiac trunk of the aorta, divides into the right and left hepatic arteries, which enter the liver's lobes. The portal vein transports blood to the liver from the pancreas, spleen, gallbladder, and entire digestive tract, except for the rectum. The portal vein subdivides and also enters the liver's lobes. Both of these afferent blood supplies taper into capillary like sinusoids, which are lined by endothelial cells and Kupffer' s cells.

The sinusoids are lined by a fenestrated endothelium that separates the hepatocytes from the bloodstream, but allows blood plasma into the space between the hepatocytes and endothelium. The blood filtering through the sinusoids comes directly from the intestines. The sinusoids also contain phagocytic cells called hepatic macrophages (Kupffer's cells), which remove bacteria and debris from the blood. The hepatic lobules are separated by a sparse connective tissue stroma. In cross-sections, the stroma is especially visible in the triangular areas where three or more lobules meet. Here there is often a **hepatic**

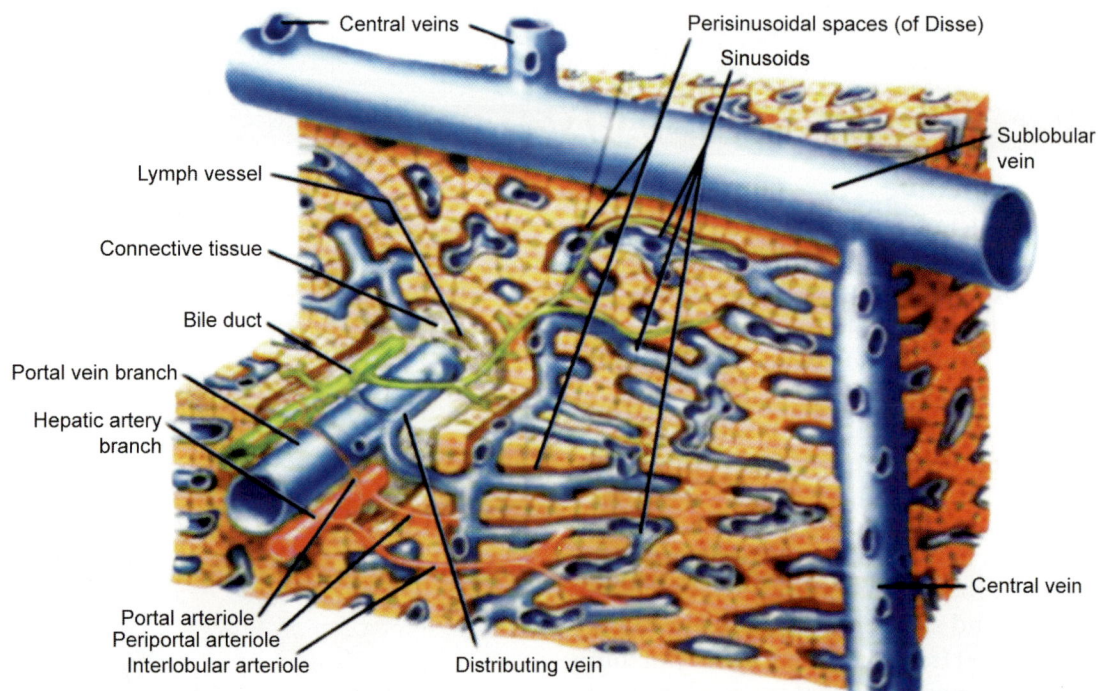

Fig. 5.2: Histological section of the liver. The hepatic lobules and their relationship to the blood vessels and bile tributaries
(Nitter,1991)

triad of two blood vessels and a bile ductule. The blood vessels are small branches of the proper hepatic artery and hepatic portal vein. Both of them supply blood to the sinusoids, which, therefore, receive a mixture of nutrientladen venous blood from the intestines and freshly oxygenated arterial blood from the celiac trunk. After filtering through the sinusoids, this blood collects in the central vein. From here, it ultimately flows into the right and left hepatic veins, which leave the liver at superior surface and drain immediately into the inferior vena cava.

After a meal, the liver removes glucose, amino acids, iron, vitamins, and other nutrients from it for metabolism or storage. It also removes and degrades hormones, toxins, bile pigments, and drugs. At the same time, the liver secretes lipoproteins, albumin, angiotensinogen, clotting factors, and other products into the blood. Between meals, it breaks down stored glycogen and releases glucose into the circulation.

The Biliary System

The liver secretes bile into narrow channels, the bile canaliculi and between sheets of hepatocytes. Bile passes from there into the small bile ductules of the triads and ultimately into the right and left hepatic ducts.

The right and left hepatic ducts exit the liver, forming the common hepatic duct, which then merges with the cystic duct of the gallbladder to form the bile duct. This bile duct then drains to the duodenum at the ampulla of Vater. Through this system, bile is formed, transported, stored, and delivered to the intestinal tract. The billiary system is shown in Fig. 5.3.

NORMAL HEPATIC PHYSIOLOGY

Hepatocytes are the main functional cells of the liver. They contribute to carbohydrate homeostasis, lipid metabolism, protein synthesis including albumin and coagulation factors, bilirubin synthesis and bile formation, drug metabolism, and abnormal biotransformation, hormone metabolism and serum enzymes.

Carbohydrate Homeostasis

The liver capacity for glycogen synthesis, storage, and metabolism is essential for maintaining normal blood glucose levels. This permits glucose homeostasis during periods of fasting or sustained exercise or subsequent to carbohydrate intake. The amount of glucose uptake or released by the liver responds to the level of hypoglycemia or hyperglycemia. Excess glucose is taken in by the hepatocytes and stored as glycogen. Glycogen is degraded (glycogenolysis) to glucose as needed to maintain blood glucose levels. The liver can store approximately 75 grams of glycogen, which supplies approximately 24 hours of glucose during times of starvation, such as the preoperative fasting period. After depletion of glycogen stores, liver gluconeogenesis becomes responsible for glucose homeostasis. Gluconeogenesis converts available protein and amino acids (alanine and glutamine) to glucose. Blood glucose level is under hormonal control. Insulin increases glycogen synthesis and decreases gluconeogenesis. The opposite effects occur with glucagon and epinephrine, which increase gluconeogenesis and inhibit glyco-genesis.

Protein Synthesis

The liver synthesizes proteins such as albumin and clotting factors. The hepatocytes also form proteins (microsomal enzymes) that are important in drug metabolism. Hepatic production of albumin is in the range of 10–15 gm daily.

Albumin

Albumin is the main protein in human serum and it:
1. Contributes the bulk of colloid oncotic (osmotic) pressure, i.e. albumin helps maintain the oncotic force necessary to restrict excessive loss of intravascular fluid into the interstitium. Osmotic pressure is essential in maintaining intravascular volume. Albumin helps maintain the oncotic force necessary to restrict excessive loss of intravascular fluid into the interstitium.
2. Albumin is also involved in protein bound transportation within the circulation. Drugs,

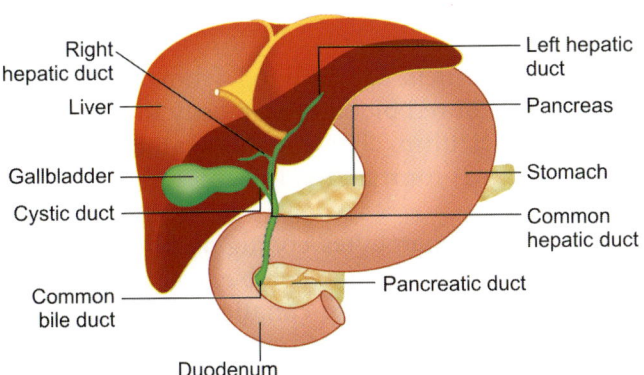

Fig. 5.3: The biliary system

hormones, and metals (calcium) bind to albumin reversibly and have their physiologic effects modified by albumin concentration.

Albumin also has a large number of reactive sites and can, therefore, reversibly binds to most drugs. If albumin production falls sufficiently, then serum levels fall below 2.5 gm/dl. The results are edema, ascites and elevation in the free-bound ratio of administered drugs. The half-life of albumin is about 20 days; therefore, hypoalbuminemia is not usually seen in acute hepatic dysfunction. Measurement of serum albumin of less than 2.5 g/dL being significant; however, malnutrition can also cause hypoalbuminemia.

Synthesis of Clotting Factors

Clotting factors V, XI, XII, XIII, and fibrinogen (non-vitamin K dependent), and II, VII, IX, and X (vitamin K dependent) are all synthesized in the liver. Factor VIII is produced by the endothelial cells. Decreased coagulation factor synthesis can be directly due to hepatocyte injury or indirectly due to decreased intestinal vitamin K absorption secondary to reduced bile production or biliary obstruction. Vitamin K supplementation may improve coagulation, if deficiency is due to biliary disorders but does not help, if hepatocellular disease exists.

The half-life of clotting factors is short (hours) compared with that of albumin (20 days). Although coagulation factor levels must fall to 20 from 30% of their normal levels before spontaneous bleeding occurs, their short half-life results in clotting abnormalities relatively early in acute liver dysfunction. The liver also clears proteins of the fibrinolytic system from the circulation. Therefore, liver dysfunction may lead to increased fibrinolysis, which combined with reduced factor production may enhance bleeding.

Prothrombin time (PT): This test measures the test taken for a clot to form in a blood sample. The prothrombin time is influenced by the presence or lack of vitamin K. The prothrombin time will take longer as a result of deficiencies in vitamin K. Severe liver disease is indicated by a prolonged prothrombin time (PT) and a decreased platelet count.

Activated partial thromboplastin time ratio (APTR): It is the time taken for thromboplastin to convert into thrombin.

Differences in normal range for different laboratories can make it difficult to compare or comment on individual test results specifically. This is due to the different brand of tests that are used and how these are interpreted. There are, however, international normal ranges that all doctors, nurses and health care professionals use an approximate guide. Interestingly, the normal values for liver function tests can vary between men and women, at different times of the day and as the person get older.

The PT, PTT (partial thromboplastin time), international normalized ratio (INR) and platelet levels should be checked. If the INR is greater than 1.5 times the normal value, replacement of clotting factors with fresh frozen plasma (FFP) is necessary. The effect of FFP is limited in duration by factor VIII which has a half-life of 4 to 8 hours; therefore, FFP is given immediately before and/or during surgery. A platelet count greater than 50,000 should be the cutoff in considering platelet transfusion before surgery.

Bleeding time can be checked to determine qualitative platelet function. If this is abnormal, one must consider both platelet and FFP transfusion.

Bilirubin Metabolism

Bilirubin

Formed from hemoglobin and the main pigment in bile (a yellow/green substance made by the liver). An increase of bilirubin causes jaundice, a yellowing of the eyes and skin in liver disease.

Bilirubin is a degradation product of hemoglobin (Figs 5.4 and 5.5). It is one of the major constituents of bile and is yellowish in color. Bilirubin is normally transported to the liver by way of the plasma. In the liver, it conjugates with glucuronic acid and is then excreted into the intestine, where it aids in the emulsification of fats and stimulates peristalsis. When liver disease is present, bilirubin tends to accumulate in the plasma because of decreased liver metabolism and transport.

Hemoglobin is catabolized from the normal degradation of red blood cells, mostly in the spleen, to form bilirubin. This is the water-insoluble (unconjugated) form and is transported to the liver by albumin.

There the hepatocytes conjugate bilirubin with glucuronic acid. The water-soluble (conjugated form) is secreted into the bile canaliculi and collected through the biliary system to enter the intestinal tract. Bile composed of bilirubin, water, bile salts, cholesterol, and phospholipids is secreted into the

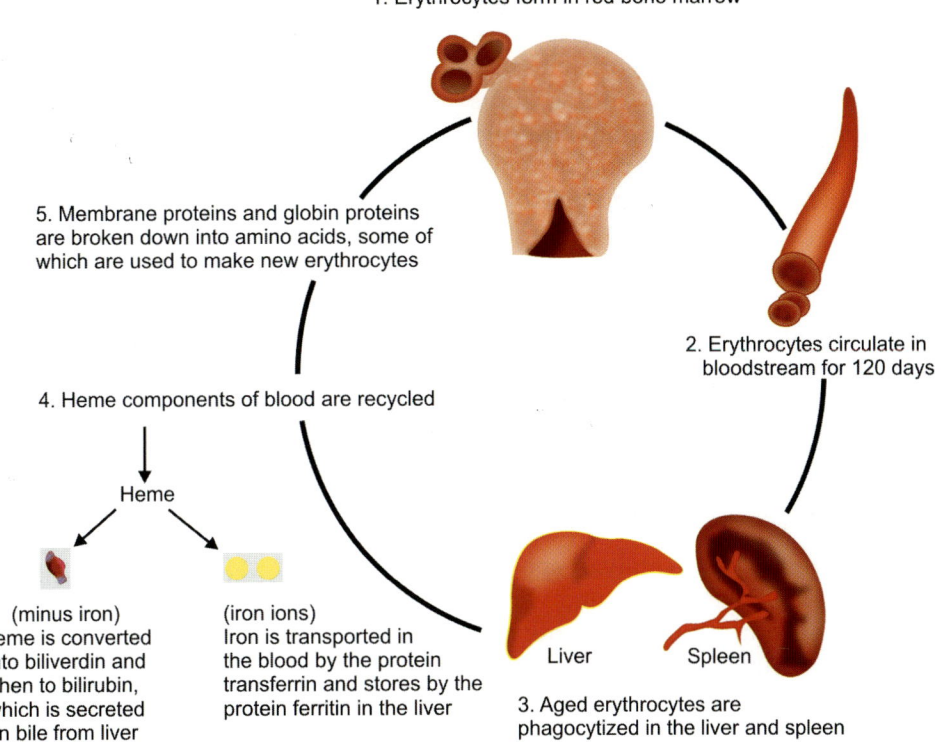

Fig. 5.4: Recycling the components of old or damaged erythrocytes. Erythrocytes have an average lifespan of about 120 days. Their molecular components are then breakdown and recycled or eliminated from the body *(Mckinley and O'Loughlin, 2006)*

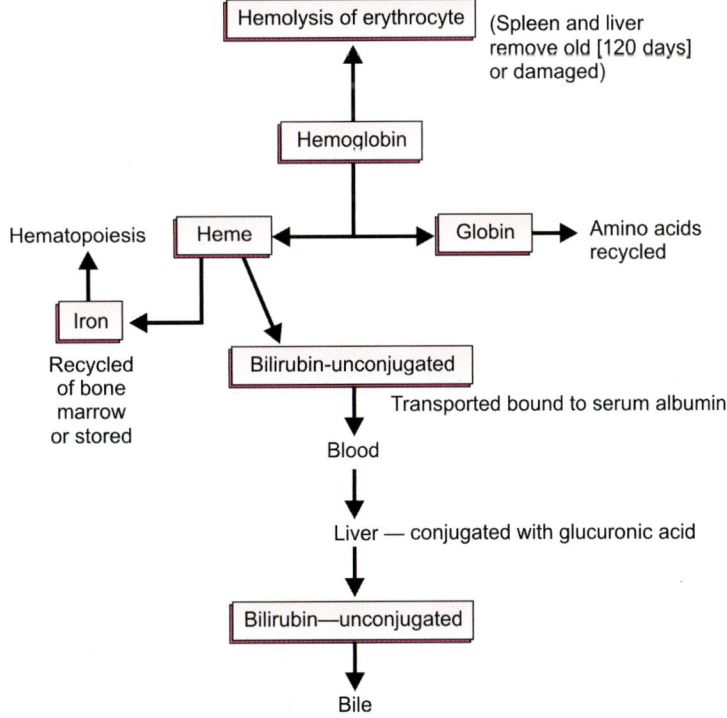

Fig. 5.5: Breakdown of hemoglobin

intestinal tract to assist with fat absorption and provide one method of drug excretion (e.g. erythromycin). Some conjugated bilirubin is resorbable from the biliary system into the circulation and accounts for the measurable conjugated portion of total serum bilirubin. The measurable unconjugated portion is due to transport of insoluble bilirubin by albumin to the liver.

Concentration of materials in the bile can lead to the eventual formation of gallstones (Fig. 5.6). Gallstones occur twice as frequently in women as in men, and are more prevalent in developed countries. Obesity, increasing age, female sex hormones, Caucasian ethnicity, and lack of physical activity are all risk factors for developing gallstones.

Serum Enzymes

Serum enzymes are proteins that catalyze specific cellular metabolic reactions. They are located within the cell and enter the circulation under normal circumstances by secretion or physiologic cell turnover. Elevations of enzyme levels occur as a result of cellular injury or disease.

Enzymes are widely distributed in organ tissues. Isoenzymes are enzymes that catalyze the same reaction. As a result of a slightly altered genetically controlled amino acid sequence, a specific isoenzyme is useful clinically to determine its tissue origin. All enzymes are released simultaneously at the time of cell injury. The persistence of plasma levels depends on the rate of enzyme release and the enzyme serum half-life. Although serum levels generally parallel the severity of cellular damage, there is no absolute correlation with biopsy proven disease severity or prognosis. Usually, acute processes are associated with higher serum levels than chronic disease. The more valuable use of the enzymes is in following trends and changes of the serum concentrations overtime.

Many drugs including those used for anesthesia, are metabolized by the liver, with liver failure, the breakdown of these drugs are slowed, and drug effects (therapeutic and toxic) can be prolonged, if the dose is not adjusted (Box 5.1).

Drugs used for anesthesia and analgesia may need to be modified in patients with severe liver diseases include non-steroidal anti-inflammatory drugs, tetracyclines, diazepams, morphine, lidocaine and beta blockers.

Hypoproteinemia occurring in association with chronic hepatic disease or alcoholism can in particular with serum albumin levels under 2.5 g%, lead to a distinct increase in the toxicity of the local anesthetic. This is especially true with compounds that demonstrate high plasma protein binding.

A particular form of proteins synthesized by the liver and secreted into the blood is plasma

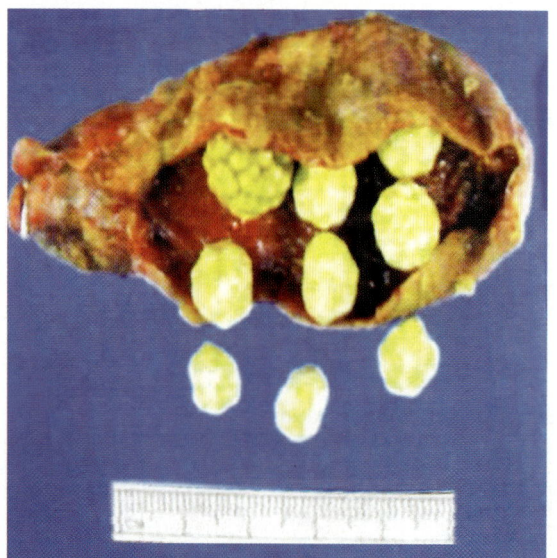

Fig. 5.6: Photo of gallstones in a gallblader *(Mckinley and O'Loughlin, 2006)*

Box 5.1: Dental drugs metabolized primarily by the liver

Local anesthetics
1. Lidocaine (xylocaine).
2. Mepivacaine (carbocaine).
3. Prilocaine (citanest).
4. Bupivacaine (marcaine).

Analgesics
1. Aspirin.
2. Acetaminophen (tylenol, datril).
3. Codeine.
4. Meperidine (demerol).
5. Ibuprofen.

Sedatives
1. Diazepam (valium).
2. Barbiturates.

Antibiotics
1. Ampicillin.
2. Tetracycline.
3. Metronidazole.
4. Vancomycin.

cholinesterase **(pseudocholinestrase)**. This plasma enzyme is responsible for metabolism and deactivation of drugs such as succinylcholine and ester local anesthetics. By breaking the ester linkages, it inactivates these drugs. Reduced hepatic synthesis of plasma cholinesterase thus may prolong the anesthetic effects of succinylcholine, although severe prolongation of muscle relaxation does not usually occur with liver disease alone. Atypical cholinesterase must be considered, if prolonged paralysis occurs.

The half-life of pseudocholinestrase is approximately 14 days. The hepatic microsomal enzyme system converts lipid-soluble drugs into more water-soluble ones that can be excreted by the kidney. Agents such as benzodiazepines, lidocaine, meperidine, morphine, and alfentanil depend on this system for elimination.

In a completely recovered patient, there are no special drug considerations. However, if a patient has chronic active hepatitis or is a carrier of HBsAg and has impaired liver function, drugs metabolized by the liver should be avoided, if possible, or the dosage decreased. As can be seen in Box 5.1, many drugs commonly used in dentistry are metabolized principally by the liver, but in other than the most severe cases of hepatic disease, these drugs can be used although in limited amounts. For example, the maximum amount of lidocaine used should be limited empirically to approximately 120 mg (three cartridges of 2%).

Drug Metabolism

Drug metabolism in the liver is controlled by the microsomal enzyme system within the smooth endoplasmic reticulum of the hepatocytes. These enzymes permit hydrolysis, oxidation, and conjugation of substances with a resultant increase in water solubility of the modified drug. The increased solubility enhances drug excretion in the urine or bile. Hepatic blood flow and plasma protein binding of the drug affect biotransformation.

Hormone Metabolism

The liver is involved in hormone metabolism. Thyroxine (T4) is activated to triiodothyronine (T3), and thyroid-binding protein synthesized in the liver. Insulin, aldosterone, antidiuretic hormone (ADH), estrogen, androgens are all inactivated by the liver. The liver may influence endocrine homeostasis during hepatic dysfunction.

Liver Function Testing

Laboratory evaluation of liver function may be considered in two main categories. Tests that measure enzymes involved in liver biotransformation reactions are commonly called **liver function tests.** This group includes laboratory tests such as serum glutamic-oxaloacetic transaminase (SGOT), serum glutamic pyruvic transaminase (SGPT), gamma-glutamyl transpeptidase (GGTP), alkaline phosphatase, and lactate dehydrogenase (LDH). The other group of laboratory values that assess **the synthetic function** of **the liver** includes prothrombin time (PT), partial thromboplastin time (PTT), serum albumin, total protein, and ammonia. Bilirubin values indicate the synthetic and excretory function.

Laboratory tests for liver function help to evaluate patients with suspected liver disease:

1. Serum asparate aminotransferase (AST, SGOT) levels rise because of damage of either liver, heart, kidney, or skeletal muscles. The AST value may also give an indication of muscle damage elsewhere in the body and in alcohol-related liver disease.

2. Serum alanine aminotransferase (ALT, SGPT) levels are most specific for hepatocellular disease. The aminotransferases are enzymes that are present in the liver cells (hepatocytes). They leak into the bloodstream when the liver cells are damaged. It indicates the degree of inflammation. These values are usually high in hepatitis—possibly 20 to 50 times higher than normal

3. Measurement of serum albumin: Albumin is a very important protein that helps keep fluid pressures in the body stable and carries many substances in the body. It gauges the severity of liver disease. Albumin may decrease (hypo-albuminemia) in chronic liver disease, particularly if the disease is getting worse, but may be decreased for other reasons such as a lack (deficiency) of protein, e.g. malnutrition. The levels may be less than 2.5 gm/dl.

4. Severe liver disease is indicated by a prolonged prothrombin time (PT) and a decreased platelet count.

5. Immunologic tests for signals of viral disease in hepatic disease.

6. Alkaline phosphatase is present in the liver, biliary and bone.

Alkaline phosphatase catalyzes phosphate reactions in an alkaline pH range. This enzyme is present in the biliary system, hepatocytes, bone, placenta, and kidney. Alkaline phosphatase exists as an isoenzyme that can be differentiated as heat stable (liver) and heat labile (bone). Alkaline phosphatase is elevated in liver dysfunction, usually associated with biliary disease. Alkaline phosphatase levels maximize during active childhood, growth, and puberty, reflecting active bone formation. In pregnancy, elevation of alkaline phosphatase occurs during the second and third trimesters, with subsequent reduction after delivery.

HEPATITIS

Oral and maxillofacial surgeons and surgical support staff are well advised to seek vaccination, if they do not already have antibodies. It is appropriate to be tested for antibodies not only before but also after vaccination to confirm that protection has been conferred, because the vaccine does not induce antibody formation in every individual.

The term hepatitis is defined non-specifically as inflammation of the liver. Hepatitis may result from a variety of causes. It may occur as a primary disease or secondarily to another disease. Examples of primary hepatitis are viral hepatitis, drug-induced hepatitis (e.g. caused by alcohol), and toxic hepatitis (e.g. caused by halothane). Examples of secondary hepatitis include that occurring with infectious mononucleosis, secondary syphilis, and tuberculosis.

Autoimmune hepatitis, often referred to as AIH, is one cause of chronic hepatitis and can be, if untreated, one of the most severe forms. The cause is not well understood, but it is believed to be the result of the immune system attacking the liver, as if the liver did not belong to the body. The cells that do damage are circulating blood cells known as lymphocytes. They behave as though the hepatocytes (liver cells) are foreign and start to destroy them. This leads to chronic hepatitis which, if untreated, will progress to cirrhosis and eventually to liver failure.

VIRAL HEPATITIS

Acute viral hepatitis is caused by at least five distinct viruses—types A, B, C, D, and E. These viruses each belong to a different family with distinct antigenic properties. They have little in common except for the target organ they infect and some epidemelogic characteristics. Hepatitis A was called infectious hepatitis, and hepatitis B was referred to as serum hepatitis. Hepatitis D, also known as delta hepatitis occurs only in association with hepatitis B. Hepatitis C and hepatitis E were known as non-A and non-B hepatitis(NANB). They were distinguished by the route of transmission. The parentrally acquired form now is known as hepatitis C, and the community-acquired form and enteric subtypes are called hepatitis E.

HEPATITIS A (HAV)

Type A hepatitis is transmitted almost exclusively by **fecal contamination of** food or water. Common sources include contaminated wells or water supply, food sources (restaurants), and shell fish beds. Because the reservoir for infection is frequently a common food or water source, hepatitis A often occurs as an epidemic. Transmission is also enhanced by poor personnel hygiene. This may be especially apparent among schoolage youngsters or food handlers, day care workers, and travelers in developing countries. Transmission by contaminated blood products is rare, occurring early during the course of the infection when titre in blood can be high and the patient is most infectious. Persons of any age may be infected; however, the disease occurs primarily in children and young adults. In general, hepatitis A tends to be of mild severity and self-limiting; it lasts a couple of weeks and often goes undiagnosed. Hepatitis A may be diagnosed by signs and symptoms such as fatigue, lymphadenopathy, gastrointestinal upset/nausea, night sweats, and possibly icteric jaundice. Of importance is the fact that no carrier state is known to exist for it. No vaccine is currently available, and recovery usually conveys immunity against reinfection.

HEPATITIS B (HBV)

Hepatitis B, sometimes called hep B or HBV, is a virus that is carried in the blood which infects and damages the liver. Hepatitis B is the most widespread form of hepatitis. It is common in South-East Asia, the Middle and far East, Southern Europe and Africa. The World Health Organization estimates that one-third of the world's population has been infected at some time and that there are approximately 350 million people who are infected long term.

NANB HEPATITIS

As previously stated, two distinct forms of non-A and non-B hepatitis have been confirmed (hepatitis C and hepatitis E).

i. Type C Hepatitis (HCV)

HCV infection is universal in occurrence. The incubation period for hepatitis CV is 15–150 days. HCV spreads through the sharing of needles (accounting for 40% of infections), parentral transmission is the major etiologic factor of post-transfusion non-A–non-B hepatitis accounting for 80 to 90% of such cases (Fig. 5.7), needle-sticks or sharp exposures on the job, from an infected mother to her baby during birth, and through heterosexual or homosexual transmission. The sexual transmission rate is quite low when compared with that for hepatitis B. HCV is similar to type B in behavior and characteristics.

Hepatitis C can be acute or chronic and the chronic rate of hepatitis C is higher. Hepatitis CV usually has a silent acute onset (80%). Only 5–10% of patients are symptomatic and experience nausea and jaundice. Thus, the occurrence of jaundice is rare. The patient has a better chance of clearing the infection in the presence of symptoms.

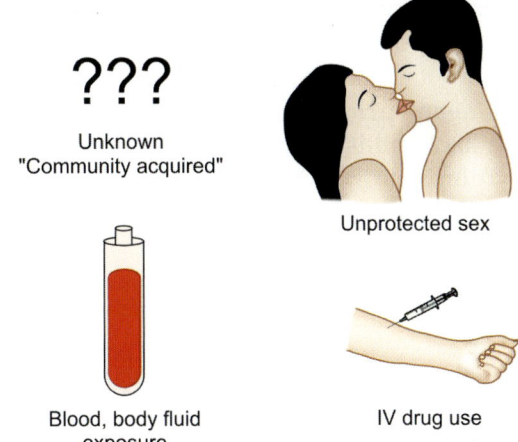

Causes of hepatitis C

Fig. 5.7: Modes of cross-infection with hepatitis C

Hepatitis C has a higher rate (55–85%) of progression to silent chronic hepatitis. Aggressive progression (70%) to chronic hepatitis occurs in the presence of coinfection with hepatitis B or HIV, at an older age, in male patients, and in the presence of alcohol use. Of chronic hepatitis patients, 20% develop cirrhosis and 2–3% of patients with cirrhosis develop liver cancer.

Hepatitis C is thus associated with a slow evolution (20–40 years) to end-stage liver disease and is the leading cause for liver transplant. Within 8 weeks from the start of the infection, anti-HCV antibody is formed. Anti-HCV antibody, unlike other antibodies, is not a protective antibody.

ii. Type E Hepatitis

The enteric form of non-A–non-B hepatitis, **hepatitis E,** resembles hepatitis A and is transmitted via fecal-oral contamination. The disease is endemic in India, Asia, Africa, and Central America.

Patients at risk for this disease include illicit drug users, health care workers exposed to blood, hemodialysis patients, and recipients of whole blood, blood cellular components, or plasma. Of interest, however, are the 40% of patients with hepatitis C that has occurred sporadically—in other words, with no identifiable risk factor for infection.

DELTA HEPATITIS

Delta hepatitis occurs only as a coinfection with acute hepatitis B or as a super-infection in carriers of hepatitis B and, therefore, is transmitted parenterally via infected blood or blood products. Hepatitis D virus needs the hepatitis B virus to survive, which means that it is only possible to have hepatitis D, if you have hepatitis B.

It is seen primarily in drug addicts and hemophiliacs and is frequently associated with more severe fulminate infections than is infection with hepatitis B alone.

VIRUS TRANSMISSION

This virus replicates predominantly in hepatocytes and to a lesser extent in stem cells in pancreas, bone marrow, and spleen. The antibody responsible for clearing the infection is anti-HBs, which signals long-term immunity.

Hepatitis B is effectively transmitted by three modes:
1. By means of parenteral contact, e.g. intravenous drug use and blood or body fluid exposure in health care workers.
2. Sexual contact (homosexual or heterosexual).
3. In a vertical manner (pre-natal transmission).

Blood

Direct products (serum plasma, factor concentrates), needle sharing, tattooing, and blood piercing. The increased risk of infection being directly related to exposure to blood, explains the reported prevalence rate of past infection among general dentists ranging from 13 to 30%, whereas that among oral surgeons is as high as 38%. Of interest is the fact that, although hepatitis B can occur at any age, statistically it is unusual in persons under the age of 15.

Hepatitis B is known as a 'blood-borne virus" (BBV) and is spread by blood to blood contact. Even a tiny amount of blood from someone who has the virus can pass on the infection, if it gets into the bloodstream. This might be an open wound, a cut or scratch, or from a contaminated needle. People who use drugs and share injecting equipment have a high risk of infection. Having a tattoo or body-piercing or even acupuncture can pose a small risk, if unsterile equipment is used.

The virus is able to survive outside the body for at least a week. This means that care should be taken not to share items such as razor or toothbrush which might be contaminated with dried blood.

All blood donations are now tested for hepatitis B, but before testing was introduced it was possible to become infected by receiving blood or blood products from an infected person. In countries where blood is not tested, blood transfusions may still be a cause of infection.

Some people transmit hepatitis B more easily than others because they have more of the virus in their bloodstream.

Saliva

The role of **saliva** in HBV transmission, except by percutaneous or permucosal routes does not appear to be significant. Even oral sex can pass on the virus. Transmission has been reported, however, as a result of a human bite. Therefore, it would appear that permucosal or percutaneous inoculation of infectious saliva is necessary for transmission of the disease.

Other Body Fluids

Although it is called a blood-borne virus, hepatitis B may be present in other body fluids such as nasopharyngeal secretions, saliva, semen and vaginal fluid, particularly if these have become contaminated with blood. Small traces have been found in sweat, tears, breast milk, urine and feces. However, most of these fluids are not regarded as infectious.

Therefore, household contact can also lead to transmission in conjunction with the sexual and parenteral routes. In fact, transmission between siblings and household contacts readily occurs through contact with skin lesions such as eczema, through sharing of potentially contaminated objects such as toothbrushes and razor blades, and occasionally by human bites. Household transmissions are probably inapparent parentral exposures to blood and saliva, over an extended period of contact with a persistent or active carrier.

Mother to Baby

Hepatitis B is usually transmitted to the baby during delivery, as the baby is exposed to the mother's blood in the birth canal. Transmission to the unborn baby does not usually occur in the uterus (before birth). Infection at birth is called "perinatal transmission" as is the most common way the virus is spread globally. Vaccination of the baby at birth prevents the majority of infections. Although small amounts of the virus have been found in breast milk, the risk from breastfeeding is not fully known and is prevented by vaccination of the newborn baby.

Work and Environment

Certain jobs can put people at risk from hepatitis because they may involve contact with infectious body

- The risk of HBV infection is more a factor of exposure to blood than of exposure to general patient contact.
- Intraorally, the greatest concentration of HBV occurs at the gingival sulcus. In most patients' mouth, the sulcus is routinely inflamed, allowing blood to mix with saliva and, thus, making saliva infectious with HBV.
- For this reason, the dental hygienist, who works primarily in the area of the gingival sulcus, has been demonstrated to be as highly at risk as the dentist, followed closely by the laboratory technician and the dental assistant.
- Additionally, the routine presence of blood in the saliva of dental patients is the reason why saliva in dentistry is considered a potentially infectious fluid and subject to universal precautions.

fluids. Healthcare workers such as doctors, dentists, nurses, and midwives are in this category, as are those who live and work in accommodation for people with severe learning difficulties.

Travel

People traveling to and working in countries where there is increased risk of hepatitis B infection are more prone to this virus infection.

Homo- and Heterosexuals

Hepatitis B can be transmitted by having penetrative sex without a condom with an infected person. Absorption of infected secretions, such as saliva or semen, through mucosal surfaces, usually follows heterosexual or homosexual contact.

Hepatitis B can cause an acute or a chronic illness. An acute illness is one that gets better quickly, usually within weeks or, at the most, a few months. A chronic illness is one that lasts more than six months, possibly for the rest of life. Sometimes symptoms come and go.

Some people have the virus in their bodies for a long time, sometimes for life, without experiencing any symptoms. They are known as carriers and may not know that they are infected. One of the more significant features of hepatitis B is the existence of a chronic carrier state that can persist for variable periods after resolution of acute disease. A carrier is defined as an individual in whose serum the HBsAg persists and is detectable for longer than 6 months, i.e. a carrier is a person who is HBsAg-positive on at least two occasions 6 months apart. Carriers develop little anti-HBs and thus remain HBsAg-positive. It is significant to note that most carriers are unaware that they have had hepatitis. An explanation for this is that

many cases of hepatitis B are apparently mild, subclinical, and nonicteric. These cases may be essentially asymptomatic or may resemble a mild viral disease and, therefore, go undetected.

Some carriers develop liver disease while others remain healthy. Most carriers are infectious, but some get rid of the virus after several years. About 25% of carriers develop serious liver disease, including chronic hepatitis and cirrhosis. After many years, a small number of them go on develop primary liver cancer, known as hepatocellular carcinoma.

Compared with hepatitis A, hepatitis B tends to have greater associated morbidity and mortality, especially in older patients. The lifetime risk of hepatitis B occurrence among the general population is low, however, certain groups have a much higher risk. Included among these are health care workers (including dentists and dental personnel), refugees, residents of mental institutions and prisons, hemodialysis patients, users of illicit drugs, male homosexuals, heterosexuals with multiple partners, and recipients of blood transfusions. Box 5.2 lists persons who are at substantial risk of contracting hepatitis B and should receive the vaccine. Note that health care workers (including dentists) are at the top of the list. It is strongly recommended that all dentists and dental personnel be inoculated with the vaccine.

Although there is no single histopathologic lesion that is characteristic of viral hepatitis, the appearances of types A, B, delta, and NANB hepatides are similar. Therefore, they will be described together. Commonly, acute viral hepatitis is characterized by degeneration and necrosis of liver cells with ballooning degeneration of the hepatocytes (Figs 5.8 and 5.9). The entire liver lobule is inflamed and consists of lymphocytes and mononuclear phagocytes.

Box 5.2: Persons at substantial risk for hepatitis B

1. Individuals with occupational risk:
   - Healthcare workers.
   - Public safety workers.
2. Clients and staff of institutions for the developmentally disabled.
3. Hemodialysis patients.
4. Recipients of certain blood products.
5. Household contacts and sex partners of HBV carriers.
6. Adopters from countries where HBV infection is endemic.
7. International travelers.
8. Illicit drug users.
9. Sexually active homosexual and bisexual men.
10. Sexually active heterosexual men and women.

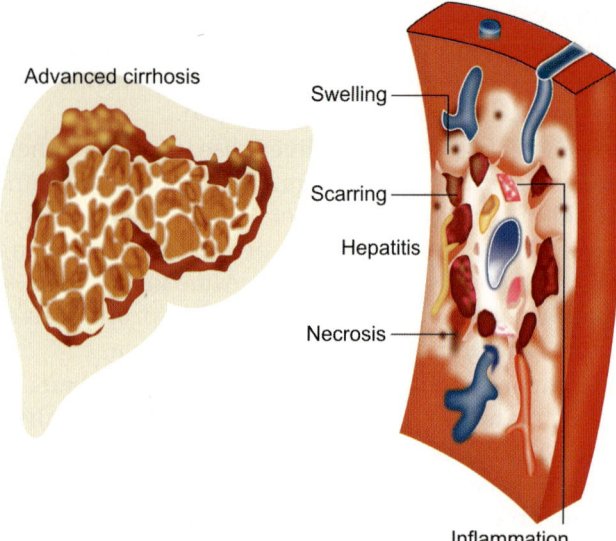

Fig. 5.8: Chronic liver destruction

Signs and Symptoms of Viral Hepatitis

Similarly, it is frequently impossible to differentiate hepatitis type by clinical appearance; therefore, it is appropriate to describe the clinical manifestations of viral hepatitis in general.

After the virus enters the body, there are no symptoms for one to six months. This is known as the incubation period. Many people never have any symptoms. Some people may only have a mild illness and are not ill enough to see a doctor. Many people, perhaps over 30%, may not know they are infected

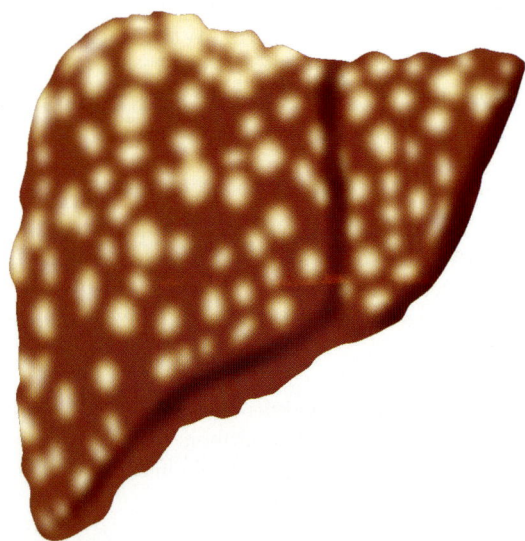

Fig. 5.9: Liver with marked inflammation from hepatitis *(Martini, 2008)*

and can pass on the virus to others. A few people develop a serious illness and need to be looked after in hospital.

There may be general symptoms such as tiredness, aches and pains, fever and/or loss of appetite, which may be diagnosed as flu. Other general symptoms may include:

- Nausea
- Stomach ache
- Diarrhea
- Jaundice

Jaundice (icterus) is commonly associated with hepatitis and is caused by an accumulation of bilirubin in the skin and mucous membrane (Fig. 5.10).

Jaundice usually becomes clinically apparent when the plasma level of bilirubin approaches 2.5 mg/100 ml (normal is less than 1 mg/100 ml). If the plasma bilirubin does not reach this level, the patient is, anicteric (without jaundice) thus explaining nonicteric hepatitis.

Phases of Acute Viral Hepatitis

There are classically three phases of acute viral hepatitis.

1. The *(prodromal)* preicteric phase usually precedes the onset of jaundice by 1 or 2 weeks and consists of anorexia, nausea, vomiting, fatigue, myalgia, malaise, fever and yellowish coloration of the sclera, lips, palate and finger nails (Fig. 5.10). With hepatitis B, 5 to 10% of patients will demonstrate serum sickness like manifestations, including arthralgia or arthritis, rash, and angioedema.

2. *Icteric* phase is heralded by the onset of clinical jaundice. Many of the non-specific prodromal symptoms may subside, but gastrointestinal

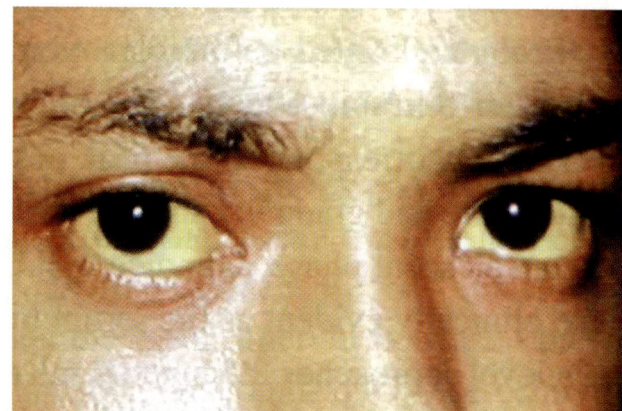

Fig. 5.10: Patient with jaundice. Note the yellow sclera

symptoms (e.g. anorexia, nausea, vomiting, and right upper quadrant pain) may increase, especially early in the phase. Hepatomegaly and spleno-megaly are frequently seen. This phase usually lasts 6 to 8 weeks.

3. During posticteric (*convalescent or recovery*) phase, the symptoms disappear, but hepatomegaly and abnormal liver function values may persist for a variable period. This phase can last for weeks or months, with recovery time for hepatitis types B and C generally being longer. The usual sequence is for recovery (clinical and biochemical) to be complete approximately 4 months after the onset of jaundice.

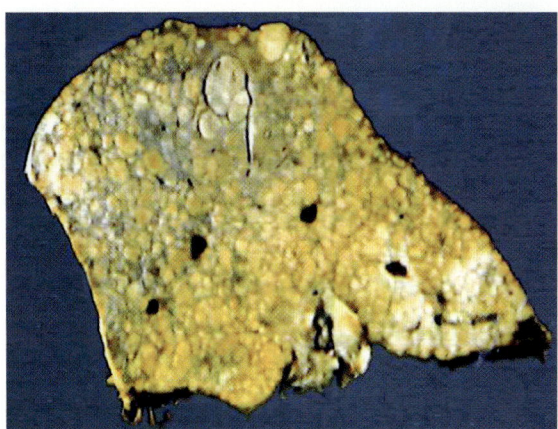

Fig. 5.11: Cirrhotic region in the liver

Cirrhosis

This is usually the result of long-term continuous damage to the liver, irregular bumps, known as nodules, replace the smooth liver tissue and the liver becomes harder. The effect of this, together with continued scarring from fibrosis, means that the liver will run out of healthy cells to support normal functions (Figs 5.11 and 5.12). This can lead to complete liver failure. In most cases, a liver transplant will be necessary.

Swollen Abdomen and Legs

Swelling of the abdomen is known as ascites (Fig. 5.13). The swelling is caused by fluid building up in the lining around the abdomen. This can happen slowly over weeks or months and can be painful, especially if the fluid becomes infected. Swelling of the legs known as peripheral edema may develop.

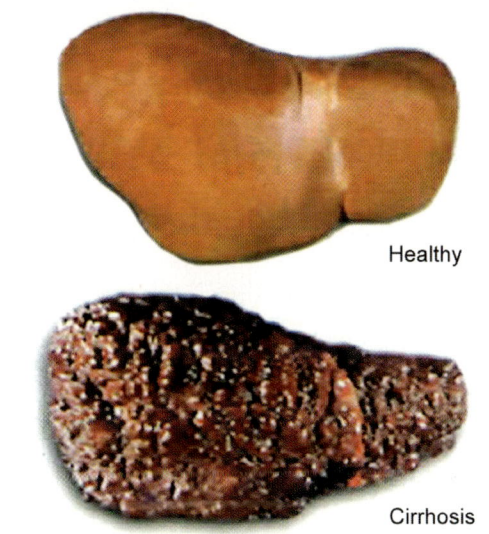

Healthy

Cirrhosis

Fig. 5.12: Topical view of normal and massive hepatocellular destruction and cirrhosis

Laboratory Findings

Liver Function Tests

Liver function tests measure the amount of substances present in the blood that might indicate damage to the liver. The laboratory studies most useful in making a diagnosis of acute viral hepatitis include the serum transaminases (aspartate aminotransferase [AST, SGOT] and alanine aminotransferase [ALT, SGPT]), serum bilirubin level, alkaline phosphatase level, WBC count, and prothrombin time. Antigen–antibody serologic tests also are of extreme importance.

The serum transaminase level will usually become elevated before elevation of the serum bilirubin occurs. The highest levels often correspond to the peak of the icteric phase and gradually subside during the

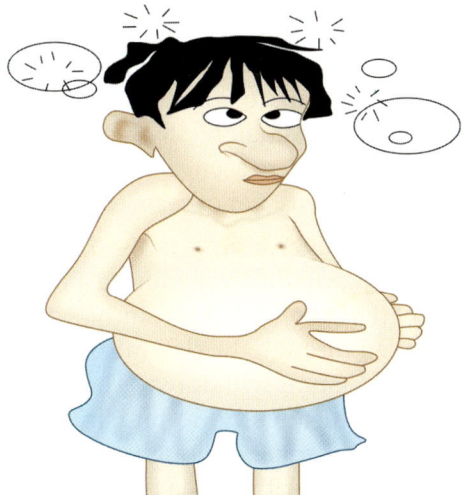

Fig. 5.13: Enlargement of the abdomen is a sign of hepatomegaly

convalscent phase. Jaundice will become clinically evident as the serum bilirubin level approaches 2.5 mg/100 ml. An elevated bilirubin level may persist after the transaminase level begins to fall. The serum alkaline phosphatase level may be mildly elevated or normal; however, this is a relatively non-specific test.

There is usually an increase in the WB count, with a relative lymphocytosis. Atypical lymphocytes are seen that are identical to those seen in infectious mononucleosis. It is important to monitor the prothrombin time because it may be elevated, especially in more extensive disease that results in hepatic cellular destruction. If the prothrombin time is severely elevated, abnormal hemostasis may be encountered.

Of the viral hepatides, types B and C are the biggest concern because both can be transmitted percutaneously, and because fulminate disease has a significant rate of mortality (up to 15% in some series). In addition, 10% of patients develop chronic liver disease (chronic active hepatitis), and patients with a history of hepatitis have a risk of liver cancer exceeding that of non-hepatitis patients.

Hepatitis B is detected by a blood test that looks for antibodies to hepatitis B. Antibodies are protein substances produced by the immune system of the body in response to invading substances (antigens) that come with the virus.

Of particular interest in hepatitis B are antigen–antibody serologic tests and their relationship to the progress of the disease.

In type C, the sensitivity and specificity of the currently available tests for anti-HCV are not well-defined. In post-transfusion cases, the mean interval between date of transfusion and anti-HCV seroconversion is approximately 18 weeks but may be 6 to 12 months. The presence of anti-HCV is an indication of infectivity not of recovery or immunity.

Liver biopsy: A liver biopsy is used to assess the amount of damage to the liver. During a liver biopsy, a tiny piece of the liver is taken for study. A fine hollow needle is passed through the skin into the liver and a small sample of tissue is withdrawn. The test is usually done under local anesthetic and may mean an overnight stay in hospital, although some people may be allowed home later the same day. As the test can be uncomfortable and there is a very small risk of internal bleeding or bile leakage, a stay of at least six to eight hours is required.

Ultrasound scan: In addition to liver biopsy, an ultrasound scan may be used. This is the same technology used to confirm all is well as in pregnancy. Gel is applied to the skin, which may feel slightly cold. A probe, like a microphone, is moved across the skin to send sound waves into the liver area. The reflected sound waves, or echoes, are picked up through the probe and used to build a screen image of the liver condition.

MEDICAL MANAGEMENT

As is the case with most viral diseases, there is no specific treatment for acute viral hepatitis. Therapy is basically palliative and supportive bed-rest may be prescribed, especially early in the course of the disease. A nutritious and high-calorie diet is advisable. Drugs metabolized by the liver are to be avoided (Table 5.1). The effectiveness of corticosteroids is doubtful in treatment of acute viral hepatitis. They are usually reserved for fulminant hepatitis. Some drugs are of value to prevent the virus from growing and causing more liver damage, e.g. interferon and pegylated interferon.

Interferons: Interferons are polypeptides secreted by cells that have been invaded by viruses. They diffuse to neighboring cells and stimulate them to produce antiviral proteins, which prevent viruses from multiplying within them. Interferon also activates natural killer cells and macrophages, which destroy infected host cells before they release more viruses. Interferons are not specific for a particular virus but provide generalized protection. They also promote the destruction of cancer cells. Pharmacologically, a drug similar to the interferon and produced by the immune system is prescribed to fight infection and to boost the immune system. It is usually given as injection three times a week for at least three months.

Pegylated interferon: It remains in the body for longer than the conventional interferon. For this reason, it requires only a single weekly injection.

The drugs that are indicated and contraindicated in hepatitis patient are mentioned in (Tables 5.1 and 5.2). The details will be discussed in prophylaxis and cross-infection.

Table 5.1: Drugs used in patients with liver disease

	Contraindicated	Used instead
Central venous system depressants	1. Barbiturates 2. Opioids 3. Phenothiazine 4. Diazepam* 5. Midazolam * 6. Propofol*	1. Pethidine 2. Benzodiazepine 3. Lorazepam * 4. Oxazepam*
General anesthetics	1. Thiopentone 2. Halothane 3. Methohexitone	1. Nitrous oxide 2. Local anesthetic 3. Isoflurane 4. Desflurane 5. Sevoflurane
Muscle relaxants	Suxamethonium	1. Atracurium 2. Cisatracurium 3. Pancuronium 4. Vecuronium 5. Curare
Analgesics	1. Aspirin 2. Codeine 3. Indometacin 4. Mefenamic acid 5. Meperidine* 6. NSAIDs 7. Opioids 8. Paracetamol/acetaminophen *	1. Codeine 2. COX-2 inhibitors 3. Celecoxibrofecoxib 4. Hydrocodone 5. Oxycodone
Antidepressants	Monoamine oxidase inhibitors	1. SSRls 2. Tricyclics*
Antimicrobials	1. Aminaglycosides 2. Azithromycin 3. Tetracycline 4. Miconazole, fluconazole, ketoconazole, itraconazole 5. Clarithromycin* 6. Clindamycin* 7. Co-amoxiclav* 8. Co-trimoxazole 9. Doxycycline 10. Erythromycin estolate 11. Metronidazole 12. Roxithromycin 13. Talampicillin	1. Amoxicillin 2. Ampicillin 3. Cephalosporins 4. Erythromycin stearate 5. Imipenem 6. Minocycline 7. Nystatin 8. Penicillins
Corticosteroids/others	1. Prednisone anticoagulants 2. Anticonvulsants 3. Biguanides 4. Diuretics 5. Liquid paraffin 6. Lomotil 7. Methyldopa 8. Oral contraceptives	Prednisolone
Local anesthetics		1. Articaine 2. Prilocaine

Table 5.2: Drugs used in patients with cirrhosis

Drugs	Used in patients with cirrhosis	Common
Acetaminophen	Yes with modifications	Acetaminophen can be given to adults with cirrhosis in divided doses of no more than 4.0 gm per day for up to 2 weeks without adverse hepatic effects. Patients should be strongly advised not to take alcohol during the period when they are using acetaminophen.
Amide local anesthetics (e.g. lidocaine, mepivacaine)	Yes with caution	Most amide local anesthetics (e.g. lidocaine, mepivacaine) are primarily metabolized (~90%) in the liver. Articaine is metabolized primarily (90–95%) in the plasma, while prilocaine is metabolized in the liver and kidneys . The serum-elimination phase of lidocaine, and of amides in general, is siginifacntly increased when there has been severe destruction of hepatic tissue. However, lidocaine has a large and rapid volume of distribution. Once lidocaine has become distributed, only 6% of that volume is present in the blood. Changes in hepatic metabolic function, and subsequently lidocaine elimination half-life, cause only a minimal elevation of the peak blood concentrations after single-dose use such as in local anesthesia, and are usually insignificant. Therefore, amide local anesthetics can be used with relative safety in the treatment of patients with cirrhosis. However, caution should still be exercised since they are at still at some degree of increased risk of developing toxic plasma concentrations. The minimum dose necessary to achieve adequate level anesthesia should be administered.
Aspirin and non-steroidal anti-inflammatory drugs (NSAIDs)	Avoid	The clearance of aspirin and NSAIDs is relatively normal in patients with chronic liver disease, but these drugs are protein bound. A decrease in serum protein concentrations may result in enhanced toxicity in as much as more free drug will be available. The antiplatelets effect of aspirin and NSAIDs in patients already susceptible to bleeding makes their use hazardous. In addition, esophageal varices, hemorrhagic gastritis, and peptic ulcers are commonly found in patients with portal hypertension. The tendency of these drugs to cause erosive lesions of the stomach and esophagus is well known, and they pose a particular threat to these patients. Prophylaxis with an antacid or histamine receptor antagonist may be considered to prevent gastritis and gastrointestinal bleeding associated with the hepatic dysfunction. However, the use of aspirin and NSAIDs in patients with cirrhosis should be avoided, if at all possible.
Benzodiazepines	Yes, with modifications	In patients with cirrhosis, hydrolytic reactions are impaired. This causes a decrease in metabolism, with subsequent accumulation of benzodiazepines (and any active metabolites, if produced) leading to excess sedation with repeated doses. It has also been suggested that, in the patient with cirrhosis, benzodiazepine receptors in the brain are more sensitive to this class of drugs, which may lead to or exacerbate hepatic encephalopathy independent of limitations in drug elimination and accumulation. If a benzodiazepine is to be used, the dosage should be decreased and given at less frequent intervals. Also, benzodiazepines without significant active metabolites (ex. alprazolam, lorazepam) are preferable over those with active metabolites (ex. diazepam).
Beta-lactam antibiotics (e.g. Penicillin, amoxicillin)	Yes	In general, antibiotics of beta-lactam group (including first-generation cephalosporins) can be used, in as much as their means of elimination are predominantly renal filtration and tubular excretion. Penicillin, ampicillin, cephalexin, and cefazolin are generally well tolerated in patients with cirrhosis.
Clindamycin	Avoid	The metabolism of clindamycin is prolonged in patients with chronic liver disease, in patients receiving clindamycin, and there is evidence suggesting that the drug contributed to the damage. Clindamycin should be avoided in patient with cirrhosis.
Macrolide antibiotics: azithromycin	Yes, with caution	Azithromycin is principally eliminated via the liver. Therefore, caution should be exercised when azithromycin is administrated to patients with impaired hepatic function. Abnormal liver functions, including cholestatic jaundice,

Contd...

Contd...

Drugs	Used in patients with cirrhosis	Common
		hepatitis, and pancreatitis have been reported infrequently in clinical trials or during post-marketing studies with azithromycin. Hepatic necrosis and hepatic failure, sometimes resulting in death, have occurred rarely.
Macrolide antibiotcs: clarithromycin	Yes, with caution	Liver function impairment alters the pharmacokinetics of clarithromycin by decreasing the amount of metabolites formed and increasing the renal clearance of parent drug; however, steady-state concentrations in patients with mild to severe hepatic function impairment do not differ from those in patients with normal hepatic function, unless there is also concurrent severe renal function impairment; no dosage adjustment is necessary in patients with hepatic function impairment, if renal function is normal.
Marcolide antibiotics: erythromycin	Yes, with caution	Erythromycin is principally excreted by the liver. The elimination half-life of both orally and parenterally administrated erythromycin has been shown to be increased in patients with impaired hepatic function due to alcoholic liver disease. Additionally, there have been reports of hepatic dysfunction, including increased liver enzymes, hepatitis, hepatocellular and cholestatic hepatitis, with or without jaundice, occurring in patients receiving oral and parenteral erythromycin products. Therefore, caution should be exercised when erythromycin is administrated to patients with impaired hepatic function.
Metronidazole	Yes, with modifications	Obstructive liver disease affects metronidazole metabolism to a greater extent than does hepatocellular liver disease. It has been recommended that if this drug is used for the patient with end-stage liver disease, 500 mg be given on a 12-hour regimen instead of the usual 6-hour regimen.
Narcotic analgesics	Yes, with modifications	Like all drugs that depress the central nervous system, narcotic analgesics may trigger or aggravate hepatic encephalopathy when used in patients with end-stage liver disease; the mechanism is not clear. Codeine is readily absorbed from the gastrointestinal tract, is rapidly distributed to body tissues, and is preferentially deposited in such organs as the spleen, kidney, and liver. Codeine (and presumably its derivatives, such as oxycodone and hydrocodone) can be used in patients with cirrhosis, but the dosage intervals need to be increased. Chronic use should be avoided. These drugs should be used with caution in combination with other drugs, such as acetaminophen, that may complete with glucuronic conjugation pathways. This system may become rapidly depleted, which can lead to the formation of hepatotoxic metabolites that may cause further injury to the already compromised liver.

DENTAL MANAGEMENT

> It is unethical to refuse dental care on the grounds that it could expose the dentist to personal risk.

The dental management of patients with history of hepatitis B begins with identification. The ideal goal is to identify potential or actual carriers of B, delta, or NANB hepatitis because they are potentially infectious. Unfortunately, this is not possible because in most instances, carriers cannot be identified by history. The inability to identify potentially infectious patients extends to AIDS and other sexually trans-mitted diseases. Therefore, it is necessary to manage all patients as though they are potentially infectious. The dental management considerations in hepatitis patients and the urgent dental care needed are mentioned in Box 5.3.

The US Public Health Service's Centers for Disease Control and the American Dental Association have published recommendations for infection control

Box 5.3: Dental management considerations in hepatitis

Urgent dental care for the patient with hepatitis

1. Consult with physician to discuss patient's status and planned dental treatment.
   No elective procedure should be undertaken in a patient with acute viral hepatitis. Do only work that is absolutely necessary.
2. Any emergency procedure in a patient with acute viral hepatitis should be undertaken only with full precautions.
3. Use isolated operatory.
4. If surgery is necessary, obtain preoperative prothrombin time and bleeding time; discuss abnormal results with physician.
5. Adhere to strict universal precautions.
6. When a choice exists, local anesthesia is preferable to general anesthesia. Many agents used for or in conjunction with general anesthesia have a degree of hepatotoxicity or are metabolized in the liver and may be poorly tolerated by the patient with acute viral hepatitis.
7. Minimize use of drugs metabolized by liver.
8. Use rubber dam when possible to minimize contact with saliva and blood.
9. Minimize aerosol production by using slow-speed handpiece when possible; use air syringe judiciously.

practice in dentistry that have become the standard of care to prevent cross-infection in dental practice. There are five categories of patients with a history of hepatitis that must be considered by the dentist. These are patients with active hepatitis, patients with a history of hepatitis, patients at a high risk for HBV infection, patients who are HBV carriers, and patients with signs or symptoms of hepatitis.

1. Patients with Active Hepatitis

Routine, elective dental care should not be performed for a patient with active hepatitis. If a patient is seen who has acute hepatitis, the physician should be contacted immediately. Unless the patient is clinically and biochemically recovered, no treatment should be rendered other than urgent care.

2. Patients with a History of Hepatitis

A primary concern of the dentist is to identify patients who are or could be carriers of type B, delta, or C hepatitis. As previously noted, however, the medical history will fail to identify up to 80% of carriers of hepatitis B and cannot be relied on for this purpose. In addition, it should be remembered that there is undoubtedly a carrier state with hepatitis C though not well-defined as yet.

Routine laboratory screening for all patients is economically impractical because of its high cost-effectiveness. Therefore, the only practical method of protection from these individuals, and other patients with undetected infectious diseases, is to adopt a strict program of clinical asepsis for *all* patients. In addition, the availability and effectiveness of the hepatitis B vaccine can further decrease the threat of hepatitis B infection. Inoculation of all dental personnel with hepatitis B vaccine is strongly urged. For those patients who provide a positive history of hepatitis, additional historical information will occasionally be of some help in determining the type of disease. For instance, if the infection occurred under age 15 years or was caused by contaminated food or water, this would suggest hepatitis A infection.

Unfortunately, this approach will not reveal a person who has had infection with both type A and type B or C in which the *B* or *C* infection was subclinical or undiagnosed. This, again, supports the adoption of universal precautions for all patients and inoculation of dental personnel with hepatitis B vaccine. An additional consideration in patients with a history of hepatitis of unknown type is to use the clinical laboratory to screen for the presence of hepatitis B surface antigen(HBsAg). This may be indicated even in patients who specifically indicate which type of hepatitis they have had, because studies have shown that historically provided information of this type is unreliable 50% of the time. We do not currently recommend screening for anti-HCV due to the uncertain specificity and sensitivity of this test.

3. Patients at High Risk for HBV Infection

As indicated, there are several groups of people who are at unusually high risk for HBV infection. Individuals who fit into one or more of these categories should routinely be screened for HBsAg before dental care is provided unless laboratory evidence exists for anti-HBs. It may seem redundant to recommend screening patients for the presence of HBsAg, because all patients are to be managed in such a manner as to prevent the transmission of infection by following the Centers for Disease Control recommendations. Even if a patient is found to be a carrier, no modifications in treatment approach would theoretically be necessary. However, this information may still be of benefit in certain situations. If a patient is found to be a carrier, the information could be of extreme importance for the modification of lifestyle.

In addition, the patient might have undetected chronic active hepatitis, which could lead to bleeding complications or drug metabolism problems. Finally, if an accidental needle stick or puncture wound occurs during treatment and the dentist is not vaccinated (or antibody titer status is unknown), it would be of extreme importance to know whether the patient was HBsAg positive, which would dictate the need for IG or HBIG vaccination.

4. Patients who are Hepatitis Carriers

If a patient is found to be a hepatitis B carrier (HBsAg positive) or to have a history of NANB hepatitis, the Centers for Disease Control recommendations should be closely followed to avoid transmission of infection. In addition, some hepatitis carriers may have chronic active hepatitis, leading to compromised liver function and interfering with hemostasis and drug metabolism. Physician consultation or laboratory screening for liver function is advised.

5. Patients with Signs or Symptoms of Hepatitis

Any patient who has signs or symptoms that suggest hepatitis, should not be treated electively but referred immediately to a physician. If emergency care becomes necessary, it should be provided as for the patient with acute disease.

Surgical Considerations in Acute and Chronic Hepatic Insufficiency

Most cases of viral hepatitis, especially type A resolve without any complications, however, occasional chronic problems do develop with hepatitis B and a significant number of cases of type C result in chronic sequelae. Approximately, 3 to 5% of patients with acute hepatitis B and 40 to 50% with acute type C will develop chronic active hepatitis. This form of hepatitis is characterized by the persistence of signs and symptoms of chronic liver disease, persistent hepatic cellular necrosis, and biochemical abnormalities for longer than 6 months. There also is a persistence of HBsAg in the serum with hepatitis B. It appears that patients who have HBsAg in their serum with the acute B infection have a greater chance than those who do not develop this form of chronic hepatitis. The chronic liver destruction and resulting fibrosis can lead to cirrhosis in cases of chronic hepatitis. The most serious complication of acute viral hepatitis is fulminant hepatitis, which sometimes occurs with hepatitis B and delta coinfection and with hepatitis C.

This is, fortunately, a rare entity and is characterized by massive hepatocellular destruction. The mortality rate approaches 80%. The complication of a persistent carrier state, which was previously discussed, is seen in 5 to 10% of cases of hepatitis B. There is noteworthy evidence that suggests a positive correlation between the chronic HBsAg carrier state and the development of hepatocellular carcinoma. There is, however, a positive correlation with chronic hepatitis C and **hepatocellular** carcinoma.

No treatment planning modifications are required for the patient who has recovered from hepatitis.

The main problems in management of patients with liver diseases are:

1. Bleeding tendency.
2. Impaired drug detoxification.
3. Infection susceptibility
4. Transmission of viral hepatitis.

In addition to:

1. Electrolytes and nutrition imbalance.
2. Ulcer therapy.
3. Renal malfunction.
4. Blood ingestion.

Patients with acute and chronic hepatic insufficiency require consideration of the consequences of their disease state during surgical treatment planning. Preoperative laboratory testing includes complete blood count, platelet count, electrolytes, glucose, albumin, total protein, bilirubin, liver function tests, and coagulation profiles. Bleeding time tests and hepatitis screens are also valuable. Presurgical management considerations include the following.

1. Bleeding Tendency

The main oral complication associated with hepatitis is the potential for abnormal bleeding in cases of significant liver damage (Fig. 5.14).

Evaluation of the patient's hemostatic ability can be determined with PT, PTT, bleeding times and platelet counts. PT and PTT values greater than 1.5 times control require correction. Before any surgery, the prothrombin time should be checked to ensure that it is less than 2.5 times normal (35 seconds), the normal is 14 seconds. If it is greater than 35 seconds, the potential for severe postoperative bleeding exists. Acute correction may be accomplished with fresh frozen plasma (FFP) with care to monitor the effects

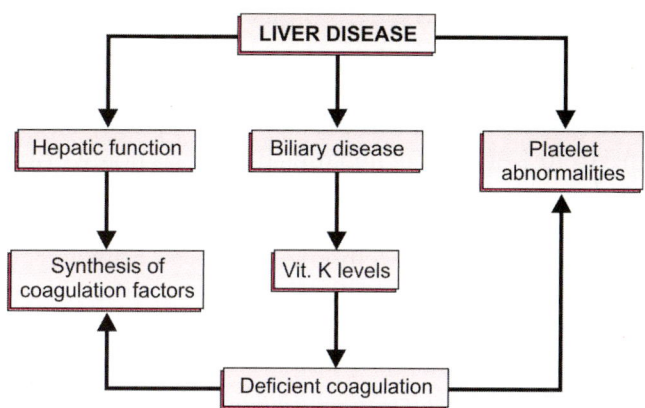

Fig. 5.14: Relation between liver diseases and defective coagulation

of volume overload. FFP contains all necessary coagulation factors. If concentrated factor VIII and factor I (fibrinogen) are needed, cryoprecipitate may be administered. The attendant risks and reactions to transfusions should be balanced against the medical need.

Vitamin K supplementation to enhance vitamin K dependent coagulation factor synthesis is recommended. Intravenous vitamin K (5–10 mg over 3–5 min) can be administered, if a deficiency is suspected and will shorten an abnormal PT in 4 to 12 hours. Fresh frozen plasma can be used temporarily to make up for a vitamin K deficiency until the parenterally administered vitamin is effective.

Hypersplenism with associated platelet sequestration may be evident in platelet counts and bleeding time studies. It is also advisable to check platelet function; severe damage can also result in decrease platelet count. The bleeding time is less than 20 minutes. Values greater may require platelet replacement and should be discussed with the physician. Correction of hypersplenic thrombocytopenia with platelet transfusions may be difficult. It may be further compounded by hepatic platelet sequestration or alcoholic suppression of platelet function and production. Generally, a platelet count of approximately 50,000/mm^3 is considered adequate in the presence of careful surgical technique. A low platelet count and a low fibrinogen level should release the question of disseminated intravascular coagulation (DIC).

Because patients with severe liver disease have problems with improper gluconeogenesis, the surgeon should closely monitor serum glucose levels.

2. Impaired Drug Detoxification

Drugs used for anesthesia and analgesia may need to be modified in the patient with hepatic disease. Drugs to avoid in patients with severe liver disease include all non-steroidal anti-inflammatory drugs, tetracyclines, pentazocaine, and atenolol. Drugs for which dosages need to be reduced include diazepam, meperidine, morphine, thiophylline, lidocaine, and most β-sympathetic antagonists (Table 5.1). Most anesthetics are generally safe in patients with hepatic disease, although some feel halothane, fentanyl, and nitrous oxide should be avoided because of their potential for causing toxicity.

3. Infection Susceptibility

Patients with hepatic insufficiency have a lowered resistance to infection owing to a variable level of reduced immunocompetence. Antibiotic prophylaxis should be considered. Selection of antibiotic coverage and dosage must consider hepatic and renal function, infection source, probable microorganisms involved, patient allergy, and any recent antibiotic use.

4. Transmission of Viral Hepatitis

Will be discussed in cross-infection.

5. Electrolytes and Nutrition Imbalance

Aberrations of electrolytes and fluid status associated with hepatic dysfunction or ascites require attention. Evaluation of nutritional status is important because malnutrition can lead to delayed wound healing and wound dehiscence.

6. Ulcer Therapy

Gastritis or previous gastrointestinal bleeding is often present. Prophylactic therapy with anti-acids is helpful to prevent exacerbation of any upper gastrointestinal bleeding or peptic ulcer disease.

7. Renal Malfunction

Hepatorenal syndrome may occur concomitant with hepatic disease. Adverse renal effects of aminoglycosides and non-steroidal anti-inflammatory medications are enhanced, if associated with hepatic insufficiency.

8. Blood Ingestion

Surgical techniques with oral procedures should minimize ingestion of blood to avoid increasing ammonia production by intestinal bacteria.

CROSS-INFECTION

Universal precautions typically include having all doctors and staff who come in contact with patient blood or secretions, whether directly or in aerosol form, wear barrier devices, including a facemask, eye protection, and gloves. Universal precaution procedures go on to include decontaminating or disposing of all surfaces that are exposed to patient blood, tissue and secretions. Finally, universal precautions mandate avoidance of touching, and thereby contaminating surfaces (e.g. the dental record, telephone) with contaminated gloves or instruments.

Cross-infection is the transmission of infectious agents between patients and staff within the clinical environment. The mouth carries a large number of potentially infective microorganisms; saliva and blood are known vectors of infection. Members of the dental team have a duty to ensure that infection control procedures are followed routinely. Potential risks include not only hepatitis and HIV, but also other viruses (e.g. herpes) and bacteria (e.g. *Streptococcus pyogenes*). Most carriers of latent infection are unaware of their condition and it is important, therefore, that the same infection control routine is adopted for all patients. The procedure that should be followed to guard against cross-infection will be discussed in some details.

Use of Disposables

One of the best ways to prevent patient-to-patient cross-contamination is to use a disposable item that never contacts a second patient. Numerous disposables are available in dentistry, including gloves, masks, gowns, surface covers, patient bibs, saliva ejector tips, air-water syringe tips, high-volume evacuator tips, prophy cups, some instruments, some burs, impression trays, fluoride gel trays, sharps containers, bio-hazard bags, and high-speed handpieces. These and other items that are manufactured as single-patient use (disposable) items should not be reused on another patient, these items were not designed for cleaning and decontamination and tend to hold contaminants in scratches of the "soft" plastic often used or melt when heat processed.

Hand Protection

Keep fingernails short with smooth, filed edges to allow thorough cleaning and to prevent glove tears. Do not wear artificial fingernails or extenders when having direct contact with patients at high risk. Do not wear hand or nail jewelry, if it makes donning gloves more difficult or compromises the fit and integrity of the glove.

The care of hands is vital to infection control; lacerated, abraded and cracked skin can offer a portal of entry for microorganisms. Gloves must be worn for all clinical procedures and treated as single-use items, so a new pair of gloves must be used for each patient.

Gloves should be donned immediately before contact with the patient and removed as soon as clinical treatment is complete. No recommendation is offered regarding the effectiveness of wearing two pairs of gloves to prevent disease transmission during oral surgical procedures. The effectiveness of wearing two pairs of gloves in preventing disease transmission has not been demonstrated. Used gloves must be disposed of as clinical waste.

Recommendations for hand care during clinical sessions include:
- Removal of rings, jewelry and watches.
- Covering all cuts and abrasions with waterproof adhesive dressings.
- Methodical hand washing using a good-quality liquid soap preferably containing a disinfectant – a full hand wash and thorough drying is recommended before donning gloves, removing gloves and washing hands after each patient (gives the hands time to recover from being covered).
- Regular use of an emollient hand cream to prevent the skin from drying, especially after every clinical session. There is a variety of gloves reliable. Those selected should be: good-quality non-sterile, and single use, worn for all clinical procedures and changed after every patient. They should be well fitting and non-powdered. The powder from gloves can contaminate veneers and radiographs, disperse allergenic proteins into the surgery atmosphere and interfere with wound healing 'hypoallergenic' and 'low protein' to reduce the possibility of allergy.

Allergic contact dermatitis is rare but, if it develops, it may be serious enough to cause the person to cease practice. If it is suspected, the advice of a dermatologist should be sought. Irritant contact dermatitis is more

common and can be avoided by careful choice of glove suitable hand disinfectant and meticulous hand care. Those with an allergy to latex can try vinyl, or wear under gloves of silk or nylon. Non-powdered gloves are advisable. Remove gloves that are torn, cut or punctured as soon as feasible, and wash hands before regloving.

Increasingly, dentists are encountering patients who are allergic to the latex itself or the chemicals used in glove manufacture. Non-latex gloves are available, but additional precautions will be needed to protect the allergic patient against contact with latex through other sources in the surgery—local anesthetic cartridges, rubber dam and protective glasses, for example.

Surface Covers of Sterilized Instruments

During use, instruments should only be placed on a sterilizable tray or impermeable disposable covering. A system of zoning high efficiency as only those areas which are likely to be contaminated need to be cleaned and disinfected with a suitable viricidal disinfectant.

Surface covers are materials impervious to moisture (e.g. thin plastic) that are used to prevent contamination of surfaces. Care is required to avoid contamination of areas which are difficult to disinfect. Surface covers should be used on surfaces that are difficult to clean and disinfect (e.g. air-water syringe buttons, dental light handles, electrical toggle switches and button, knurled handles, sink faucets, difficult-to-reach areas). A routine use of small surface cover for the head rest or longer one to cover also any control buttons on the side of the chair is of value.

Surgery Clothing

There is no consensus view on whether surgery clothing should have short or long sleeves. Short sleeves will allow the forearms to be washed as part of the hand washing routine. Long-sleeved coats or tunics will protect the skin of the arms against splatter. This is important, if skin is cracked or abraded (as a result of eczema, for example). Long sleeves, however, are more likely to become contaminated during clinical sessions and could cause a breach in infection control. Surgery clothing should be made of a material that can be machine washed with a suitable detergent at a temperature of 65°C to eradicate any potential microbial contamination.

Aerosol

Reducing the amount of spray and spatter that exit patient's mouth during care, reduces the number of microbes contaminating the dental team. This is accomplished by the use of high-volume suction, wear gloves, eye protection, and masks and flush aspirators and tubing carefully daily with a recommended disinfecting agent.

The rubber dam and high-volume evacuation have been shown to reduce greatly the number of microbes in dental aerosols generated during operative procedures, and saliva ejection keeps saliva from accumulating in the mouth.

Eyewear and face-shields with adequate side protection prevent spatter from patient's mouth or splashes of contaminated solutions and chemicals from contacting the eyes.

Similar to protective eyewear, facemasks prevent spatter from patient's mouth or splashes of contaminated solutions and chemicals from contacting the mucous membranes of the mouth and nose. A secondary protective aspect of a mask is a reduction in the inhalation of airborne particles. Recommendations to change the mask after 20 minutes in aerosol or 60 minutes in nonaerosol environments are based on studies observing wetness and wicking through masks.

Inoculation Injuries

Inoculation injuries are the most likely route for transmission of blood-borne viral infections in dentistry. The definition of an inoculation injury includes all incidents where a contaminated object or substance breaches the integrity of the skin or mucous membranes or comes into contact with the eyes. The following are typical examples:
- Sticking or stabbing with a used needle or other instrument.
- Splashes with a contaminated substance to the eye or other open lesion. Cuts with contaminated equipment.
- Bites or scratches inflicted by patients.

Inoculation injuries must be dealt with promptly and correctly:
- The wound should be allowed to bleed and washed thoroughly with running water.
- Where there is reason to be concerned about the possible transmission of infection, the injured person should seek urgent advice according to the local arrangements in place on what follow-up action, including serological surveillance, is necessary. Ideally, all practices should have formal links with an occupational health service, so that management of sharps injuries is undertaken promptly and according to accepted national protocols.

The risk of acquiring HIV infection following an inoculation injury is small. If the injury is risk-assessed as significant for transmission of HIV and the source patient is HIV infected, the use of anti-retroviral drugs taken prophylactically as soon as possible after exposure, ideally within 1h, is recommended. Post-exposure prophylaxis (PEP) involves the use of a short course (4 weeks) of treatment with anti-retroviral drugs in an attempt to reduce even further the risk of infection with HIV following exposure.

Factors associated with HIV transmission:
- Deep injury to the healthcare worker.
- Visible blood on the device causing injury.
- Device previously placed in source patient's vein or artery.
- Source patient within last 60 days of life (i.e. late-stage AIDS).

Blood Spillages

If blood is spilled, either from a container or as a result of an operative procedure, the spillage should be dealt with as soon as possible. The spilled blood should be completely covered either by disposable towels, which are then treated with 10,000 ppm sodium hypochlorite solution, or by sodium dichloroisocyanurate granules. At least 5 mm must elapse before the towels, etc. are cleared and disposed of as clinical waste. The dental health care worker who deals with the spillage must wear appropriate protective clothing, which will include household gloves, protective eyewear and a disposable apron and, in the case of an extensive floor spillage, protective footwear. Good ventilation is essential.

Disposal of Clinical Waste

All wastes in the practice should be segregated into clinical and non-clinical waste:
- Clinical waste is waste that is contaminated with blood, saliva or other body fluids and may prove hazardous to any person coming into contact with it.
- Clinical waste sacks must be no more than three-quarters full, have the air gently squeezed out to avoid bursting when handled by others, labeled and tied at the neck, not knotted.
- Sharps waste (needles and scalpel blades) must be sealed in puncture-proof containers, which must be labeled before disposal.
- Local anesthetic cartridges, whether partially discharged (hazardous) or fully discharged, must always be disposed of via the sharps' container.

- Sharps' containers should be disposed of when no more than two-thirds full.
- Clinical waste and sharps waste must be stored securely before collection for final disposal.
- Usually by high-temperature incineration.
- Clinical waste must only be collected for disposal by a waste carrier. When waste is collected for disposal, a transfer note must be completed and signed by both parties. The transfer note provides the dentist with evidence that the waste will be disposed of in the correct manner.
- Repeated transfers of the same kind of waste between the same parties can be covered by one transfer note for up to 1 year but a copy must be kept for 2 years.

Some primary care trusts have local arrangements for the collection and disposal of clinical waste; otherwise arrangements for the collection of clinical waste should be made with a private contractor.

Partially used local anesthetic cartridges are regarded as hazardous waste and are subject to additional disposal controls; when the waste is collected, consignment notes must be completed and kept for 3 years. If a local anesthetic cartridge is fully discharged, however, it is not regarded as hazardous waste and can be disposed of as clinical waste via the sharps' container. If partially discharged local anesthetic cartridges are disposed of via the sharps' container, the container must be disposed of as hazardous waste.

Amalgam-filled extracted teeth cannot be discarded via the sharps' container, as amalgam must not be incinerated. These teeth should be disposed of with waste amalgam but care should be taken as the teeth will be contaminated with blood.

Waste collection agencies often produce special containers for the disposal of amalgam-filled teeth. It is possible to send amalgam-filled teeth (and non-filled teeth) through the post to universities for teaching and research purposes but the patient's consent must be obtained first (and recorded in the clinical records). It is important to ensure that extracted teeth that are sent through the post are first decontaminated and packaged securely to avoid the package being split open during transit. Some dental schools provide a container and disinfectant suitable for decontamination, storage and transport.

A dentist who fails to dispose of waste in a safe manner will face prosecution by the authorities and may be liable to proceedings for serious professional

misconduct. Clinical waste and hazardous waste must never be disposed of at local refuse tips or landfill sites.

DECONTAMINATION OF INSTRUMENTS AND EQUIPMENT

All instruments contaminated with oral and other body fluids must be thoroughly cleaned and sterilized after use. Instruments selected for a treatment session but not used must be regarded as contaminated. There are three stages to the decontamination process:

i. Pre-sterilization cleaning,
ii. Sterilization and
iii. Storage.

Manufacturers are now required to provide instructions for the decontamination of their equipment—these instructions should be followed. It is worth checking with the manufacturers prior to purchase that equipment can be used for the purpose intended and decontaminated by the methods used in the practice. A systematic approach to the decontamination of instruments after use will ensure that dirty instruments are segregated from clean.

I. Presterilization Cleaning

Used instruments are often heavily contaminated with blood and saliva and must be completely cleaned before sterilization. Instruments can be cleaned by hand, in an ultrasonic bath or using an instrument washer/disinfector— do check with the manufacturer that instruments can withstand ultrasonic cleaning and automated processing. Ultrasonic cleaners and washer/disinfectors are preferred over hand cleaning instruments as they are more efficient and contact with contaminated instruments is kept to a minimum thereby reducing the likelihood of inoculation injuries.

Hand cleaning of dental instruments is the least efficient cleaning method. If this method is used, however, the instruments should be fully immersed in a sink prefilled with warm water and detergent, and a long-handled kitchen-type brush used to remove debris. Instruments should be washed under water with the sharp end of the instrument held away from the body; extra care must be taken when cleaning instruments that are sharp at both ends. Thick waterproof household gloves must be worn to protect against accidental injury and protective eyewear to shield against splashing. The brush used to remove debris from the instruments should be cleaned and autoclaved at regular intervals—at the end of each clinical session, for example. Cleaned brushes should be stored dry.

After cleaning, all instruments must be examined thoroughly and, if there is residual debris, recleaned.

Ultrasonic cleaners should be used and serviced according to the manufacturer's instructions and should contain a detergent not a disinfectant—disinfectant solutions alone can precipitate proteins and make them resistant to removal. Do check with the manufacturer's recommendations. The liquid in the ultrasonic cleaners should be disposed off at the end of each clinical session and more often, if it appears heavily contaminated. Ultrasonic cleaners with baskets are preferred. The cleaning cycle should not be interrupted to add further instruments. At the end of each day, the ultrasonic cleaner must be emptied, cleaned and left dry.

Washer/disinfectors designed for cleaning instruments are now available and, if used, the manufacturer's instructions should be followed. Washer/disinfectors are more efficient at presterilization cleaning than ultrasonic cleaners and hand cleaning but must not be used as a substitute for sterilization procedures.

II. Sterilization

The method of choice for the sterilization of all dental instruments is autoclaving. Sterilization should be performed at the highest temperature compatible with the instruments in the load. For dental instruments and equipment, autoclaves should reach a temperature of 134–137°C for 3 min. New autoclaves should have an integral printer to allow the parameters reached during the sterilization cycle to be recorded for routine monitoring. Hot air ovens, ultraviolet light, boiling water and chemiclaves are not recommended for sterilizing dental instruments and equipment.

Effective sterilization depends on steam condensing on all surfaces of the instruments in the load to be autoclaved, so it is essential that instruments be placed to allow free circulation of steam; the autoclave chamber must not be overloaded. The sterilization process is impaired or prevented by air remaining in the chamber or trapped in the load items. Air is removed from the autoclave chamber by either being displaced downwards by steam or evacuating the air to create a vacuum before steam is introduced into the chamber. For many years, downward-displacement autoclaves were the only autoclaves used in a dental surgery; they are still considered an acceptable means of sterilizing dental instruments and equipment.

More recently, however, vacuum-phase autoclaves have become available to dentists in general practice.

Dentists considering purchasing a vacuum-phase autoclave should ensure that it is capable of sterilizing the intended load items (various types are available and not all are suitable for processing dental equipment). The autoclave should be equipped only with cycles providing a pre-sterilization vacuum stage to minimize the possibility of an incorrect cycle being selected and a consequent failure to sterilize the load.

Processing wrapped instruments in a conventional downward-displacement autoclave may result in inadequate air removal and failure to sterilize. Wrapped instruments and instruments in pouches must be sterilized using a vacuum-phase autoclave.

There continues to be some debate about the effective decontamination of handpieces. In theory, a vacuum-phase autoclave will remove the air from the lumen of a dental handpiece, allowing steam to penetrate. The presence of lubricating oil, however, may compromise the sterilization process. Current opinion is that effective pre-sterilization cleaning of dental handpieces and subsequent processing in a properly functioning downward-displacement autoclave is acceptable.

All autoclaves must be regularly serviced and maintained according to the manufacturer's reco-mmendations and periodically inspected (usually annually) to ensure the integrity of the associated pipe work. Vacuum-phase autoclaves are more complicated than conventional steam sterilizers and require more vigorous testing by the user to demonstrate that they function correctly . If you are considering purchasing a vacuum-phase autoclave, you must be aware of all the user tests that you will be required to perform and record on a regular basis. Your service and maintenance agreement should cover the anticipated response time in the event that the autoclave breaks down or malfunctions.

At the end of each day, the residual water should be drained from the autoclave chamber and reservoir, which should then be cleaned and left open to dry over-night. Many autoclaves now incorporate a facility for draining residual water. A drain valve can be retrofitted to many autoclaves that do not have an integral drainage device. As a last resort, the high-volume suction unit may be used (if it is conveniently placed). If this is necessary, the autoclave should not be moved or lifted unless it can be done safely and without risk of injury.

It is important that the water used in the autoclave should contain no minerals that may cause damage and, to ensure the integrity of the sterilization cycle, it should be free of pathogens and endotoxins (pyrogenfree).

Successful sterilization depends upon the consistent reproducibility of sterilizing conditions:

- Autoclaves must be validated before use and their performance monitored routinely (by periodic testing, including daily and weekly user tests).
- The equipment must be properly maintained according to the manufacturer's instructions.
- Correct operation of the autoclave must be checked whenever the autoclave is used by recording the readings (physical parameters) on the autoclave's instruments or printout at the beginning of each clinical session.
- The readings should be compared with the recommended values, if any reading is outside its specified limits, the sterilization cycle must be regarded as unsatisfactory, irrespective of the results obtained from chemical indicators, and the autoclave cycle checked again. If the second cycle is unsatisfactory, the autoclave should not be used until the problem has been rectified by an engineer.
- Autoclave logs and printouts should be retained for inspection and monitoring—to demonstrate that the autoclave is performing within the recommended parameters.

Chemical and biological indicators do not demonstrate sterility of the load. Chemical indicators serve only to distinguish loads that have been processed in an autoclave from those that have not. Biological indicators are of limited value in moist-heat sterilization and can only be regarded as additional to the measurement of physical parameters.

III. Instrument Storage

Sterilized instruments should be stored in dry, covered conditions—trays with lids are now available for this purpose. Sterilized instruments should not be stored in a disinfectant or antiseptic solution. Pouches can be useful for storing infrequently used instruments such as extraction forceps and elevators. Pouches with a clear side allow instruments to be easily identified before opening.

The instruments necessary for treatment should be selected prior to the treatment session. If additional instruments are needed during treatment, care must be taken to avoid the cross-contamination of other instruments. Tray systems can help with this.

Unlike most viruses, the hepatitis virus is exceptio-nally resistant to desiccation and chemical dis-infectants, including alcohols, phenols, and quaternary ammonium compounds. Therefore, the hepatitis B virus is difficult to avoid, particularly when oral surgery is being performed.

Fortunately, means of inactivating the virus include halogen-containing disinfectants (e.g. iodophor, hypochlorite), formaldehyde, ethylene oxide gas, all types of properly performed heat sterilization, and irradiation. These methods can be used to minimize the spread of hepatitis from one patient to another (Table 5.3).

DECONTAMINATION OF HANDPIECES

If a cleaning machine is not used, the following protocol should be adopted for the pre-sterilization cleaning of handpieces:

• Leave the bur in place during cleaning to prevent contamination of the handpiece bearing. Clean the outside of the handpiece with detergent and water—never clean or immerse the handpiece in disinfectant. Remove the bur.

• If recommended by the manufacturer, lubricate the handpiece with pressurized oil until clean oil appears out of the chuck and clean off excess oil.

• Sterilize in an autoclave.

• If recommended by the manufacturer, lubricate the handpiece after sterilization and run it briefly before use to clear excess lubricant. The oil used for presterilization cleaning/lubrication should not be the same as used for post-sterilization lubrication; two tips should be used and the nozzle changed between applications.

DECONTAMINATION OF IMPRESSION MATERIALS AND PROSTHETIC AND ORTHODONTIC APPLIANCES

The responsibility for ensuring impressions and appliances have been cleaned and disinfected prior to dispatch to the laboratory lies solely with the dentist:

• Immediately on removal from the mouth, the impression or appliance should be rinsed under running water to remove saliva, blood and debris.

• Continue the process until it visibly clean. If an appliance is grossly contaminated, it should be cleaned in an ultrasonic bath containing detergent and then rinsed.

• The impression or appliance should be disinfected according to the manufacturer's recommendations. Materials such as sodium hypochlorite (household bleach) may no longer be suitable for disinfecting impressions unless specifically recommended by the manufacturer.

• Disinfectants should not be sprayed on to the surface of the impression; it lessens the effectiveness and creates an inhalation risk. Immersion of the impression is recommended.

• The impression or appliance should be rinsed again in water before sending to the laboratory accompanied by a confirmation that it has been disinfected.

The manufacturer's recommendations for the dilution of the disinfectant and immersion time must be followed.

Table 5.3: Suitable methods for sterilizing common dental Instruments and items

	Steam autoclave	Dry heat oven	Chemical vapor	Ethylene oxide
General hand instruments				
Stainless steel	1	1	1	2
Carbon steel	3	1	1	2
Mirrors	2	1	1	2
Burs				
Steel	2	1	1	2
Carbon steel	3	1	1	2
Tungsten-carbide	2	1	2	2
Stones				
Diamond	2	1	1	2
Polishing	1	2	1	2
Sharpening	2	1	2	2
Polishing wheels and disks				
Rubber	2	4	3	2
Garnet and cuttle	4	3	3	2
Rag	1	2	2	2

Contd...

Contd...

	Steam autoclave	Dry heat oven	Chemical vapor	Ethylene oxide
Rubber dam equipment				
Carbon or carbide steel clamps	3	1	1	2
Stainless steel clamps	I	1	1	2
Punches	3	1	1	2
Plastic frames	3	4	4	2
Metal frames	1	1	1	2
Impression trays				
Aluminium metal, chrome plated	1	1	1	2
Custom acrylic resin	4	4	4	2
Plastic (discarding is preferred)	4	4	4	2
Fluoride gel trays				
Heat-resistant plastic	1	4	3	2
Non-heat-resistant plastic	4	4	4	2
Orthodontic pliers				
High quality stainless	1	1	1	2
Low quality stainless	4	1	1	2
With plastic parts	4	4	3	1
Endodontic instruments				
Reamers and files, broaches, stainless metal handles	1	1	1	1
Non-stainless metal handles	4	1	1	1
Stainless with plastic handles	3	3	3	1
Pluggers and condensers	1	1	1	2
Glass slabs	1	2	1	2
Dappen dishes	1	2	1	2
Handpieces				
High speed	3	3	3	2
Low-speed straight	3	3	3	2
Prophy angles	2	2	2	2
Contra-angles	4	4	4	2
Radiographic equipment				
Plastic film holders, columating devices	3	4	4	2
Stainless steel surgical instruments	1	1	2	2
Ultrasonic scaling tips	2	4	4	2
Electrosurgical tips and handles	4	4	4	4
Needles				
Disposable (do not reuse)	4	4	4	4
Reusable	2	2	4	4

* 1, indicates preferred method with minimum risk of damage; 2, indicates that materials should withstand treatment with minimum risk of damage; 3, indicates that treatment is usually not suitable and may damage materials, manufacturer should be consulted; 4, indicates that materials are likely to be damaged or process may be ineffective.

Chemical protection of certain nonstainless instruments may permit steam autoclaving. A rust-preventive dip (1% sodium nitrate) is recommended before sterilization.

Steel burrs may be sterilized in hot endodontic sterilizer for 15 to 20 seconds at 475°F (246°C), but the process may not be suitable for carbide burrs.

Some common latch-type contra-angles cannot withstand repeated heat sterilization; short, heat sterilizable contra-angle handpieces are now available.

INFECTION CONTROL CHECKLIST

At Start of Day/Session

- Fill the autoclave reservoir and run the autoclave for a complete cycle.
- Record the sterilization parameters reached in your autoclave logbook.
- Compare these with the manufacturer's recommended parameters.

Before Patient Treatment

- Ensure that all equipment has been sterilized or adequately disinfected (if it cannot be sterilized).
- Put disposable coverings in place where necessary.
- Place only the appropriate instruments on bracket table.
- Set out all materials and other essential instruments.
- Update patient's medical history.

During Patient Treatment

- Treat all patients as potentially infectious.
- Wear gloves, masks and protective eyewear and protective clothing.
- Provide eye protection for patient.
- Wash hands before gloving; a new pair of gloves must be used for each patient.
- Change gloves immediately, if they are torn, cut or punctured. Use rubber dam to isolate where appropriate.
- Use high-volume aspiration.

- Ensure good general ventilation of the treatment area. Handle sharps carefully and only re-sheath needles using a suitable device.

After Patient Treatment

- Dispose of sharps via the sharps' container.
- Segregate and dispose of clinical waste.
- Clean and inspect all instruments to ensure visibly clean before placing in an ultrasonic cleaning machine or washer/disinfect or,
- Sterilize cleaned instruments using an autoclave and store covered. Clean and disinfect all contaminated work surfaces.
- Clean and disinfect impressions and other dental appliances before sending to laboratory. Prepare surgery for next patient.

At the End of Each Session

- Dispose of all clinical waste from the surgery area.
- Clean and disinfect all work surfaces thoroughly.
- Disinfect the aspirator, its tubing and the spittoon.
- Clean the chair and the unit.
- Empty and clean ultrasonic cleaning machine and leave to dry.

At the End of the Day

Drain autoclave chamber and water reservoir to remove all residual water and leave to dry.

PROPHYLAXIS OF VIRAL HEPATITIS

Prophylaxis against hepatitis B is effectively accomplished by using the hepatitis B vaccine. Originally, the vaccine was derived from pooled donor plasma; however, this form is no longer available. Currently, two vaccines are licensed for use and both are produced by recombinant DNA technology. The vaccine is administered in three doses over a 6 months period and results in an effective antibody response in more than 90% of adults and 95% of infants, children, and adolescents. This conversion rate is based upon injections given in the deltoid muscle, since injections administered in the buttocks resulted in only 81% of recipients developing effective antibody liters. Individuals who have received the vaccine in the buttocks should have serologic confirmation of their antibody titer status.

The duration of immunity and the need for booster doses remain somewhat uncertain. The vaccine is intended for use not in mass inoculations but rather in selected target populations who are at high risk for contracting hepatitis B.

Immunoglobulin (Ig), is an antibody, a defensive gamma globulin found in the blood plasma, body secretions, and some leukocyte membranes. Once released by a plasma cell, antibodies render antigens harmless.

Prophylaxis of viral hepatitis is the preferred form of treatment and is accomplished by administering either early post-exposure immune globulins or post-exposure hepatitis B vaccine.

Immune serum globulin (IG) is a pool of antibodies collected from human plasma that is free of HBsAg. This sterile solution contains antibodies against both hepatitis A and hepatitis B.

Another type of IG is called **hepatitis B IG (HBIG)** and is specially prepared from preselected plasma that is high in titers of **anti-HBs.** Administration of both IG and HBIG is safe and is not associated with transmission of the AIDS virus. In hepatitis A, IG given either before exposure or shortly after exposure is effective in preventing clinical infection.

Hepatitis A and E Vaccinations

Hepatitis A infection can be prevented with the hepatitis A vaccine , which is given in two doses, 6–18 months apart. The vaccine is recommended for children in day-care settings, cafeteria workers, and those traveling to areas with a high risk of transmission.

Of adults vaccinated, 94–100% develop antibodies 1 month after the first injection, and 100% of the vaccinated adults develop protective antibodies after the second dose. Hepatitis A vaccine gives life-long immunity. Immune globulin (IG) is given after the first dose to travelers who plan to travel in less than 1 month after the first dose of the vaccine. There is no vaccine for hepatitis E.

If a vaccinated individual sustains a needle stick or puncture wound contaminated with blood from a patient known to be HBsAg positive, it is recommended that the vaccinated individual be tested for an adequate titer of anti-HBs, if unknown, and, if levels are inadequate, immediately receive an injection of HBIG and a vaccine booster dose. If the antibody titer is adequate, nothing further is required. If an unvaccinated individual sustains an inadvertent percutaneous or permucosal exposure to hepatitis B immediate administration of HBIG and initiation of the vaccine are recommended.

A question also arises concerning dentists who are carriers of HBsAg. As of this writing, there have been nine reported outbreaks since 1974 of hepatitis B traceable to carrier dentists or oral surgeons. In each instance, the practitioner was found to be seropositive for HBsAg **did not use gloves during dental or surgical procedures.** None of the practitioners was aware of his chronic infections. Two patients have died as a result of these infections. It is interesting to note that almost all these reported outbreaks occurred before the increased awareness of transmission of blood-borne pathogens took place in the late 1980s.

Hepatitis B Vaccine

The hepatitis B virus has the most serious risk of transmission for unvaccinated dentists, their staffs, and their patients. It is usually transmitted by the introduction of infected blood into the bloodstream of a susceptible person; however, infected individuals may also secrete large amounts of the virus in their saliva, which can enter an individual through any moist mucosal surface or epithelial (skin or mucosal) wound. Minute quantities of the virus have been found capable of transmitting disease (only 10^5 to 10^7 virions/mL of blood).

Transmission can occur by inoculation or inhalation. The following recommendations should be followed:

1. Universal precautions: A standard cross-infection control policy for all patients. This is advisable because it may not be possible to distinguish the healthy carrier. Also, an effective policy will decrease the risks to the dentist and his staff, as well as being a practice-builder.
2. Carriers of blood-borne viruses (hepatitis, HIV) can be treated in general dental practice, provided routine procedures are implemented vigorously.
3. Patients with manifestations of immunosuppression should be referred for specialist hospital care.
4. All staff should be trained in cross-infection control and every practice must have a written infection control policy.

PRACTICE INFECTION CONTROL POLICY

Infection control is of prime importance in dental practice. It is essential to the safety of dentists, their patients, and their families. Every member of staff will receive training in all aspects of infection control, including decontamination of dental instruments and equipment, and the following policy must be adhered to at all times. If there is any aspect that is not clear, please ask.

You might not be the only person who is unclear and it is useful to discuss the policy frequently to ensure that all dentists understand its implications. Remember, any of your patients might ask you about the policy, so make sure you understand it.

1. All staff must be immunized against hepatitis B and record of their hepatitis B seroconversion held by the practice owner. For those who do not

seroconvert, or cannot be immunized, medical advice and counseling will be sought. In these cases, it may be necessary to restrict their clinical activities.

2. The practice provides protective clothing, gloves, eyewear and masks that must be worn by dentists and assistant during all operative procedures. Protective clothing worn in the surgery should not be worn outside the practice premises.

3. Before donning gloves, hands must be washed. Using any glove that becomes damaged must be replaced and a new pair of gloves must be used for each patient.

4. Before sterilization, reusable instruments should be cleaned either by placing in ultrasonic cleaner or washer/disinfector or by washing in a designated area by hand under water using a long-handled brush. Inspect instruments for residual debris and reclean, if necessary. Instruments are then rinsed under running water before being sterilized using an autoclave. Heavy-duty gloves and eye protection must be worn when handling and cleaning used instruments. All instruments that have been potentially contaminated must be sterilized. Single-use items must not be decontaminated and reused.

5. Sterilized instruments should be stored in covered trays/pouches.

6. Working areas that have instruments placed on them during treatment will be kept to a minimum, clearly identified and, after each patient, cleaned with (detergent) and disinfected using.

7. Needles should be resheathed only using the resheathing device provided. Needles, scalpel blades, LA cartridges, burs, matrix bands, etc. shall be disposed of in the yellow sharps container. This must never be more than two-thirds full.

8. All clinical wastes must be placed in the appropriate sacks or bins provided in each surgery. The sack must be securely fastened when three-quarters full and stored in the designated area.

9. All dental impressions must be rinsed until visibly clean and disinfected using (as recommended by the manufacturer) and labeled as 'disinfected' before being sent to the laboratory. Technical work being returned to the laboratory should also be disinfected and labeled.

10. In the event of an inoculation injury, the wound should be allowed to bleed, washed thoroughly under running water and covered with a waterproof dressing. The incident should be immediately discussed with to assess whether further action is needed. Advice on post-exposure prophylaxis can be obtained from record the incident in the accident book.

11. Any spillages involving blood or saliva or mercury will be reported.

12. Anyone developing a reaction to protective gloves or a chemical must inform immediately.

In addition to preventing patient-to-patient spread, the dentist and staff also need to take precautions to protect themselves from contamination, because several instances have occurred in which dentists have been the primary source of a hepatitis B epidemic (Box 5.4).

Members of the dental staff should receive hepatitis B vaccinations, which have been shown to reduce an individual's susceptibility to hepatitis B infection effectively, although the longevity of protection has not been definitively determined.

Office-cleaning personnel and commercial laboratory technicians can be protected by proper segregation and labeling of contaminated objects and by proper disposal of sharp objects. Recognition of

Box 5.4: Methods designed to limit the spread to hepatitis viruses

From infected patient to other patients
- Use disposable materials.
- Disinfect surfaces.
  - A. With halogen compounds
    1. Iodophores.
    2. Hypochlorite (bleach).
  - B. With aldehydes.
    1. Formaldehyde.
    2. Glutraldehyde.
- Sterilize reusable instruments.
  - A. With heat.
  - B. With ethylene oxide gas.
- Use disposable materials

From infected patient to dental staff
- Learn to recognize individuals likely to be carriers.
- Use barrier techniques (gloves, facemasks, eye protection) during surgery when handling contaminated instruments.
- Promptly dispose sharp instruments into well-labeled protective containers. Dispose needles immediately after use or resheathing in-use instruments. Use an instrument to place a scalpel blade on take one off a blade handle. Administer hepatitis V vaccine.

all individuals known to be carriers of hepatitis B and C would aid in knowing when special precautions were necessary.

Two single antigen-hepatitis B vaccines are licensed in a number of countries for persons of any age. The vaccine is given in three doses at 0,1, and 6 months. The second dose is given 1 month after the first dose and the third is given 5 months after the second dose. If the series is interrupted after the first dose, the second dose should be given immediately. The third dose should be given at least 2 months after the second. A delayed third dose should be given immediately.

When the vaccine is given according to the protocol of 0, 1, and 6 months, 30–50% protection occurs after the first dose. 50–75% protection occurs after the second dose and 90% protection occurs after the third dose.

HIV patients may need several more shots, beyond the routine three, to gain immunity. Individuals who do not respond to the primary vaccine series may have to complete a second three-dose series and be tested subsequent to that.

All clinical staff should be vaccinated against the common illnesses. All those involved in clinical procedures must be vaccinated against hepatitis B. If an inoculation injury is sustained before completion of the course, follow-up action, including boosters and tests for hepatitis B markers, is essential. The hepatitis B vaccine is effective in preventing infection in individuals who produce specific antibodies to the hepatitis B surface antigen (anti-HBs). UK experts recommend that anti-HBs level of >100 mIU/ml will provide protection against hepatitis B infection. It is now clear that immunological memory is produced in those who respond to the primary course of the vaccine (>100 mIU/ml).

Protection against infection is maintained, even if antibody concentrations at the time of exposure have declined. Anti-HBs levels must be measured 2–4 months after completion of the immunization course.

A single booster dose 5 years after completion of the primary course is recommended for all healthcare workers who have contact with blood, blood-stained fluids and patients' tissues. Pre- and post-testing at the time of a booster is not required, if the individual responded to the primary course of the vaccine.

Not everyone will respond to the vaccine, however, some because they are true non-responders, others because they carry the virus. Those who fail to respond should undergo further investigation to establish, if test markers of hepatitis B infection are present. Investigation to establish infection should take place before booster doses of the vaccine are given in an attempt to achieve anti-HBs levels of at least 100 mIU/ml. True vaccine non-responders may remain susceptible to infection and it is essential that inoculation injuries be followed up with tests for hepatitis B markers where appropriate.

Hepatitis B Postvaccination Testing

Testing for antibody response is not indicated after completion of the injections at 0, 1 and 6 months. Post-vaccination testing after completion of the routine series or interrupted series may be indicated in the following:

1. *Healthcare workers (HCW):* HCW coming in close contact with blood or body fluids may be tested 1–2 months after the last dose.

2. *Chronic hemodialysis patients:* Chronic hemodialysis patients may be tested 1–2 months after the last dose.

3. *Sex partners of hepatitis B-infected persons:* Sex partners of hepatitis B-infected persons may be tested 1–2 months after the last dose.

4. *Infants born to hepatitis B-infected mothers:* Infants born to hepatitis B-infected mothers may be tested at 9–15 months of age.

Hepatitis B infection in pregnant women may result in severe disease for the mother and chronic infection in the newborn. Although infants can receive active/passive immunization at birth, vaccination should not be withheld from a pregnant woman, if she is likely to be at risk from contracting hepatitis B infection. Many women have discovered at a later date that, at the time of receiving the vaccine, they were pregnant. In these instances, the vaccine caused no harm to themselves or their children. The vaccine also does not affect fertility and does not prevent breastfeeding.

6

Kidneys

- Anatomy
- Physiology (Glomerular Filtration)
- Chronic Renal Failure
  - Renal Dialysis
  - Dental Management of Chronic Renal Failure
  - Renal Transplant

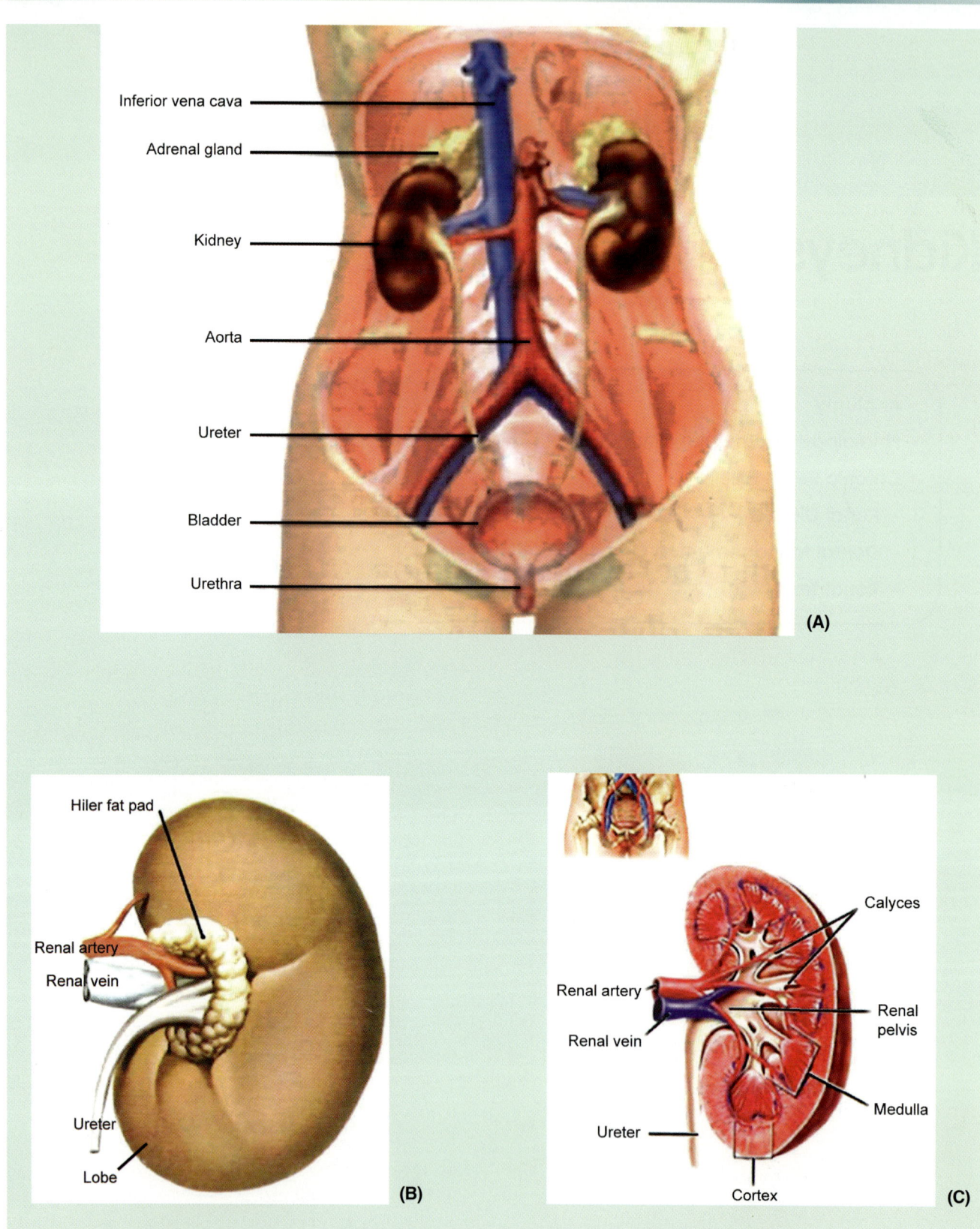

Plate VI: The urinary system, frontal view (**A** and **B**) and section (**C**) showing gross anatomy of the kidney

ANATOMY

The gross anatomy of the kidney is illustrated in Plate VI-A and B. The kidneys lie against the posterior abdominal wall at the level of vertebrae T12 to L3. The right kidney is slightly lower than the left because of the space occupied by the liver above it (Plate VI-A). Each kidney weighs about 160 g and measures about 12 cm long, 5 cm wide, and 2.5 cm thick– about the size of a bar of bath soap. The lateral surface is convex while the medial surface is concave and has a slit, the hilum, where it receives the renal nerves, blood vessels, lymphatic vessels, and ureter (Fig. 6.1).

The left adrenal gland rests on the superior pole of that kidney, while the right adrenal gland is more medial, between the hilum and pole. The kidneys, adrenal glands, ureters, and urinary bladder are retroperitoneal– they lie between the peritoneum and body wall. The urinary system consists of six organs: two kidneys, two ureters, the urinary bladder, and the urethra.

Functions of the Kidneys

The kidneys play vital role in the maintenance of normal body fluid volumes and in the composition of the extracellular fluid components. Although the adult kidney weighs approximately 150 g with both kidneys accounting for only 0.5% of the total body weight, yet they receive almost 25% of the cardiac output. Nearly one-quarter of the blood volume perfuses the kidneys each minute. There are normally more than 2 million

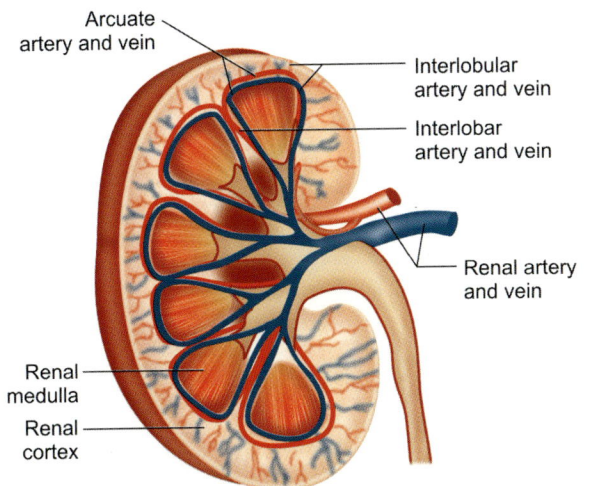

Fig. 6.1: Renal circulation. The larger blood vessels of the kidney

functioning nephron that regulate total body water and solute concentrations.

The kidney performs numerous essential functions:

1. Excretion of metabolic waste products, drugs and hormones. Metabolism constantly produces a variety of waste products that can poison the body, if not eliminated. The most fundamental role of the kidneys is to eliminate these wastes.

2. Regulating the acid-base balance.

3. Monitoring body concentrations of water and sodium. Homeostatically regulate the volume and composition of the body fluids.

4. The kidneys act as endocrine organs for the synthesis of hydroxycholecalciferol (active vitamin D), erythropoietin, renin and prostaglandins, and are target organs for parathyroid hormone and aldosterone.

All of the following processes are aspects of kidney function:

- They filter blood plasma, separate wastes from the useful chemicals, i.e. filtering small molecules and ions from the blood and eliminate these wastes while returning the rest to the bloodstream.

- They regulate blood volume and pressure by eliminating or conserving water as necessary.

- They regulate the osmolarity of the body fluids by controlling the relative amounts of water and solutes eliminated. They secrete the enzyme renin, which activates hormonal mechanisms that control blood pressure and electrolyte balance.

- They secrete the hormone *erythropoietin*, which controls the red blood cell count and oxygen-carrying capacity of the blood.

- They function with the lungs to regulate the PCO_2 and acid-base balance of the body fluids.

- They contribute to calcium homeostasis through their role in synthesizing calcitriol (vitamin D).

- They detoxify free radicals and drugs with the use of peroxisomes.

In times of starvation, they carry out gluconeogenesis; they deaminate amino acids (remove the –NH_2 group), excrete the amino group as ammonia (NH_3) and synthesize glucose from the rest of the molecule.

PHYSIOLOGY (Glomerular Filtration)

It is a process in which water and some solutes in the blood plasma pass from the capillaries of the glomerulus into the capsular space of the nephron (Fig. 6.2). The nephron consists of a: Bowman's capsule and glomerulus. The glomerulus is a capillary network within the Bowman's capsule. Blood leaving the glomerulus passes into a second capillary network, proximal convoluted tubule. This, by active transport, reabsorbs all the glucose, and amino acids, and most of the uric acid and inorganic salts. The active transport of Na^+ out of the proximal tubule is controlled by angiotensin 2.

The active transport of phosphate $(PO_4)_2$ is regulated (suppressed by) the parathyroid hormone. As these solutes are removed, a large volume of the water follows them by osmosis loop of Henle. Here water continues to leave by osmosis because the interstitial fluid is very hypertonic from the active transport of Na^+ out of the tubular fluid distal convoluted tubule. Here more Na^+ is reclaimed by active transport, and still more water follows by osmosis collecting tubule.

Here there is a final adjustment of the Na^+ and water content of the body, and the surplus or waste molecules and ions are left to flow out as urine, which passes to the pelvis of the kidney, from where it flows to the bladder and periodically, onto the outside.

URINE AND RENAL FUNCTION TEST

I. Urine Analysis

Urine analysis—physical and microscopic examination are of value. Concerning the kidneys, no two fluids are as valuable for this purpose as blood and urine. Urinalysis, the examination of the physical and chemical properties of urine is, therefore, one of the most routine procedures in medical examinations. The principal characteristics of urine and certain tests used to evaluate renal function are described here.

Composite and Properties of Urine (Table 6.1)

The basic composition and properties of urine are as follows.

Appearance: Urine varies from almost colorless to deep amber, depending on the body's state of hydration. The yellow color of urine is due to **urochrome,** a pigment produced by the breakdown of hemoglobin from expired erythrocytes. Pink, green, brown, black, and other colors result from certain foods, vitamins, drugs, and metabolic diseases. Urine is normally clear but turns cloudy upon standing because of bacterial growth.

Pus in the urine **(pyuria)** makes it cloudy and suggests kidney infection. Blood in the urine (hematuria) may be due to a urinary tract infection,

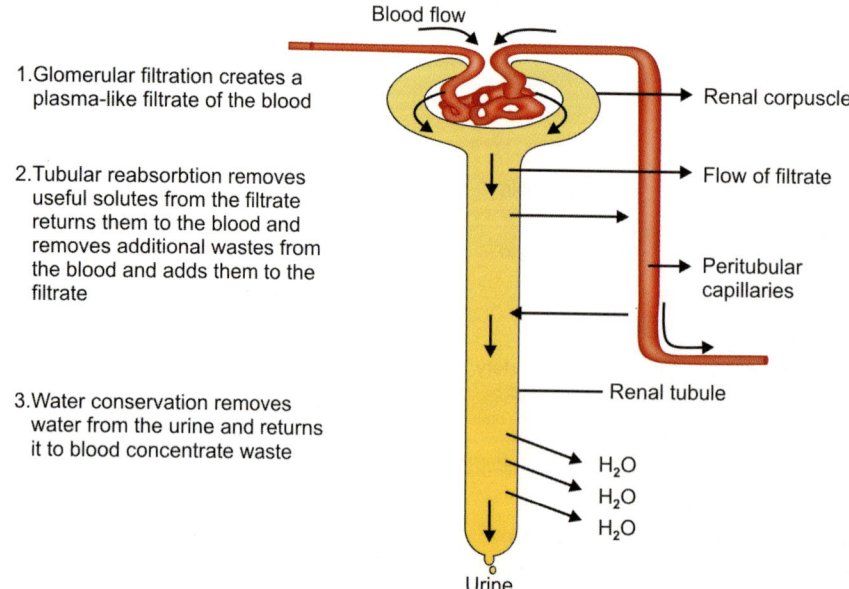

1. Glomerular filtration creates a plasma-like filtrate of the blood

2. Tubular reabsorbtion removes useful solutes from the filtrate returns them to the blood and removes additional wastes from the blood and adds them to the filtrate

3. Water conservation removes water from the urine and returns it to blood concentrate waste

Blood flow

Renal corpuscle

Flow of filtrate

Peritubular capillaries

Renal tubule

H_2O
H_2O
H_2O

Urine

Fig. 6.2: Basic steps in the formation of urine *(Saladin, 2003)*

trauma, or kidney stones. Cloudiness or blood in a urine specimen sometimes, however, simply indicates contamination with semen or menstrual fluid.

Odor: Fresh urine has a distinctive but not repellent odor. As it stands, however, bacteria multiply, degrade urea to ammonia, and produce the pungent odor typical of stale wet diapers. Asparagus and other foods can impart distinctive aromas to the urine. Diabetes mellitus gives it a sweet, "fruity" odor of acetone. A "mousy" odor suggests phenylketonuria (PKU), and a "rotten" odor may indicate urinary tract infection.

Specific gravity: This is a ratio of the density (g/mL) of a substance to the density of distilled water. Distilled water has a specific gravity of 1.000, and urine ranges from 1.001 when it is very dilute to 1.028 when it is very concentrated. Multiplying the last two digits of the specific gravity by a proportionality constant of 2.6 gives an estimate of the grams of solid matter per liter of urine. For example, a specific gravity of 1.025 indicates a solute concentration of 25 × 2.6 = 65 g/L.

Osmolarity: Urine can have an osmolarity as low as 50 mosm/L in a very hydrated person or as high as 1,200 mosm/L in a dehydrated person. Compared with the osmolarity of blood (300 mOsm/L), then, urine can be either hypotonic or hypertonic under different conditions.

pH: The pH of urine ranges from 4.5 to 8.2 but is usually about 6.0 (mildly acidic).

Chemical composition: Urine averages 95% water and 5% solutes by volume. Normally, the most abundant solute is urea, followed by sodium chloride, potassium chloride, and lesser amounts of creatinine, uric acid, phosphates, sulfates, and traces of calcium, magnesium, and sometimes bicarbonate (Table 6.1).

Urine contains a trace of bilirubin from the breakdown of hemoglobin and related products, and urobilin, a brown oxidized derivative of bilirubin. It is abnormal to find glucose, free hemoglobin, albumin, ketones, or more than a trace of bile pigments in the urine; their presence is sometimes an indicator of disease.

Urine volume: An average adult produces 1 to 2 L of urine per day. An output in excess of 2 L/day is called diuresis or **polyuria**[1]. Fluid intake and some drugs can temporarily increase output to as much as 20 L/day. Chronic diseases such as diabetes can do

Table 6.1: Properties and composition of urine

Physical properties		
Specific gravity	1.001–1.028	
Osmolarity	50–1. 200 mosm/L	
pH	6.0 (range 4.5–8.2)	
Solute	Concentration	Output (g/day)*
Inorganic ions		
Chloride	533 mg/dL	6.4 g/day
Sodium	333 mg/dL	4.0 g/day
Potassium	166 mg/dL	2.0 g/day
Phosphate	83 mg/dL	1 g/day
Ammonia	60 mg/dL	0.68 g/day
Calcium	17 mg/dL	0.2 g/day
Magnesium	13 mg/dL	0.1 6 g/day
Nitrogenous waste		
Urea	1.8 g/dL	21 g/day
Creatinine	150 mg/dL	1.8 g/day
Uric acid	40 mg/dL	0.5 g/day
Urobilin	125 µg/dL	1.52 mg/day
Bilirubin	20 µg/dL	0.24 mg/day
Other organics		
Amino acids	288 µg/dL	3.5 mg/day
Ketones	17 µg/dL	0.21 mg/day
Carbohydrates	9 µg/dL	0.11 mg/day
Lipids	1.6 µg/dL	0.02 mg/day

Typical values for a reference male.

* Assuming a urine output of 1.2 L/day

so over a long term. **Oliguria**[2] is an output of less than 500 mL/day, and **anuria**[3] 1 is an output of 0 to 100 mL/day. Low output can result from kidney disease, dehydration, circulatory shock, prostate enlargement, and other causes. If urine output drops to less than 400 mL/day, the body cannot maintain a safe, low concentration of wastes in the blood plasma. The result is azotemia.

Diuretics: Diuretics are chemicals that increase urine volume. They are used for treating hypertension and congestive heart failure because they reduce the body's fluid volume and blood pressure. Diuretics work by one of two mechanisms—increasing glomerular filtration or reducing tubular reabsorption. For example, caffeine, in the former category, dilates the afferent arteriole and increases glomerular filtration rate (GFR). Alcohol, in the latter category, inhibits antidiuretic hormone (ADH) secretion. Also in the latter category are many osmotic diuretics, which reduce water reabsorption by increasing the

---

1. *Poly = many, much;* 2. *Oligo = few, a little;* 3. *An = without*

osmolarity of the tubular fluid. Many diuretic drugs, such as furosemide (Lasix), produce osmotic dieresis by inhibiting sodium reabsorption.

II. Renal Function Tests

"Renal profile-blood urea nitrogen, serum creatinine, serum electrolytes".

Creatine clearance test: The glomerular filtration rate (GFR) is calculated from creatinine clearance, i.e. plasma creatine levels. In healthy, the normal level is $120/$ ml/min/1.73 m^2 for women and $130/$ml/ min/ 1.73 m^2 for men.

RENAL INSUFFICIENCY

Renal insufficiency is a state in which the kidneys cannot maintain homeostasis due to extensive destruction of their nephrons. Some causes of nephron destruction include:

- Chronic or repetitive kidney infections.
- Trauma from such causes as blows to the lower back or continual vibration from machinery.
- Prolonged ischemia and hypoxia, as in some long-distance runners and swimmers.
- Poisoning by heavy metals such as mercury and lead and solvents such as carbon tetrachloride, acetone, and paint thinners. These are absorbed into the blood from inhaled fumes or by skin contact and then filtered by the glomeruli. They kill renal tubule cells.
- Blockage of renal tubules with proteins small enough to be filtered by the glomerulus–for example, myoglobin released by skeletal muscle damage and hemoglobin released by a transfusion reaction.

- Atherosclerosis, which reduces blood flow to the kidney.
- Glomerulonephritis, an autoimmune disease of the glomerular capillaries. Nephrons can regenerate and restore kidney function after short-term injuries. Even when some of the nephrons are irreversibly destroyed, others hypertrophy and compensate for their lost function. Indeed, a person can survive on as little as one-third of one kidney. When 75% of the nephrons are lost, however, urine output may be as low as 30 mL/hr compared with the normal rate of 50 to 60 mL/hr. This is insufficient to maintain homeostasis and is accompanied by azotemia and acidosis. Uremia develops when there is 90% loss of renal function. Renal insufficiency also tends to cause anemia because the diseased kidney produces too little erythropoietin (EPO), the hormone that stimulates red blood cell formation.

CHRONIC RENAL FAILURE

Twenty-five percent of the circulating blood perfuses the kidney each minute. Ultrafiltrate, the precursor of urine, is produced at a rate of about 125 mL/min in the nephrons.

Early stage renal disease (ESRD) manifests when 50 to 74% of the 2 million nephrons lose function.

The nephron includes the glomerulous, tubules, and vasculature. Various diseases affect different segments of the nephron at first, but the entire nephron eventually is affected (Fig. 6.3). For example, hypertension affects the vasculature first, whereas glomerulonephritis first affects the glomeruli.

The early phase of end-stage renal disease (ESRD) is usually asymptomatic, where there is sudden extreme reduction in glomerular filtration rate. There is decreased ability of the kidney to perform its excretory, endocrine, and metabolic functions beyond compensatory mechanisms. This stage is called *renal insufficiency* or acute renal failure. If the reduction in renal effusion is untreated more than a few hours, irreversible tubular necrosis will occur and the disease then progresses to a frank renal failure or *end-stage renal failure.*

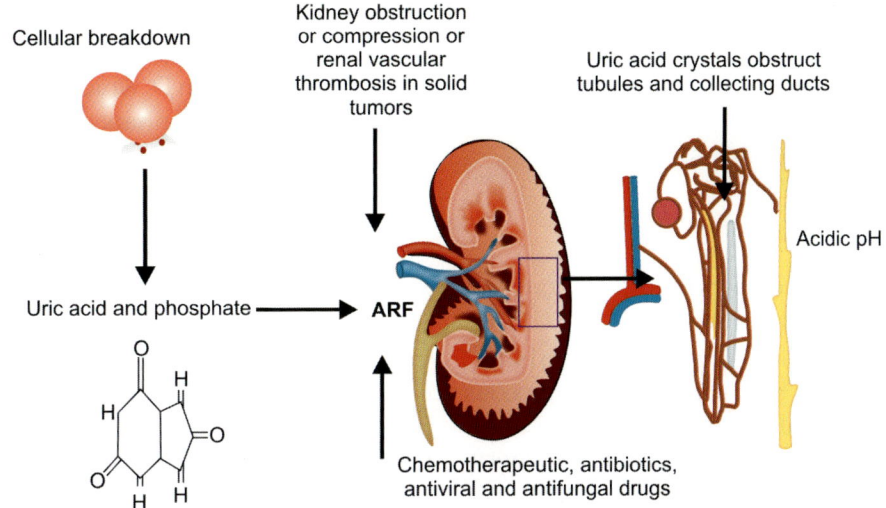

Cellular breakdown

Kidney obstruction or compression or renal vascular thrombosis in solid tumors

Uric acid crystals obstruct tubules and collecting ducts

Acidic pH

Uric acid and phosphate → **ARF**

Chemotherapeutic, antibiotics, antiviral and antifungal drugs

Fig. 6.3: Various diseases affect different segments of the nephron

The end-stage renal disease is a bilateral progressive, and chronic deterioration of nephrons that results in uremia and ultimately leads to death. The most common known causes of ESRD are diabetes mellitus, hypertension, chronic glomerulonephritis, polycystic kidney disease, and systemic lupus erythematosus. Renal failure results in a syndrome known as uremia. Uremia has adverse influences on the cardiovascular, gastrointestinal, neuromuscular, skeletal, hematologic and dermatologic systems. The common sequelae of uremia include anemia, bleeding problems, hypertension, electrolyte and fluid imbalance, and altered drug metabolism.

Clinical Features of Chronic Renal Failure

Clinical features of chronic renal failure are described in Box 6.1.

Laboratory Findings of Chronic Renal Failure

Laboratory findings of chronic renal failure are discussed in Table 6.2.

Oral Complications of Chronic Renal Failure

1. Xerostomia (dry mouth) decreased salivary flow usually develops due to the restricted fluid intake necessitated by decreased urinary output.
2. Caries prevalence.
3. Parotid gland infection: The gingiva looks pale, poorly defined and not well demarcated from the vestibular mucosa. This could be attributed to anemia resulting from decreased erythropoietin production by the diseased kidney with consequent diminished red cell production and anemia. Necrotizing ulcerative gingivitis (NUG)

Box 6.1: Clinical features of chronic renal failure

1. *Metabolic*
   - Nocturia and polyuria
   - Thirst
   - Raised serum urea, creatine, lipids and uric acid
   - Glycosuria
   - Electrolyte disturbance
   - Secondary hyperparathyroidism
2. *Cardiovascular*
   - Hypertension
   - Congestive heart failure
   - Pericarditis
   - Cardiomyopathy
   - Atheroma
3. *Gastrointestinal*
   - Anorexia
   - Nausea and vomiting
   - Hiccup
   - Peptic ulcer and gastrointestinal bleeding
4. *Neuromuscular*
   - Weakness and lassitude
   - Drowsiness leading to coma
   - Headaches
   - Disturbances of vision
   - Tremor
5. *Dermatological*
   - Pruritus
   - Bruising
   - Hyperpigmentation
6. *Hematological*
   - Bleeding
   - Anemia
   - Lymphopenia
7. *Immunological*

Table 6.2: Laboratory findings of chronic renal failure

Urea	Raised
Creatine	Raised
Potassium	Raised
Phosphate	Raised
Calcium	Low
Hemoglobin	Low

and periodontitis have been found in increased prevalence in these patients.

4. The development of submucosal bruising, petechiae, ecchymosis, hematoma and spontaneous gingival bleeding following injection of local anesthesia, oral surgery or periodontal surgery. These abnormal reactions develop due to the reduced platelet count and adhesiveness and capillary fragility commonly encountered in uremic patients.
5. Calcified extraction wounds (socket sclerosis).
6. Edema secondary to decreased osmotic pressure from loss of protein may be observed.
7. Fungal infections. Candidiasis is more frequent when salivary flow is diminished. Soft, white slightly elevated plaques are seen in the buccal mucosa, gingiva, floor of the mouth, and palate. The plaques can usually wiped away with a gauze leaving either a normal or erythematous area.
8. Loosening, drifting and even loss of teeth.
9. Enlarged tongue with abnormal metallic taste sensation.
10. Halitosis
11. Enamel hypoplasia, brownish discoloration or staining of teeth and altered eruption of teeth.

Bone Osteodystrophy

Bone osteodystrophy is a term used to describe a variety of bone changes occurring in the bone secondary to chronic renal failure and chronic hemodialysis. With decreasing nephron function, there is decreased glomerular filtration, which results in an increased level of serum phosphate. Because phosphate is the driving force of bone mineralization, the excess phosphate tends to cause serum calcium to be deposited in bone, leading to a decreased serum calcium level. In response to low serum calcium, the parathyroid glands are stimulated to secrete parathormone(PTH), which results in a secondary hyperparathyroidism.

The parathormone (PTH): (1) inhibits the tubular reabsorption of phosphate; (2) stimulates the renal production of vitamin D, which is necessary for calcium metabolism; and(3) enhances vitamin D absorption from the intestine. However, an additional defect in ESRD is the inability of that failing kidney to synthesize 1,25-dihydroxycholecalciferol, the active metabolite of vitamin. As a result, there is decreased intestinal absorption of calcium and a sustained high level of secretion of PTH. PTH, tumor necrosis factor, and interleukin 1 activate bone remodeling and mobilize calcium from the bones and promote the excretion of phosphate. This leads to osteomalacia (increased unmineralized bone matrix), osteitis fibrosa (bone resorption lytic lesions and marrow fibrosis), and osteosclerosis (enhanced bone density) in varying degrees, as well as to impaired bone growth in children.

With renal osteodystrophy, there is also a tendency for spontaneous fractures with slow healing, myopathy, aseptic necrosis of the hip, and extraosseous calcifications. Concerning the jaw bones, a triad of radiographic features occurs. This triad includes: total or partial loss of lamina dura, demineralization of bone, and localized radiolucent lesions. This triad appears most frequently in the mandibular molar region superior to the mandibular canal.

- Loss of lamina dura is a pathognomonic sign of hyperparathyroidism.
- Alternations in normal trabecular pattern and generalized mineralization of the jaws and other bones have been described by different terms as 'ground glass', 'granular', 'chalky', 'salt and pepper', 'pepper pot skull', and 'peau d'orange' (Fig. 6.4). Hyperparathyroidism secondary to chronic renal failure is associated with loss of cortical bone outlining the hard palate, sinuses, nose and orbits. Widened irregular nutrient canal is commonly seen in these cases.

Late in the course of hyperparathyroidism, circumscribed radiolucencies, or cyst-like lesions is a dominant radiographic manifestation in the jaw and other bones. This radiolucent lesion is known as brown tumor, osteitis fibrosa systica, tumor of hyperparathyroidism, and von Recklinghausen's disease of bone. Brown tumor represents foci of bone rarefaction filled with hemorrhage and granulation tissue with accumulation of macrophages and giant cells, making this lesion histologically distinguishable from giant cell granuloma.

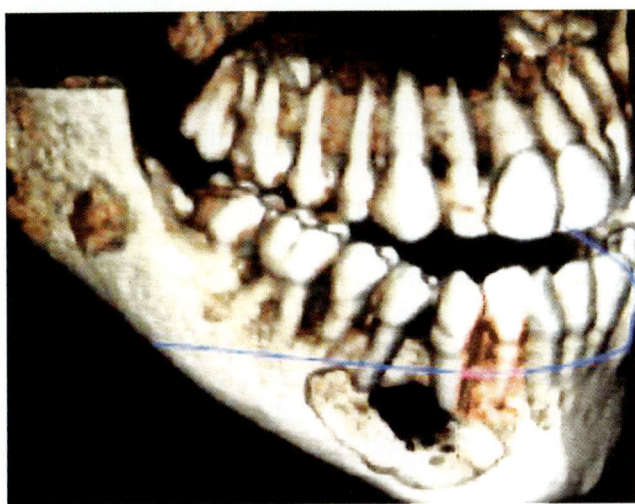

Fig. 6.4: Osteodystrophy secondary to chronic renal failure. The figure reveals generalized demineralization of the jaws, loss of lamina dura, localized radiolucent lesions and the bone appears as ground glass, chalky, and granular and mutiple radiolucent lesions

Temporomandibular joint may also be affected by bone abnormalities in cases of osteodystrophy. TMJ changes include decreased bone density, subcortical osteolysis, irregularities of the contour of the articular surfaces and glenoid fossa. The patient complains of joint pain due to the development of 'erosive arthritis'. Complete resorption of the condyle with resultant acquired maxillofacial deformity has been reported.

As the disease progresses, conservative medical management becomes inadequate, and either artificial filtration of the blood by dialysis or transplantation of a kidney is required.

RENAL DIALYSIS

Dialysis is the separation of some solute particles from others by diffusion through a selectively permeable membrane, **Hemodialysis.** Is the process of separating wastes from the bloodstream and sometimes adding other substances to it (such as drugs and nutrients) by circulating the blood through a machine with a selectively permeable membrane, used to treat cases of renal or hepatic insufficiency.

Dialysis is a procedure for artificially clearing wastes from the blood when the kidneys are not adequately doing so, dialysis is a medical procedure that artificially filters the blood.

The procedure can be accomplished by either hemodialysis or peritoneal dialysis.

Hemodialysis (Fig. 6.5)

Blood is pumped from the radial artery to a dialysis machine (artificial kidney) and returned to the patient

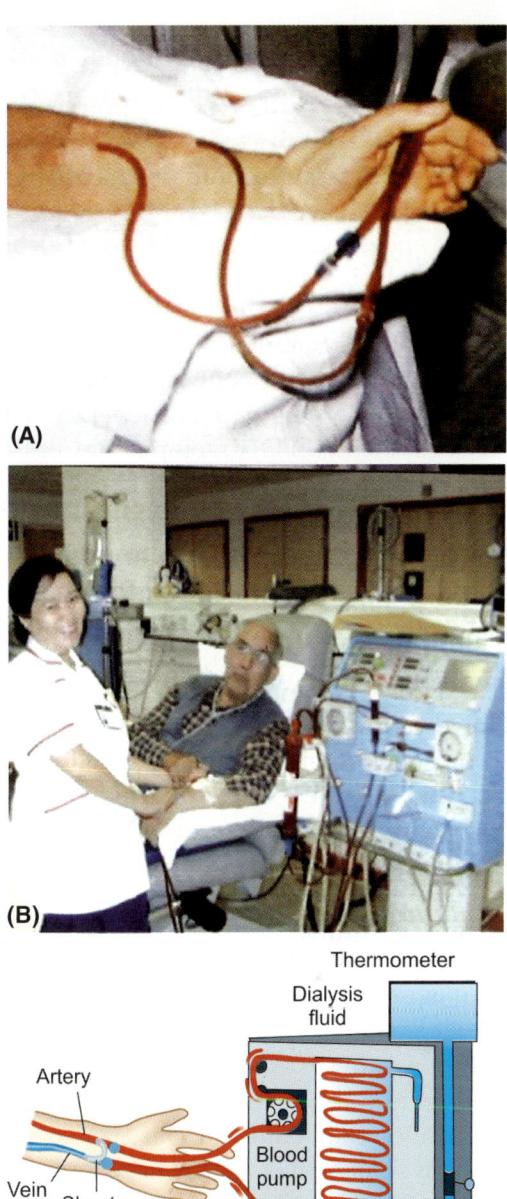

Fig. 6.5: Hemodialysis. **(A)** Vascular access for long-term hemodialysis is usually provided through a surgically created arteriovenous fistula. Blood leaves the patient through the distal needle to pass through the dialyzer before returning to the patient through the proximal needle. Patients usually become adapt at inserting their own needles. **(B** and **C)** Blood is pumped into a dialysis chamber, where it flows through selectively permeable dialysis tubing surrounded by dialysis fluid. Blood leaving the chamber passes through a bubble trap to remove air before it is returned to the patient's body. The dialysis fluid picks up excess water and metabolic wastes from the patient's blood and may contain medications that diffuse into the blood

by way of a vein. In the dialysis machine, the blood flows through a semipermeable cellophane tube surrounded by dialysis fluid. Urea, potassium, and other solutes that are more concentrated in the blood than in the dialysis fluid diffuse through the membrane into the fluid, which is discarded. Glucose, electrolytes, and drugs can be administered by adding them to the dialysis fluid so they will diffuse through the membrane into the blood. People with renal insufficiency also accumulate substantial amounts of body water between treatments, and dialysis serves also to remove this excess water. Patients are typically given erythropoietin (EPO) to compensate for the lack of EPO from the failing kidneys.

The technique requires the surgical creation of a permanent arteriovenous fistula (shunt), usually at the wrist, that is readily accessible to cannulation with a large-gauge needle. The surgically created AV shunt (radial artery to cephalic vein) facilitate arterial and venous cannulation during dialysis runs. The patient is 'plugged in' to the hemodialysis machine at the fistula site, and blood is passed through the machine, filtered, and returned to the patient. Heparin is administered during the procedure to prevent clotting and keep both the infusion lines and the dialysis machine tubing patent. The arm containing the arteriovenous shunt should be protected from application of the blood pressure cuff or the introduction of intravenous medications. As inflated blood pressure cuff or tourniquet could collapse the shunt and render it non-useful. Likewise, the complication of phlebitis from IV medications could produce a clot that could jeopardize the shunt.

Hemodialysis patients typically have three sessions per week for 4 to 8 hours per session. Hemodialysis is carried out at home or as an outpatient. In addition to inconvenience, hemodialysis carries risks of infection and thrombosis. Blood tends to clot when exposed to foreign surfaces, so an anticoagulant such as **heparin** is added during dialysis. Unfortunately, this inhibits clotting in the patient's body as well, and dialysis patients sometimes suffer internal bleeding.

Arteriovenous fistula: An artery and a vein are joined together through an anastomosis using the patient's own vasculature, and it takes an average of about 4–6 weeks for the fistula to mature. Fistulas are usually created in the arm and it is extremely important for the patient not to use that arm for blood pressure monitoring or IV/IM injections.

Peritoneal Dialysis

A procedure called *continuous ambulatory peritoneal dialysis* (CAPD) is more convenient (Fig. 6.6). It can be carried out at home by the patient, who is provided with plastic bags of dialysis fluid.

Fluid is introduced into the abdominal cavity through an indwelling catheter. Here, the peritoneum provides over 2 m² of blood-rich semipermeable membrane. The fluid is left in the body cavity for 15 to 60 minutes to allow the blood to equilibrate with it; then it is drained, discarded, and replaced with fresh dialysis fluid. The patient is not limited by a stationary dialysis machine and can go about most normal activities. CAPD is less expensive and promotes better morale than conventional hemodialysis, but it is less efficient in removing wastes and it is more often complicated by infection.

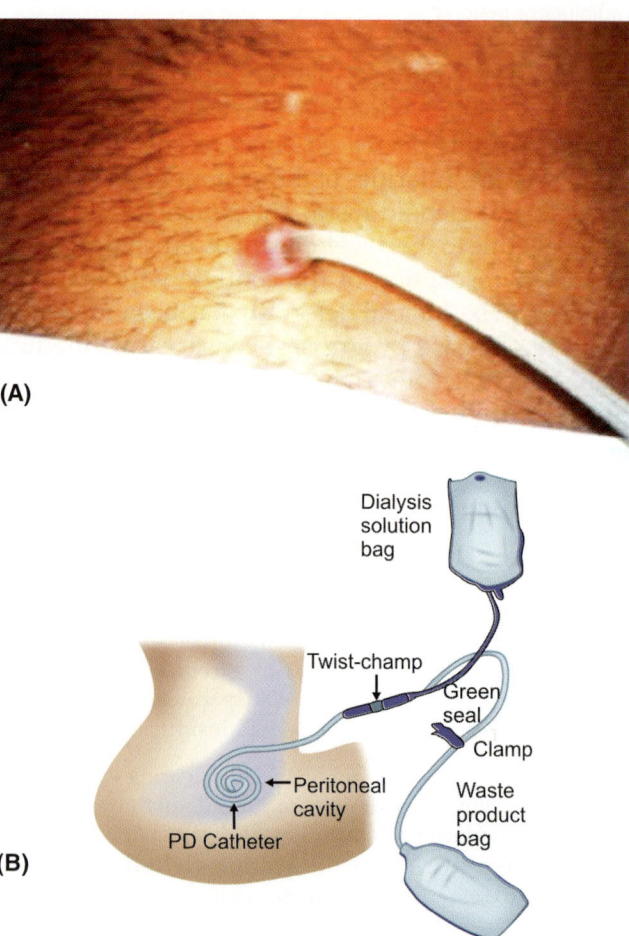

(A)

(B)

Fig. 6.6: Chronic ambulatory peritoneal dialysis catheter in the abdominal wall A and B, *(Lewis SM, Heitkemper MM, Dirksen SR: Medical Surgical Nursing, 6 ed, Louis Mosby)*

It is a slower procedure than hemodialysis and is less often used especially on long-term basis. It is helpful as acute therapy, such as in cases of acute renal failure, patients requiring only occasional dialysis, or with suddenly discovered advanced chronic renal failure. It is accomplished by inserting a catheter through the abdominal wall into the peritoneum and installing the dialysis fluid. This allows the solutes to diffuse from peritoneal capillaries to the dialysis fluid in the peritoneal cavity. After a short time, the fluid is then drained from the cavity through the catheter. Many of the precautions necessary with hemodialysis are not necessary with peritoneal dialysis as vascular access is not required. The advantages of peritoneal dialysis are its relatively low cost, ease of performance, reduced likelihood of infectious disease transmission, and lack of anticoagulation. Disadvantages include the need for frequent sessions, risk of peritonitis, and its significant lower effectiveness than hemodialysis.

Complications of Dialysis

The complications associated with chronic hemodialysis are:

1. Improper serum calcium concentration, which contribute to the development of muscle tetany, oversecretion of parathyroid hormone. Regulation of the serum calcium level can be achieved with calcium supplementation or the use of dialysate containingg calcium.
2. There is a risk of developing hepatitis B and C and the human immunodeficiency virus (HIV) because these patients have usually had multiple blood exposures.
3. Leukocytic abnormalities. Decrease of both number and function of lymphocytes, and impaired functions of neutrophils (chemotaxis, phagocytosis, enhanced bacterial activity).
4. Abnormal bleeding. Patients with early stage renal failure (ESRD) have bleeding tendencies because of:
   a. Altered platelet aggregation
   b. Decreased platelet factor III activity.
   c. Abnormal platelet destruction by mechanical trauma involved in performing arteriovenous shunt.
   d. Heparin administered during dialysis: Therefore, the hematologist should first be consulted and pretreatment screening for bleeding disorders should be performed including bleeding time and platelet count. A

hematocrit level and a hemoglobin count also should be obtained to assess the status of anemia.
5. Infection of the arteriovenous fistula, which may result in septicemia, septic emboli and infective endocarditis.

Susceptibility to infection represents a major problem in patients with renal disease because of the associated defective mechanism, impaired B cell function, and decreased cell-mediated immunity, together with general debilitation. Patients receiving hemodialysis showed higher incidence of developing infective endocarditis than those with rheumatic heart disease. The plausible explanation of this finding is that the surgically created arteriovenous fistulas are potentially susceptible to infection (endarteritis) resulting from a dentally induced bacteremia, and are a source of emboli that can cause infective endocarditis.

Oral diseases and dental manipulation create bacteremias. Periodontal diseases, endodontically treated teeth, oral ulcers, and dental procedures all can induce bacteremia. Therefore, every effort should be taken to eliminate the sources of dental infections by:

1. Good home oral care.
2. Regular use of antifungal and antimicrobial mouth wash.
3. Prophylactic antibiotic coverage to reduce the chance of septicemia and endocarditis before any dental manipulation. The suggested antibiotic prophylaxis against the development of bacterial endocarditis in patients receiving hemodialysis include:
   - The drug of choice is vancomycin (1.0 g) infused one hour during dialysis the day before dental treatment. Because of the renal impairment, this antibiotic will protect the patient for up to seven days, or amoxicillin (3.0 g per mouth) one hour before the dental procedure; a second dose is not needed, or
   - Erythromycin ethylsuccinate (800 mg) or erythromycin stearate (1.0 g by mouth) two hours before the dental procedure, or clindamycin (300 g by mouth) one hour before the dental procedure. Then 150 mg six hours after the initial dose.
   - Benzylpenicillin has a significant potassium content and may be nephrotoxic and may, therefore, be contraindicated. Tetracyclines can

worsen nitrogen retention and acidosis in cases of chronic renal failure. Cephalosporins should be avoided as they are nephrotoxic, similarly NSAIDs are nephrotoxic drugs. Tetracyclines, cephalosporins, and NSAIDs are accumulated in the body when there is impaired renal drug excretion, and can produce encephalopathy.

Because patients undergoing hemodialysis are exposed to multiple blood exposure and because of the immunosuppression, there is a great risk of developing hepatitis B and C and the human immuno-deficiency virus (HIV). The patient should be encouraged to undergo periodic testing for hepatitis infectivity and HIV antibodies.

DENTAL MANAGEMENT OF CHRONIC RENAL FAILURE

Dental treatment is best carried out on the day after dialysis, when there has been maximal benefit from dialysis and the effect of the heparin has worn off (Box 6.2).

The risk of bleeding tendencies in uremic patients dictates that the dentists have local (topical thrombin,

Box 6.2: Dental management of end-stage renal disease

Under conservative care

- Consultation with physician is advised.
  - Avoid dental treatment, if disease is poorly controlled or advanced
- Screen for bleeding disorder before surgery (bleeding time, platelet count, hematocrit, hemoglobin)
- Monitor blood pressure closely
  - Pay attention to good surgical technique avoid nephrotoxic drugs (acetaminophen in high doses, aspirin, non-steroidal anti-inflammatory drugs)
- Adjust dosage of drugs metabolized by the kidney
- Manage orofacial infections aggressively with culture and sensitivity test
- Consider hospitalization for severe infection or major procedure

Receiving hemodialysis

- Same as conservative care recommendations

Plus

- Concern of the arteriovenous (AV) shunt
  - Low risk for infective endarteritis and endocarditis
  - Consultation with physician
  - Avoid blood pressure cuff and IV medications in arm with shunt
- Avoid dental care on day of treatment (especially within first 4 hours afterward); best treated one day after
- Screen for HBsAg before any treatment; treat as potential carrier

microfibrillar collagen, suture). Should bleeding be prolonged, systemic (desmopressin 0.3 µg/kg over 30 minutes) hemostatic agents should be available during surgical procedures. Desmopressin may provide hemostasis for up to 4 hours. If fails, cryoprecipitate (a plasma derivative rich in factor VIII, fibrinogen, and fibrinoectin) may be effective, has a peak effect at 4–12 hours and lasts up to 36 hours. Conjugated estrogens may aid hemostasis: the effect takes 2–5 days to develop, but persists for 30 days.

Platelet transfusions are used infrequently because of risk of immunogenic sensitization.

Aspirin and non-steroidal anti-inflammatory drugs potentiate uremic platelet defects— thus, these antiplatelet drugs should be avoided. These drugs also aggravate gastrointestinal irritation (Table 6.3).

Nephrotoxic Drugs

Drugs excreted primarily by the kidney, and nephro-toxic drugs should be avoided, e.g. tetracyclines, aminoglycosides, aspirin, non-steroidal anti-inflam-matory drugs, and acetaminophen.

The frequency and dosage of dental drug administration require adjustment during uremia for reasons beside nephrotoxicity and renal metabolism. For example: A low serum albumin value reduces the number of binding sites for circulating drugs, thus enhancing drug effects. Drugs removed during hemodialysis are those with low binding capacity to plasma proteins. However, uremia may greatly alter the normal degree of protein binding, and a drug such as phenytoin but normally has high protein binding exhibits lower plasma protein binding during uremia and is available to a greater extent for dialysis removal. Drugs with high lipid affinity have high tissue binding and are not available for dialysis removal.

1. Uremia can modify hepatic metabolism of drugs (increasing or decreasing clearance).
2. Certain drugs (antiacids) can affect acid-base or electrolyte balance.

Anxiolytic Drugs

Although nitrous-oxide and diazepam are antianxiety drugs that require little modification for use in patients with early-stage renal disease (ESRD), the hematocrit or hemoglobin concentration should be measured before intravenous sedation to ensure adequate oxygenation. Drugs that depress the central nervous system (barbiturates, narcotics) are best avoided in the

Table 6.3: Drug modification in patients with chronic renal failure

Safe (no dosage change usually required)	Fairly safe (dosage change only in severe renal failure)	Less safe (dosage reduction indicated in mild renal failure)	Avoid (best avoided in any patient with renal failure)
Azithromycin	Ampicillin	Aciclovir	Aminoglycosides
Cloxacillin	Amoxicillin	Cephalosporins	Cephaloridine
Doxycycline	Benzylpenicillin	Ciprofloxacin	Cephalothin
Flucloxacillin	Clindamycin	Etafloxacin	Gentamicin
Fucidin	Co-trimoxazole	Fluconazole	Sulphonamides
Minocycline	Erythromycin	Levofloxacin	Tetracyclines
Metronidazole	Ketoconazole	Ofloxacin	Pethidine and
Rifampicin	Lincomycin	Vancomycin	Opioids
Lidocaine	Phenoxymethyl	NSAIDs and	
Paracetamol	Penicillin	Aspirin	
Acetaminophen	Codeine		
Diazepam			
Midazolam			

Glomerular filtration rate (GFR): Severe renal failure— GFR< 10 mL/min; moderately severe renal failure— GFR < 25 mL/min; mild renal failure—GFR < 50 mL/min.

presence of uremia, because the blood-brain barrier may not be intact, and excessive sedation may result.

Local Anesthesia

Patients receiving dialysis are not contraindicated for simple outpatient dental procedures (e.g. extraction of teeth). These patients are not generally a problem under local anesthesia.

The use of lidocaine (xylocaine) with epinephrine is not contraindicated. Local anesthesia is safe. A small percentage of an administered local anesthetic dose is eliminated from the blood unchanged, in its active form, through the kidney. Reports have cited values for urinary excretion as 3% for lidocaine, less than 1% for prilocaine, 1% for mepivacaine, less than 1% for etidocaine. The patients requiring renal dialysis represents a relative contraindication to the administration of large doses of local anesthetics. Such patients are ambulatory between dialysis appointments and visit the dental office for treatment. Undetoxified local anesthetic may accumulate in the blood of the patient, producing clinical signs and symptoms (usually mild) of local anesthetic overdose.

Conscious Sedation

Relative analgesia may be used. The veins of the forearms and the saphenous veins are lifelines for patients on regular hemodialysis. If it is necessary to give intravenous sedation, or take the blood, other veins

such as those at or above the elbow should be used because of the risk of consequent fistula infection or thrombophlebitis. Midazolam is preferable to diazepam because of the lower risk of thrombophlebitis.

General Anesthesia

Chronic renal failure is invariably complicated by anemia, which is a contraindication to general anesthesia, if the hemoglobin is below 10 g/dl. Induction with thiopentone followed by very light general anesthesia with nitrous oxide is generally the technique of choice. Euflurane is metabolized to potentially organic fluoride ions and, therefore, should be avoided, if other nephrotoxic agents are used concurrently. Isoflurane and sevoflurane are probably safer.

RENAL TRANSPLANT

The patient requiring surgery after renal or other major organ transplantation is usually receiving a variety of drugs to preserve the function of the transplanted tissue. These patients receive corticosteroids and may need supplemental corticosteroids in the perioperative period. Most of these patients also receive immunosuppressive agents that may cause otherwise self-limiting infections to become severe.

Therefore, more aggressive use of antibiotics and early hospitalization for infections are warranted.

The patient's primary care physician should be consulted concerning the need for prophylactic antibiotics. Cyclosporine A, an immunosuppressive drug administered after organ transplantation, may cause gingival hyperplasia. The dentist performing oral surgery should recognize this so as not to wrongly attribute gingival hyperplasia entirely to hygiene problems. Patients who have had renal transplants occasionally have problems with severe hypertension. Vital signs should be obtained before oral surgery is performed (Box 6.3).

Box 6.3: Management of patient with renal transplant*

1. Defer treatment until primary care physician or transplant surgeon clears patient for dental care.
2. Avoid use of nephrotoxic drugs.
3. Consider use of supplemental corticosteroids.
4. Monitor blood pressure.
5. Consider hepatitis B screening before dental care. Take hepatitis precautions, if unable to screen for hepatitis.
6. Watch for presence of cyclosporine A-induced gingival hyperplasia. Emphasize importance of oral hygiene.
7. Consider use of prophylactic antibiotics, particularly for patients on immunosuppressive agents.

* Most of these recommendations apply to patients with other transplant organs, the clinician should avoid the use of drugs toxic to that organ

7

Diabetes Mellitus

- Anatomy
- Physiology
- Type I
- Type II
- Diagnosis
- Hypoglycemic Coma
- Hyperglycemic Coma
- Management of Coma in Diabetic Patient
- Oral manifestations of Diabetes Mellitus
- Complications of Diabetes Mellitus
- Dental Management of Diabetes Mellitus

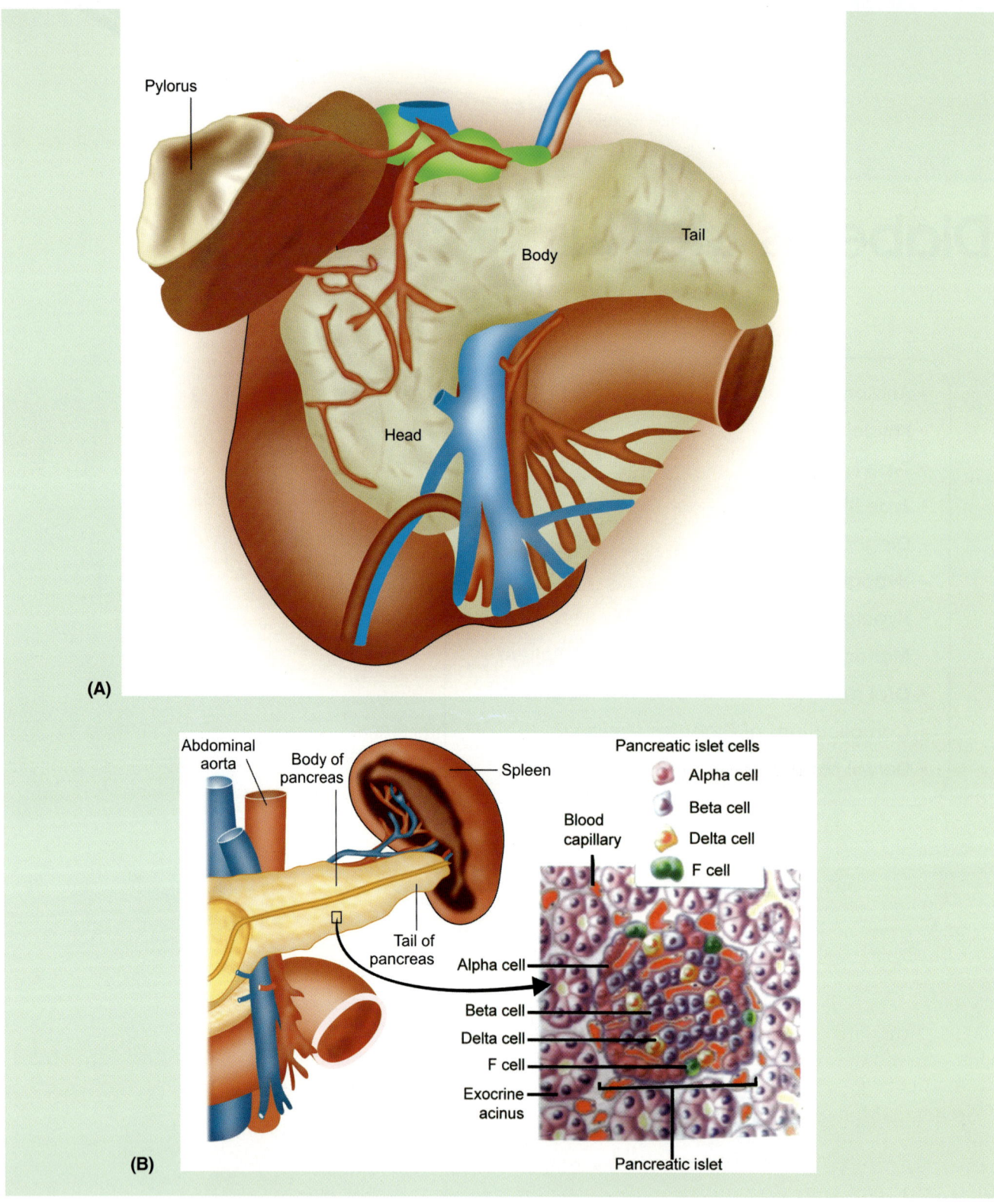

Plate VI: The pancreas. **(A)** Gross anatomy and relationship to the duodenum and other nearby organs, notice the head, body, and blunt tail of the pancreas. **(B)** Light micrograph of alpha, beta and delta and other cells of a pancreatic islet amid the exocrine acini *(Forbes and Jackson, 2003)*

Insulin is a signal to the body that it has been fed and a mean for the maintenance of glucose homostasis. Insulin is called a hypoglycemic hormone because it lowers the blood glucose levels.

Terminology related to glucose and glycogen metabolism:
  Glycogenesis: The synthesis of glycogen by polymerizing glucose.
  Gluconeogenesis: The synthesis of glucose from non-carbohydrates such as fats and acids. Catabolic (breakdown) reactions
  Glycolysis: The splitting of glucose into two molecules of pyruvic acid in preparation for anaerobic fermentation or aerobic respiration.
  Glycogenolysis: The hydrolysis of glycogen to release free glucose or glucose-1-phosphate.

Poorly controlled diabetes are regarded as truly compromised hosts with an increased susceptibility to infection. Repeated, frequent infection breach the protective tegument, and diabetic microvascular disease and peripheral neuropathy both lead to infection and delayed wound healing.

The second line of defense is impaired as well. The granulocytes and monocytes chemotactic activity is abnormal, thus explaining the delayed inflammatory response. Phagocytic adherence, phagocytosis, and bactericidal function of granulocytes are reduced because of impaired glucose metabolism of these cells.

Diabetes mellitus is the most common endocrine disorder characterized by abnormal glucose metabolism and persistently raised blood glucose level (hyperglycemia) that results from absolute deficiency in insulin secretion; a reduction in the biologic effectiveness of insulin or both. The body needs 200 gm of carbohydrates per day to maintain a glucose level without gluconeogenesis, thus preventing hypoglycemia and ketoacidosis.

PANCREAS

ANATOMY

The pancreas is a spongy retroperitoneal gland located retroperitoneally, inferior and dorsal to the greater curvature of the stomach (Fig. 7.1). It has a globose head encircled by the duodenum, a midportion called the body, and a blunt, tapered tail on the left (Plate VII-A). It is approximately 15 cm long and 2.5 cm thick.

The pancreas is both an endocrine and exocrine gland. Most of it is an exocrine digestive gland, which secretes 1,200 to 1,500 mL of pancreatic juice per day. The pancreatic juice includes trypsin which digests dietary protein, pancreatic amylase, which digests starch; pancreatic lipase, which digests fat; and ribonuclease and deoxyribonuclease, which digest RNA and DNA, respectively.

Scattered through the exocrine tissue are endocrine cell clusters called pancreatic islets (islets of Langerhans) (Plate VII-B). There are 1 to 2 million islets, but they constitute only about 2% of the pancreatic tissue. The islets secrete at least five hormones and paracrine products, the most important of which are insulin, glucagon, and somatostatin.

PHYSIOLOGY

Normal fasting blood glucose levels for venous blood range from 70 to 120 mgm%. A fasting blood glucose level of 140 mgm/100 mL on two or more occasions is adequate for the diagnosis of diabetes mellitus.

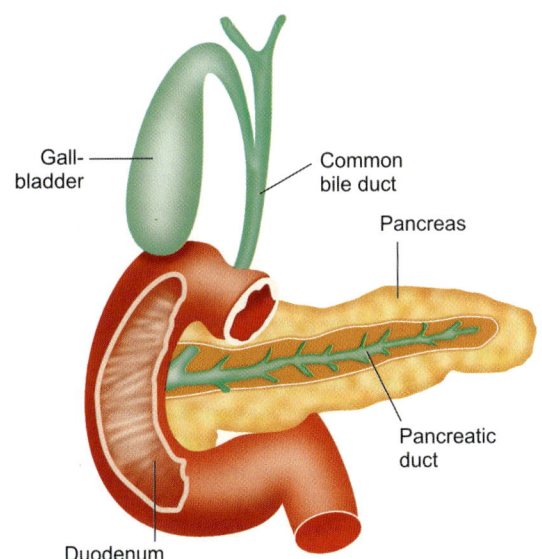

Fig. 7.1: The pancreatic ducts and their orifices

Diabetes can be managed by maintaining control overdiet, physical activity and administering oral antidiabetic drugs and insulin, as needed.

Insulin

Insulin is called a hypoglycemic hormone because it lowers the blood glucose levels.

Insulin is the most important factor in the regulation of blood glucose level. It is synthesized in B-0 cells of the pancreas (Fig. 7.2) and rapidly secreted in the blood in response to elevation in blood-sugar levels, e.g. after a meal. There are 8 to 15 microunits of insulin per milliliter of blood. This increases to 100 microunits under stimulation by protein, lipids, sugar ingestion and surgery. Insulin remains in the circulation for only

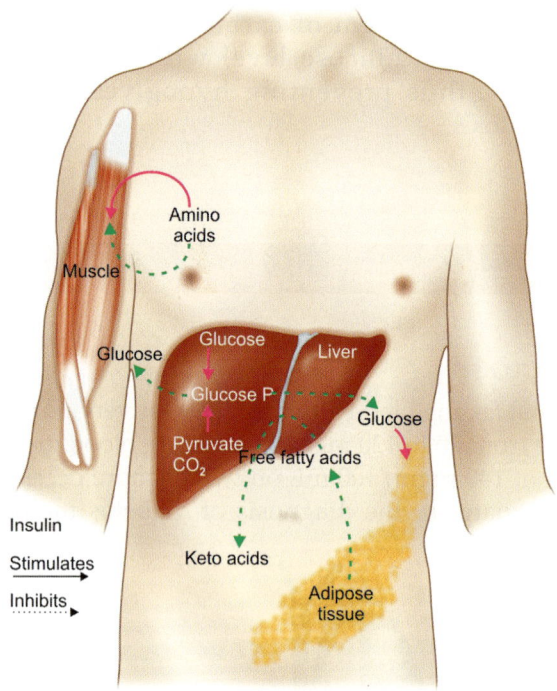

Fig. 7.2: Functions of insulin. Insulin is a fuel-storage hormone. The major fuels used by cells are glucose, fatty acids, and ketoacids derived during fatty acid metabolism. Some cells preferentially use glucose as their fuel (e.g. neurons), whereas other cells preferentially use fatty acids (e.g. skeletal muscle). Ketoacids can be used by many cells when glucose and fatty acids are not readily available (e.g. fasting). Insulin stimulates the uptake of glucose into cells, where it is stored in the form of glycogen (especially in the liver and skeletal muscle). It also stimulates fat synthesis and inhibits lipolysis, thus storing fatty acids as triglycerides (fatty acid metabolism to ketoacids is also inhibited). Finally, insulin stimulates the uptake of amino acids into cells and their storage as protein. The net effect is that blood levels of glucose and ketoacids decrease *(Netter's: Atlas of Human Physiology, 1991)*

several minutes, then it interacts with target tissues and binds with cell surface insulin receptors.

When we digest a meal and the level of glucose and amino acids in the blood rises. In such times of plenty, insulin stimulates cells to absorb glucose and amino acids from the blood and especially stimulates muscle and adipose tissue to store glycogen and fat. Essentially, insulin stimulates cells to store excess nutrients for later use, and it suppresses the use of already-stored fuels. The stored nutrients are then available for use between meals and overnight. Thus after a meal, the high blood level of insulin tells the body's cells to absorb and store any fuel that is not immediately required for metabolic needs. In the fasting state, low insulin level tells the body that no food is entering, and that storage forms of nutrients should be utilized for fuel in the different organs. However, some cells and organs do not depend on insulin for glucose uptake as the kidneys, brain, liver, and red blood cells.

Insulin stimulates the synthesis of glycogen, fat, and protein and thus promotes cell growth and differentiation. Insulin also promotes the liver's synthesis of glycogen from the absorbed glucose. Insulin also antagonizes the effects of glucagon.

Thus, insulin produces a decrease in the blood glucose level, preventing its loss through, urinary excretion. Insulin is needed for muscle, fat, and liver to utilize glucose from the blood; therefore, these tissues are described as being insulin-dependent.

They require its presence to enable glucose to cross the cell membrane, even in hyperglycemic states. Without insulin, the cell membranes of cells of these tissues are impermeable to glucose. In the absence of insulin, these cells breakdown triglycerides into fatty acids, which the body can use as an alternative energy source. This process gives rise to hyperglycemia state known as diabetes ketoacidosis. By contrast, the central nervous system and renal cortex can utilize glucose from the blood without insulin, i.e. can transfer glucose across cell membrane without insulin.

In the fasting stage, decreased blood sugar levels (hypoglycemia) inhibit insulin secretion. The lack of glucose utilization by many of the cells of the body leads to cellular starvation. The body cells require glucose, however, two mechanisms exist through which it is made available:

1. The body breaks down glycogen stores in the liver into glucose through a process called **glycogenolysis, and**

Box 7.1: Factors encourages the development of hyper-glycemia

Weight gain	Pregnancy (gestational diabetes)
Thyroid medication	Corticosteroid therapy
Lack of exercise	Hyperthyroidism
Epinephrine therapy	Acute infection
Fever	

2. The amino acids are converted into glucose through a process called **gluconeogenesis.** The patient often will increase the intake of food but in many cases still lose weight.

The goal of these mechanisms is to provide the CNS with the minimal glucose level required to maintain normal function.

The patient with uncontrolled diabetes is deprived of insulin or its action but will continue to use carbohydrates at the usual rates in the brain and nervous system because insulin is not required by these tissues. However, other tissues in the body are unable to take glucose into the cells or use it at a normal rate. Increased production of glucose may occur from glycogen and from protein; thus the rise in blood glucose in diabetic persons results from a combination of underutilization and overproduction.

Factors that encourages the development of hyperglycemia are mentioned in Box 7.1. Factors that decrease the requirements for insulin are: weight loss, increased exercise, termination of pregnancy, termination of other drug therapies (epinephrine, thyroid, corticosteroid), and recovery from an infection or fever. Most common cause is inadequate food intake. To summarize, insulin possesses the following functions:

1. Promotes the uptake of glucose into the body cells, i.e. it transfers glucose from the blood to insulin-dependent tissues.
2. Promotes storage of glucose in the liver as glycogen.
3. Promotes uptake of fatty acids and proteins into the cells and their subsequent conversion into storage forms (triglycerides and amino acids), i.e. it stimulates triglyceride synthesis from fatty acids.
4. Insulin suppresses glycogenolysis, lipolysis, and proteolysis, thus preventing ketosis.

Glucagon

The functions of insulin are opposite to those of glucagon, the two hormones usually work in concert to maintain a normal blood glucose concentration. Glucagon is secreted by alpha (α) cells when blood glucose concentration falls between meals (Figs 7.3 and 7.4).

In the liver, it stimulates gluconeogenesis, glycogenolysis, and the release of glucose into circulation. In adipose tissue, it stimulates fat catabolism and the release of free fatty acids. Glucagon is also secreted in response to rising amino acid levels in the blood after a high-protein meal. By promoting amino acid absorption, it provides cells with raw material for gluconeogenesis.

Somatostatin

Somatostatin is secreted by the delta cells when blood glucose and amino acids rise after a meal. Somatostatin travels briefly in the blood and inhibits various digestive functions, but also acts locally in the pancreas

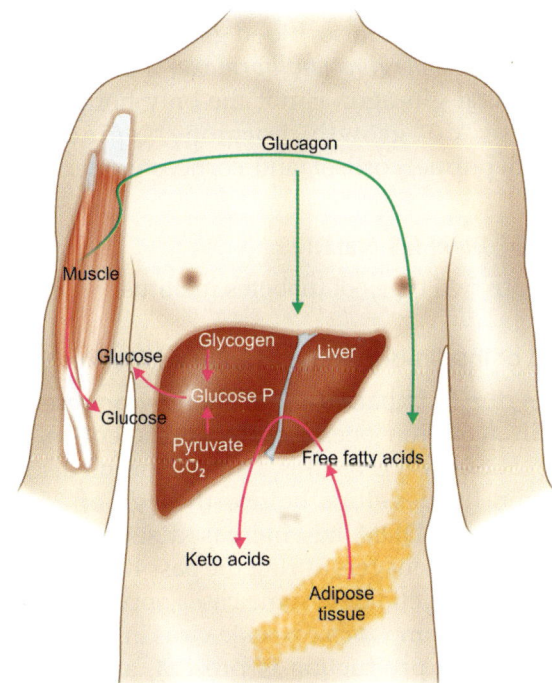

Fig. 7.3: Glucagon is a fuel mobilization hormone. It acts on the liver to breakdown glycogen and stimulates hepatic gluconeogenesis from amino acids. The effect of these actions is to increase the blood glucose concentration. Glucagon acts also on adipose tissue to stimulate lipolysis and the release of fatty acids. Metabolism of the fatty acids by the liver produces keto acids. Amino acids are released from muscle in response to glucagons and are converted to glucose in the liver by gluconeogenesis. The net effect of glucagon is that glucose fatty acids, and keto acid levels in the blood increase *(Netter's: Atlas of Human Physiology, 1991)*

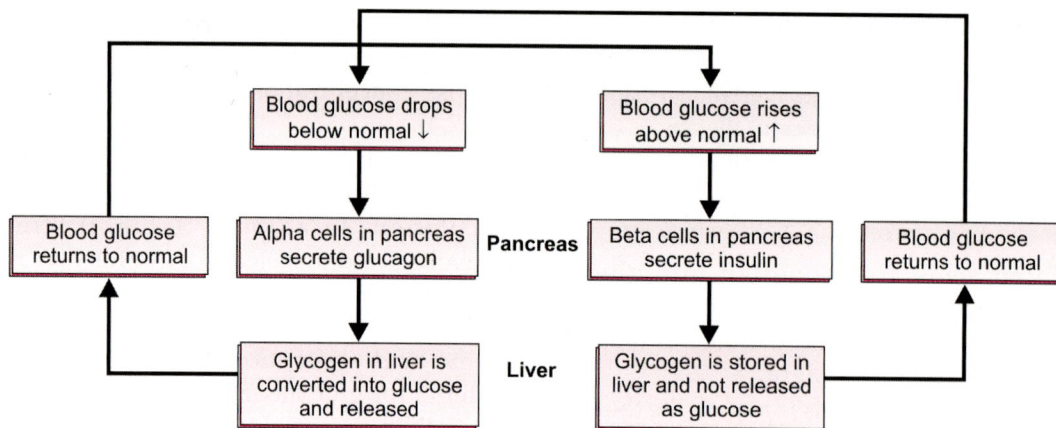

Fig. 7.4: Glucagon and insulin regulation. Negative feedback mechanism regulating the secretion of glucagon and insulin. Note that both the pancreas and liver are involved

as a *paracrine* secretion—a chemical messenger that diffuses through the tissue fluid to target cells a short distance away. Somatostatin inhibits the secretion of glucagon and insulin by the neighboring and cells. Any hormone that raises blood glucose concentration is called a *hyperglycemic hormone*. You may have noticed that glucagon is not the only hormone that does; so do growth hormone, epinephrine, norepinephrine, cortisol, and corticosterone.

TYPES OF DIABETES MELLITUS

There are two types of diabetes mellitus.

Type I or Insulin-dependent Diabetes Mellitus (IDDM)

This is due to impaired production by or absence of insulin secretion because of insufficient mass of pancreatic islet B cells. It is a ketosis-prone disorder. It generally develops before the age of 25. The incidence of IDDM has increased several fold in children and teenagers during the past 40 years. There may be a viral etiology; some cases appear to follow an attack of mumps or a coxackie virus infection. Little or no insulin production is present, and anti-islet antibodies are usually detectable early in the disease (Fig. 7.5).

This is suggestive of an autoimmune etiology. The onset is relatively acute, typically with thirst, polyuria (especially at night), hunger and loss of weight.

The process of lipolysis is activated with increased production of acetoacetate which is converted to the other ketone bodies, hydroxybutyrate and actone. These cause acidosis and thus hyperventilation. Ketone bodies also appear in the urine (ketonuria).

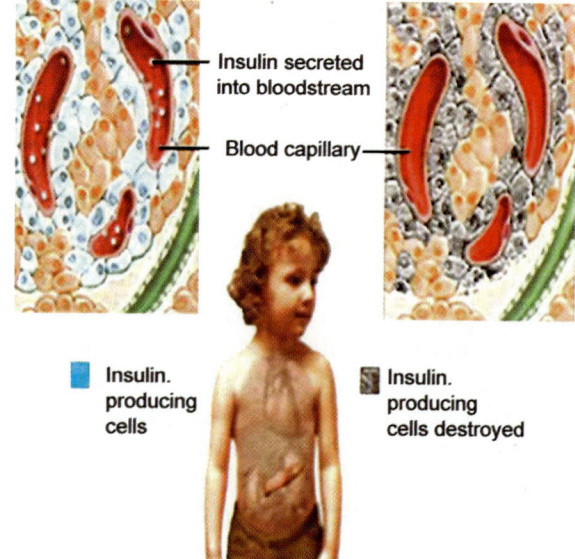

Insulin secreted into bloodstream

Blood capillary

Insulin. producing cells

Insulin. producing cells destroyed

Fig. 7.5: Type I diabetes

Insulin is required daily for treatment, for life, and diet must be controlled.

Type II or Non-insulin-dependent Diabetes Mellitus (NIDDM)

Occurs due to altered number and affinity of peripheral insulin receptors. Patients with NIDDM have both decreased insulin secretion and impaired insulin action (Fig. 7.6). It is non-ketosis prone disorder. Non-insulin-dependent diabetes mainly affects obese, middle-aged patients, often with a family history of diabetes.

The cause of type II diabetes are several, and while the genetic basis has been difficult to identify, it is clear

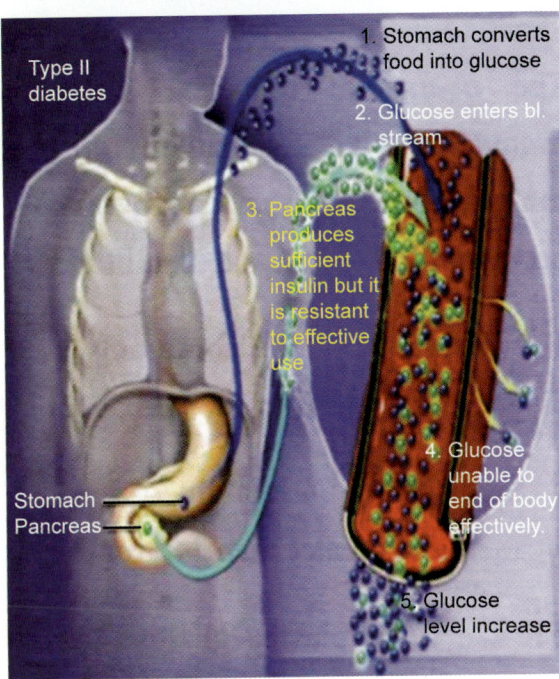

Type II diabetes

1. Stomach converts food into glucose

2. Glucose enters bl. stream

3. Pancreas produces sufficient insulin but it is resistant to effective use

4. Glucose unable to end of body affectively

Stomach

Pancreas

5. Glucose level increase

Fig. 7.6: Diabetes type II

that subtypes result from mutations in the glucokinase gene, changes in insulin signaling molecules, defective phosphatidyl-inositol kinase or other mechanisms. The diagnosis of diabetes in type II disease is gradual, but otherwise features are similar to type I diabetes. Most patients with this type of diabetes can be managed on diet and oral hypoglycemic drugs and though some may need insulin, they are often resistant.

There appear to be a good correlation between the status of the beta cells and the clinical severity of the diabetes. In the early stage of IDDM, the islets of Langerhans may be enlarged and there is a lymphocytic infiltrate, which suggests the possibility of an autoimmune response. Later, the islets become smaller, and essentially no insulin is produced. By contrast, most individuals with NIDDM are able to produce some insulin. However, the primary defect in IDDM appears to be a defect in insulin secretion.

Cortisol secretion often is increased in type I diabetic in response to the stress of the disease, leading to protein breakdown and difficulty incorporating amino acids into protein. The result is conversion of amino acids to glucose and a loss of body nitrogen in the urine.

As the inability to utilize glucose progresses, the type I diabetic person shifts to fat metabolism. Body fat stores are mobilized, and the glycerol portion of

the triglyceride is separated and converted to glucose. The fatty acids are metabolized through the Krebs cycle; but if excessive fat breakdown continues, the ability of the breakdown product acetyl coenzyme A, to be processed through the Krebs cycle fails. There is an excess of acetone and beta-hydroxybutyric acid, which builds up in concentration in body fluids and are excreted in the urine.

Glucagon secreted by the alpha cells of the pancreas opposes insulin and serves in a catabolic way. It activates glycogen breakdown. Glucagon is a rapid counter-regulator of insulin; it attempts to maintain normal glucose levels. Ketoacidosis is thus promoted by low insulin with high glucagons, which usually is also being seen.

Diagnosis of Diabetes Mellitus

The course of diabetes is variable. Many insulin-treated patients are liable to hypoglycemia, due to an imbalance between food intake and insulin therapy.

The criteria which are commonly used to diagnose diabetes include (Box 7.2):

1. Two fasting plasma glucose measurements of greater than 140 mg/dL, or
2. Two-hour plasma glucose measurement after 75 g of oral glucose of greater than 200 mg/dL, with one other value during glucose tolerance test exceeding 200 mg/dL, or
3. Presence of diabetic ketoacidosis.
4. The patients typically have polyuria, polydipsia, polyphagia, and glycosuria.

The usual daily production of insulin by a lean adult is 33 units; approximately 3 to 5 units are needed for each meal whereas the basal insulin requirement is about lU/h. The ketosis-prone diabetic produces less than 10% of the average daily insulin requirements, but the typical NIDDM patient produces an average of 15 U/24 h. IDDM patients, in contrast to those with NIDDM, have a high rate of systemic problems. The lack of glucose utilization by many of the cells of the body leads to cellular starvation. The patient will often increase the intake of food but in many cases still loose weight.

COMAS OF DIABETES

Hypoglycemic Coma

Hypoglycemic coma is usually the result of failure to take food, or over dosage of insulin, hypoglycemic drugs or alcohol. It is increasing in frequency with

Box 7.2: Symptoms of diabetes

1. IDDM
a. Cardinal symptoms—common
  • Polydipsia
  • Polyuria
  • Polyphagia
  • Weight loss
  • Loss of strength
b. Other symptoms
  • Recurrence of bed wetting
  • Repeated skin infections
  • Marked irritability
  • Headache
  • Drowsiness
  • Malaise
  • Dry mouth

2. NIDDM
a. Cardinal symptoms—much less common
b. Usual symptoms
  • Slight weight loss or gain
  • Urination at night
  • Vulvar pruritus
  • Blurred vision
  • Decreased vision
  • Paresthesia
  • Loss of sensation
  • Impotence
  • Postural hypotension

the trend towards tighter metabolic control of diabetes. The brain has priority over glucose, which it utilizes for energy. The remainder of its energy is derived from lactates and glycerol. Actually, the bodily need for glucose is decreased during starvation because glycogen is broken down. By the 16th hour of starvation, glycogen stores are depleted, and gluconeogenesis becomes the source of glucose. Therefore, ketoacidosis results because of beta-hydroxybutyric acid and acetoacetic acid, formed from fats and proteins.

Hypoglycemic coma is of rapid onset and may resemble fainting. There is adrenaline release, often with anxiety, irritability and disorientation, before consciousness is lost. Occasionally, the patient may convulse. The pulse is strong and bounding, and the skin sweaty.

Hyperglycemic (Diabetic Ketoacidotic) Coma

Hyperglycemic coma is the result of a relative or absolute deficiency of insulin and, in patients under treatment, may be precipitated by several factors. Diabetic coma usually has a slow onset over many hours, with increasing drowsiness and signs of (Box 7.3):

1. Dehydration (dry skin, weak pulse, hypotension).
2. Acidosis (deep breathing).
3. Ketosis (acetone smell on breath, vomiting).

Hyperglycemia leads to glucose excretion in the urine, which results in an increase in urinary volume. The increased fluid lost through urine may lead to dehydration and loss of electrolytes.

Box 7.3: Comparative features of hypo- and hyperglycemic comas and their management

Hypoglycemic coma—diabetes usually known	*Hyperglycemic coma—diabetes may be unrecognized*
Too much insulin or	Too little insulin,
Too little food or	Infection or
Too much exercise or alcohol	Myocardial infarction
Adrenalin release causes	
Sweaty warm skin	Vomiting
Rapid pounding pulse	Hyperventilation
Dilated (reacting) pupil	Ketonuria
Anxiety, tremor, aggression	Acetone breath
Tingling around the mouth	
Cerebral hypoglycemia causes	*Osmotic diuresis and polyuria cause*
Confusion, disorientation, Aggression	Dehydration, hypotension
Headache	Tachycardia
Dysarthria	Dry mouth and skin
Unconsciousness	Abdominal pain
Focal neurological signs, e.g. fits	

Management of Coma in Diabetic Patient

If possible, take blood for glucose measurement and if there is any doubt about the cause never give insulin but immediately give glucose as a diagnostic test. This will cause little harm in hyperglycemic coma but will improve hypoglycemic coma. Insulin, by contrast, can cause severe brain damage or kill a hypoglycemic patient. Hypoglycemia must be quickly corrected or brain damage can result. If the patient is conscious immediately give 10 g sugar or equivalent glucose solution by mouth. If the patient is comatosed, take a blood sample estimation (2 mL blood in a yellow cap bottle containing fluoride) and give 10–20 mL of 20–50% sterile dextrose intravenously. On arousal, the patient should be given glucose orally.

If it is certain that collapse is due to hyperglycemic ketoacidotic coma, the first priority is to establish an intravenous infusion line and start rapid rehydration. Blood should be taken for baseline measurements of glucose, electrolytes and pH. Insulin is then started either 20 units i.m. stat. Then 6 units hourly, or 6 U/h as an i.v. infusion. The intravenous infusion is required to correct dehydration, and electrolyte (especially potassium) losses, and to facilitate the administration of insulin. Medical help should be obtained as soon as possible.

ORAL MANIFESTATIONS OF DIABETES MELLITUS

The oral manifestations of uncontrolled diabetes may include xerostomia, infection, poor healing, increased incidence and severity of periodontal disease, and burning mouth syndrome. The oral findings in patients with uncontrolled diabetes most likely relate to the excessive loss of fluids through urination, the altered response to infection, the microvascular changes, and possibly the increased glucose concentration in saliva.

The effects of hyperglycemia lead to increased amounts of urine which depletes the extracellular fluids and reduces the secretion of saliva, and this results in the complaint of dry mouth and occasionally there is swelling of the salivary glands (sialosis), possibly due to autonomic neuropathy. An increase in the rate of dental caries has been reported in young diabetic patients and would appear to be related to reduced salivary flow. The parotid saliva of persons with uncontrolled diabetes has been reported to contain a slight increase in the amount of glucose. The glucose concentration in parotid saliva from non-

diabetic individuals varies from 0.22 to 1.69 mg/dl, whereas the glucose concentration in parotid saliva from persons with uncontrolled diabetes has been reported to range from 0.22 to 6.33 mg/dl. The effect of this slight increase on the incidence of dental caries and other oral conditions in diabetic patients remain to be established.

1. Several studies have reported an increased incidence and severity of gingival inflammation, periodontal abscesses, and chronic periodontal disease in diabetic patients. This has been attributed to small blood vessel changes in the gingival tissues consisting of flattening of the endothelial cells and narrowing of the lumina.
2. Glossitis. The tongue may show glossitis and alternations in filiform papillae or (it is said) there may be burning sensations in the absence of physical changes.
3. Diabetic neuropathy may lead to oral symptoms of tingling, numbness, burning, or pain caused by pathologic changes involving nerves in the oral region.
4. Oral fungal infections may be found in the uncontrolled diabetic patient including moniliasis. The oral mucosal lichenoid reactions may result from the use of chlorpropamide and some other antidiabetic agents. However, the 'Grinspan syndrome' (diabetes, lichen planus and hypertension) may be purely coincidental associations of common disorders probably related to drug use.
5. Healing is delayed in individuals with uncontrolled diabetes and that they are more prone to various oral infections following surgical procedures. Infection causes an increase in glucagons secretion thus promoting tissue breakdown with cachexia and muscle wasting.

COMPLICATIONS OF DIABETES MELLITUS

The complications of diabetes are associated with the vascular system and the peripheral nervous system (Box 7.4).

Vascular complications: The vascular complications result from two pathologic changes, microangiopathy and arteriosclerosis. The vessel changes (microangiopathy) include thickening of the intima, endothelial proliferation, lipid deposition, and accumulation of para-aminosalicylic acid-positive material. These changes are seen throughout the body but have particular clinical importance when they occur in the retina and small vessels of the kidney.

Box 7.4: Complications of diabetes mellitus

1. Ketoacidosis (type I diabetes)
2. Hyperosmolar non-ketotic coma (type II diabetes)
3. Diabetic retinopathy—blindness, cataracts
4. Diabetic nephropathy—renal failure
5. Accelerated atherosclerosis
   Coronary heart disease
   Stroke
   Ulceration and gangrene of feet
6. Diabetic neuropathy
   Dysphagia
   Gastric distension
   Diarrhea
   Impotence
   Muscle weakness, cramps
   Numbness, tingling, deep burning pain
7. Early death

Arteriosclerosis: It occurs earlier, and is more widespread, and more severe in diabetic than in non-diabetic persons. Hyperglycemia appears to play a role in the evolution of arteriosclerotic plaques. Uncontrolled diabetics have increased levels of low-density lipoprotein (LDL) cholesterol and reduced levels of high-density lipoprotein (HDL) cholesterol. Attainment of normal glycemia often will improve the LDL/HDL ratio. Arteriosclerosis increases the risk of ulceration and gangrene of the feet (Figs 7.7 and 7.8), hypertension, renal failure, coronary insufficiency, myocardial infarction, and stroke.

Retinal complications: Diabetic retinopathy consists of microaneurysms, retinal hemorrhages, retinal edema, and retinal exudates. Diabetic retinopathy is a leading cause of blindness.

Renal complications: Diabetic nephropathy leads to end-stage renal disease in 30 to 40% of individuals with IDDM.

Renal failure occurs in only 5% of individuals with NIDDM. However, because NIDDM is much more common, the number of persons with renal failure is equal for the two types of diabetes. Renal failure is a leading cause of death in patients with IDDM. Twenty percent of all patients using dialysis are diabetic. The microangiopathy in the kidney usually involves the capillaries of the glomerulus.

Neuropathic complications: Diabetics have more complaints concerning nerve disease than any other chronic complication, and there is growing evidence that hyperglycemia is a major factor in the onset and progression of diabetic nephropathy. Increased uptake of glucose by Schwann cells leads to the production of intracellular sorbitol, which attracts water into the cell and may cause cellular injury and nerve dysfunction. In the extremities, diabetic neuropathy may lead to muscle weakness, muscle cramps, a deep burning pain, tingling sensation, and numbness.

In addition, tendon reflexes, two point discrimination, and position sense may be lost. Oral paresthesia and burning tongue are caused by this complication.

Autonomic nervous system: Diabetic nephropathy may involve autonomic nervous system: Esophageal dysfunction may cause dysphagia; stomach involvement may cause a loss of motility, with massive gastric distension; and involvement of small intestine may result in nocturnal diabetic diarrhea. There may also be sexual impotence and bladder dysfunction.

Diabetic ulcer and wound healing: Diabetes mellitus is a chronic systemic disease that affects most

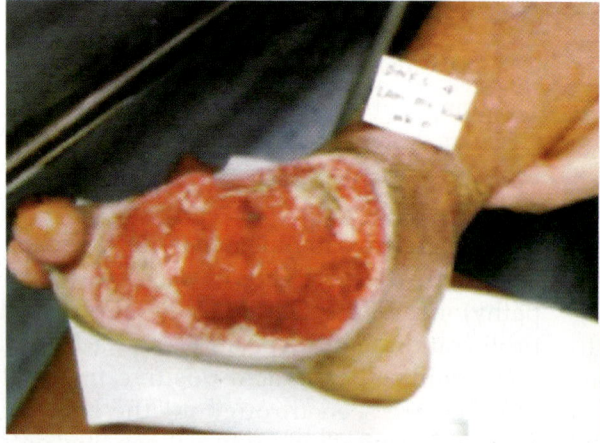
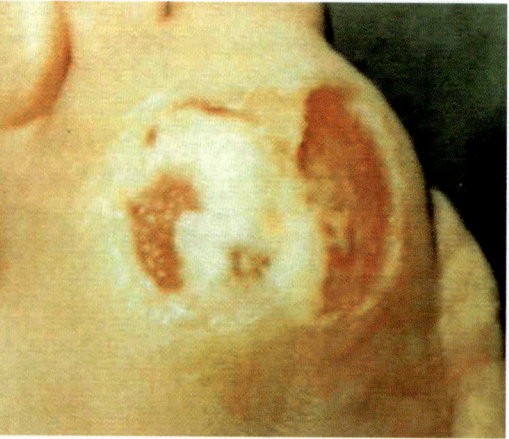

Fig. 7.7: Chronic ulceration in diabetes mellitus affecting weight-bearing areas of the foot *(Forbes and Jackson 2003)*

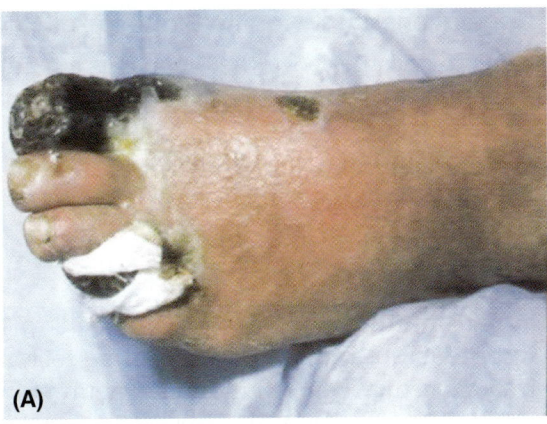 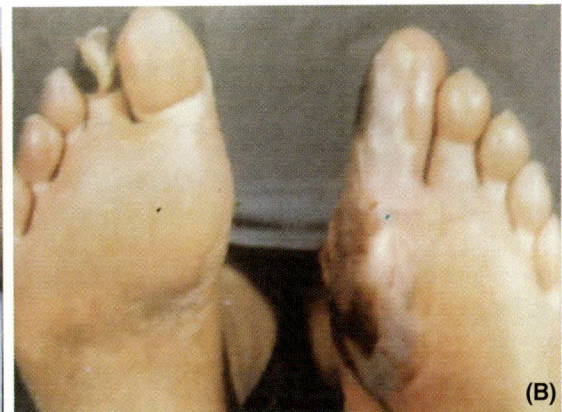

Fig. 7.8: (A) Gangrene of the foot is a common complication of chronic diabetes. **(B)** In this patient, "wet" gangrene has developed in the hallux of the left foot. Ulceration and gangrene of the foot are commonly the result of a combination of diabetic neuropathy with large or small vessel disease, or both

systems of the body, in particular peripheral vascular disease, neuropathy, infection, and impaired healing. **Diabetic ulcers** have always been defined in conjunction with the triad of **neuropathy, ischemia, and infection** (Figs 7.7 and 7.8). Vascular changes, such as impairment of blood flow, and neurogenic abnormalities in diabetic patients are closely related. Infection plays a major role in the duration of such ulcers and is believed to be fostered by abnormalities in neutrophil function as a result of insulin deficiency.

Several factors have been defined that contribute to a reduction in the healing potential of such patients after minor injuries. These factors are reduced hyperemic response to injury, a defect in the inflammatory response leading to impaired migration of neutrophils and macrophages, and abnormalities in the release and action of several growth factors and neuropeptides.

Hyperglycemia and ketoacidosis delay the migration of granulocytes in the area of injury and decrease phagocytic activity and facilitate the growth of certain microorganisms. The vascular wall changes lead to vascular insufficiency, which can result in decreased blood flow to an area of injury and could hamper granulocytic mobilization as well as reduce oxygen tension. The end results of these effects, and others are to render the patient with uncontrolled diabetes much more susceptible to infection once it is established, and to delay the healing of traumatic and surgical wounds.

DENTAL MANAGEMENT OF DIABETES MELLITUS

"It is better to err toward hyperglycemia thus preventing ketosis. The effects of stress and trauma may raise insulin requirements and precipitate ketosis".

Insulin dose needs to be adjusted, if oral intake will be impaired after the procedure.

Rarely, a patient will be admitted to the hospital for complicated extractions to have good control of the blood sugar levels. Transient periods of hyperglycemia tolerated better than periods of hypoglycemia. After extensive treatment, make sure the patient checks his glucometer readings at least 4 times a day and adjusts his insulin dose accordingly. Involvement of the patient's physician is a good idea before any problems develop.

Precautions required during oral surgery in diabetics depend mainly on:

1. The type and severity of the diabetes and complications such as autonomic neuropathy that may predispose to hypotension or cardiac arrest (Box 7.5).
2. The degree of control of the diabetes.
3. The type of the anesthetic agent.
4. The extent of surgery.
5. The extent of interference with normal feeding postoperatively.

Type I diabetes presents the more significant challenge to the well-being of a surgical patient. Patients are usually lean and have had this disease since their youth. Those with long-standing IDDM cannot go without diabetic ketoacidosis (DKA) occurring. Hormones that increase during periods of physiologic stress, including cortisol, catecholamines, and glucagon act to counter the effects of insulin, producing a stress-induced glucose intolerance, even in many healthy nondiabetic patients. This is why

Box 7.5: Screening for diabetes in the dental office

1. Selection of patient
2. On each of the days before screening, patient's diet should contain 250 to 300 g of carbohydrate.
3. Overnight fast before screening.
4. Have patient come to dental office for 8:30 to 9:00 AM appointment on day of testing (no breakfast)
   a. Fasting blood glucose test:
      1. Make wound on finger pad with sterile blood lancet.
      2. Drop blood onto reagent end of Dextrostix.
      3. Wash blood off after 1 minute.
      4. Using color chart, estimate blood glucose level.
   b. 2-hour postprandial blood glucose:
      1. Have patient ingest 75 g of glucose (Glucola).
      2. 2 hours later, obtain blood sample and test as above.
      3. Refer patient to physician if:
         a. Fasting blood glucose is 140 mg/dl 100 or higher.
         b. 2-hours postprandial blood glucose is 200 mg/dl or higher.

IDDM patients who depend on exogenous administration of their insulin commonly have increased insulin requirements from preoperative emotional stress, intraoperative anesthetic stress, and postoperative wound and emotional stress. Studies have shown that elevated blood glucose not only impairs wound healing but also can depress leukocyte and pancreatic B cell function, which are reasons, in addition to prevention of diabetic ketoacidosis (DKA), for appropriate insulin supplementation during and after surgery. The reader is referred to Chapter 15, "D": Diabetes, page 440.

Local Anesthesia for the Diabetic Patient

Surgery combined with anesthetic agents causes a 70% increase in blood sugar. Dental disease and treatment may disrupt the normal pattern of food intake and can interfere with diabetic control. Treatment is best carried out just after breakfast and routine antidiabetic medication, to allow the diabetic to have lunch. Diabetic patients can tolerate minor surgical procedures, such as single extractions under local anesthetic, without problems. The dose of adrenaline used in dental local anesthetic solution is unlikely to increase blood glucose levels significantly. The essential requirement is to avoid hypoglycemia but to keep hyperglycemia below levels which may be harmful because of delayed wound healing or phagocyte dysfunction. The desired whole blood glucose levels are therefore 120–180 mg/dl (3–5 mmol/l).

General Anesthesia for the Diabetic Patient

General anesthesia for the diabetic is a matter for the specialist anesthetist since it may be complicated especially by:

1. Hypoglycemia.
2. Chronic renal failure.
3. Ischemic heart disease
4. Autonomic neuropathy.

Autonomic neuropathy can lead to postural hypotension and impaired ability to respond to hypoglycemia. Severe autonomic neuropathy carries a risk of cardiorespiratory arrest, if a general anesthetic is given.

A brief general anesthetic can be given without special precautions apart from monitoring the urine sugar before the operation and on recovery, at 2-hourly intervals. However, such patients must have the anesthetic in hospital, so that if ketonuria develops, blood sugar levels can be rapidly estimated. Not all such patients are necessarily well controlled. In this case, or if more major surgery is planned, the patient should be admitted to hospital and the following precautions should be taken:

a. Before the operation, the patient should be put on soluble insulin and stabilized. Insulin may need to be given twice or three times daily, and control is confirmed by estimation of blood sugar (fasting, midday, and before the evening meal).

b. The operation should be carried out early in the morning and booked first in the list, so that any delays in the operation schedule will not impair diabetic control.

c. At 8.00 to 9.00 a.m., blood should be taken for glucose estimation and an intravenous infusion set up giving glucose l0 g, soluble insulin 2 units and potassium 2 m mol/h, until normal oral feeding is resumed—at which time the patient can be returned to the preoperative insulin regimen. Get the patient out of ketoacidosis, correct any electrolyte imbalance and rehydrate well before surgery.

d. Blood-glucose should be monitored at 2–4 hourly intervals until the patient is feeding normally.

Infectious agents grow well in sugar. Therefore, a hyperglycemic state leads to susceptibility to infections. Orofacial infections should be vigorously treated as they may precipitate ketosis. Drugs such as aspirin and steroids must be avoided.

8

Adrenal Glands

- Anatomy
- Physiology
  - i. Adrenal Medulla
  - ii. Adrenal Cortex
    - – Cortisol
    - – Pharmacological Action
- Prescription of Corticosteroid Drugs
- Complications of Systemic Corticosteroid Therapy
  - ◆ Pathophysiology of Suppression of Adrenal Functions
  - ◆ Prevention of Adrenal Crises
  - ◆ Management of Acute Adrenal Insufficiency
  - ◆ Hypersecretion
    - – Cushing's Syndrome
  - ◆ Hyposecretion
    - – Addison's Disease
  - ◆ Suggested Dental Outlines

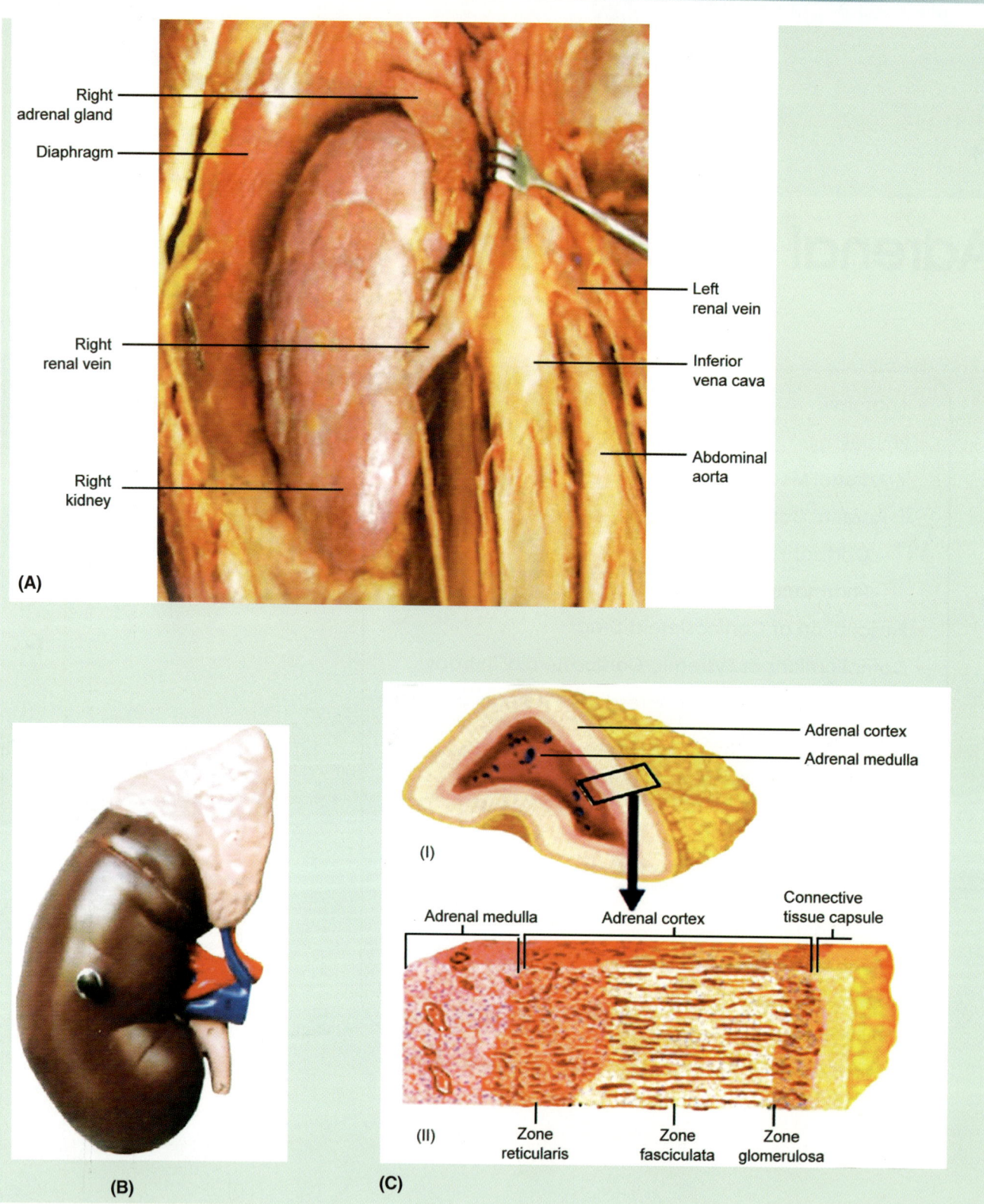

Plate VIII: Adrenal gland. **(A)** The adrenal gland is a two-part gland that secretes stress-related hormones. The adrenal cortex produces steroid hormones and the adrenal medulla (modified sympathetic ganglion) produces epinephrine and norepinephrine. The plate shows Cadaver photo. **(B)** The adrenal glands rest like hat on the superior pole of each kidney. **(C)** Histology, the cortex and medulla components of the suprarenal gland

ANATOMY

The adrenal (suprarenal) gland rests like a hat on the superior pole of each kidney (Plate VIII). In adults, the adrenal is about 5 cm (2 in) long, 3 cm (1.2 in) wide, and weighs about 4 g; it weighs about twice this much at birth. Its inner core, the *adrenal medulla*, is a small portion of the total gland. Surrounding it is a much thicker *adrenal cortex*.

PHYSIOLOGY

The secretory products of the adrenal glands are illustrated in Table 8.1.

I. Adrenal Medulla

The adrenal medulla produces epinephrine and norepinephrine. The medullary cells actually are the postganglionic elements of the sympathetic division of the autonomic nervous system, but as endocrine cells, they release epinephrine and norepinephrine into the blood rather into a synaptic cleft.

The adrenal medulla is usually discussed as a part of the sympathetic nervous system. It arises from the neural crest and is not fully formed until the age of three. It is actually a sympathetic ganglion consisting

Table 8.1: Secretory products of the adrenal glands

Adrenal cortex	Adrenal medulla
Glucocorticoids	Epinephrine*
Cortisol*	Norepinephrine
Corticosterone	Dopamine
Mineralocorticoids	
Aldosterone*	
Dexycorticosterone	
Sex hormones	
Dehydroepiandoslerne	
Androstenedone	

* *Principal secretory products*

of modified neurons, called *chromajfin cells,* that lack dendrites and axons. These cells are richly innervated by sympathetic preganglionic fibers and respond to stimulation by secreting catecholamines (epinephrine and norepinephrine) and dopamine.

About three-quarters of the output is epinephrine. Epinephrine accounts for 70 to 80% of the medullary secretions. **The regulation of adrenal medullary secretions is illustrated in** Fig. 8.1. The relative magnitude and effects of epinephrine and norepinephrine are illustrated in Fig. 8.2 and Table 8.2.

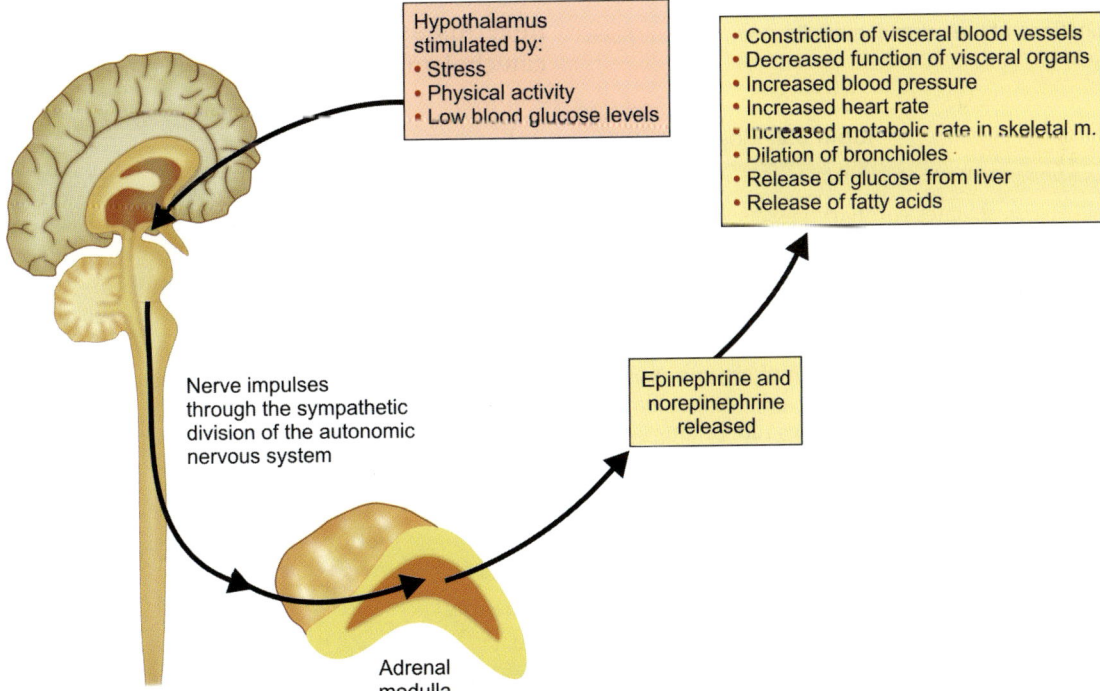

Fig. 8.1: Regulation of adrenal medullary secretions. Stimulation of the hypothalamus by stress, physical activity, or low blood glucose levels causes action potentials to travel through the sympathetic nervous system to the adrenal medulla. In response, the adrenal medulla releases epinephrine and smaller amounts of norepinephrine, which has several effects on the body to prepare it for physical activity

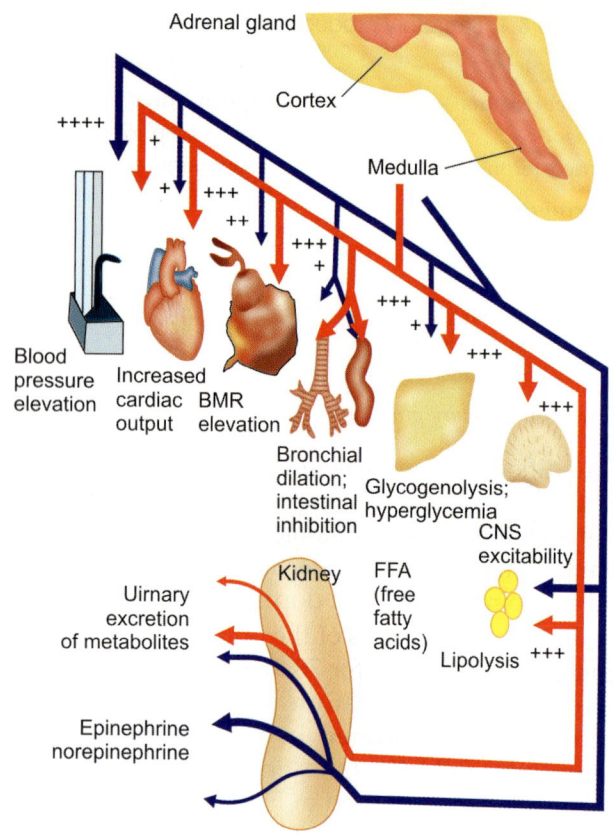

Fig. 8.2: Functions of the adrenal medulla *(Netter's: Atlas of Human Physiology, 1991)*

These hormones supplement the effects of the sympathetic nervous system, but their effects last much longer (about 30 min.) because the hormones circulate in the blood. They prepare the body for physical activity in several ways. They raise the blood pressure and heart rate, increase circulation to the skeletal muscles, increase pulmonary airflow, and inhibit such temporarily in essential functions as digestion and urine formation (Figs 8.1 and 8.2). They stimulate *glycogenolysis* (hydrolysis of glycogen to glucose) and *gluconeogenesis* (the synthesis of glucose from amino acids and other substrates), thus raising the blood glucose level. In order to further ensure an adequate supply of glucose to the brain, epinephrine inhibits insulin secretion and thus, the uptake and use of glucose by the muscles and other insulin-dependent organs. Thus, epinephrine has a glucose-sparing effect, sparing it from needless consumption by organs that can use alternative fuels to ensure that the nervous system has an adequate supply. The use of adrenaline in dental office is mentioned in *Chapter 15, "A": Adrenegic Drug, page 434.*

The medulla and cortex are not as functionally independent as once thought. The boundary between them is indistinct and some cells of the medulla extend into the cortex. When stress activates the sympathetic nervous system, these medullary cells secrete catecholamines that stimulate the cortex to secrete

Table 8.2: Major effects of epinephrine and norepinephrine

Organ or function	Effects of epinephrine	Effects of norepinephrine
Heart and blood vessels	Dilates coronary vessels; dilates arterioles in skeletal muscles; increases heart rate and cardiac output.	Dilates coronary vessels; causes vasoconstrictions in other orgnas; increases heart rate and cardiac output.
Blood pressure	Raises blood pressure because of increased cardiac output and peripheral vasoconstriction.	Raises blood pressure because of peripheral vasoconstriction.
Muscles	Inhibits contraction of smooth muscles of digestive system, producing relaxation; dilates respiratory pathways; decreases rate of fatigue in skeletal muscle; increases respiratory rate.	Relaxes smooth muscle of gastrointestinal tract.
Metabolism	Stimulates glycogenelysis (the breakdown of glycogen to glucose) in liver and muscles, which elevate concentrations of blood glucose and muscle lactic acid; increases oxygen consumption; enhances lipid metabolism; inhibits insulin release from pancreas; providing a ready supply of fatty acids for fuel for skeletal muscles and making glucose available, especially to skeletal muscles and central nervous system during emergencies.	Enhances lipid metabolism and release of free fatty acids from adipose tissue.

corticosterone. Table 8.2 shows major effects of epinephrine and norepinephrine.

II. Adrenal Cortex

The adrenal cortex has three layers of glandular tissue—an outer zona glomerulosa, a thick middle zona fasciculata and an inner zona reticularis (Plate VIII). The cortex synthesizes more than 25 steroid hormones known collectively as the corticosteroids, or corticoids. The three tissue layers secrete, in the same order, the following corticosteroids (Table 8.1):

1. *Mineralocorticoids* (zona glomerulosa only), which act on the kidneys to control electrolyte balance. The principal mineralocorticoid is aldosterone, which promotes Na⁺retention and K⁺excretion by the kidneys.

2. *Glucocorticoids* (mainly zona fasciculata), especially cortisol (hydrocortisone); corticosterone is a less potent relative. Glucocorticoids stimulate fat and protein catabolism, gluconeogenesis, and the release of fatty acids and glucose into the blood. This helps the body adapt to stress and repair damaged tissues. Glucocorticoids also have an anti-inflammatory effect and are widely used in ointments to relieve swelling and other signs of inflammation. Long-term secretion, however, suppresses the immune system for reasons shown in the discussion of stress.

3. *Sex steroids* (mainly zona reticularis), including weak androgens and smaller amounts of estrogens. Androgens control many aspects of male development and reproductive physiology. Adrenal estrogen (estradiol) is of minor importance to women of reproductive age because its quantity is small compared to estrogen from the ovaries. After menopause, however, the ovaries no longer function and the adrenals are the only remaining estrogen source. Both androgens and estrogens promote adolescent skeletal growth and help to sustain adult bone mass.

Cortisol (Cortisone)

"Allows the body to adapt to stress"

The adrenal cortices of normal adults secrete about 30 mg cortisol daily. During periods of extreme stress, this figure has been reported to approach 300 mg. Cortisol secretion normally follows a diurnal pattern.

Peak levels of plasma cortisol occur at about the time of awakening in the morning and lowest in the afternoon and evening. Anticipation of surgery or an athletic event is usually accompanied by only minimal increase in cortisol secretion, but surgery itself is one of the most potent activators of the hypothalamic-pituitary-adrenal (HPA) axis. The greatest response is found to occur in the immediate postoperative period, however, and can be reduced by morphine like anlgesics or by local anesthesia.

Pharmacological Action (Fig. 8.3)

1. *Carbohydrate metabolism:* Cortisone promotes the process of gluconeogenesis, the formation of glucose from the amino acids of protein precursors. It also possesses an anti-insulin properties. As a result, hyperglycemia may occur which could lead to glycosuria.

2. *Protein metabolism:* Cortisone has a catabolic effect leading to negative nitrogen balance, osteoporosis and excess secretion of uric acid.

3. *Fat metabolism:* Cortisone influences the rate of absorption and prolonged administration produces abnormal deposition of fat particularly in the face (Moon's face).

4. *Anti-inflammatory effect:* Cortisone is a powerful anti-inflammatory compound. It inhibits fibrous tissue formation and the process of inflammatory reaction. It masks the infection.

5. *Antirheumatic effect:* Cortisone inhibits the enzyme hyaluronidase which regulates and controls the formation of collagen tissue, it controls the permeability of the capillaries and the synovial membrane.

6. *Healing of wounds:* Cortisone highly delays the healing of wounds due to inhibition of fibrous tissue.

7. *Inhibition of antibody formation:* Cortisone inhibits antibody formation. It is extremely useful whenever it is desirable to depress the process of antibody formation as in transplantation of heterogenous tissues or organs (transplantation of corneal grafts in corneal ulcers, in kidney or liver transplantation).

8. *Anti-allergic properties:* Cortisone and its analogues have anti-allergic effect and suppress the hypersensitivity reactions.They inhibit the antigen–antibody reaction.

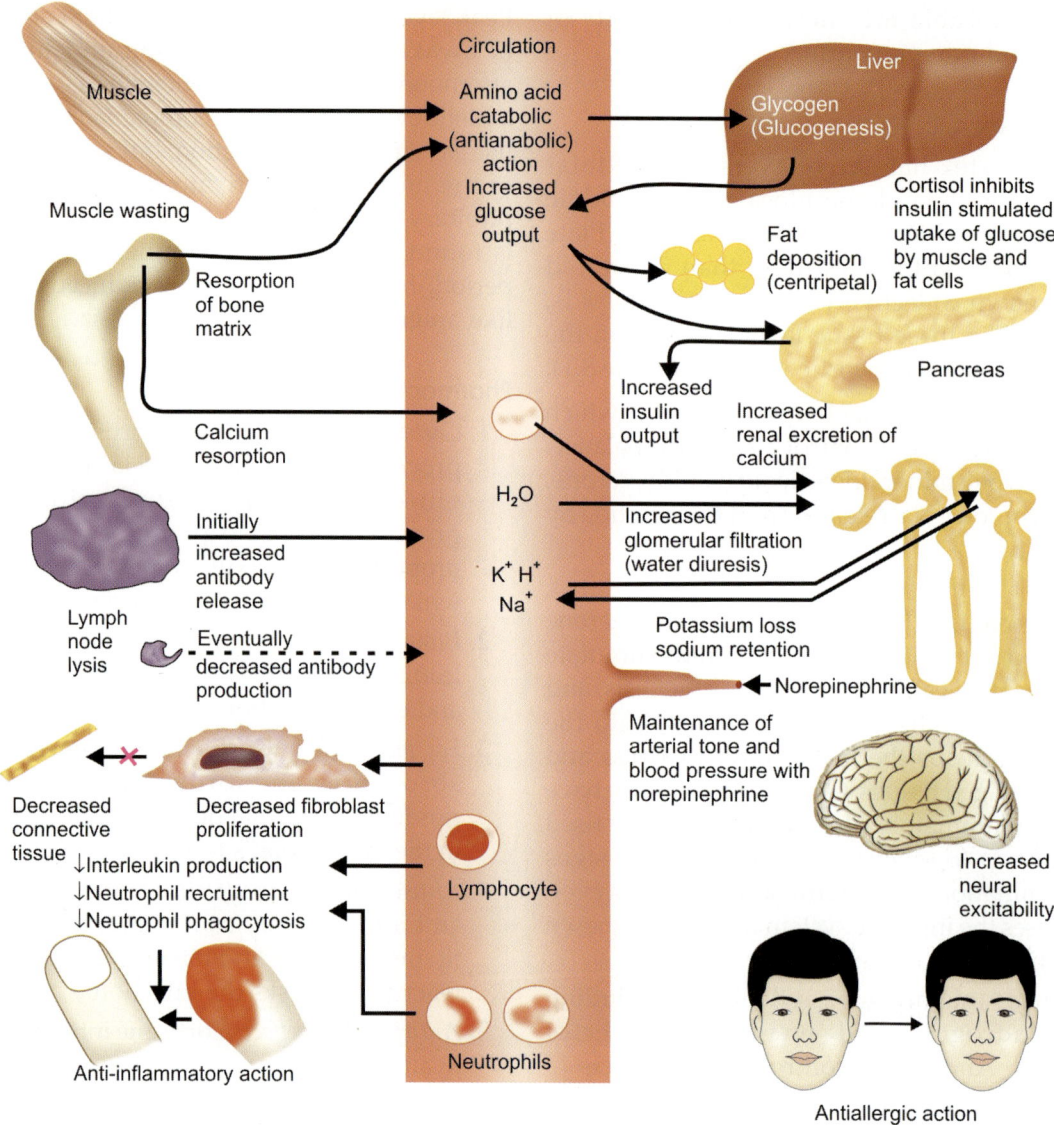

Fig. 8.3: Actions of cortisol. Cortisol has many direct and indirect actions. It causes muscle weakness, fat deposition, hyperglycemia, insulin resistance, osteoporosis, suppression of the immune response (anti-inflammatory), and reduced production of connective tissue that can lead to poor wound healing. At higher levels, it can exhibit mineralocorticoid actions and cause Na+ retention and enhanced K+ and H+ excretion by the kidneys. Cortisol is also necessary for the normal production of epinephrine by the adrenal medulla *(Netter's: Atlas of Human Physiology, 1991)*

9. *Lymphopenic effect:* It inhibits the activity of the lymphatic system producing lymphopenia and reduction in the size of the lymph nodes.
10. *Eosinophilic effect:* It reduces the number of circulating eosinophils.

PRESCRIPTION OF CORTICOSTEROID DRUGS

Glucocorticoid drugs are widely prescribed to replace missing hormones (in Addison's disease, or after adrenalectomy), for immunosuppression, or for the symptomatic relief of a wide variety disorders. Corticosteroids vary tremendously in their potency as anti-inflammatory agents. As a rough guide, 3 mg of dexamethasone, 3 mg betamethasone, 20 mg prednisone and 80 mg hydrocortisone are about equipotent. Synthetic glucocorticoids are used in the treatment of the aforementioned diseases, however, they differ in potency relative to cortisol and in their duration of action. Box 8.1 illustrates the systemic uses of corticoids.

Box 8.1: Systemic uses of corticoids

1. *Cardiovascular diseases:* Shock.
2. *Eye diseases:* Conjunctivitis, glaucoma, keratitis, rhinitis.
3. *Gastrointestinal tract diseases:* Colitis, hepatitis.
4. *Hemopoietic diseases:* Anemia, leukemia, lymphoma, purpura.
5. *Infection and inflammation:* Meningitis, thyroiditis.
6. *Mesenchymal diseases:* Arthritis, rheumatoid, rheumatic fever, lupus erythematosus.
7. *Pulmonary diseases:* Emphysema, silicosis, sarcoidosis.
8. *Mucocutaneous diseases:* Dermatitis, drug eruptions, pemphigus
9. *Renal disorders:* Nephritic syndrome, renal transplants.
10. *Miscellaneous conditions:* Bell's palsy, dental and general surgery, angioneurotic edema, asthma, dermatitis, transfusion reactions. Urticaria and insect bites.

COMPLICATIONS OF SYSTEMIC CORTICOSTEROID THERAPY

Long-term systemic use of corticosteroids can cause many side effects (Boxes 8.2 and 8.3), often beginning soon after the start of treatment. The most significant effect is suppression of ACTH secretion, leading to adrenal atrophy and failure to respond to stress (Fig. 8.4). Corticosteroids in high doses also cause a significant morbidity or mortality, particularly from infection, perforated or bleeding peptic ulcers, diabetes and hypertension and their complications. However, the more immediately obvious effects are of cushingoid weight gain around the face (moon face), buffalo hump, thin translucent skin, and hirsutism. In children, there may be growth retardation.

These complications may be reduced but not abolished, if steroids are given on alternate days. Thus, once the desired therapeutic effect of the steroid is

Box 8.2: Side effects of corticosteroids after long-term systemic use

- Glucocorticoid therapy reduces resistance to infection mainly as a result of its effect on the leukocyte responses. The patient may activate silent endogenous infections and have increased difficulty in combating acquired infections.
- Minor localized infections may spread, and usually nonpathogenic organisms may cause disease.
- Glucocorticoids suppress acute and chronic inflammatory responses, alternate immunologic responses, impair the intracellular killing and delay wound healing processes.
- Blood lymphocytes in corticosteroid-treated patients produce fewer immunoglobulins than normal cells; a direct result is a suppression of antibody levels.

Box 8.3: Complications of systemic corticosteroid therapy

Metabolic suppression	Hypothalamic-pituitary-adrenal suppression, or growth retardation.
	Loss of sodium and potassium
	Osteoporosis
	Fat redistribution (moon face and buffalo hump)
Diabetes mellitus	Impaired glucose tolerance
Immuno suppressive	Increased susceptibility to infections
Cardiovascular	Hypertension
	Myocardial infarction
	Cerebrovascular accidents
Gastrointestinal	Peptic ulcer
Neurological	Mood changes
	Psychosis
	Cataracts
Dermatological	Acne
	Striae
	Bruising
	Neoplasm

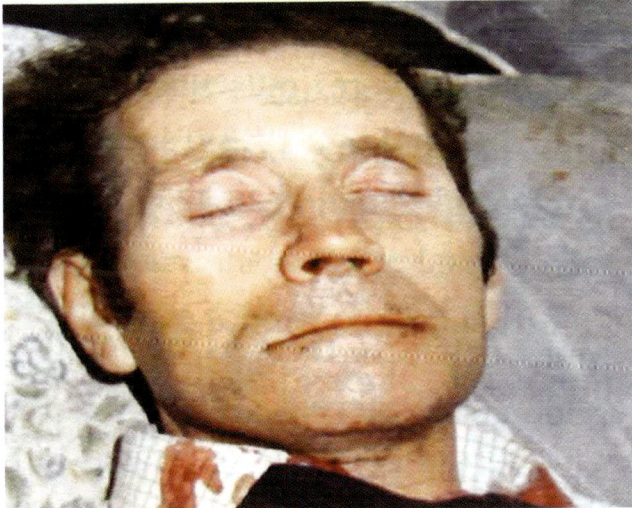

Fig. 8.4: Steroid collapse. This patient, taking only 5 mg prednisolone daily, was given brief sedation for an extraction. Adrenal suppression resulted in collapse and despite considerable doses of corticosteroid and fluid supplementation the patient did not recover fully for 48 hours. *(Cawson RA, Odel EW: Cawson's Essentials of Oral Pathology and Oral Medicine 7th ed., Churchill-Livingstone 2002)*

achieved by daily administration, there should be a transition to giving the entire 48-hour dose as a single early morning dose on alternate days. This is because it is generally presumed that the suppression is more likely with supraphysiologic doses taken daily over an extended period.

The rationale for the alternate day regimen is that the cortisol level normally is high in the morning, so a dose given at that time does not tend to suppress ACTH abnormally, whereas on the off-day, the HPA axis can function normally and produce endogenous steroids. The result is less adrenal suppression than is seen with daily therapy.

Since systemic corticosteroids cause the greatest risk of adrenocortical suppression, it is obvious, therefore, topical steroids should always be used in preference to systemic steroids provided that the desired therapeutic effect is achievable.

However, there can also be adrenocortical suppression from extensive application of steroid skin preparation, particularly if occlusive dressings are use.

Similar comments can be made concerning the use of inhaled corticosteroids, if given in frequent and high doses.

Pathophysiology of Suppression of Adrenal Functions

Corticosteroids are an essential part of the body's response to physiologic or psychologic stresses. The physiologic stresses include traumatic injuries, surgery, infection, acute changes in environmental temperature, severe muscular exercise or burns. Psychologic stress, such as that seen in fearful dental chair may also precipitate adrenal crises.

At times of stress there is normally increased corticosteroid production and the size of the response is related to the degree of stress. In the absence of such a response, there is rapidly developing hypotension, collapse and death, i.e. should the patient be stressed, adrenal suppression that results from exogenous corticosteroids may prevent the normal release of increased amounts of endogenous glucocorticoids needed to help the body meet the elevated metabolic demands.

The hypothalamus is an overall control of adrenocortical function by producing releasing factors that stimulate the pituitary to release adreno-corticotropic hormone (ACTH or corticotropin). ACTH stimulates the production of adrenal corticosteroids. Circulating steroids control hypothalamic activity by negative feedback mechanism.

The function of the hypothalamic-pituitary-adrenocortical axis (HPA) is disrupted, if the pituitary or adrenal cortex ceases to function as a result of trauma, surgery, or disease, or if exogenous corticosteroids are given. Administration of corticosteroids results in negative feedback to the hypothalamus, reduced ACTH secretion and consequent adrenocortical atrophy. The adrenal cortex is then unable to produce the necessary steroid response to stress, and acute adrenal insufficiency (adrenal crisis) is precipitated.

Suppression of the HPA axis becomes deeper as the dose of steroids exceeds physiologic levels (more than 7.5 mg/day of prednisolone), but especially if treatment is prolonged. However, adrenal function may even be suppressed for up to a week after cessation of steroid treatment lasting only 5 days. If steroid treatment is for longer periods, adrenal function may be suppressed for at least 30 days and perhaps for 2–24 months after the cessation of treatment. Adrenal suppression is less when the exogenous steroid is given on alternate days or as a single morning dose (rather than as divided doses through the day). Corticotropin (ACTH) was formerly used in the hope of reducing adrenal suppression, but the response is variable and unpredictable, and wanes with time.

The administration of exogenous glucocorticoids to a patient with functional adrenal cortices may produce adrenocortical hypofunction. The factors influencing the return of adrenal function after exogenous glucocorticoid therapy are:

1. Dose of glucocorticosteroid administered.
2. Duration of course of therapy.
3. Frequency of administration.
4. Time of administration.
5. Route of administration.

Steroids should then be prescribed under the following conditions:

1. There should be no contraindications such as hypertension.
2. The smallest effective dose should be given.
3. The steroid is best given in the morning on alternate days.
4. The patient must be given a warning card and told of the dangers of withdrawal and side effects.
5. There should never be abrupt withdrawal of the steroid.
6. The dose should be increased, if there is illness, infection, trauma, or operation.

Patients who are to be on steroids should have baseline evaluation of their:

1. Weight.
2. Blood pressure.

3. Chest radiograph.
4. Blood glucose.

Prevention of Adrenal Crises

As in many other emergencies, the best treatment is prevention. Patients on, or who have been on, corticosteroid therapy within the past 30 days are at risk from adrenal crisis, and those who have been on them during the previous 24 months may be at risk, if they are not given supplementary corticosteroids before and during the periods of stress.

1. Patients should be warned of this danger and should carry a steroid card indicating the dosage and the responsible physician (Box 8.4) carried at all times by patients on systemic corticosteroids in view of the danger of an adrenocortical crisis and collapse if the patient is subjected to trauma, stress or anesthesia.

2. The Rule of Two's: Adrenocortical function is likely to be suppressed, if a patient is on corticosteroid therapy. In other words, the patient should receive supportive therapy if; he/she has received a dose of 20 mg or more of cortisone or its equivalent daily via the oral or parenteral route for a continuous period of 2 weeks or longer within 2 years of dental therapy.

Evidence indicated that it may take up to 9 months to achieve full recovery of full adrenal function following prolonged exogenous therapy in patients with normal cortices. In stressful situations, there is normally an increased release of glucocorticoids from the adrenal cortices. The hypothalamic-pituitary-adrenocorticoid axis

Box 8.4: Steroid warning card

I am a patient on steroid treatment
Which must not be stopped abruptly, and in case of intercurrent illness may have to be increased.

Instructions

1. **Do not stop** taking the steroid drug except on medical advice. Always have a supply in reserve. In case of feverish illness, accident, operation (emergency or otherwise), diarrhea or vomiting, the steroid treatment must be continued. Your doctor may wish to have a **larger dose** or an **injection** at such times.
2. If the tablets cause indigestion consult your doctor at once.
3. Always carry this card while receiving steroid treatment and show it to any doctor, dentist, nurse, or midwife whom you may consult.
4. You must still tell any new doctor, dentist, nurse or midwife that you have had steroid treatment.

mediates this increase; which normally results in a rapid elevation of glucocorticoid blood levels. Most cases of mortality and major morbidity that accompany adrenal insufficiency are usually secondary to hypotension or hypoglycemia.

In this concern, the rule of Two's has to be respected. The patient who gives a history of taking or who has taken any of the steroids should be fortified by an additional dose of the drug preceding the appointment.

3. Minor operations under local anesthesia may be covered by giving oral steroids 2–4 hours pre- and postoperatively (100 mg hydrocortisone, or 20 mg prednisolone, or 4 mg dexamethasone) or better by giving intravenous hydrocortisone immediately before operation. Intravenous hydrocortisone must be immediately available for use, if the patient collapses or the blood pressure falls. Topical corticosteroids for use in the mouth are unlikely to have any systemic effect but predispose to oral candidiasis.

4. General anesthesia must be given only in hospital by a specialist anesthetist. Cover should be provided, by giving at least 100–200 mg hydrocortisone sodium succinate intramuscularly or intravenously (with the premedication) and then 6-hourly for a further 24–72 hours. The blood pressure must also be carefully watched during surgery and especially during recovery, and steroid supplementation given immediately, if the blood pressure starts to fall. Corticosteroids given by intramuscular injection are more slowly absorbed and reach lower plasma levels than when given intravenously or orally.

5. Aspirin and other non-steroidal anti-inflammatory agents should be avoided as they may increase the risk of peptic ulceration in those on corticosteroids. Osteoporosis introduces the danger of fractures when handling the patient.

Management of Acute Adrenal Insufficiency (Table 8.3)

Acute adrenal insufficiency is a true medical emergency in which the victim is in immediate danger

Table 8.3: Management of acute adrenal insufficiency

Minimal stress	Double the daily dose. This is typical for an oral surgery appointment.
Moderate stress	100 mg hydrocortisone daily
Severe stress	200 mg hydrocortisone daily

The patient's physician should be contacted to adjust the dose of steroids.

due to glucocorticoid (cortisol) insufficiency. Mental confusion, muscle weakness, intense pain in the abdomen, lower back and legs, extreme fatigue, nausea and vomiting, and hypotension. Peripheral vascular collapse (shock), and ventricular asystole (cardiac arrest) are the usual cause of death, however, hypotension and hypoglycemia are the usual complications of adrenal crisis. Acute adrenal insufficiency should be **suspected** in patients who exhibit mental confusion, nausea, vomiting, diarrhea, abdominal pain, weakness, fatigue, weight loss, hyperpigmentation (skin, mucous membrane) and who currently are receiving glucocorticoids or have received 20 mg or more cortisone (or its equivalent) via oral or parenteral administration for 2 weeks or longer within the past 2 years.

When acute adrenal insufficiency develops:

1. Lay the patient flat with the legs raised.
2. Give 200 mg hydrocortisone intravenously.
3. Summon medical assistance.
4. Take blood for glucose and electrolyte estimation.
5. Give glucose, if there is hypoglycemia (25 g orally or intravenously).
6. Put up an intravenous infusion of normal saline or glucose-saline. Give 1 liter over 2 hours together with 200 mg hydrocortisone sodium succinate, repeating this at 4–6 hourly intervals as required and monitor the blood pressure.
7. Control of pain and infection is particularly important and steroid supplementation must be continued for at least 3 days after the blood pressure has returned to normal. Refer to Chapter 15, "I" Adrenal Insufficiency, page 447.

HYPER- AND HYPOSECRETION OF CORTISOL

  i. Cushing's syndrome—excess of cortisol.
 ii. Addison's disease—lack of cortisol

I. Hypersecretion

Clinically, cortisol hypersecretion is referred to as Cushing's syndrome, a condition that can normally be corrected through surgical removal of part or all of the adrenal gland. Hypersecretion of cortisol leads to increased fat deposition in certain areas, such as the face and the upper back. (often called a buffalo hump), abdominal striae, elevates blood pressure, and alters blood cells distribution (eosinopenia and lympho-penia). Other findings may include glucose intolerance (e.g. diabetes mellitus), heart failure, osteoporosis and bone fractures, impaired healing, and psychiatric disorders (mental depression, mania, anxiety disorders, cognitive dysfunction, and psychosis). Hypersecretion of cortisol usually does not result in the acute life-threatening situation that is noticed with acute cortisol deficiency.

Also hypersecretion of cortisol or the administration of high doses of this hormone results in osteoporosis. This occurs because of the excessive protein catabolism which inhibits new bone formation, while at the same time glucocorticoids inhibit the activity of vitamin D and increase glomerular infiltration. These activities lead to a loss of calcium and demineralization of bone. Clinically, there may be collapse of vertebrae, pathologic hip fracture, and skeletal deformities.

Cushing's Syndrome
(American physician Harvey Gushing 1869–1939)

Cushing's syndrome is a complex of symptoms and signs consequent upon a persistent and inappropriate elevation of glucocorticoid levels.

The most common cause of Cushing's syndrome is iatrogenic, due to the administration of steroids for a number of conditions as shown before. The next most common cause is hypersecretion of ACTH from the pituitary gland and is referred to as Cushing's disease. Over 90% of these patients have a microadenoma of the pituitary gland. Other causes of Cushing's syndrome include excess secretion of cortisol from an adrenocortical tumor, and rarely ectopic ACTH secretion from a variety of tumors, particularly of the bronchus or an adrenal carcinoma.

Cushing's disease can occur at any age, and is more common in females, with a sex ratio of approximately 10:1. All the signs and symptoms mentioned before in hyperadrenalism are present in Cushing's syndrome, particularly the moon-shaped faces, and the buffalo hump appearance of the upper back (Figs 8.5 to 8.8).

Classically, the face is rounded and is described as "moon". The cheeks appear prominent and flushed, giving a descriptive robust appearance (Fig. 8.8). There is generalized obesity, particularly of the trunk and this has been described as a 'Lemon on matchsticks'. The skin appears thin, fragile, extensive bruising, and shows multiple purple striae (Figs 8.9 to 8.11). There is a great susceptibility to infection and poor wound healing. In children, there is arrested growth and in

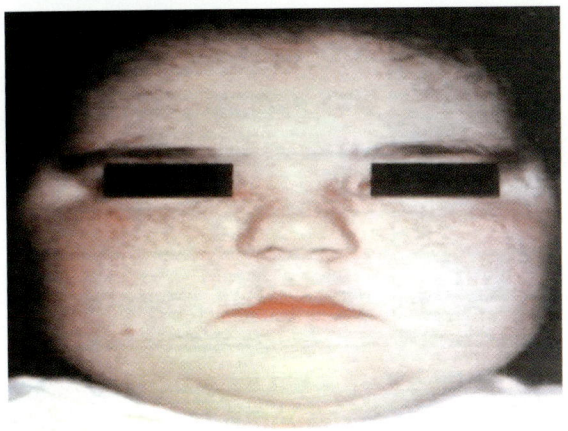

Fig. 8.5: Cushing's syndrome. The rounded face features (moon's face) of this patient are due to the abnormal deposition of fat, which is induced by excess of corticosteroid hormone

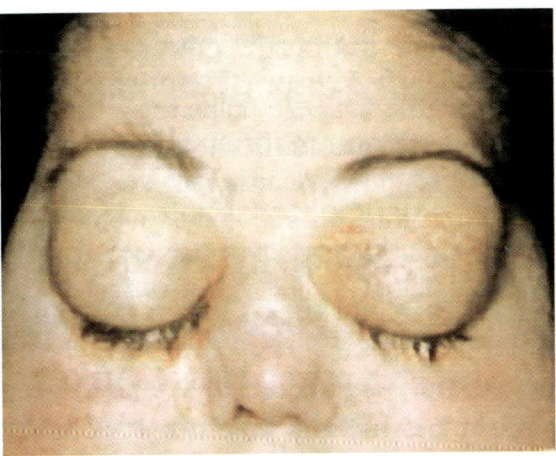

Fig. 8.6: Facial features of Cushing's syndrome

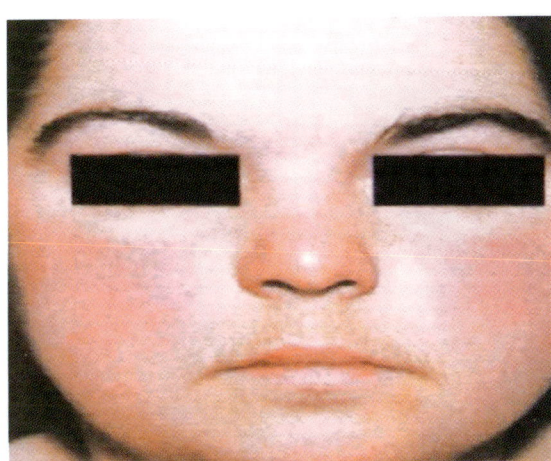

Fig. 8.7: The typical facial features of Cushing's syndrome. The patient has a moon face with erythema and hirsuties. Identical appearances may result from corticosteroid therapy

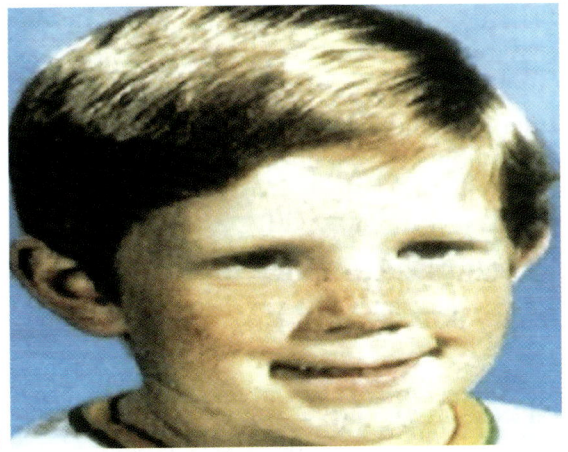

(A)

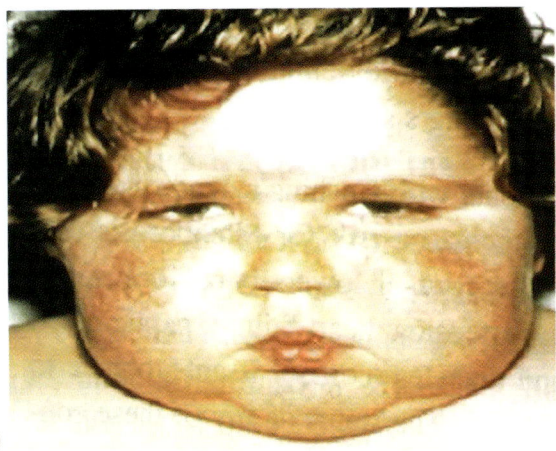

(B)

Fig. 8.8: Cushing syndrome. **(A)** Patient before the onset of the syndrome. **(B)** The same boy, only 4 months later, showing the moon face characteristic of Cushing's syndrome. *(Saladin: Anatomy and Physiology: The Unity of Form and Function. 3rd ed. McGraw-Hill Co. 2003)*

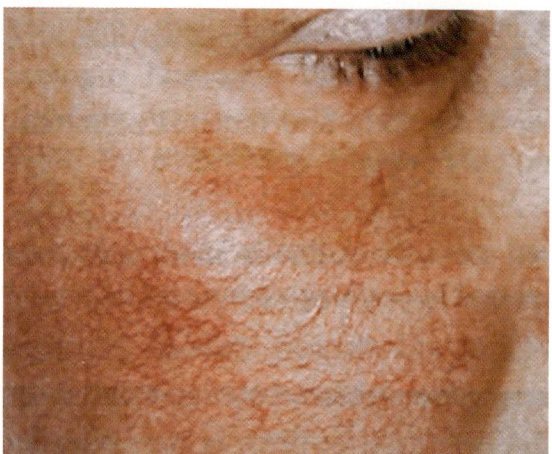

Fig. 8.9: Cushing's syndrome is associated with typical thin skin and fragile blood vessels. Bruising commonly results from very minor trauma

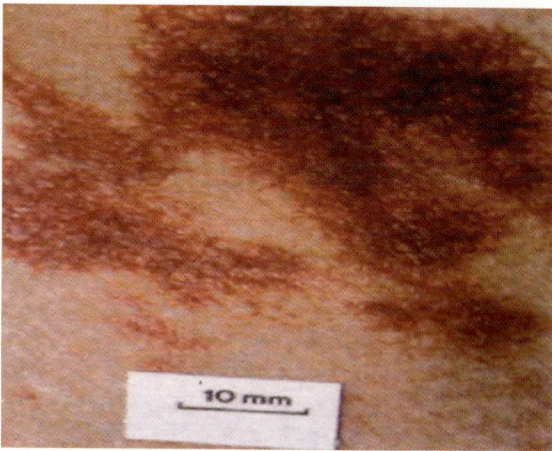

Fig. 8.11: Thin, fragile skin in Cushing's syndrome and blood vessels fragility have resulted in extensive bruising

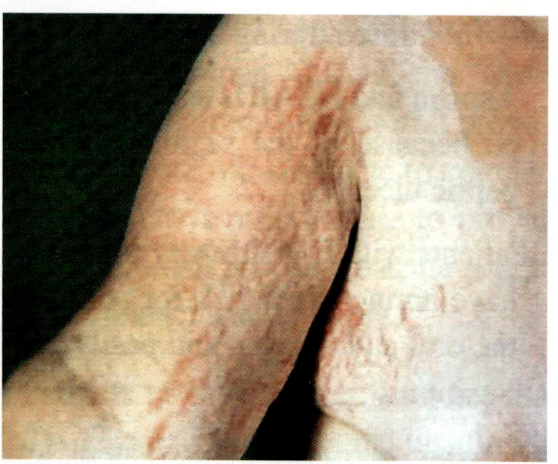

Fig. 8.10: Cushing's syndrome. This patient has typical purple striae on the breast and arm, associated with thinning of the skin

girls, there is masculinization. Hypertension is common in all age groups, about one-third of patients have associated diabetes and hypercalciuria may result in renal stones. Osteoporosis also occurs in all age groups and may result in spontaneous fractures, particularly of the axial skeleton.

Dental Precautions

The following are dental alerts associated with Cushing's syndrome:

1. Patients with Cushing's syndrome have an increased risk for osteoporosis (because cortisol lowers bone formation), hypertension, heart failure, peptic ulcer, and diabetes (cortisol is antagonistic to insulin). The status of any of these conditions when present must be assessed and dental management accordingly modified following the disease/condition-specific suggested.

2. The blood pressure should be routinely monitored during dentistry.

3. Aspirin and NSAIDs should be avoided because of the high incidence of peptic ulcer.

4. Patients with Gushing's syndrome also have an increased risk for periodontitis, oral candidiasis, and easily bleeding gums.

5. Excess steroids in the system lower the immune system activity and this increases the risk of infections and poor wound healing.

6. The practitioner should also provide adequate antibiotic coverage for 5–7 days following a major surgical procedure to promote the healing process.

7. The practitioner should assess and treat the oral cavity for oral and esophageal candidiasis when present.

8. Generalized osteoporosis can also affect the mandible and patients with dentures may need frequent adjustments.

II. Hyposecretion of Cortisol

Adrenal insufficiency first was recognized by Addison in 1844, thus primary adrenocortical insufficiency is called Addison's disease. It develops as a result of atrophy of the adrenal cortices and failure of secretion of cortisol and aldosterone. Today renal and adrenal surgeries are important factors in the development of primary adrenocortical insufficiency.

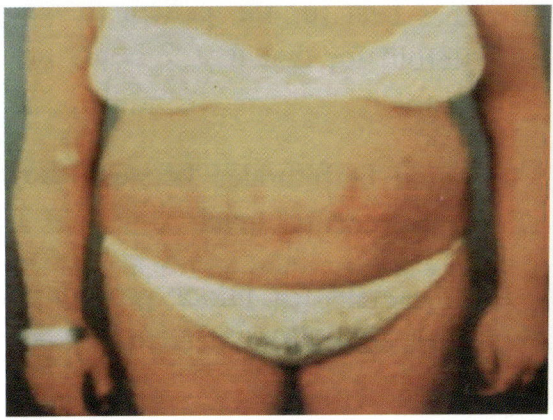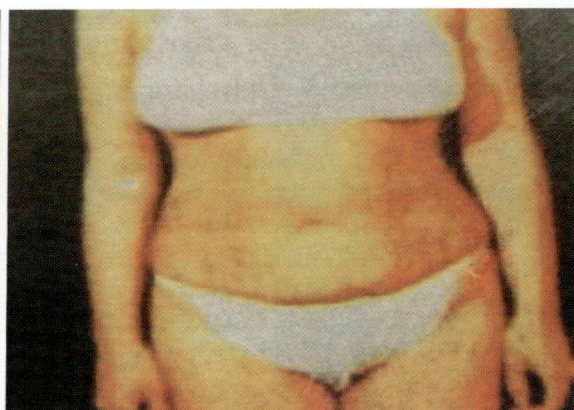

Fig. 8.12: Cushing's syndrome. **(A)** Clinical features of a patient with Cushing's disease before treatment. **(B)** The same patient 1 year after the successful removal of an ACTH-secreting pituitary microadenoma by transsphenoidal surgery

Addison's Disease

The term adrenal insufficiency signifies a reduced ability of the adrenal cortex to produce cortisol to meet physiologic demands. The most common complaints of patient with hypoadrenalism are weakness, fatigue, and abnormal pigmentation of the skin and mucous membranes (Fig. 8.13).

Lack of cortisol predisposes to hypotension and hypoglycemia and adrenal crisis. Lack of aldosterone leads to Na depletion, reduced extracellular volume and hypotension, i.e. there is excessive loss of sodium chloride and water in urine and the retention of potassium due to deficient secretion of sodium retaining hormones, particularly aldosterone; as a result hemo-concentration, hypotension and dehydration occur. Anorexia and weight loss are additional common findings.

If a patient with Addison's disease is challenged by stress (e.g. illness, infection, surgery), an adrenal crisis may be precipitated. This medical emergency manifests as severe exacerbation of the patient's condition, including sunken eyes, profuse sweating, hypotension, weak pulse, cyanosis, nausea, vomiting, weakness, headache, dehydration, fever, dyspnea and myalgia. If not treated rapidly, the patient may develop hypothermia, severe hypotension, hypoglycemia, and circulatory collapse that can result in death.

Suggested Dental Outlines

1. Patient's with Addison's disease have to be compensated with steroids to fight the stress associated with infection; inflammation; excessive bleeding; post-procedure starvation; pre- and postoperative pain (very high-risk factor); and trauma associated with surgery, due to lack of cortisol and aldosterone.

2. The dentist must consult with the patient's physician during the above mentioned circumstances and provide adequate steroid coverage to compensate for the stress. Failure to provide coverage will precipitate acute adrenal insufficiency and collapse.

3. Patients taking steroids for more than 2 weeks may have adrenal insufficiency and consequently require additional steroid coverage for up to 2 years after treatment.

4. Oral infections must be aggressively treated in the Addison's disease patient to prevent hypoadrenal crisis or acute adrenal insufficiency from happening.

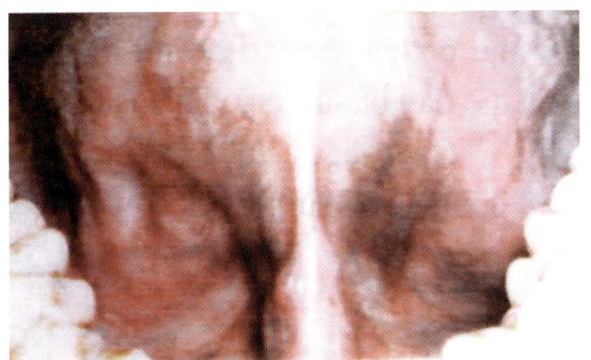

Fig. 8.13: Addison's disease. Diffuse pigmentation of the floor of the mouth and ventral tongue in a patient with Addison's disease

5. Addison's patient benefit when given stress management with benzodiazepines or O_2 + N_2O because stress reduction decreases cortisol demand.

6. It is best to treat the patient as the first appointment of the day because the cortisol secretion is at its highest in the morning between 2 and 8 am. Cortisol secretion is lowest toward the end of the day.

7. Individuals working the night shift have a circadian rhythm reversal' and maximum cortisol release occurs during early evening', when they are awake.

8. If the patient is currently on steroids, it is best for the patient to take the steroid for that day, 2 hours prior to dentistry.

9. Avoid barbiturates because they decrease cortisol level.

10. Typically for minor procedures, no extra steroids are needed.

11. For major procedures, give 25–40 mg prednisolone PO, one hour prior to treatment on the day of surgery and taper over 2 days. Alternatively, you can give 100–150 mg IV/IM hydrocortisone, one hour prior to the procedure, if the patient has to be nil-by mouth on the day of surgery. This is followed by a taper back to baseline within 48 hours, once surgery is completed.

9

Thyroid and Parathyroid Glands

Thyroid Gland
   Anatomy
   Physiology

- Hyperthyroidism
   Dental Aspects
   Dental Management

- Hypothyroidism
   Cretinism
   Myxedema
   Dental Management

Parathyroid Glands
   Anatomy and Physiology

- Hyperparathyroidism
   Frequency and Incidence
   Etiology/Pathophysiology
   Signs and Symptoms
   Management
- Hypoparathyroidism
   Pathophysiology
   Dental Aspects

THYROID GLANDS

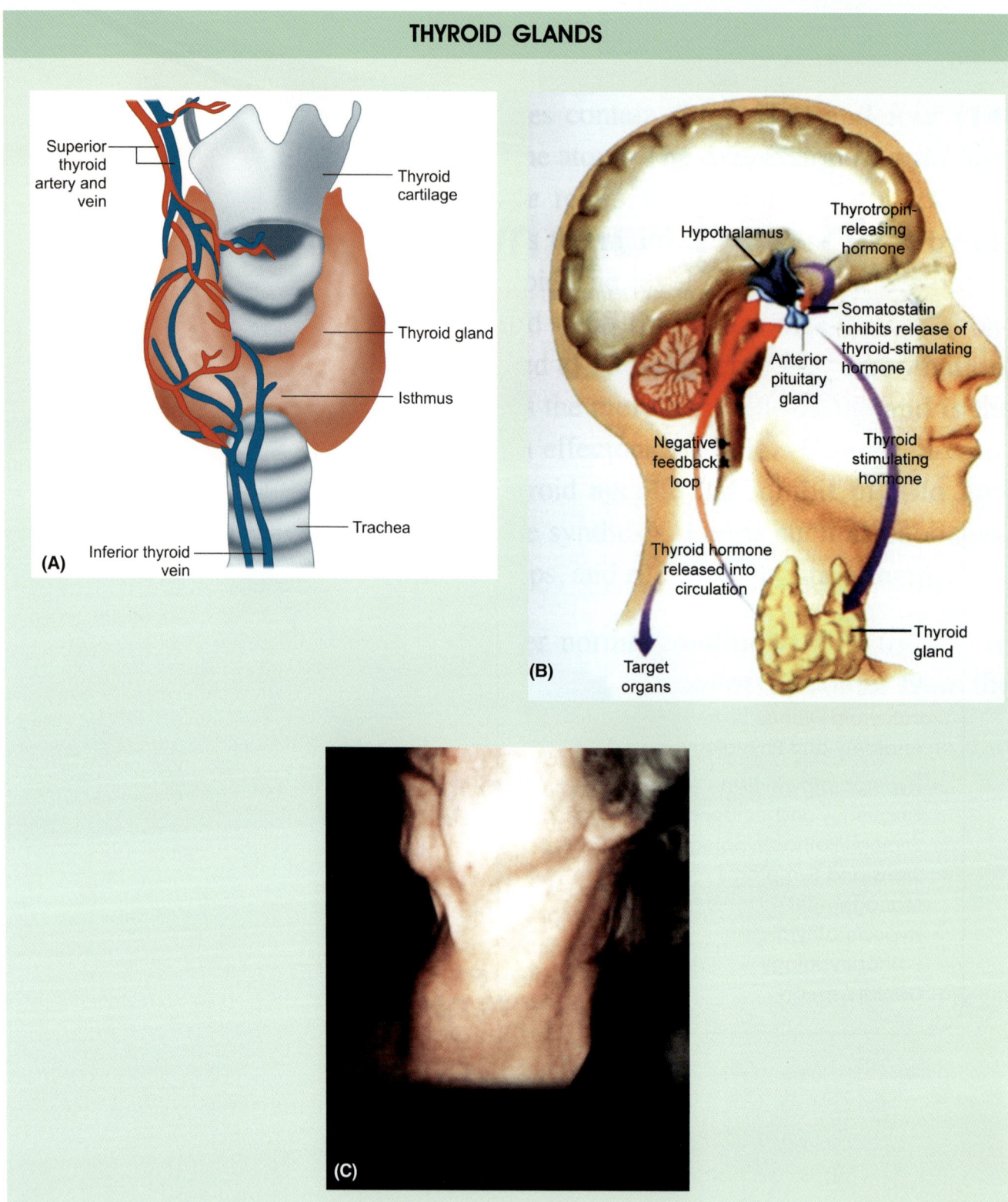

Plate IX: (A) The thyroid gland: Gross anatomy. **(B)** A negative feedback loop exists between the thyroid gland, the anterior pituitary gland and hypothalamus to prevent the oversecretion of hormones *(Marini et al, 2008)*. **(C)** Diffuse midline neck enlargement of the thyroid gland due to Graves' disease (goiter) *(Little et al, 2008)*

ANATOMY

The thyroid gland is the largest endocrine gland; it weighs 20 to 25 g and receives one of the body's highest rates of blood flow per gram of tissue. It is wrapped around the anterior and lateral aspects of the trachea, immediately below the larynx. It consists of two large lobes, one on each side of the trachea, connected by a narrow anterior *isthmus* (Plate IX-A).

PHYSIOLOGY

Histologically, the thyroid is composed mostly of sacs called thyroid follicles (Fig. 9.1). Each is filled with a protein-rich colloid and lined by a simple cuboidal epithelium of follicular cells. These cells secrete two main thyroid hormones—T3 or triiodothyronine, and thyroxine, also known as T4 or tetraiodothyronine. These names refer to the fact that the two hormones contain three (T3) and four (T4) iodine atoms.The expression *thyroid hormone* refers to T3 and T4 collectively. T4 is the main hormone secreted by the thyroid. The level of T4 in the peripheral blood is 60 times that of T3. T4 is converted to T3 peripherally by deiodination. T3 is the more active hormone and is the main effector principle. Goitrins are antithyroid agents that inhibit thyroid hormone synthesis. Foods such as cabbages, turnips, and rutabagas contain them.

Under normal conditions, 10 to 20% of the circulating pool of T3 comes from the thyroid gland and the rest comes from the monoiodination of T4. In cases of hyperthyroidism, 30 to 40% of circulating T3 comes from the thyroid.

The conversion of T4 to T3 can be inhibited by fasting, illness, steroids, and certain drugs (e.g. propylthiouracil). Iodine must be available for the synthesis of T4 and T3. The inorganic form of iodine as used by the gland comes from the peripheral degradation and deiodination of thyroid hormone and the diet. The minimum daily requirement of iodine is about 75 mg, and a typical 2800 calorie daily intake will contain some 700 mg of iodine.

The binding plasma proteins are thyroid-binding globulin (TBG), thyroid binding prealbumin (TBPA), and thyroid binding albumin (TEA). TBPA binds only to T4. TEA binds poorly to both T4 and T3. TBG binds both T4 and T3 but has less affinity for T3. Therefore, the free circulating level of T3 (FT3) is nearly 10 times greater than the free level of T4 (FT4).

Under normal conditions, thyrotropin-releasing hormone (TRH) is released by the hypothalamus in response to external stimuli (stress, illness, metabolic demand, and low levels of T3 and to a lesser degree T4). TRH stimulates the pituitary to release the thyroid-stimulating hormone (TSH), which causes the thyroid gland to secrete T4 and T3.

Blood levels of T3 and T4 are controlled through a servofeedback mechanism mediated by the hypothalamic-pituitary-thyroid axis (Plate IX-B, Fig. 9.2). Increased or decreased metabolic demand appears to be the main modifier of the system. Drugs, illness, thyroid disease, and pituitary disorders can affect the control of this balance. Recent findings also show that age has some effect on the system.

The sites of action for thyroid hormones are the cell nucleus, mitochondria, cell membrane, adrenergic receptor pathway, and tyrosine metabolic pathway. In the adrenergic receptor pathway, the thyroid hormones increase the number of receptors and amplify the beta adrenergic signal. The tyrosine

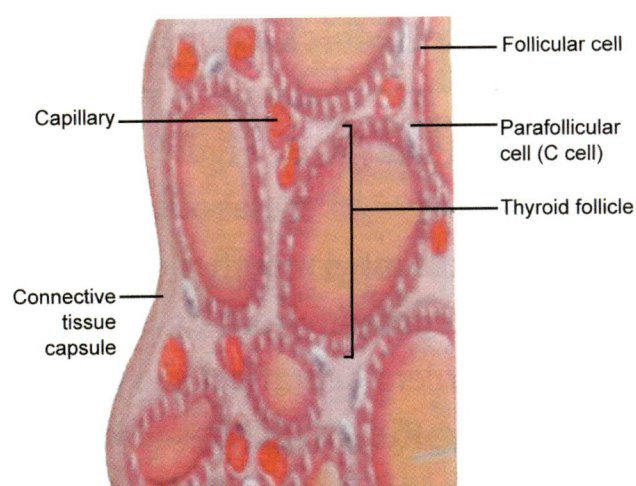

Fig. 9.1: The thyroid gland—Histology

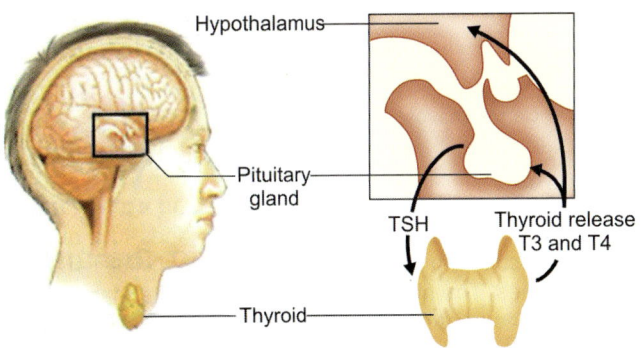

Fig. 9.2: The hypothalamic-pituitary-thyroid axis

metabolic pathway is modified by the hormones to increase alternate adrenergic neurotransmitters. Calcitonin is involved, along with parathyroid hormone and vitamin D, in regulating serum calcium and phosphorus levels and skeletal remodeling.

Thyroid hormone (TH) is secreted in response to TSH from the pituitary. The primary effect of TH is to increase the body's metabolic rate. As a result, it raises oxygen consumption and has a **calorigenic effect.** It increases heat production. TH secretion rises in cold weather and thus helps to compensate for increased heat loss. To ensure an adequate blood and oxygen supply to meet this increased metabolic demand, thyroid hormone also raises the heart rate and contraction strength and raises the respiratory rate. It accelerates the breakdown of carbohydrates, fats, and protein for fuel and stimulates the appetite. Thyroid hormone promotes alertness, bone growth and remodeling, the development of the skin, hair, nails, and teeth, and fetal nervous system and skeletal development (Fig. 9.3). It also stimulates the pituitary gland to secrete growth hormone.

Calcitonin is another hormone produced by the thyroid gland. It comes from (calcitonin) cells, also called *parafollicular cells,* found in clusters between the thyroid follicles. Calcitonin is secreted when blood calcium level rises. Calcitonin lowers the calcium and phosphate concentration in the blood, in direct contrast to the action of parathyroid hormone secreted by the parathyroid glands, which increases blood calcium. It promotes calcium deposition and bone formation by stimulating osteoblast activity. Calcitonin is important mainly to children. Calcitonin is secreted when the blood calcium concentration rises too high, and it lowers the concentration by two principal mechanisms (Fig. 9.4):

1. *Osteoclast inhibition:* Within 15 minutes after it is secreted, calcitonin reduces osteoclast activity by as much as 70%, so osteoclasts liberate less calcium from the skeleton.

2. *Osteoblast stimulation:* Within an hour, calcitonin increases the number and activity of osteoblasts, which deposit calcium into the skeleton. Calcitonin plays an important role in children but has little effect in most adults. The osteoclasts of children are highly active in skeletal remodeling and release 5 g or more of calcium into the blood each day. By inhibiting this activity, calcitonin can significantly lower the blood calcium level in

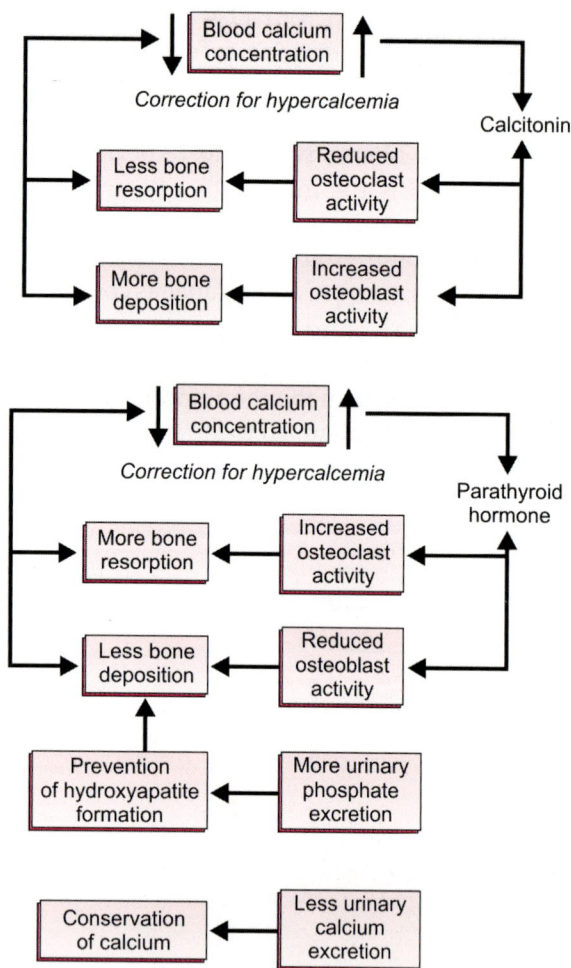

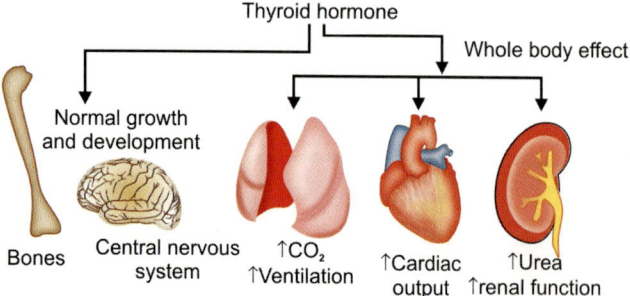

Fig. 9.3: Thyroid hormone action (T4) is converted to triiodothyronine (T3) at target tissues. T3 binds to a nuclear receptor, resulting in transcription of a host of a cellular proteins and enzymes. The net effect is an increase of metabolic rate and O_2 consumption. These effects are associated with increased heart, lung, and kidney function. T3 is also important for normal growth and development

Fig. 9.4: Negative feedback loops in calcium homeostasis. **(A)** The correction of hypercalcemia by calcitonin. **(B)** The correction of hypocalcemia by parathyroid hormone

children. In adults, however, the osteoclasts release only about 0.8 g of calcium per day. Calcitonin cannot change adult blood calcium very much by suppressing this minor contribution. Calcitonin deficiency is not known to cause any adult disease. Calcitonin may, however, prevent bone loss in pregnant and lactating women, and it is useful for reducing bone loss in osteoporosis.

Thyroid gland dysfunction may occur either through overproduction (hyperthyroidism) or underproduction (hypothyroidism) of thyroid hormones. In both instances, the observed clinical manifestations may encompass a broad-spectrum, ranging from subclinical dysfunction to acute life-threatening situations. Fortunately, most patients with thyroid dysfunction suffer the milder forms of the disease.

HYPERTHYROIDISM (THYROTOXICOSIS)

The term thyrotoxicosis refers to an excess of T4 and T3 in the bloodstream. This excess may be caused by ectopic thyroid tissue, Graves' disease, multinodular goiter, thyroid adenoma, or pituitary disease involving the anterior portion of the gland. Graves' disease will be discussed here as a model for other conditions that can result in similar clinical manifestations.

Hyperthyroid patients exhibit exaggerated responses to vasoactive drugs and catecholamines and may be prone to cardiac arrhythmias.

Signs and Symptoms

The clinical features of thyrotoxicosis are illustrated in Fig. 9.5. The clinical picture in Graves' disease is a swelling of varying dimensions of the neck region (Figs 9.6 to 9.8 and Box 9.1). The direct and indirect effects of the excessive thyroid hormones is manifested as follows (Fig. 9.5, Box 9.1).

1. Thyroid hormones produce an increase in the body energy consumption and an elevation of the basal metabolic rate. The increased use of energy results in fatigue and weight loss.
2. The patient's skin is warm and moist, the complexion rosy, and the patient may blush readily. Palmer erythema may be present, profuse sweating is common, and excessive melanin pigmentation of the skin occurs in many patients; however; pigmentation of the oral mucosa has not been reported. The patient's hair becomes fine and friable, and the nails soften.
3. Most patients show eye-changes: Retraction of the upper eye-lid, a bright eye stare, lid lag, and jerky movements of the lids. The exopthalmos may be unilateral during initial phases of the disease but

Box 9.1: Clinical findings in the patient with thyrotoxicosis

Skeletal system
- Increased bone turn over
- Rate of resorption exceeds that of formation
- Osteoporosis (common in elderly)

Cardiovascular system
- Palpitations
- Tachycardia
- Arrhythmias (10 to 15% atrial fibrillation)
- Cardiomegaly
- Congestive heart failure
- Angina, myocardial infarction

Gastrointestinal system
- Weight loss—may have increased appetite
- Decreased absorption of vitamin A
- Pernicious anemia (3%)

Central nervous system
- Anxiety, restlessness
- Sleep disturbances
- Emotional liability
- Impaired concentration
- Weakness
- Tremors (hands, fingers, tongue)

Skin
- Erythema
- Hyperpigmentation
- Thin fine hair, areas of alopecia
- Soft nails—may lift from distal bed

Eyes
- Retraction of upper lid, exopthalmos
- Corneal ulceration, ocular muscle weakness

Others
- Increased risk of diabetes mellitus
- Decreased serum cholesterol level
- Increased risk of thrombocytopenia

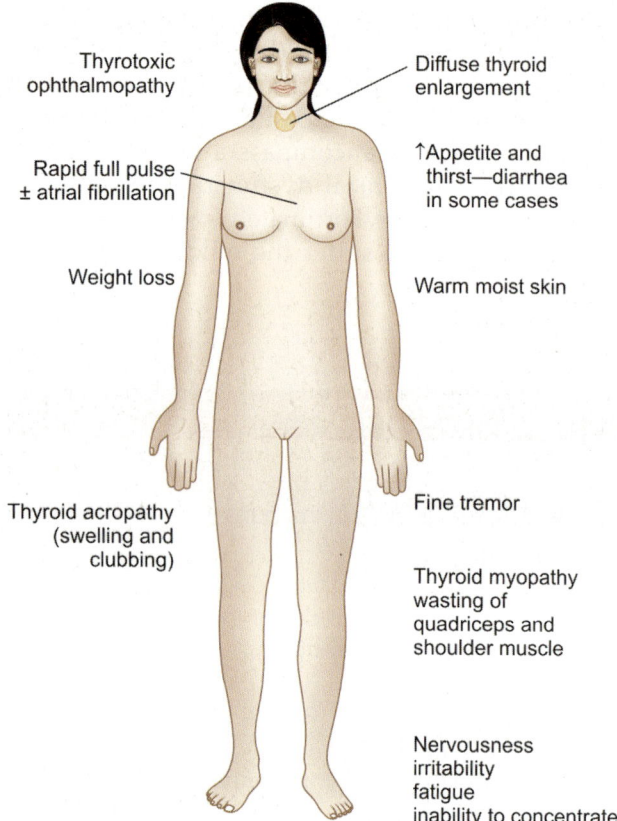

Thyrotoxic ophthalmopathy

Diffuse thyroid enlargement

Rapid full pulse ± atrial fibrillation

↑Appetite and thirst—diarrhea in some cases

Weight loss

Warm moist skin

Thyroid acropathy (swelling and clubbing)

Fine tremor

Thyroid myopathy wasting of quadriceps and shoulder muscle

Nervousness irritability fatigue inability to concentrate

Fig. 9.5: Clinical features of thyrotoxicosis

usually progresses to bilaterality (Figs 9.9 and 9.11). Corneal ulceration, optic neuritis, and ocular muscle weakness may develop as complications in these patients.

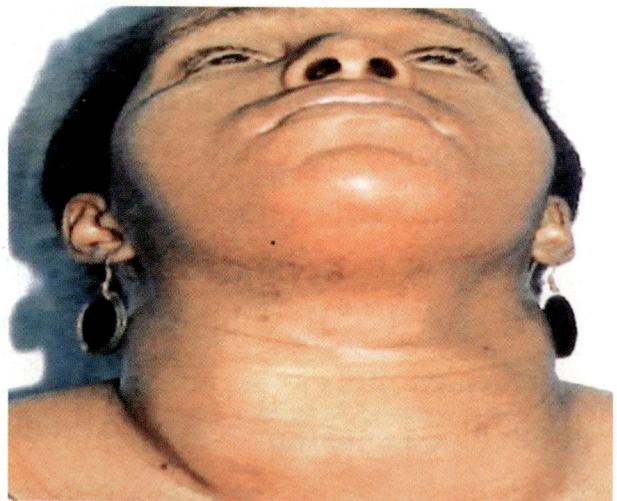

Fig. 9.6: Multinodular goiter. *(From Swartz MH, Textbook of Physical Diagnosis: History and Examination, 5th ed. Philadelphia, Saunders, 2006)*

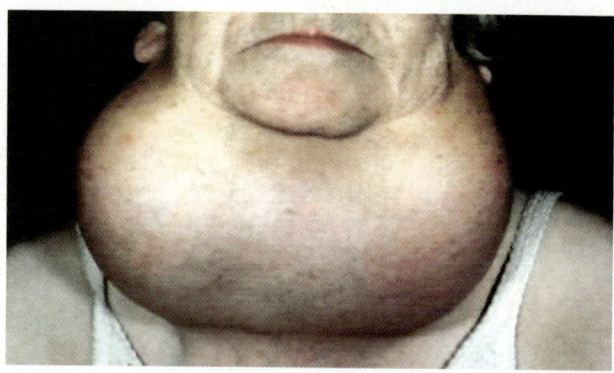

Fig. 9.7: Endemic goiter. The thyroid gland is hypertrophied as a result of iodine deficiency leading to TSH hypersecretion. *(Saladin: Anatomy and Physiology: The Unity of Form and Function. 3rd ed. McGraw-Hill Co. 2003)*

4. Cardiovascular findings in hyperthyroid patients are related to the direct actions of thyroid hormones on the myocardium. They are characterized by a hyperdynamic, electrically excitable state. Also the increased metabolic activity caused by excessive hormone secretion increases circulatory demands and increased cardiac workload, increased stroke volume and heart rate often develop in addition to widened pulse pressure, resulting in patient's complaining of palpitation.

Supraventricular cardiac dysrhythmias develop in many patients. Congestive heart failure may occur and often is somewhat resistant to the effects of digitalis. Patients with untreated or

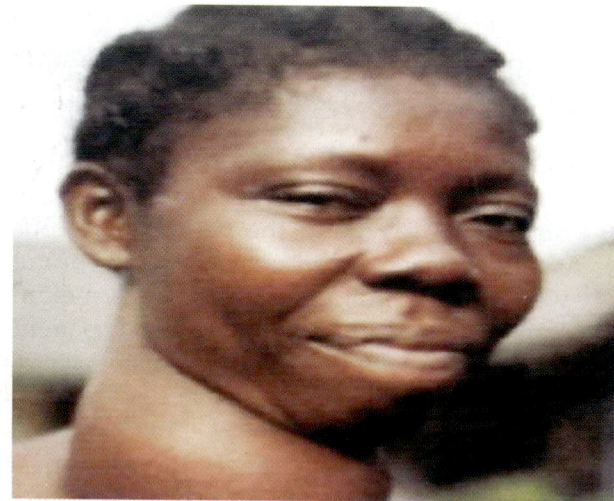

Fig. 9.8: Endemic goiter is caused by dietary iodine deficiency *(McKliney and O'Loughlin, 2006)*

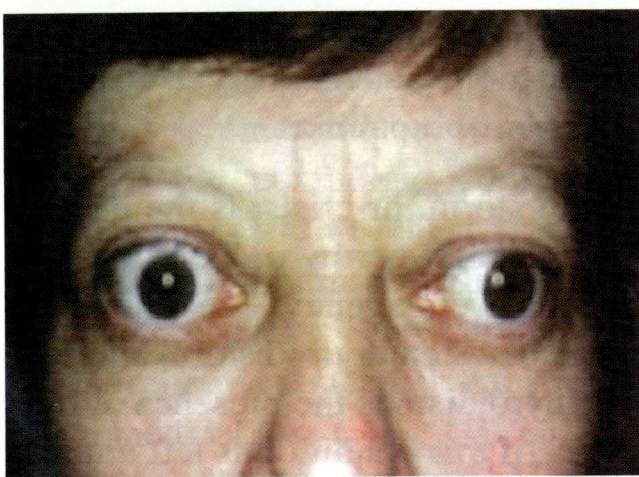

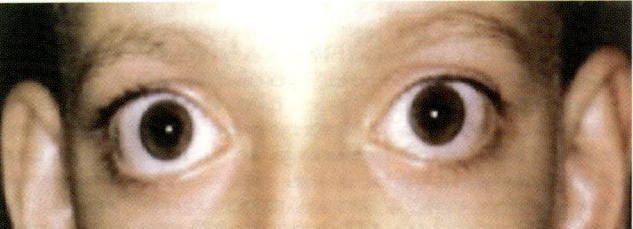

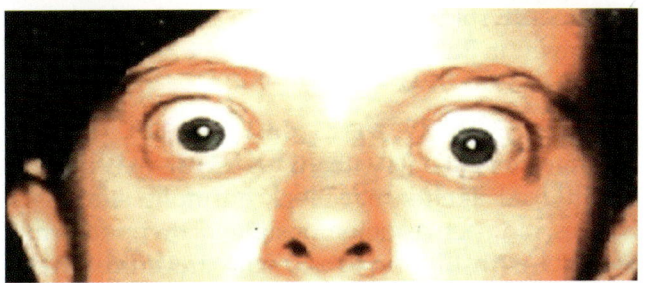

Fig. 9.9: Individuals with Graves' disease (hyperthyroidism) exhibit exopthalmos, bulging and protruding eyeballs resulting from an increase in volume of the orbital contents *(A. Goldman L, Ausiello D Cecil. Textbook of Medicine, 22 ed. Philadelphia, Saunders, 2004. B. Seidel H. Mosby's Guide to Physical Examination. 4th ed. St. Louis, Mosby, 1999)*

Fig. 9.11: Proptosis in Graves' disease results from enlargement of muscles and fat within the orbit as a result of mucopolysaccharide infiltration *(A. From goldman L, Ausiello D. Cecil Textbook of Medicine, 22nd ed. Philadelphia, Saunders, 2004. B. From Seidel H, Mosby's guide to Physical Examination, 4th ed. St. Louis, Mosby, 1999)*

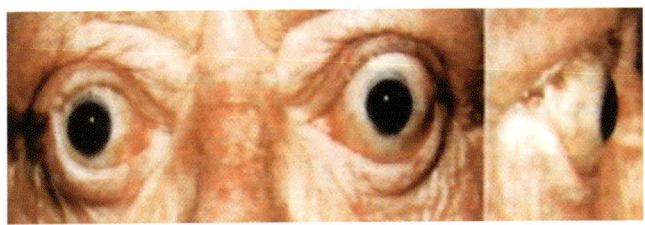

Fig. 9.10: Lid retraction is a common eye sign in Graves' disease. It is recognized when the sclera is visible between the lower margin of the upper lid and the cornea *(McKliney and O'Loughlin, 2006)*

not sit still and a realways moving. A tremor of the hands and tongue, along with lightly closed eyelids, is often present; and a generalized muscle weakness may lead to the patient's complaining of easy fatigability.

incompletely treated thyrotoxicosis are highly sensitive to the actions of epinephrine or other pressor amines, and these agents must not be administered to them; however, once the patient is well-managed from a medical stand-point, these agents can be resumed.

5. Dyspnea not related to the congestive heart failure may occur in some patients. The respiratory effect is caused by reduction in the vital capacity secondary to weakness of the respiratory muscles.

6. Weight loss even with an increased appetite is a common finding. Anorexia, nausea and vomiting are rare but, when they occur, may be the forerunners of thyroid storm.

7. Thyrotoxic patients tend to be nervous and often show a great deal of emotional liability, losing their tempers easily and crying often; severe psychic reactions may occur. These patients can

8. Thyrotoxic patients have an increased excretion of calcium and phosphorus in their urine and stools, and radiographs demonstrate increased bone loss. The serum levels of alkaline phosphatase are usually normal. The bone age of young individuals is advanced.

9. The individual red blood cells in patients with thyrotoxicosis are usually normal; however, the red blood cell mass is enlarged to carry the additional oxygen needed for the increased metabolic activities.

10. The increased metabolic activities associated with thyrotoxicosis lead to increased secretion and breakdown of cortisol; however, serum levels remain within normal limits.

11. Hyperthyroidism decreases liver function. Jaundice may appear but is readily eliminated through treatment of thyrotoxicosis.

12. Because of the variable degree of liver dysfunction associated with thyrotoxicosis, all drugs and medications metabolized primarily in the liver should be administered judiciously and in smaller-than-normal doses. Because of the effects

of atropine and epinephrine on the heart and cardiovascular systems, their use is contraindicated in severely hyperthyroid individuals. Refer to Chapter 15, "G" Graves' disease, page 445.

Laboratory Findings

The T4 and T3, TBG, and TSH tests are used as a screen for hyperthyroidism. The normal value for these tests are shown in Table 9.1.

Medical Management

Treatment of patients with thyrotoxicosis may involve antithyroid agents that block hormone synthesis, iodides, radioactive iodine, or subtotal thyroidectomy. Patients with thyrotoxicosis who are untreated or incompletely treated may develop thyrotoxic crisis, a serious but fortunately rare complication that may occur at any age and has an abrupt onset.

Thyroid storm, or crisis, is the end point of untreated hyperthyroidism. It is a life-threatening emergency. The primary difference between thyroid storm and severe hyperthyroidism is the presence of hyperpyrexia; if this condition is left untreated, the body's temperature may reach a lethal level (105°F or higher) within 24 to 48 hours. In this severe hypermetabolic state, the body's demand for energy overtaxes the cardiovascular system, which helps produce the clinical signs and symptoms of cardiac dysrhythmias, CHF, and acute pulmonary edema. The thyroid storm patient also exhibits profound delirium, vomiting, diarrhea, and dehydration.

Thyrotoxic crisis occurs in less than 1% of the patients hospitalized for thyrotoxicosis. Most patients who develop thyrotoxic crisis have goiter, wide pulse pressure, eye signs, and long history of thyrotoxicosis. Precipitating factors are infections, trauma, surgical emergencies, and operations. Early symptoms are

Table 9.1: Results for thyroid function tests

Test	Normal range
T4	5 to 12 mg/dl
T3	80 to 200 ng/dl
rT3	10 to 60/dl
TBG	12 to 30 mg/l
TSH	Less than 5 mu/l
FT4	1.3 to 3. 8 ng/dl
FT3	260 to 480 png/dl
RAIU	10 to 25% per 24 hours

extreme restlessness, tremor, nausea, vomiting, and abdominal pain; fever, profuse sweating, marked tachycardia, pulmonary edema, and congestive heart failure soon develop. The patient appears to be in a stupor, and coma may follow. Severe hypotension develops, and death may occur. These reactions appear to be associated, at least in part, with adrenocortical insufficiency. It can be brought on, in the face of thyrotoxicosis, by sources of metabolic stress including infection, trauma, and general anesthesia in an inadequtely prepared patient.

Immediate treatment for the patient in a thyrotoxic crisis consists of large doses of antithyroid drugs (200 mg of propylthiouracil), potassium iodide, propranolol (to antagonize the adrenergic component), hydrocortisone (100 to 300 mg), IV glucose solution, vitamin B complex, wet packs and ice packs. Start cardiopulmonary resuscitation, if needed, and seek immediate medical aid.

Dental Aspects of Hyperthyroidism

Once the thyrotoxic patient is under good medical management, the dental treatment plan will be unaffected. Pain, anxiety, trauma or general anesthesia may precipitate a thyroid crisis in the untreated patient with hyperthyroidism (Box 9.2). Thyroid crisis (thyrotoxic crisis) is dangerous and characterized by anxiety, tremor and dyspnea and can go on to ventricular fibrillation. An acute oral infection could precipitate a crisis. It may also be precipitated by premature cessation of antithyroid treatment. Medical assistance is essential as treatment of a crisis requires the use of potassium iodide and propylthiouracil, and propranolol or chlorpromazine.

If a crisis occurs, the dentist should be able to recognize what is happening, begin emergency treatment, and seek immediate medical assistance. The patient can be cooled with cold towels, given an injection of hydrocortisone (100 to 300 mg), and started on an IV infusion of hypertonic glucose (if equipment is available). Vital signs must be monitored and cardiopulmonary resuscitation initiated, if necessary. Patients with extensive dental caries or periodontal disease, or both, can be treated after medical management of the thyroid problem has been affected. The hyperthyroid patient is especially at risk from general anesthesia because of the risk of precipitating dangerous dysrhythmias. General anesthesia must not, therefore, be given in the dental surgery until the

Box 9.2: Dental management of the thyrotoxic patients

1. Detection of undiagnosed disease
   a. Signs
   b. Symptoms
   c. Referral for medical diagnosis and treatment
2. Patient with diagnosed disease
   a. Determination of original diagnosis
   b. Past history
   c. Present medication
   d. Assessment of clinical status (symptoms, signs, thyroid tests)
   e. Referral for reevaluation, if signs and symptoms found
   f. Consultation prior to starting dental treatment
3. Avoidance of following in untreated or poorly treated patient
   a. Surgical procedures
   b. Acute infection
   c. Epinephrine and other pressor amines (in local anesthetics, gingival retraction cords)
4. Recognition and management of initial therapy for thyrotoxic crisis
   a. Seeking of medical aid
   b. Wet packs, ice packs
   c. Hydrocortisone (100 to 300 mg)
   d. IV glucose solution
   e. Cardiopulmonary resuscitation
5. Patient under good medical treatment
   a. Avoidance of acute oral infection
   b. Treatment of all chronic oral infections
   c. Implementation of normal procedures and management

disease is treated. If needed urgently, general anesthesia should be given by a specialist anesthetist in hospital.

Patients with untreated hyperthyroidism may be also difficult to deal with as a result of heightened anxiety and irritability. The sympathetic overactivity may lead to fainting, but although the risks of giving adrenaline–containing local anesthesia in moderate amounts are more theoretical than real, however, it is generally claimed that the use of epinephrine or other pressor amines in local anesthetics, gingival retraction cords, or to control bleeding must be avoided in the untreated or poorly treated thyrotoxic patients. Uncontrolled hyperthyroid patients are exquisitely sensitive to both endogenous and exogenous (injected) catecholamines, and they often present with concomitant hypertension and arrhythmias. The excessive release of thyroid hormone can potentiate both the pressor and myocardial effects of epinephrine. However, the well-treated thyrotoxic patients present no problem in this regard and may be given normal concentrations of these vaso-constrictors. If there is anxiety on this score, prilocaine with felypressin can be given but is not known to be safer. Povidine-iodine and similar compouds are best avoided. Sedation is desirable since anxiety may precipitate a thyroid crisis.

HYPOTHYROIDISM

Hypothyroid patients may respond in an exaggerated manner to sedative and narcotic agents, necessitating, in extreme instances, respiratory support until such drugs are metabolized or eliminated.

Thyroid failure usually occurs as a result of diseases of the thyroid gland (primary hypothyroidism), pituitary gland(secondary), or hypothalamus (tertiary). Primary hypothyroidism is the most common. It may develop as a result of idiopathic atrophy of the thyroid gland or following total thyroidectomy or ablation after radioactive iodine therapy used for the management of hyperthyroidism. Thyroid hypofunction occurs 3 to 10 times more frequently in females than males, with the greatest incidence between the ages of 30 and 60 years.

Hypothyroidism is a clinical state in which the body's tissue do not receive an adequate supply of thyroid hormones.

Clinical signs and symptoms of hypothyroidism are related to the age of the patient at the time of onset and to the degree and duration of the hormonal deficiency.

A deficiency of thyroid hormone during fetal or early life can produce a clinical syndrome known as **cretinism** in infants and children—childhood hypothyroidism (Figs 9.12 and 9.13).

Neonatal cretinism is characterized by dwarfism, overweight, broad flat nose, wide-set eyes, thick lips, large protruding tongue, poor muscle tone, pale skin, stubby hands, retarded bone age, delayed eruption

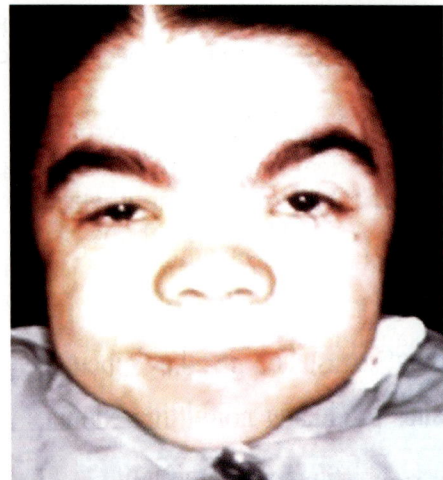

Fig. 9.12: Cretinism

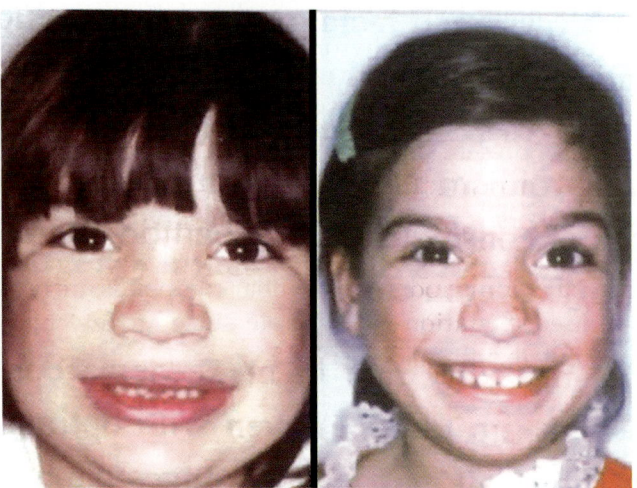

Fig. 9.13: Hypothyroidism. **(A)** The facial appearance of this 9-year-old child is due to the accumulation of tissue edema secondary to severe hypothyroidism. **(B)** Same patient after one year of thyroid hormone replacement therapy showing the return of facial appearance. Note the eruption of the maxillary permanent teeth. *(From Neville B, Danm DD, Allen CM, et al. Oral and Maxillofacial pathology, 2nd ed. Philadelphia, Saunders, 2002)*

adults leads to the deposition of a glycosamino-glycogen ground substance in the subcutaneous tissues producing nonpitting edema, fatigue, lethargy, cold intolerance, myalgias, and arthralgia. The skin may be dry and scaly, hair loss of the outer third of the eyebrows, and facial puffiness of eyelids with periorbital edema are common (Figs 9.14 and 9.15). Severe unmanaged hypothyroidism ultimately may

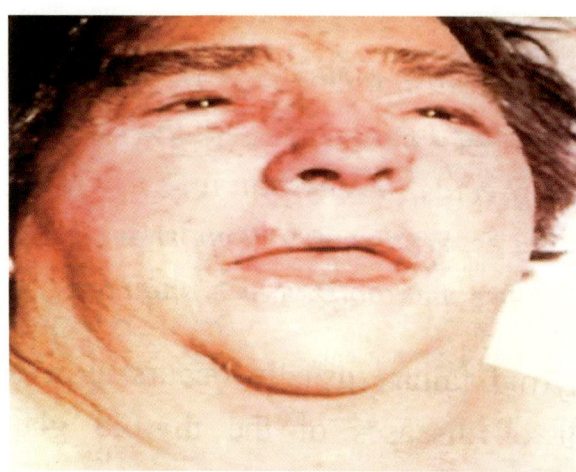

Fig. 9.14: Clinical hypothyroidism showing characteristic non-pitting edematous changes in the skin of the face. Note the dry puffy facial appearance and coarse hair *(Courtesy Paul W. Ladenson MD. The Johns Hopkins University and Hospital, Baltimore, MD. In Seidel HM, Ball JW, Dains JE, Benedict GW. Mosby's Guide to Physical Examination, 6th ed. St. Louis, Mosby, 2006)*

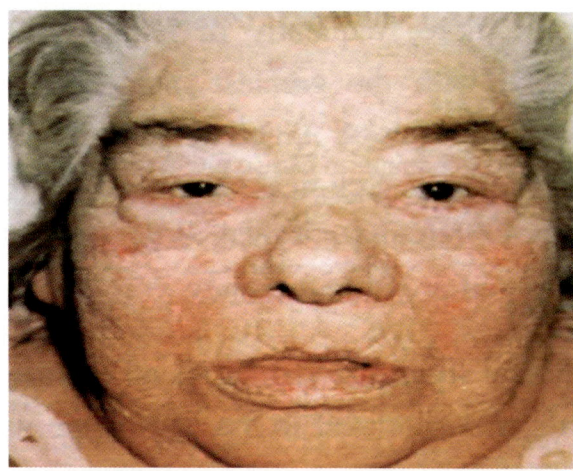

Fig. 9.15: Gross clinical hypothyroidism produces characteristic non-pitting edematous changes in the skin of the face, giving rise to a characteristic clinical appearance. Note the dry, puffy facial appearance and the coarse hair. This patient was admitted with hypothermia. Her skin was cold and she showed mental apathy

of teeth, malocclusion, a hoarse cry, umbilical hernia, and mental retardation that can be avoided with early detection and treatment.

In adults, hypothyroidism is often caused by autoimmune destruction of the thyroid hormones known as Hashimoto thyroiditis or iatrogenic factors such as, radioactive iodine therapy or surgery for the treatment of hyperthyroidism.

Severe hypothyroidism that develops in an adult is called **myxedema.** Decreased thyroid hormone in

induce the loss of consciousness, a condition known as **myxedema coma.**

The mortality rate in myxedaema coma is high (up to 50%) even with optimum treatment. It may lead to congestive heart failure, pericardial effusion, ascites, and mental changes. Myxedema coma is a decompensated state precipitated by stress which may be fatal. Treatment of hypothyroidism is with chronic replacement therapy with sodium L-thyroxin.

In general, the patient with mild symptoms of untreated hypothyroidism is not in danger when receiving dental therapy (Box 9.3). Central nervous system depressants (including diazepam), opioid analgesics (including codeine), other tranquilizers and general anesthetic sedatives may cause an exaggerated response in patients with mild to severe hypothyroidism. Once the hypothyroid patient is under good medical care, no special problems are presented in terms of dental management.

Box 9.3: Dental management of the hypothyroid patient

1. Detection of undiagnosed disease
   a. Symptoms
   b. Signs
   c. Referral for medical diagnosis and treatment
2. Patient with diagnosed disease
   a. Assessment of clinical status (symptoms, signs, thyroid tests)
   b. Referral for re-evaluation
3. Avoidance of the following in untreated or poorly treated patient
   a. Surgical procedures
   b. Oral infections
   c. CNS depressants (narcotics, barbiturates, etc.)
4. Recognition and management of initial stages of myxedematous coma
   a. Seeking of immediate aid
   b. Hydrocortisone (100 to 300 mg)
   c. Artificial respiration
5. Patient under good medical management
   a. Avoidance of acute oral infections
   b. Implementation of normal procedures and management

Hypothyroidism and Local Anesthetics

Use the following guidelines for local anesthetics:

1. *Uncontrolled hypothyroid patient:* Do not use epinephrine in the uncontrolled hypothyroid patients. The epinephrine will stay in the system longer because the BMR is decreased, plus epinephrine can tax as sluggish heart.
2. *Controlled hypothyroid patient:* Use xylocaine with epinephrine, but limit it to 2 carpules.

Hypothyroid and Sedatives, Hypnotics and Narcotics

1. The uncontrolled patient will have exaggerated response to narcotics and barbiturates.
2. Do not use diazepam (valium), codeine, or other sedatives hypnotics, or narcotics in the uncontrolled hypothyroid patient, because myxedema coma can occur.
3. The controlled hypothyroid patient can get diazepam (valium), tylenol, or other sedatives, hypnotics, or narcotics (Table 9.2).

Table 9.2: Common signs and symptoms of thyroid diseases

Hypothyroidism	Hyperthyroidism
Fatigue	Fatigue
Weight gain	Weight loss
Cold intolerance	Heat intolerance
Skin dry	Skin moist (hyperhidrous)
Hair dryness and/or loss	Hair fine and silky
Depression	Nervousness
Dementia	Insomnia
	Tremor
Muscle cramps and myalgia	Muscle weakness
	Dyspnea
Bradycardia	Tachycardia
	Palpitations
Constipation	Hyperdefecation
Infertility	
Edema	
Menestrual irregularity (hypermenorrhea common)	Menestrual irregularity (hypermenorrhea common)

PARATHYROID GLANDS

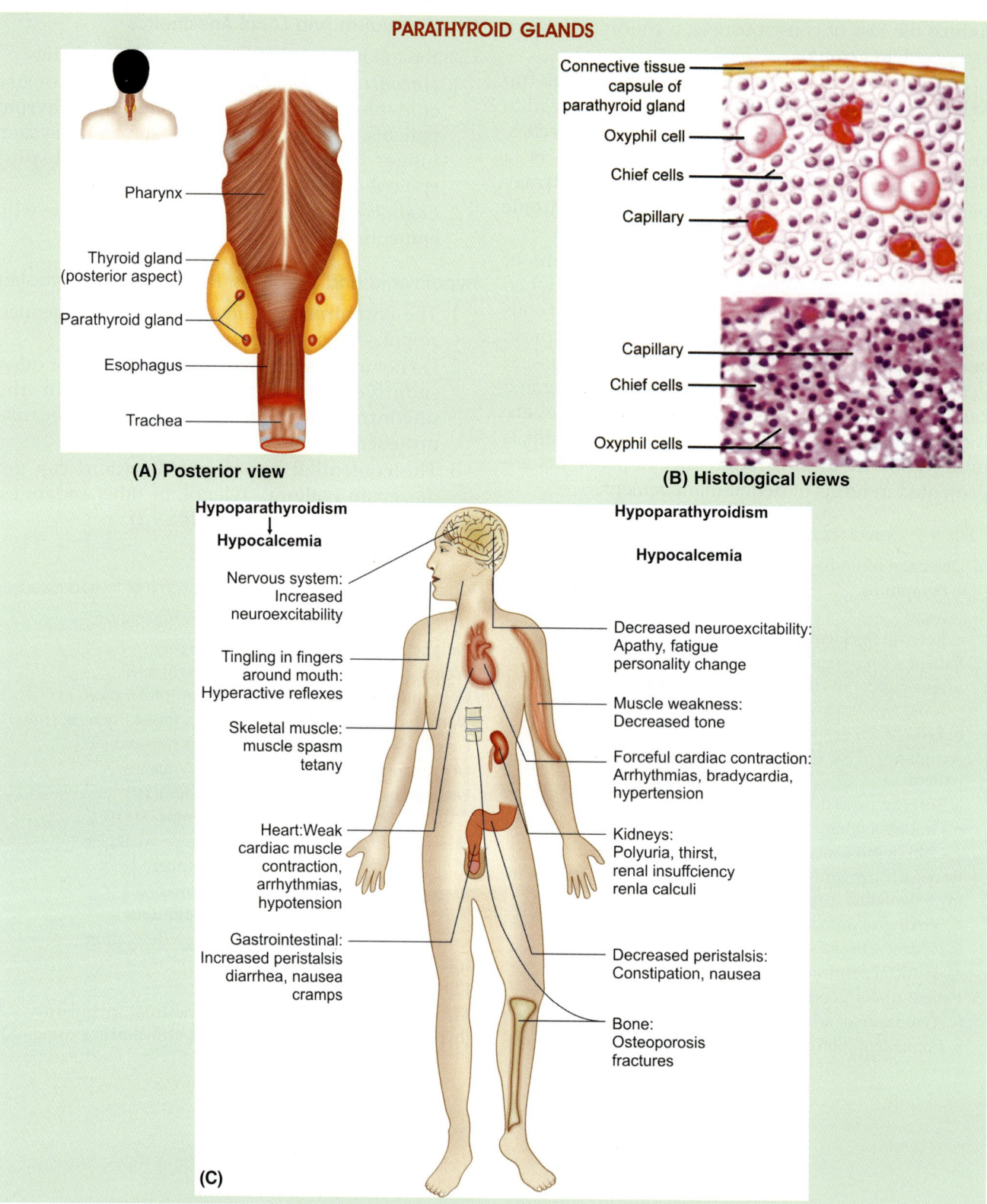

(A) Posterior view

Pharynx

Thyroid gland (posterior aspect)

Parathyroid gland

Esophagus

Trachea

(B) Histological views

Connective tissue capsule of parathyroid gland

Oxyphil cell

Chief cells

Capillary

Capillary

Chief cells

Oxyphil cells

(C)

Hypoparathyroidism
↓
Hypocalcemia

Nervous system: Increased neuroexcitability

Tingling in fingers around mouth: Hyperactive reflexes

Skeletal muscle: muscle spasm tetany

Heart:Weak cardiac muscle contraction, arrhythmias, hypotension

Gastrointestinal: Increased peristalsis diarrhea, nausea cramps

Hypoparathyroidism

Hypocalcemia

Decreased neuroexcitability: Apathy, fatigue personality change

Muscle weakness: Decreased tone

Forceful cardiac contraction: Arrhythmias, bradycardia, hypertension

Kidneys: Polyuria, thirst, renal insuffciency renla calculi

Decreased peristalsis: Constipation, nausea

Bone: Osteoporosis fractures

Plate X: Parathyroid glands. **(A)** The parathyroid glands are four small nodules attached to the capsule of the thyroid gland on its posterior surface. Parathyroid gland is composed of chief cells and oxyphil cells. **(B)** Common effects of parathyroid hormone imbalances (*Gould, 2006*)

Anatomy and Physiology

The parathyroid glands are partially embedded in the posterior surface of the thyroid (Fig. 9.16). There are usually four, each about 3 to 8 mm long and 2 to 5 mm wide. The parathyroid glands produce parathyroid hormone (PTH) which regulates a normal plasma calcium level by acting on the kidneys, gastrointestinal tract and bone.

The normal control of calcium metabolism is illustrated in Fig. 9.17. These glands release parathyroid hormone (PTH) when the blood calcium is too low. A mere 1% drop in the blood calcium level doubles the secretion of PTH. Calcium metabolism depends upon a series of factors serving together to maintain the integrity of the skeleton, and to control the neuro-muscular excitability so that tetany does not occur. Among these factors must be included, the amount of calcium and phosphorus in the diet, the efficiency with which calcium is absorbed from the jejunum, the concentration of the serum proteins to which calcium is bound, the pH of the blood which in turn determines the proportion of the calcium in serum held in the ionized state and the renal function (Fig. 9.18). Finally, the parathyroid hormone, thyrocalcitonin and calciferol (vitamin D), are important factors.

In normal circumstances, parathyroid hormone is secreted in response to a fall in the concentration of

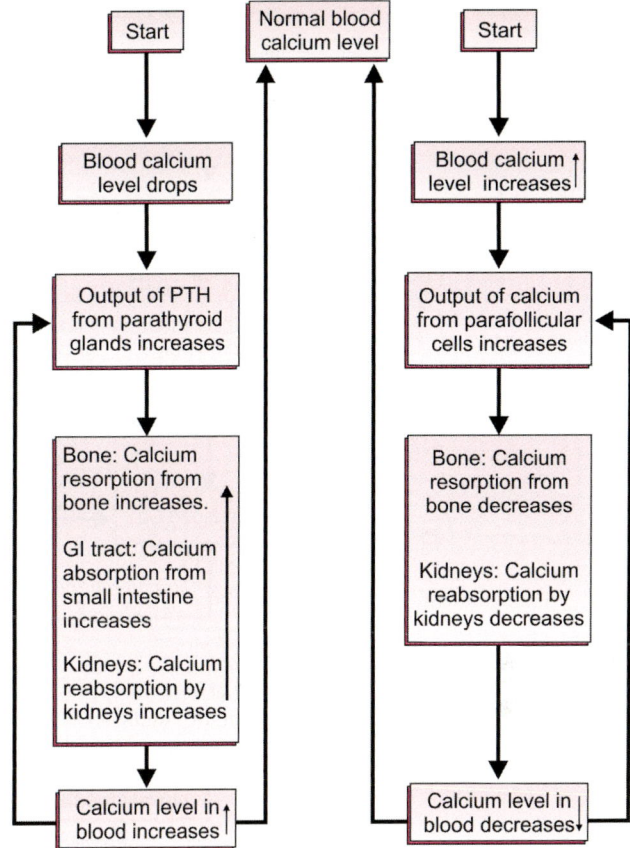

Fig. 9.17: Regulation of calcium levels by parathyroid hormone (PTH) and calcitonin (Ct)

serum calcium, and the hormone prevents this fall by mobilizing calcium (and normally phosphorus) from bone. It increases the excretion of phosphorus by the kidney. Calciferol enhances the absorption of calcium, raises its concentration in serum, and facilitates its deposition in bone. Calciferol also increases the excretion in urine.

PTH raises the blood calcium level by four mechanisms (Fig. 9.17):

1. PTH binds to receptors on the osteoblasts, stimulates them to secrete osteoclast-stimulating factor, and this in turn raises the osteoclast population and promotes bone resorption.
2. PTH promotes calcium reabsorption by the kidneys.
3. PTH promotes the final step of calcitriol synthesis in the kidneys, thus enhancing the calcium raising effect of calcitriol.
4. PTH inhibits collagen synthesis by osteoblasts, thus inhibiting bone deposition.

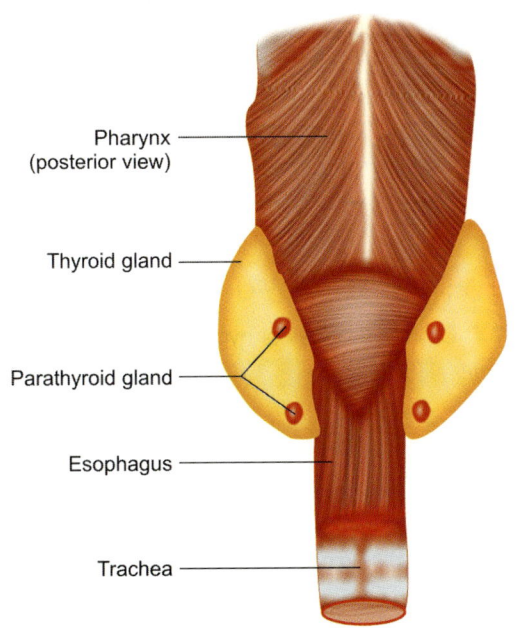

Fig. 9.16: The parathyroid glands

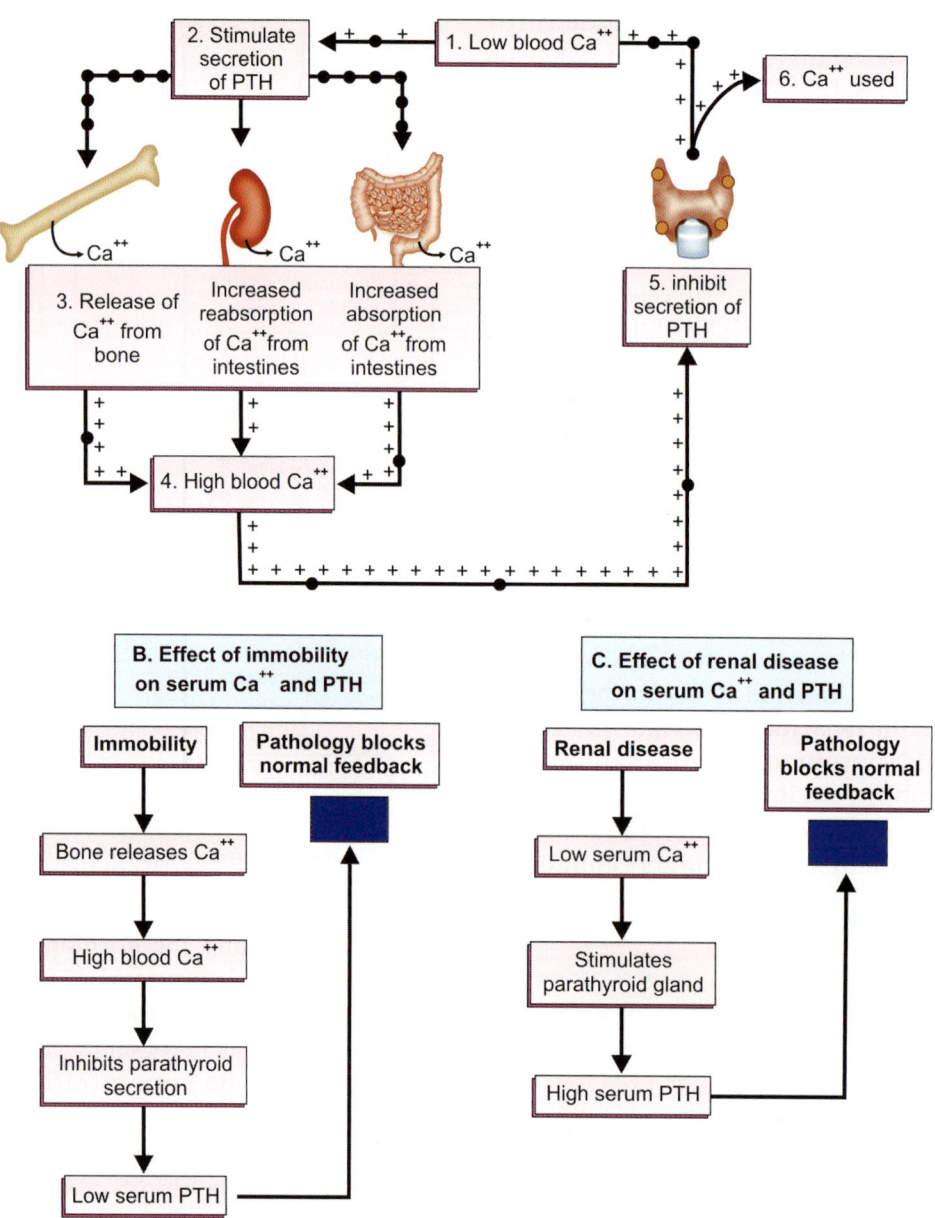

A. Normal control and feedback of calcium

Fig. 9.18: Calcium and PTH relationships; PTH + Ca$^{++(GOULD)}$

Notwithstanding these normal effects of PTH, the intermittent secretion (or injection) of PTH at low levels can cause bone deposition. PTH can, therefore, increase or decrease bone mass, depending on other factors such as exercise, stress on the bones, calcium and phosphate availability, and the action of vitamin D and other hormones.

Deficiency of this vitamin and of the parathyroid hormone, together or separately, may be associated with depression of the concentration of calcium in serum. Either in excess will produce hypercalcemia

Box 9.4: Clinical features of hypo- and hyperparathyroidism

Hypothyroidism	Hyperthyroidism
Tetany	Renal stones
Epilepsy	Nephrocalcinosis
Candidiasis	Bone resorption
Cataracts	Peptic ulcer, pain
Psychiatric disorders	Psychiatric disorders
Dental defects	Polyuria
	Constipation
	Hypertension
	Weakness
	Acute pancreatitis

which, if severe and not treated vigorously, may lead to death in uremia. Thyrocalcitonin is probably a physiological antagonist to the thyroid hormone and depresses the level of the serum calcium.

The clinical signs and symptoms of hyperthyroidism as compared to hypothyroidism are illustrated in Box 9.4.

HYPERPARATHYROIDISM

The main features are hypercalcemia, renal disease and, less commonly, skeletal disease. Most patients have renal calcifications and often hypertension, dysrhythmias and peptic ulceration. Bone pain, pathological fractures, giant cell tumors and bone rarefaction also are features of hyperparathyroidism.

Incidence

Hyperparathyroidism ranks third among the incidence of endocrine disorders behind diabetes mellitus and hyperthyroidism. It occurs in 30 of every 100,000 patients. This disorder may occur at any age but it predominantly affects those in their 40s and 50s, with a female-to-male ratio of 3 to 1.

Etiology/Pathophysiology

Hyperparathyroidism may be due to over-production of parathormone often by an adenoma in the parathyroid glands (primary hyperparathyroidism), or secondary to conditions that reduce calcium levels in the blood, such as chronic renal disease or prolonged dialysis or severe malabsorption (secondary hyperparathyroidism).

Hyperparathyroidism is most commonly a disease of postmenopausal women. Where increased levels of parathormone are present, calcium is mobilized from the bony skeleton to raise blood levels of calcium. In the primary form of the disease, this leads to hypercalcemia, and renal calculi may develop, if the problem is not identified and, less commonly, skeletal disease.

Signs and Symptoms

Hyperparathyroidism often is asymptomatic, however, some patients will complain of or exhibit a variety of symptoms including the following: Mental depression, confusion, lethargy, muscle weakness, nausea and vomiting, peptic ulceration, renal calculi, anorexia, and skeletal demineralization. The signs and symptoms may be vague and nonspecific, and the disease may elude diagnosis for some time.

Bone changes consist of either a subtle generalized reduced bone density (osteoporosis) or mottled areas of radiolucency, subperiosteal erosions (Fig. 9.19), thinning of the cortical plates and the medullary bone (osteitis fibrosa cystic) (Fig. 9.20).

In the jaws, the mandible is more commonly affected by such lesions than the maxilla., cyst-like spaces known as "Brown tumors" may develop either unilaterally or bilaterally. This has given rise to the other name of this condition, osteitis fibrosa cystic. In the mandible, the presence of a Brown tumor may give rise to expansion of the outer and/or the inner cortical plates of bone. Radiographs reveal a well-circumscribed area of unilocular or multilocular radiolucency with a less defined lamina dura surrounding it than

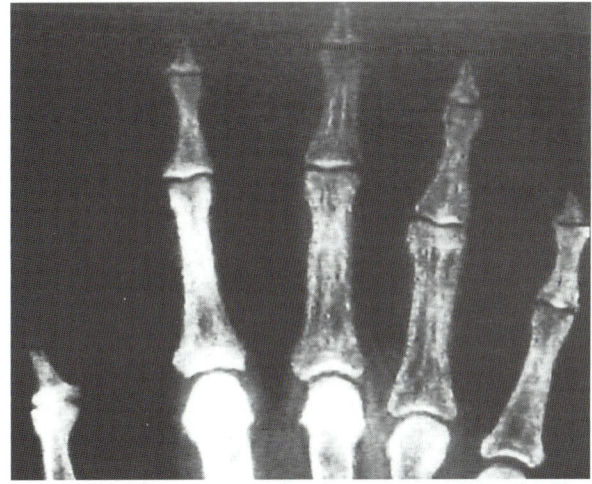

Fig. 9.19: Hyperparathyroidism. There are subperiosteal erosions along the cortical surfaces of the middle and distal phalanges, especially obvious in the index finger, and gross resorption of the distal phalanges *(Forbes and Jackson, 2003)*

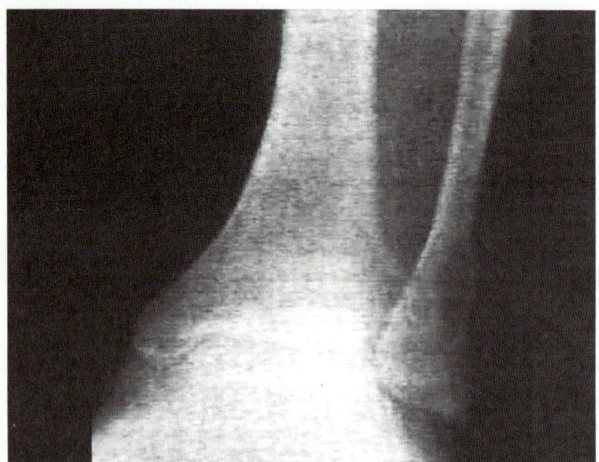

Fig. 9.20: Hyperparathyroidism. A solitary bone cyst (brown tumor) in the fibula of a patient with a large parathyroid adenoma. It is important to remember hyperparathyroidism in the differential diagnosis of bone cysts and tumors *(Forbes and Jackson, 2003)*

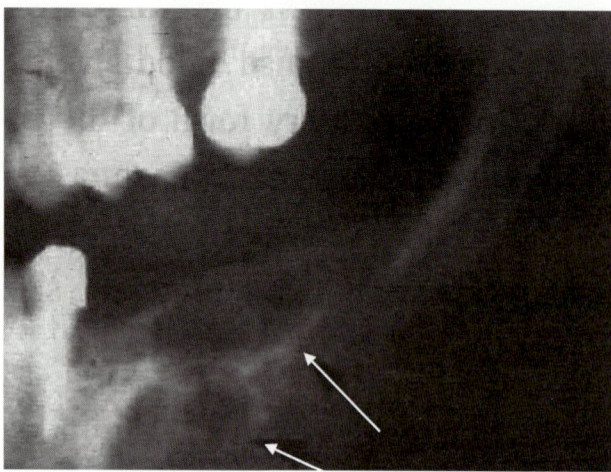

Fig. 9.22: Hyperparathyroidism: Well-defined cystic radiolucencies

is normally found in a true cystic lesion (Figs 9.21, 9.22 and *see* Fig. 6.4). The outline may have a scalloped margin and some authorities also describe a lack of definition of the lamina dura around all the standing teeth (Fig. 9.23). This, in fact, is difficult to discern and tends to be a rather subjective finding. The bone in these tumors is resorbed by vascular fibrous tissue with multinucleated giant cells. Panoramic and periapical radiographs are the ideal imaging methods to evaluate jaw changes that may occur with the disorder.

Occasionally, the soft tissue of the brown tumor may grow through the upper border of the alveolar process and appear as a dark red or purple-colored mass under the oral mucosa. The lesion is usually non-painful but may be tender to palpation. An incision biopsy of the lesion reveals the typical histological appearance of fibrous vascular tissue with large numbers of multinucleated giant cell tumors. Microscopically, they are identical to central giant cell granuloma (Fig. 9.24). Serum biochemistry will reveal elevated parathormone levels and, in the primary form of the disease, this will be accompanied by a raised serum calcium and lowered phosphate level. Primary hyperparathyroidism is normally treated surgically by removal of usually an adenoma of the parathyroid gland. The bone lesions usually resolve spontaneously following this surgery.

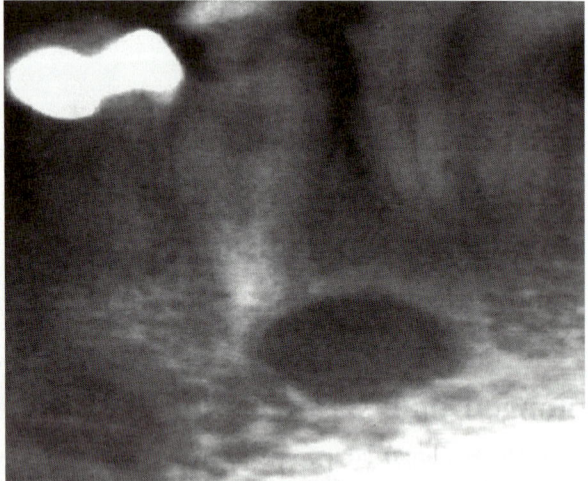

Fig. 9.21: Lytic lesion in the anterior mandible of a patient with hyperparathyroidism

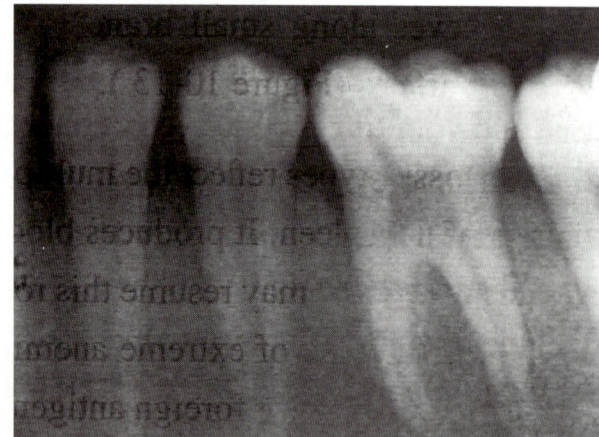

Fig. 9.23: Hyperparathyroidism. Radiograph of mandibular alveolar process demonstrating generalized lack of bone density, indistinct trabecular pattern, and loss of the normally distinct lamina dura surrounding roots of the teeth

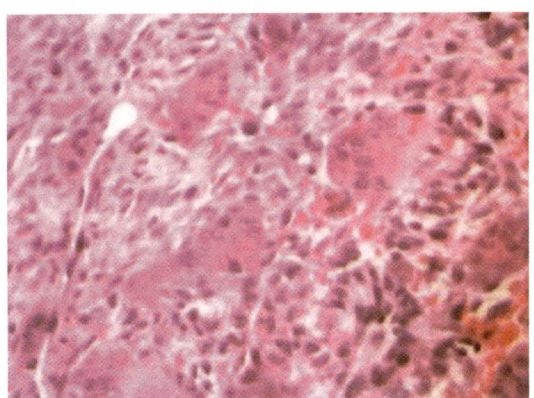

Fig. 9.24: Hyperparathyroidism. This high power photomicrograph of a Brown tumor of hyperparathyroidism shows scattered multinucleated giant cells within a vascular and proliferative fibroblastic background

The plasma calcium may be high and the phosphate level low. Alkaline phosphatase is raised, reflecting increased osteoblastic activity in response to bone resorption. Radiological changes in the early stages include demineralization or subperiosteal erosions in the phalanges (Fig. 9.19).

Management

Primary hyperparathyroidism is treated with parathyroidectomy with a 90% success rate. Those patients refractory to or not surgical candidates are managed medically with oral phosphate supplements, estrogen therapy, and calmodulin to decrease serum calcium. The secondary form is treated by correcting the underlying medical condition.

HYPOPARATHYROIDISM

Hypoparathyroidism may be caused by a congenital lack of the four parathyroid glands, following surgery (thyroidectomy) or radiation in the neck region, or as a result of autoimmune disease.

Pathophysiology

Hypocalcemia (low serum calcium levels) affects nerve and muscle function in different ways (Fig. 9.17). Hypocalcemia does not weaken skeletal muscle contractions because sufficient calcium is stored in skeletal muscle cells. Cardiac muscle cells, on the other hand, do not have large stores of calcium but rely instead on calcium from the blood for contraction, so hypocalcemia weakens cardiac contraction.

Low serum calcium levels increase the excitability of nerves, leading to spontaneous contraction of skeletal muscle. This causes muscle twitching and spasms, commonly known as **tetany.** The classic features of tetany include numbness and tingling of arms and legs, facial twitching (Chvostek's sign, contracture of the facial muscles upon tapping over the facial nerve), carpopedal spasms (Trousseau's sign,

contracture of the hands and fingers on occluding the arm with a cuff) and even laryngeal stridor (Box 9.5).

Box 9.5: Dental aspects of hypoparathyroidism

Oral manifestations of idiopathic (congenital) hypoparathyroidism may include enamel hypoplasia, shortened roots with osteodentine formation, delayed eruption and sometimes chronic mucocutaneous candidiasis which can be resistant to antimycotic treatment. There may be facial paresthesia and facial twitching caused by tetany (Chvostek's sign)

• Dental management may be complicated by:
  1. Tetany.
  2. Epilepsy.
  3. Psychiatric problems or mental handicap.
  4. Hypoadrenocorticism or other endocrinopathies such as diabetes mellitus
  5. Dysrhythmias

10

Diseases of the Immune System

I. The Lymphatic System
Origin of Lymph
Functions of Lymph
Components of the Lymphatic System
Lymphatic Circulation
Lymphedema

II. The Immune Response
Introduction
Types of Immunity
Innate Immunity
Acquired Immunity
Functions of the Immune System
Components of the Immune System
Properties of Immunity
Immune Responses

III. Upsets of the Immune Response
• **A. Autoimmune Diseases**
Rheumatoid Arthritis
Pathophysiology
Signs and Symptoms
Progression of Rheumatoid Arthritis
Laboratory Features
Treatment

• **B. Immunodeficiency States**
Categories of Immunodeficiency
Diseases which Suppress the Response
Drugs which Suppress the Immune Response
Acquired Immunedeficiency Syndrome
(AIDS), Human Immunodeficiency Virus
(HIV)
Introduction

Incidence
Pathology
Mode of Transmission
Signs and Symptoms
Oral Manifestations
Medical Treatment
Dental Treatment
Infection Control

• **C. Hypersensitivity (Allergy)**
Introduction
Pathophysiology and Complications
Type of Hypersensitivities
i. Type I hypersensitivity
Pathophysiology
Atopy
Anaphylaxis
Pathophysiology
Signs and Symptoms
Skin Tests
Hay Fever
Angioneurotic Edema
Allergic Reactions to Local Anesthesia
ii. Type II Hypersensitivity
Pathophysiology
Blood Transfusion
iii. Type III Hypersensitivity
iv. Type IV Hypersensitivity
Tissue and Organ Transplant Rejection
Cells Responsible for Prevention of Organ
Rejection
Dental Protocol for Organ Transplant Patient

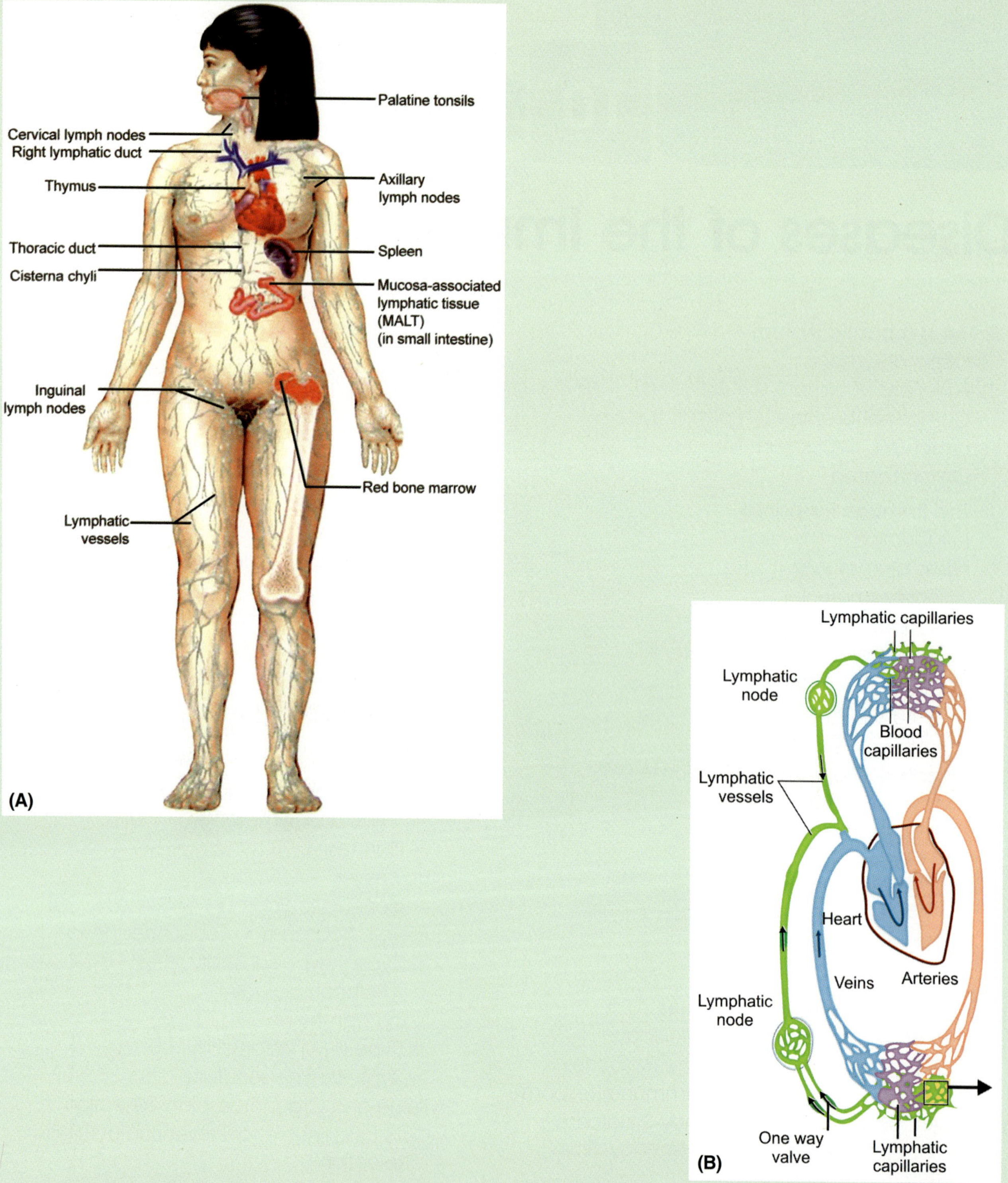

Plate XI: (A) Major components of the lymphatic system. The lymphatic system vessels, and lymphatic organs that work together to pick up and transport interstitial fluid back to the blood and mount an immune response when needed. **(B)** Relationship of the blood vessels and lymphatic vessels (green). Excess fluid and proteins in the tissue spaces enter lymphatic capillaries and return to the venous system by lymphatic vessels. Arrows indicate direction of fluid flow *(Mcklincy and Loughlin, 2006)*

I. THE LYMPHATIC SYSTEM

Lymph is usually a clear, colorless fluid, similar to blood plasma but low in protein. Its composition varies substantially from place to place. The **lymphatic system** (Plate XI) is composed of a network of vessels that penetrate nearly every tissue of the body, and a collection of tissues and organs that produce immune cells.

ORIGIN OF LYMPH

Lymph originates in microscopic vessels called lymphatic capillaries. These vessels penetrate nearly every tissue of the body but are absent from the central nervous system, cartilage, bone, and bone marrow. They are closely associated with blood capillaries, but unlike them, they are closed at one end (Fig. 10.1 A).

A lymphatic capillary consists of a sac of thin endothelial cells that loosely overlap each other like the shingles of a roof. The cells are tethered to surrounding tissue by protein filaments that prevent the sac from collapsing. Unlike the endothelial cells of blood capillaries, lymphatic endothelial cells are not joined by tight junctions. The gaps between them are so large that bacteria and other cells can enter along with the fluid. The overlapping edges of the endothelial cells act as valve-like flaps that can open and close. When tissue fluid pressure is high, it pushes the flaps inward (open) and fluid flows into the lymphatic capillary. When pressure is higher in the lymphatic capillary than in the tissue fluid, the flaps are pressed outward (closed).

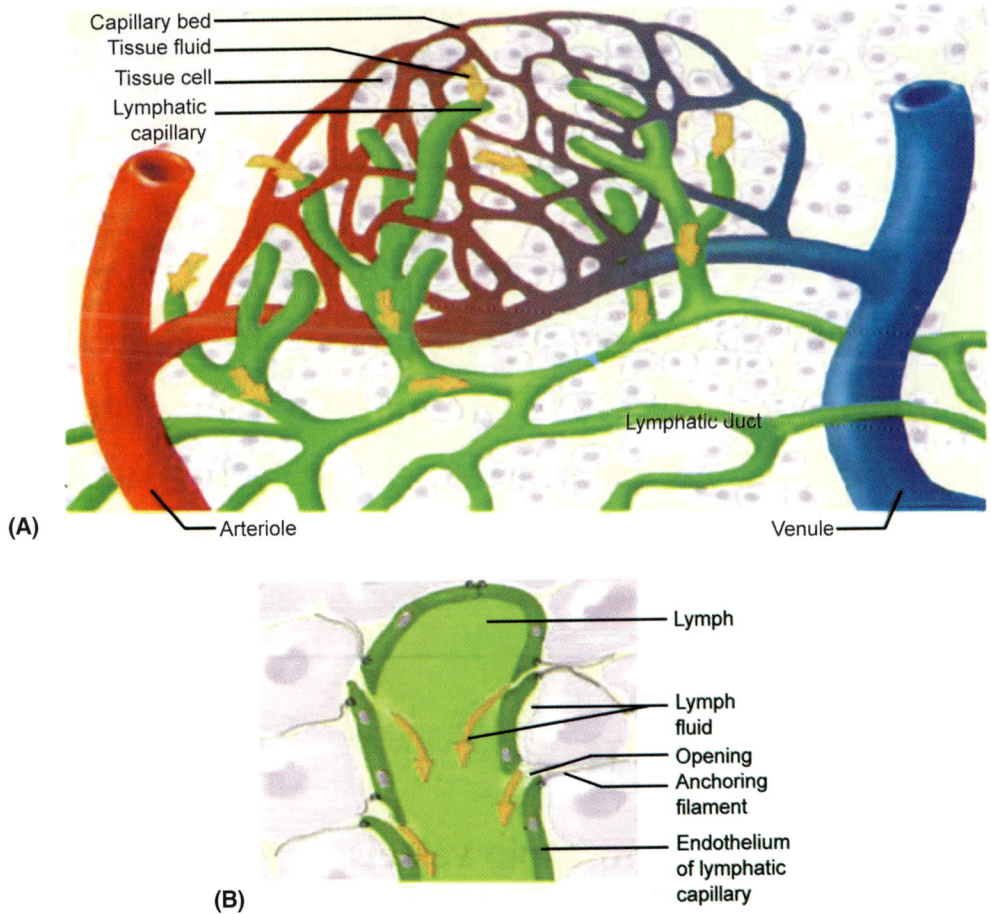

(A)

Capillary bed
Tissue fluid
Tissue cell
Lymphatic capillary
Lymphatic duct
Arteriole
Venule

(B)

Lymph
Lymph fluid
Opening
Anchoring filament
Endothelium of lymphatic capillary

Fig. 10.1: Lymphatic capillaries. **(A)** Relationship of the lymphatic capillaries to a bed of blood capillaries. **(B)** Uptake of tissue fluid by a lymphatic capillary *(Saladin, 2003)*

FUNCTIONS OF LYMPH

The lymphatic system has three functions:

1. *Fluid recovery:* Fluid continually filters from the blood capillaries into the tissue spaces. The blood capillaries reabsorb most of it, but by no means all. Each day, they lose an excess of 2 to 4 L of water and one-quarter to one-half of the plasma protein. The lymphatic system absorbs this excess fluid and returns it to the bloodstream by way of the lymphatic vessels (Figs 10.2 and 10.3). If not for this fluid recovery, the circulatory system would not have enough blood to function properly and causes a rapid and potentially fatal decline in blood volume.

2. *Immunity:* As the lymphatic system recovers excess tissue fluid, it also picks up foreign cells and chemicals from the tissues. On its way back to the bloodstream, the fluid passes through lymph nodes, where immune cells stand guard against foreign matter. When they detect it, they activate a protective immune response.

One of the functions of the lymphatic system is the production, maintenance, and distribution of lymphocytes. Lymphocytes are produced and stored within lymphoid organs, such as the spleen, thymus, and bone marrow. These cells are vital to the body's ability to resist or overcome infection and disease. Lymphocytes respond to the presence of: (1) invading pathogens, such as bacteria or viruses; (2) abnormal body cells, such as virus-infected cells or cancer cells and (3) foreign proteins, such as the toxins produced by some bacteria. Lymphocytes attempt to eliminate these threats or render them harmless through a combination of physical and chemical actions.

Lymphocytes respond to specific threats, such as bacterial invasion of a tissue, by mounting a defense against that specific type of bacterium. Such a specific defense of the body is known as an immune response. Immunity is the body's ability to resist infection and disease through the activation of specific defenses.

3. *The distribution of hormones, nutrients, and waste products from their tissues of origin to the general circulation.* Substances unable to enter the bloodstream directly may do so by way of lymphatic vessels. For example, lipids absorbed by the digestive tract do not often enter the bloodstream through capillaries. They reach the bloodstream only after they have traveled along lymphatic vessels.

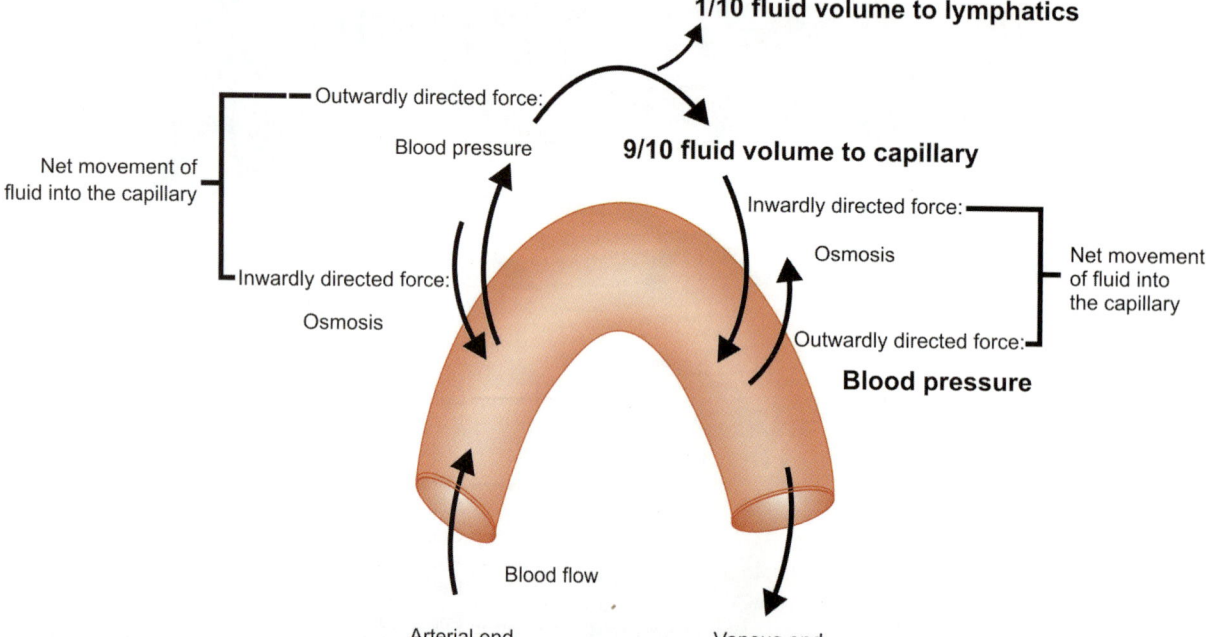

Fig. 10.2: At the arteriolar end of the capillary, the forces causing fluid to leave the capillary are greater than forces attracting fluid into it. At the venous end of the capillary, the blood pressure is decreased, making the forces that attract fluid into the capillary greater than the forces that cause fluid to leave the capillary. Approximately nine-tenths of the fluid is returned to the capillary at its venous end. The remaining one-tenth of the fluid volume enters the lymphatic capillaries *(Seeley et al, 1996)*

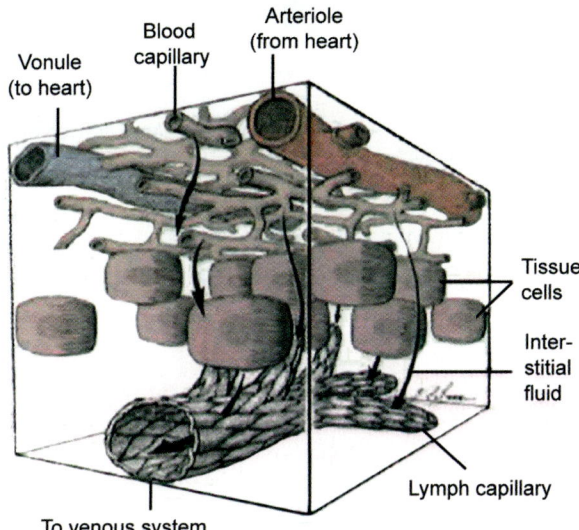

Vonule (to heart)
Blood capillary
Arteriole (from heart)
Tissue cells
Inter-stitial fluid
Lymph capillary
To venous system

Fig. 10.3: Lymph formation and drainage. Movement of fluid from blood capillaries into tissues and from tissues into lymphatic capillaries to form lymph *(Seeley et al, 1996)*

COMPONENTS OF THE LYMPHATIC SYSTEM

The components of the lymphatic system as listed in Table 10.1 include:

i. *Lymphatic vessels,* which transport the lymph.

ii. *Lymphatic cells* composed of aggregates of lymphocytes and macrophages that populate many organs of the body.

iii. *Lymphatic organs,* in which these cells are especially concentrated and which are set off from surrounding organs by connective tissue capsules.

The tissues of the thymus gland and bone marrow, where stem cells develop into lymphocytes are called *central lymphoid tissues.* The newly formed lymphocytes, still inactive, can eventually migrate via the blood to the *peripheral lymphoid tissues*—lymph nodes, spleen, the gut-associated lymphoid tissue, which include aggregated unencapsulated lymph nodules in the small intestine, appendix, tonsils, and adenoid. There they react with foreign antigens and become activated.

I. Lymphatic Vessels

Lymphatic vessels form in the embryo by budding from the veins, so it is not surprising that the larger ones have a similar histology. They have a *tunica interna* with an endothelium and valves, a *tunica media* with elastic fibers and smooth muscle, and a thin outer *tunica externa.* Their walls are thinner and their valves are more numerous than those of the veins. Lymph takes the following route from the tissues back to the bloodstream:

- Lymphatic capillaries.
- Collecting vessels.
- Six lymphatic trunks.

Table 10.1: Components of the lymphatic system

Structure	Major functions
Lymphatic capillaries	Collect excess fluid from tissues
Lymphatic vessels (collecting vessels)	Carry lymph from lymphatic capillaries to vein in neck
Lymph nodes	Situated along collecting lymphatic vessels; filter foreign material from lymph.
Axillary nodes	Drain arms, most of thoratic wall, breasts, upper abdominal wall.
Supratrochlear nodes	Drain hands, forearm.
Cervical nodes	Drain scalp, face, nasal cavity, pharynx.
Intestinal nodes	Drain abdominal viscera.
Inguinal nodes	Drain legs, external genitalia, lower abdominal wall.
Lilac nodes	Drain pelvic viscera.
Lumbar nodes	Drain pelvic viscera.
Tonsils	Destroy foreign substances at upper entrances of respiratory and digestive systems.
Spleen	Filters foreign substances from blood, manufactures phagocytic lymphocytes, stores red blood cells, releases blood to body in case of extreme blood loss.
Thymus gland	Forms antibodies in newborn; involved in initial development of immune system; site of differentiation of lymphocytes into T cells; produces thymosin.
Aggregated unencapsulated lymph nodules (Peyer's patches)	Respond to antigens in intestine by generating plasma cells that secrete antibodies.

- Two collecting ducts.
- Subclavian veins.

The lymphatic capillaries converge to form **collecting vessels** (Fig. 10.4).

These often travel along side veins and arteries and share a common connective tissue sheath with them. Numerous lymph nodes occur along the course of the collecting vessels, receiving and filtering the lymph. The collecting vessels converge to form larger **lymphatic trunks,** each of which drains a major portion of the body.

The lymphatic trunks converge to form two collecting ducts, the largest of the lymphatic vessels: (1) The right lymphatic duct (Figs 10.5 and 10.6) begins in the right thoracic cavity with the union of the right jugular, subclavian, and bronchomediastinal trunks. It receives lymphatic drainage from the right arm and right side of the thorax and head and empties into the **right subclavian vein.** (2) The thoracic duct, on the left, is larger and longer. It begins as a prominent sac in the abdominal cavity called the cisterna chyli and then passes through the diaphragm and up the

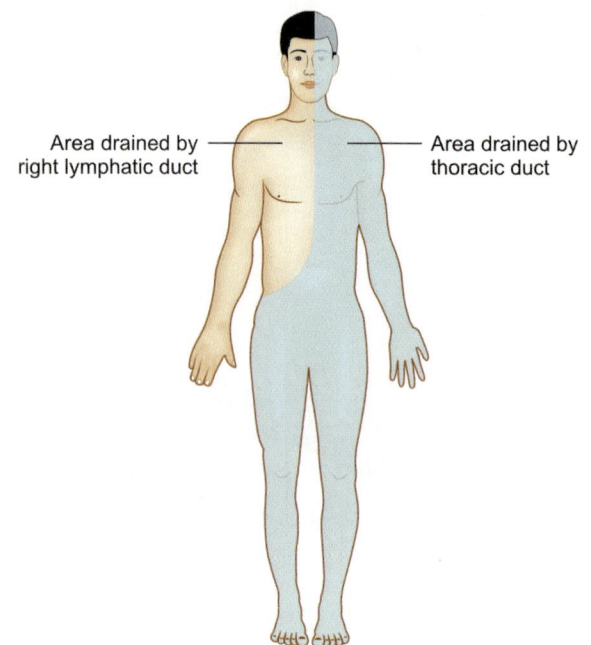

Fig. 10.5: The lymphatic ducts. The thoracic duct carries lymph that originates in tissues inferior to the diaphragm and from the left side of the upper body (blue area). The right lymphatic duct drains the right half of the body superior to the diaphragm (white area)

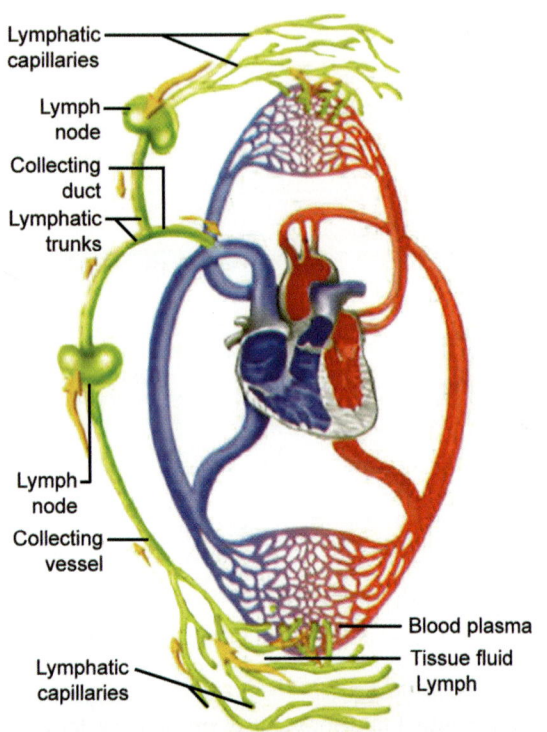

Fig. 10.4: Fluid exchange between the circulatory and lymphatic systems. Blood capillaries lose fluid to the tissue spaces. The lymphatic system picks up excess tissue fluid and returns it to the bloodstream

mediastinum. It receives lymph from all parts of the body below the diaphragm and from the left arm and left side of the head, neck, and thorax. It empties into the left subclavian vein. The principal lymphatic trunks are the *lumbar, intestinal, intercostal, bronchomediastinal, subclavian,* and *jugular trunks* (Fig. 13.6). Their names indicate their locations and parts of the body they drain; the lumbar trunk also drains the lower extremities. Thus, there is a continual recycling of fluid from blood to tissue fluid to lymph and back to the blood.

II. Lymphatic Cells

Lymphatic tissues are composed of a variety of lymphocytes and other cells which play a role in the immune system. These include:

1. *T lymphocytes (T cells):* These are so-named because they develop for a time in the thymus and later depend on thymic hormones. The T-stands for *thymus-dependent* (Fig. 10.7). There are several subclasses of T.

2. *B lymphocytes (B cells):* These are named for an organ in chickens (the *bursa of Fabricius*) in which they were first discovered. When activated, B cells

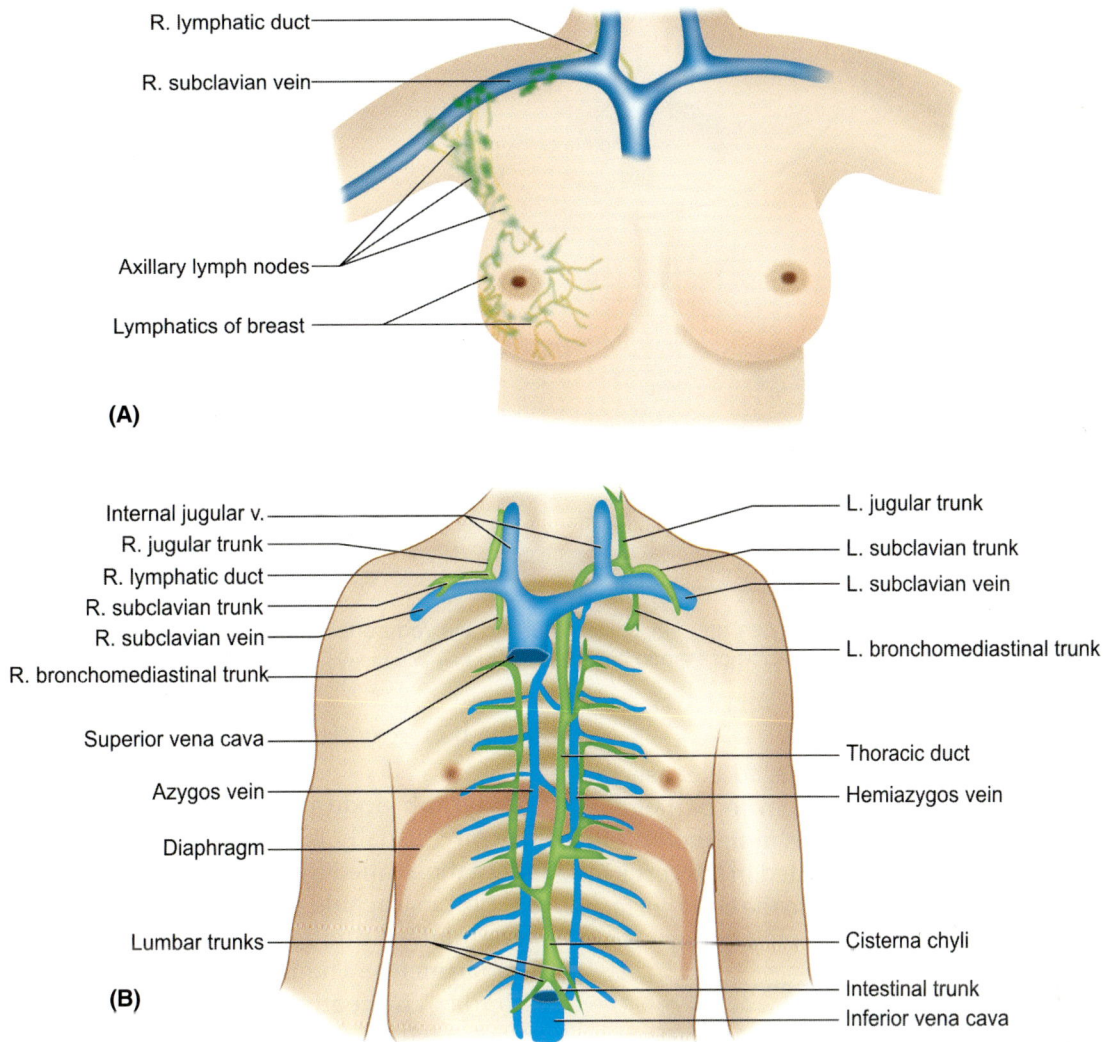

Fig. 10.6: Lymphatic drainage of the thoracic region. **(A)** Drainage of the right mammary and axillary regions. **(B)** Drainage of the right lymphatic duct and thoracic duct into the subclavian vein *(Saladin, 2003)*

differentiate into *plasma cells,* which produce circulating **antibodies,** the protective gamma globulins of the body fluids.

3. *Macrophages:* These cells, derived from monocytes of the blood, phagocytize foreign matter **(antigens)** and "display" fragments of it to certain T cells, thus alerting the immune system to the presence of an enemy. Macrophages and other cells that do this are collectively called antigen-presenting cells (APCs).

4. *Dendritic cells:* These are APCs found in the epidermis, mucous membranes, and lymphatic organs. (In the skin, they are often called *Langerhans cells.)*

5. *Reticular cells:* These are branched cells that contribute to the stroma (connective tissue framework) of the lymphatic organs and act as APCs in the thymus. (They should not be confused with reticular *fibers,* which are fine branched collagen fibers common in lymphatic organs.)

III. Lymphatic Organs

In contrast to the diffuse lymphatic tissue, lymphatic organs have well-defined anatomical sites and at least partial connective tissue capsules that separate the lymphatic tissue from neighboring tissues. These organs include the lymph nodes, tonsils, spleen and thymus (Plate XI).

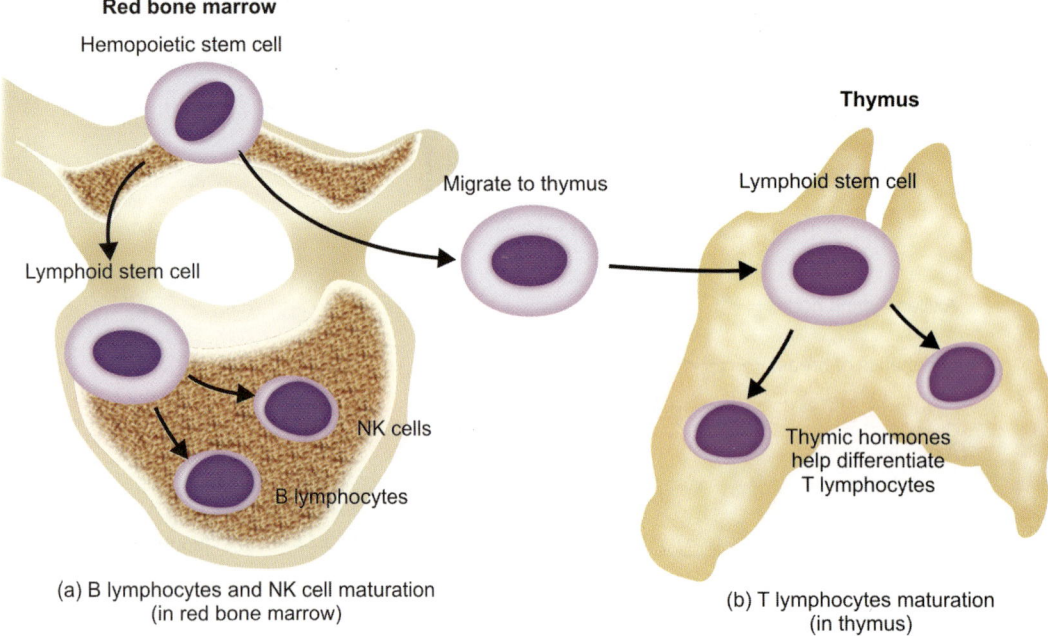

Red bone marrow

Hemopoietic stem cell

Migrate to thymus

Thymus

Lymphoid stem cell

Lymphoid stem cell

NK cells

B lymphocytes

Thymic hormones help differentiate T lymphocytes

(a) B lymphocytes and NK cell maturation
(in red bone marrow)

(b) T lymphocytes maturation
(in thymus)

Fig. 10.7: Lymphopoiesis. **(A)** B lymphocytes and NK cells mature in the red bone marrow. **(B)** T lymphocytes mature and differentiate in the thymus under the influence of thymic hormones *(McKliney and Louglin, 2006)*

A. *Lymph Node*

Lymph nodes serve two functions: to cleanse the lymph and alert the immune system to pathogens. There are hundreds of lymph nodes in the body (Fig. 10.8). They are especially concentrated in the cervical, axillary, and inguinal regions close to the body surface, and in thoracic, abdominal, and pelvic groups deep in the body cavities. Most of them are embedded in fat.

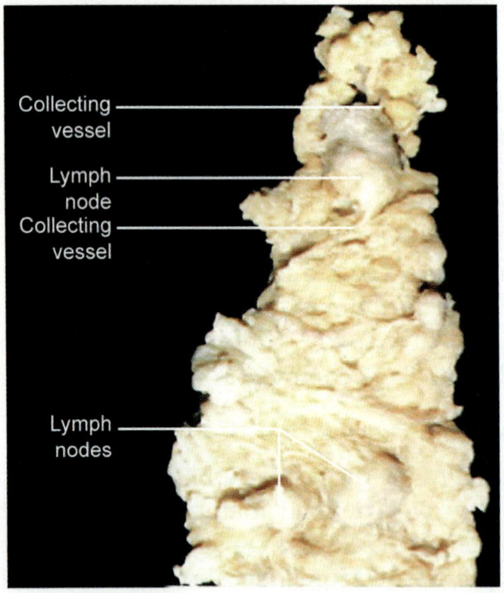

A lymph node is an elongated or bean-shaped structure, usually less than 3 cm long, often with an indentation called the *hilum* on one side. It is enclosed in a fibrous capsule with extensions (trabeculae) that incompletely divide the interior of the node into compartments. The interior consists of a stroma of reticular connective tissue (reticular fibers and reticular cells) and a parenchyma of lymphocytes and antigen-presenting cells. Between the capsule and parenchyma is a narrow space called the *subcapsular sinus*, which contains reticular fibers, macrophages, and dendritic cells.

The parenchyma is divided into an outer *cortex* and, near the hilum, an inner *medulla* (Fig. 10.9). The cortex consists mainly of ovoid lymphatic nodules. When the lymph node is fighting a pathogen, these nodules acquire light-staining germinal centers where B cells multiply and differentiate into plasma cells. The medulla consists largely of a branching network of *medullary cords* composed of lymphocytes, plasma cells, macrophages, reticular cells, and reticular fibers. The cortex and medulla also contain lymph-filled sinuses continuous with the subcapsular sinus.

Several **afferent lymphatic vessels** lead into the node along its convex surface. Lymph flows from

Collecting vessel

Lymph node

Collecting vessel

Lymph nodes

Fig. 10.8: Lymph nodes. Several collecting vessels evident leading to and from the upper lymph node *(Saladin, 2003)*

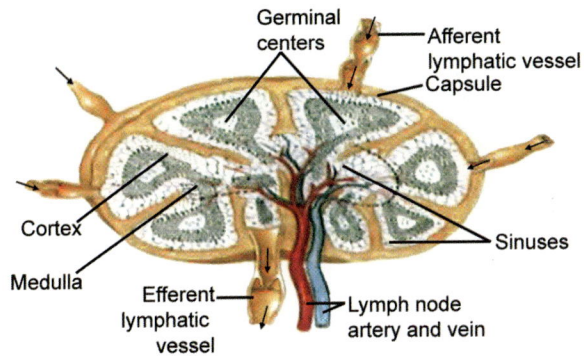

Fig. 10.9: The structure of a bisected lymph node. The arrows indicate the direction of the lymph flow. Mature B cells and T cells in the cortex and medulla remove antigens from the lymph and initiate immune responses *(Martini et al, 2008)*

these vessels into the subcapsular sinus, percolates slowly through the sinuses of the cortex and medulla, and leaves the node through one to three **efferent lymphatic vessels** that emerge from the hilum. No other lymphatic organs have afferent lymphatic vessels; lymph nodes are the only organs that filter lymph as it flows along its course. The lymph node is a "bottleneck" that slows down lymph flow and allows time for cleansing it of foreign matter. The macrophages and reticular cells of the sinuses remove about 99% of the impurities before the lymph leaves the node. On its way to the bloodstream, lymph flows through one lymph node after another and thus becomes quite thoroughly cleansed of most impurities.

When a lymph node is under challenge from a foreign antigen, it may become swollen and painful to the touch— a condition called lymphadenitis. Physicians routinely palpate the accessible lymph nodes of the cervical, axillary, and inguinal regions for swelling. Lymph nodes are common sites of metastatic cancer because cancer cells from almost any organ can break loose, enter the lymphatic capillaries, and lodge in the nodes. Cancerous lymph nodes are swollen but relatively firm and usually painless. Lymphadenopathy is a collective term for all lymph node diseases.

B. Tonsils

There are three main sets of tonsils: (1) A single medial pharyngeal tonsil (adenoids) on the wall of the pharynx just behind the nasal cavity, (2) a pair of palatine tonsils at the posterior margin of the oral cavity, and (3) numerous lingual tonsils, each with a single crypt, concentrated in a patch on each side of the root of the tongue (Figs 10.10 and 10.11). The palatine tonsils are the largest and most often infected. Their surgical removal, called tonsillectomy, used to be one of the most common surgical procedures performed on children, but it is done less often today.

The tonsils are patches of lymphatic tissue located at the entrance to the pharynx, where they guard against ingested and inhaled pathogens. Each is covered by an epithelium and has deep pits called tonsillar crypts lined by lymphatic nodules. The crypts often contain food debris, dead leukocytes, bacteria, and antigenic chemicals. Below the crypts, the tonsils are partially separated from underlying connective tissue by an incomplete fibrous capsule.

C. Spleen

The spleen is the body's largest lymphatic organ. It measures about 12 cm in length and is purplish in color. It is located inferior to the diaphragm on the left side of the body, it rests on portions of the stomach, left kidney, and large intestine (Fig. 10.12). It has a medial hilum penetrated by the splenic artery and vein and lymphatic vessels.

The parenchyma is divided into an outer *cortex* and, near the hilum, an inner *medulla*. The cortex consists mainly of ovoid lymphatic nodules. When the lymph node is fighting a pathogen, these nodules acquire light-staining **germinal centers** where B cells multiply and differentiate into plasma cells. The medulla

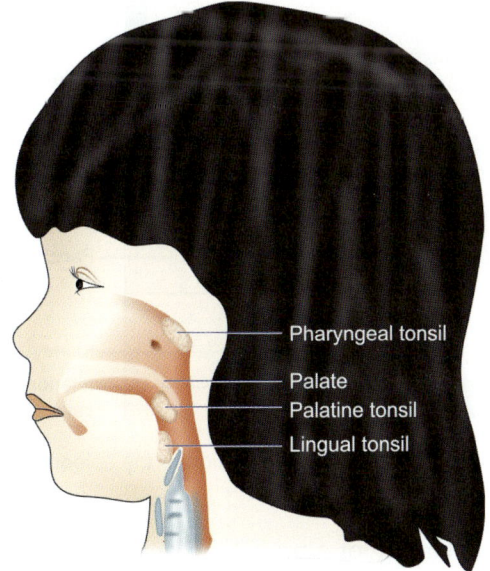

Fig. 10.10: The tonsils are lymphoid nodules in the wall of the pharynx. A single pharyngeal tonsil (the adenoids) lies above the paired palatine and lingual tonsils. Each tonsil contains germinal centers where lymphocyte divisions occur *(Martini et al, 2008)*

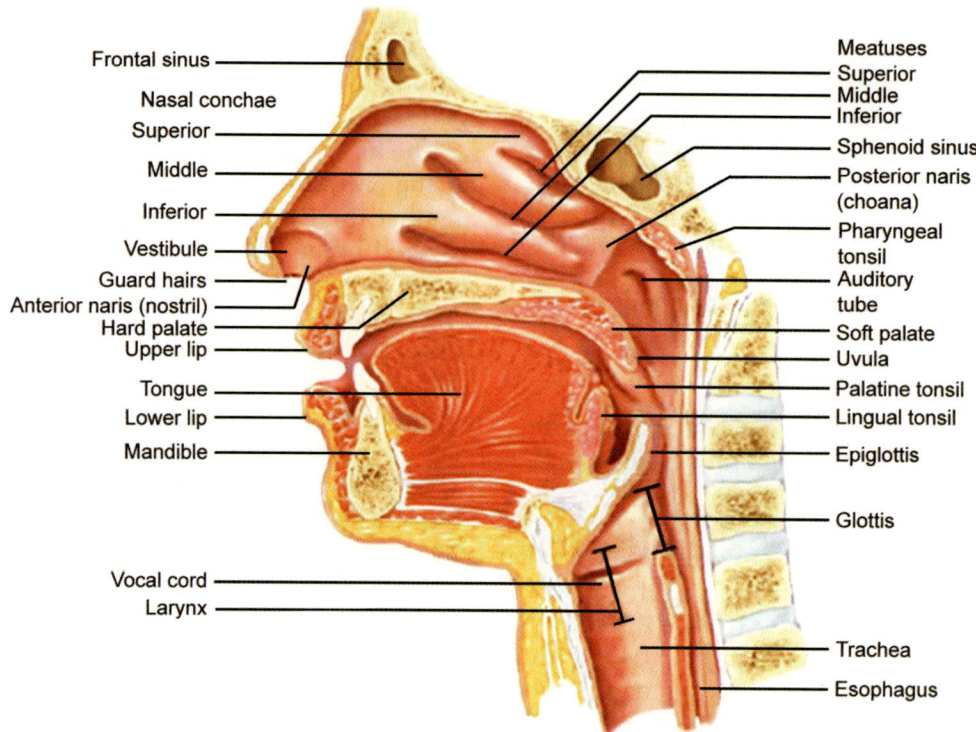

Fig. 10.11: Anatomy of the respiratory tract showing the anatomic locations of the tonsils

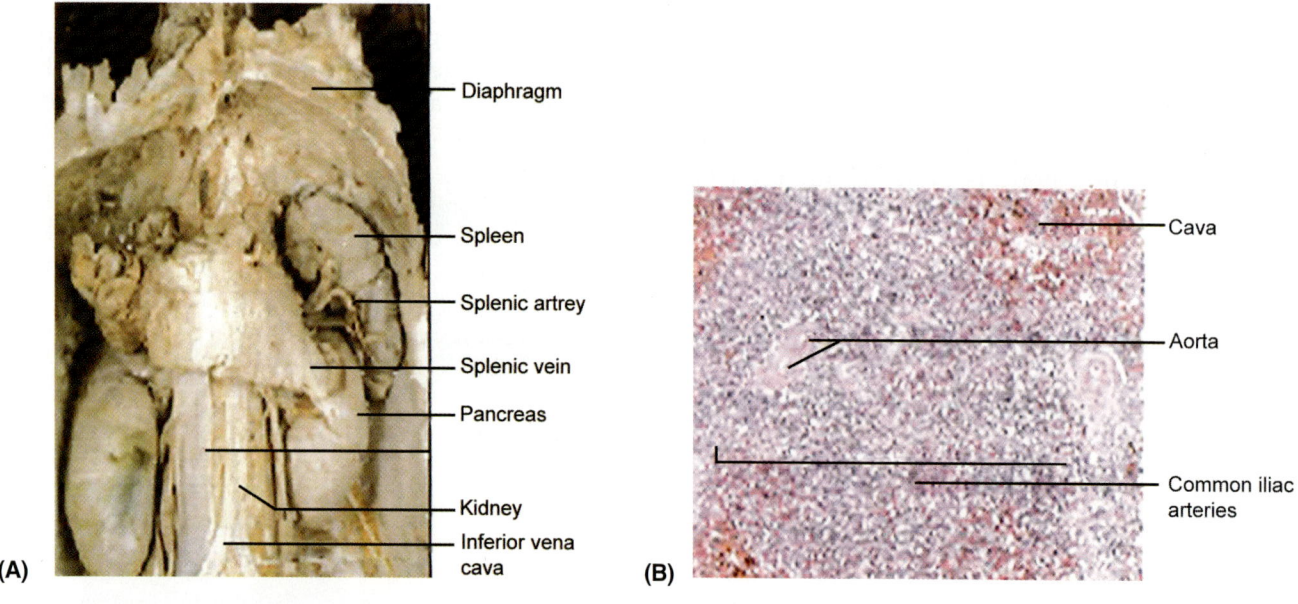

Fig. 10.12: The spleen. **(A)** Position of the spleen in the upper left quadrant of the abdominal cavity, **(B)** Histology *(Saladin, 2003)*

consists largely of a branching network of *medullary cords* composed of lymphocytes, plasma cells, macrophages, reticular cells, and reticular fibers. The cortex and medulla also contain lymph-filled sinuses continuous with the subcapsular sinus.

The spleen contains two specialized types of lymphoid tissues named for their appearance in fresh specimens (not in stained sections): red pulp, which consists of sinuses gorged with concentrated erythrocytes, and white pulp, which consists of

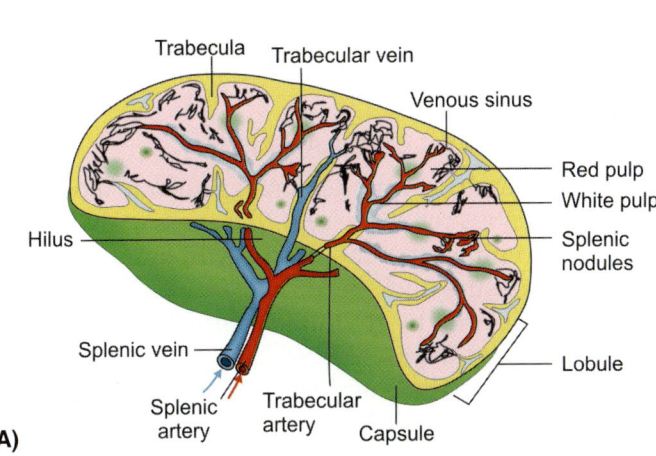

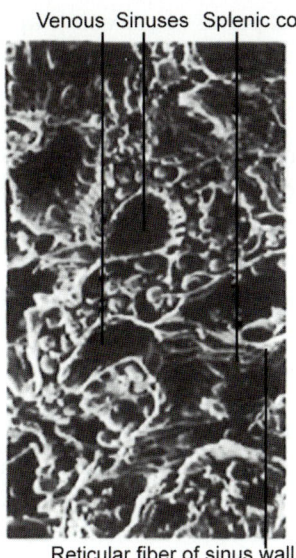

Fig. 10.13: Spleen. **(A)** Drawing of the spleen showing blood flow (colored arrows) through the white pulp to the venous sinuses in the pulp. Note that the white pulp consists of nodules and lymphocytes, while the red pulp is an open mesh with venous sinuses running through it. **(B)** Scanning electron micrograph of a section through the spleen. X 1100 *(Wynsberghe et al, 1995)*

lymphocytes and macrophages aggregated like sleeves along small branches of the splenic artery (Fig. 10.13).

These two tissue types reflect the multiple functions of the spleen. They produce blood cells in the fetus and may resume this role in adults in the event of extreme anemia. They monitor the blood for foreign antigens, much like the lymph nodes do for the lymph. Lymphocytes and macrophages of the white pulp are quick to detect foreign antigens in the blood and activate immune reactions. The splenic capillaries are very permeable; they allow RBCs to leave the bloodstream, accumulate in the sinuses of the red pulp, and reenter the bloodstream later. The spleen is an "erythrocyte grave yard"—old, fragile RBCs rupture as they squeeze through the capillary walls into the sinuses. Splenic macrophages phagocytize their remains, just as they dispose of blood-borne bacteria and other cellular debris. The spleen also compensates for excessive blood volume by transferring plasma from the bloodstream into the lymphatic system.

The spleen is highly vascular and vulnerable to trauma and infection. A ruptured spleen can hemorrhage fatally, but is difficult to repair surgically. Therefore, a common procedure in such cases is its removal, *splenectomy*. A person can live without a spleen, but is somewhat more vulnerable to infections. The main functions of the spleen are:

1. Filtering blood.
2. Manufacturing phagocytic lymphocytes and monocytes. It also contributes to the functioning of the cardiovascular and lymphatic systems as follows:
   A. Macrophages, which are abundant in the spleen, help remove damaged or dead erythrocytes and platelets, microorganisms, and other debris from the blood as it circulates through the spleen. Macrophages also remove iron from the hemoglobin of old red blood cells and return it to the circulation for use by the bone marrow in producing new red blood cells.
   B. Antigens in blood entering the spleen activate lymphocytes that develop into cells that produce antibodies are otherwise involved in the immune reaction.
3. The spleen produces red blood cells during fetal life. In later life, it stores newly formed red blood cells and platelets and releases them into the bloodstream as they are needed.
4. Because the spleen contains a large volume of blood, it serves as a blood reservoir. If the body looses blood suddenly, the spleen contracts and adds blood to the general circulation. The spleen

is capable of releasing approximately 200 mL of blood into the general circulation in one minute.

D. Thymus

The thymus is a member of both the lymphatic and endocrine systems. It houses developing lymphocytes and secretes hormones that regulate their later activity. It is located between the sternum and aortic arch in the superior mediastinum. The thymus is very large in the fetus and grows slightly during childhood, when it is most active.

After age 14, however, it begins to undergo involution (shrinkage) so that it is quite small in adults (Fig. 10.14). In the elderly, the thymus is replaced almost entirely by fibrous and fatty tissue and is barely distinguishable from the surrounding tissues. The fibrous capsule of the thymus gives off trabeculae that divide the parenchyma into several angular lobules. Each lobule has a cortex and medulla populated by T lymphocytes.

Reticular epithelial cells seal off the cortex from the medulla and surround blood vessels and lymphocyte clusters in the cortex. They thereby form a *blood-thymus barrier* that isolates developing lymphocytes from foreign antigens. After developing in the cortex, the T cells migrate to the medulla, where they spend another 3 weeks. There is no blood thymus barrier in the medulla; mature T cells enter blood or lymphatic vessels here and leave the thymus. In the medulla, the reticular epithelial cells form whorls called *thymic corpuscles,* useful for identifying the thymus histologically but of no known function. Besides forming the blood-thymus barrier, reticular epithelial cells secrete hormones called thymosins, thymulin, and thymopoietin, which promote the development and action of T cells. If the thymus is removed from newborn mammals, they waste away and never develop immunity.

LYMPHATIC CIRCULATION

Lymph flows under forces similar to those that govern venous return, except that the lymphatic system has no pump like the heart. Lymph flows at even lower pressure and speed than venous blood; it is moved primarily by rhythmic contractions of the lymphatic vessels themselves, which contract when stretched by lymph. The lymphatic vessels, like the veins, are also aided by a skeletal muscle pump that squeezes them and moves the lymph along. Also like the medium veins, lymphatic vessels have valves that prevent lymph from flowing backward. Since lymphatic vessels are often wrapped with an artery in a common sheath, arterial pulsation may also rhythmically squeeze the lymphatic vessels and contribute to lymph flow. A thoracic (respiratory) pump aids the flow of lymph from the abdominal to the thoracic cavity as one inhales, just as it does in venous return. Finally, at the point where the collecting ducts join the subclavian veins, the rapidly flowing bloodstream draws the lymph into it. Considering these mechanisms of lymph flow, it should be apparent that physical exercise significantly increases the rate of lymphatic return. The lymphatic circulation can be described as follow:

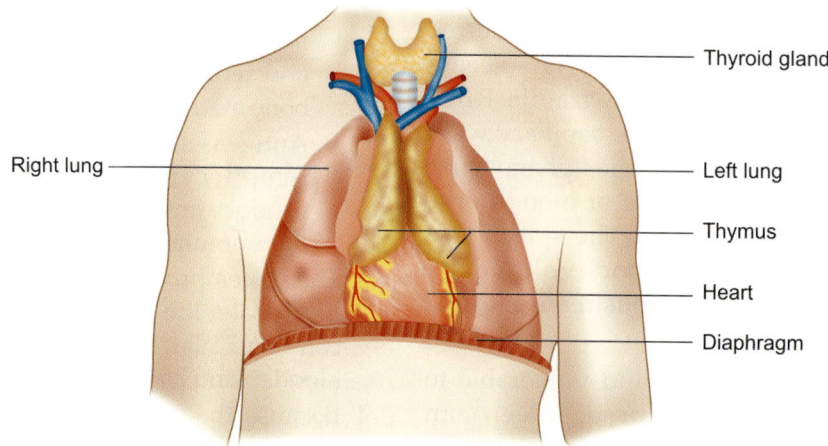

Fig. 10.14: The thymus is a bilobed lymphatic organ that is most prominent in children. In adult, the thymus is atrophied and often barely noticeable *(McKinely and O'Loughlin 2006)*

1. It begins with blind-ending capillaries containing one-way minivalves at the terminus, into which excess interstitial fluid flows as pressure builds up in the tissues.
2. The lymphatic capillaries join to form larger vessels with valves to ensure a one-way flow of fluid, similar to the network of veins. Flow depends on pressure arising from movement of surrounding skeletal muscle and organs.
3. Lymphatic vessels are interrupted periodically by lymph nodes, at which point the lymph is filtered and more lymphocytes may enter the lymph en route to the general circulation.
4. The vessels of the upper right quadrant of the body empty into the right lymphatic duct, which returns the lymph into the general circulation via the right subclavian vein.
5. The remainder of the lymphatic vessels drain into the thoracic duct in the upper abdomen and thoracic cavity. This duct drains into the left subclavian vein.
6. Lymphatic capillaries in the intestinal villi absorb and transport most lipids as chylomicrons.

LYMPHEDEMA (EDEMA = SWELLING)

The lymphatic system, is a system of one-way vessels that collect fluid from the tissues and return it to the bloodstream. Lymphedema occurs when fluid filters into a tissue faster than it is resorbed.

Lymphedema refers to an accumulation of interstitial fluid that occurs due to interference with lymphatic drainage in a part of the body. As the interstitial fluid accumulates, the affected area swells and becomes painful. It often shows as swelling of the face, fingers, abdomen, or ankles but also affects internal organs, where its effects are hidden from view. If the lymphedema is left untreated, the protein rich interstitial fluid may interfere with wound healing and can even contributes to an infection by acting as a growth medium for bacteria. It has fuor fundamental causes.

1. Obstructed Lymphatic Drainage

There are several causes of obstructive lymphoedema (Fig. 10.15):
• Any surgery that requires removal of a group of lymph nodes (e.g. breast cancer surgery when the axillary lymph nodes are removed) puts an individual risk for lymphedema.

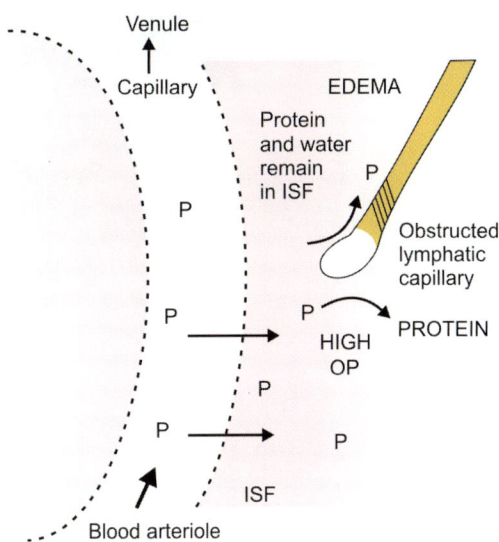

Fig. 10.15: Lymphatic obstruction. P protein, HP hydrostatic pressure, OP osmotic pressure, ISF interstitial fluid, IVF intravascular fluid

• The spread of malignant tumors within the lymph nodes and/or lymphatic vessels can obstruct lymphatic drainage.
• Radiation therapy may cause scar formation that interferes with lymphatic drainage.
• Trauma or infection of the lymph vessels obstructs lymphatic drainage.

2. Reduced Capillary Reabsorption

Capillary reabsorption depends on oncotic pressure, which is proportional to the concentration of blood albumin. A deficiency of blood albumin (hypoprotcinemia) produces edema because the capillaries osmotically reabsorb even less of the fluid that they give off. Since blood albumin is produced by the liver, liver diseases such as cirrhosis tend to lead to hypoproteinemia and edema. Edema is commonly seen in regions of famine due to dietary protein deficiency. Hypoproteinemia also commonly results from severe burns, radiation sickness, and kidney diseases that allow protein to escape in the urine.

3. Increased Capillary Filtration

This results from increases in capillary BP or permeability. Poor venous return, for example, causes pressure to back up into the capillaries. Congestive heart failure and incompetent heart valves can impede venous return from the lungs and cause pulmonary edema. Systemic edema is a common problem when a person is confined to bed

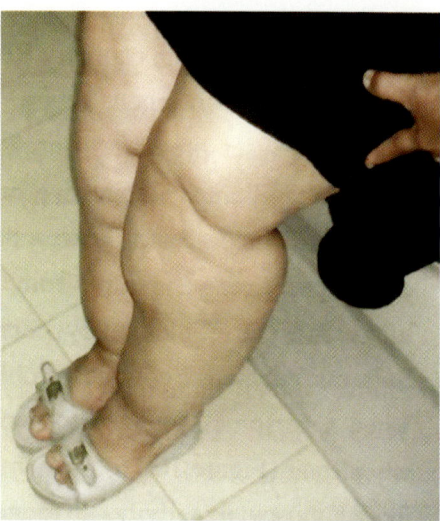

Fig. 10.16: Elephantiasis of the extremities. Confinement to a bed or wheelchair causes blockage of the flow of the lymph and recovery of tissue fluid. The resulting chronic edema leads to fibrosis and elephant-like thickening of the skin. The scrotum of men and breasts of women are often similarly affected

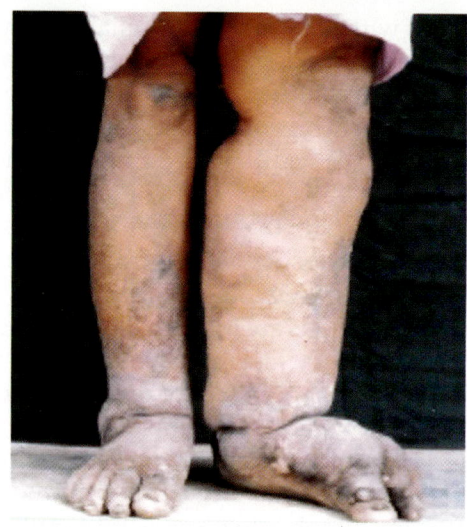

Fig. 10.17: Elephantiasis, a tropical disease caused by lymphatic obstruction. Mosquito-borne round worms infect the lymph nodes and block the flow of lymph and recovery of tissue fluid. The resulting chronic edema leads to fibrosis and elephant-like thickening of the skin. The extremities are typically affected as shown here; the scrotum of men and breasts of women are often similarly affected *(Saladin, 2003)*

or wheelchair (Fig. 10.16), with insufficient muscular activity to promote venous return. Kidney failure leads to edema by causing water retention and hypertension. Histamine causes edema by dilating the arterioles and making the capillaries more permeable. Capillary permeability also increases with age, which puts older people at risk of edema.

In severe edema, so much fluid may transfer from the blood vessels to the tissue spaces that blood volume and pressure drop so low as to cause circulatory shock. Furthermore, as the tissues become swollen with fluid, oxygen delivery and waste removal are impaired and tissue necrosis may occur. Pulmonary edema presents a threat of suffocation, and cerebral edema can produce headaches, nausea, and sometimes seizures and coma.

4. Worm Bites

Millions of individuals in South Asia and Africa have developed lymphoedema as a result of infection by thread-like parasitic filarial worms. Lymphatic filariasis is a type of lymphoedema whereby filarial worms lodge in the lymphatic system, live and reproduce there for years, and eventually obstruct lymphatic drainage. Some filarial worms gain entrance to the body through cracks in the skin of the foot are seen.

However, mosquitoes are the most common vector for transmitting filariasis. Once the mature worms have entered the body, they become permanent

residents. An affected body part can swell to many times its normal size. In these extreme cases, the condition is known also as *elephantiasis* (Figs 10.17 and 10.18). Patients are treated with antiparasitic medications to kill the filarial worms, although the damage to the lymphatic system may be irreversible. Lymphoedema has no cure, but it can be controlled. Patients may wear compression stockings or other compression garments to reduce swelling and assist interstitial fluid return to the circulation. Certain exercise regimens may improve lymphatic drainage as well.

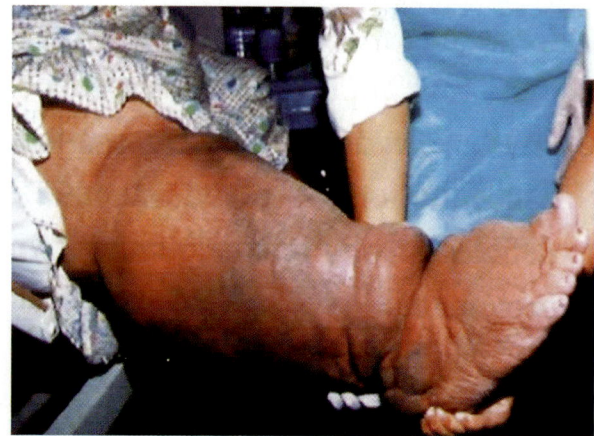

Fig. 10.18: Elephantiasis (lymphatic filariasis) of the lower limb *(McKline and Louglin, 2006)*

II. THE IMMUNE RESPONSE *(IMMUNO = FREE)*

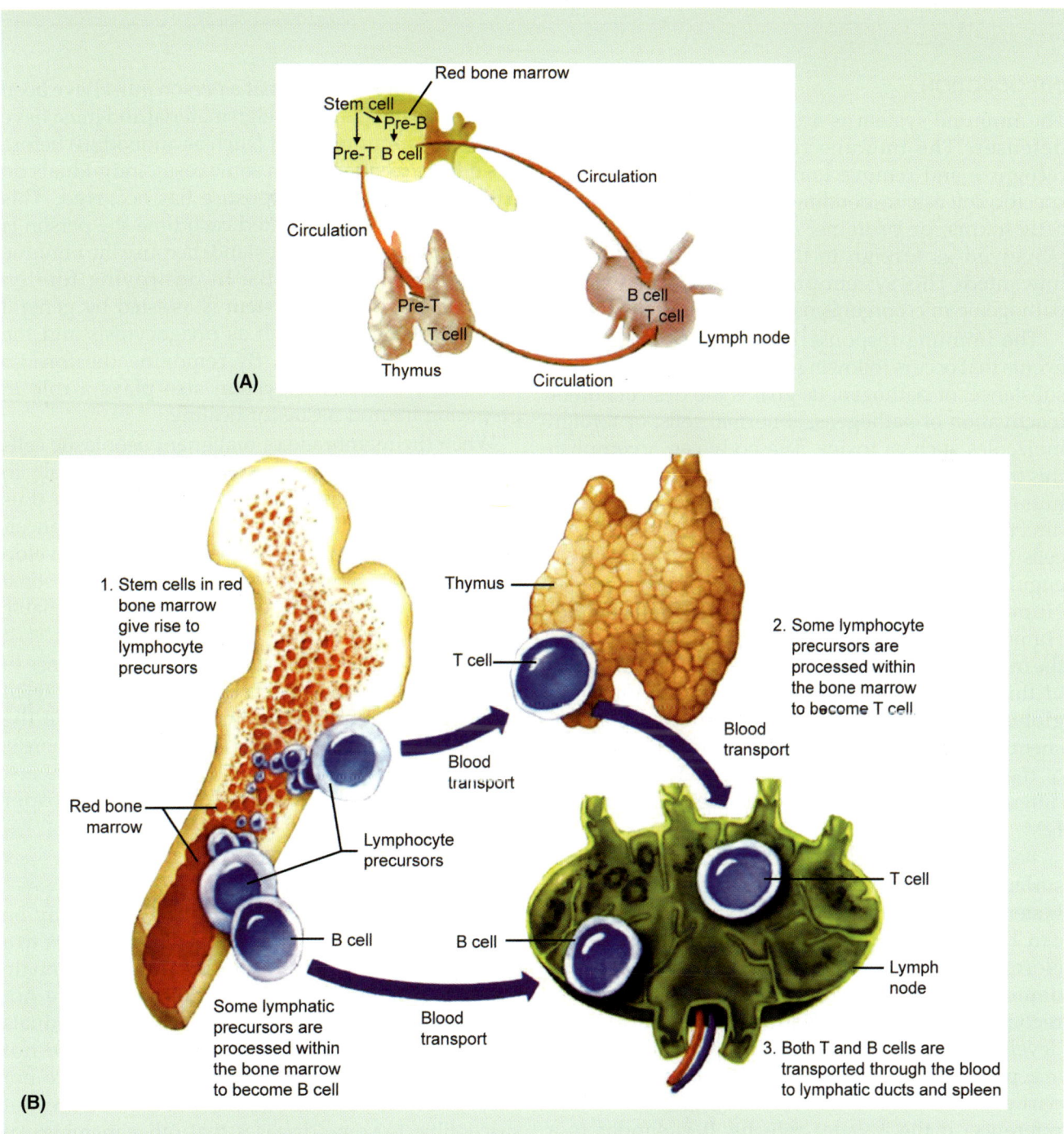

(A)

(B)

Plate XII: (A) Origin and processing of B and T cells. Both B and T cells originate from stem cell in red bone marrow. B cells are processed from pre-B cells in the red marrow, whereas T cells are processed from pre-T cells in the thymus. Both B and T cells circulate to other lymphatic tissues, such as lymph nodes. *(Seeleyetal,1996).* **(B)** Bone marrow releases relatively unspecialized lymphocytes precursors, which after processing specialize as T cells (T lymphocytes) or B cells (B lymphocytes). Note that in the fetus, the medullary cavity contains red marrow *(Shier et al, 2009)*

The immune system is not an organ system but a group of widely distributed cells that recognize foreign substances and act to neutralize or destroy them.

The immune system "learns" to distinguish self- from nonself-antigens prior to birth; thereafter, it normally attacks only nonself-antigens.

INTRODUCTION

The immune system is a major part of the body's defenses. The immune response is intended to recognize and remove undesirable material. It is a specific defense, responding to particular substances, cells toxins, or proteins, and so forth, which are perceived as foreign to the body and, therefore, unwanted. This system protects us from invading pathogenic microorganisms and cancer.

The immune response is a complex cascade of events that occurs following activation by an invading substance, or pathogen. Its goal is the destruction or inactivation of pathogens, abnormal cells, or foreign molecules such as toxins. The body can accomplish this through two mechanisms, cellular immunity and humoral immunity. Cellular immunity involves a direct attack on the foreign substance by specialized cells of the immunity system. These cells physically engulf and deactivate or destroy the offending agents. Humoral immunity is much more complicated. Humoral immunity is basically a chemical attack on the invading substance. The principal chemical agents of this attack are antibodies, also called immunoglobulins(Igs). Antibodies are a unique class of chemicals that are manufactured by specialized cells of the immune system called B cells. There are five different classes of antibodies—IgA, IgD, IgE, IgG, and IgM.

Because of unique antigens, often protein, on the surface of an individual cell, that person's immune system can distinguish self from non-self (foreign) and can thus detect and destroy unknown material. Normally, the immune system ignores "self" cells, demonstrating tolerance. The immune system recognizes a specific invader antigen as foreign, develops a specific response to that particular antigen (e.g. production of matching antibody), and stores that particular response in its **memory cells** for future reference, if the invader returns. It is similar to a surveillance system warning of attack and the subsequent mobilization of an army defense. For example, lymphoid tissues in the pharynx, such as tonsils and adenoids, can capture antigens in foreign material that is inhaled or ingested and process the

immune response. Note that a person must have been exposed to the specific foreign material and must have developed immunity to it (such as antibodies) before this defense is effective. In some cases, individuals do not realize that prior exposure has occurred. This response is usually repeated each time the person is exposed to a particular substance because the immune system has memory cells. In destroying foreign material, the immune system is assisted by general defense mechanisms such as phagocytosis and the inflammatory response. By removing the foreign material, the immune system also plays a role in preparing injured tissue for healing.

When the membrane of malignant neoplastic cells is abnormal, the immune system may be able to identify these cells as "foreign" and remove them, thus playing an important role in the prevention of cancer. It has been noted that individuals frequently develop cancer when the immune system is depressed for some reason. However, not all cancer cells are identifiable as foreign, therefore, may not be removed.

The immune system directs the correct response to an antigen, but also has built-in controls to prevent excessive response. Two limiting factors are the removal of the causative antigen during the response, and the short lifespan of the chemical messengers. Tolerance to self-antigens prevents improper responses.

TYPES OF IMMUNITY

Resistance to disease may be innate, or it may be acquired in several different ways. The resistance to a disease, which is present at birth, is called innate resistance. Some individuals and species are not susceptible to diseases that infect other individuals or species. For example, human beings are not susceptible to canine distemper, and dogs are not susceptible to tetanus. Some individuals are not susceptible to some diseases that other members of their species are susceptible to. In a sense, innate resistance is not considered in some texts as an immunity, since it does not involve the specific defenses of the immune response. As listed in Box 10.1 and Fig. 10.19, immunity, as a state of protection from

Box 10.1: The immune system*

1. Nonspecific
  a. Mechanical reflexes
  • Coughing, sneezing
  • Earwax
  • Sphincter control of bladder
  b. Secretions of bactericidal substances
  • Stomach acid
  • Action of cilia
  • Enzymes in tears and saliva
  c. Phagocytic cells
  • Neutrophils
  • Monocytes
  • Macrophages
  d. Circulating chemicals
  • Complement
  • Interferon

2. Specific
  a. Humoral immunity
  • Proection against bacterial infection
  • Clones of B lymphocytes
  • Recognition of chemical configuration
  • Production of antibodies by plasma cells
  • Eradication of antigen
  b. Cellular immunity
  • Protection against viral infection—tuberculosis, leprosy.
  • Transplant rejection
  • Production of cytokines by T lymphocytes
  • Eradication of antigen

Modified from Thomson NC, Kirkwood EM, Levers RS. In Thomson NC, et al (eds). Handbook of Clinical Allergy. Oxford, Blackwell Scientific, 1990, pp 1–36.

infectious disease, has both a less specific or innate and a more specific or acquired component.

Innate Immunity (Natural Immunity)

Innate immunity is genetically predetermined. It is present at birth and has no relation to previous exposure to a particular antigen. All humans are born with some innate immunity.

Innate immunity provides the first line of defense against infection and is not specific to a particular pathogen. It consists of four types of defensive barriers (Fig. 10.19).

1. Physical barriers, e.g. skin, mucous membrane.
2. Inflammatory barriers, e.g. leakage of fluid containing chemical mediators.
3. Chemical barriers, e.g. lysozyme, complement, interferon and others.
4. Phagocytic barriers, e.g. neutrophils, macrophages.

Acquired Immunity

The immune response consists of two steps (Fig. 10.20):
1. A primary response occurs when a person is first exposed to an antigen. During exposure, the antigen is recognized and processed, and subsequent development of antibodies or sensitized T lympho-cytes is initiated. This process may take several days or weeks and can be monitored using serum antibody titer. Following the initial rise in liter, the level of antibody falls.

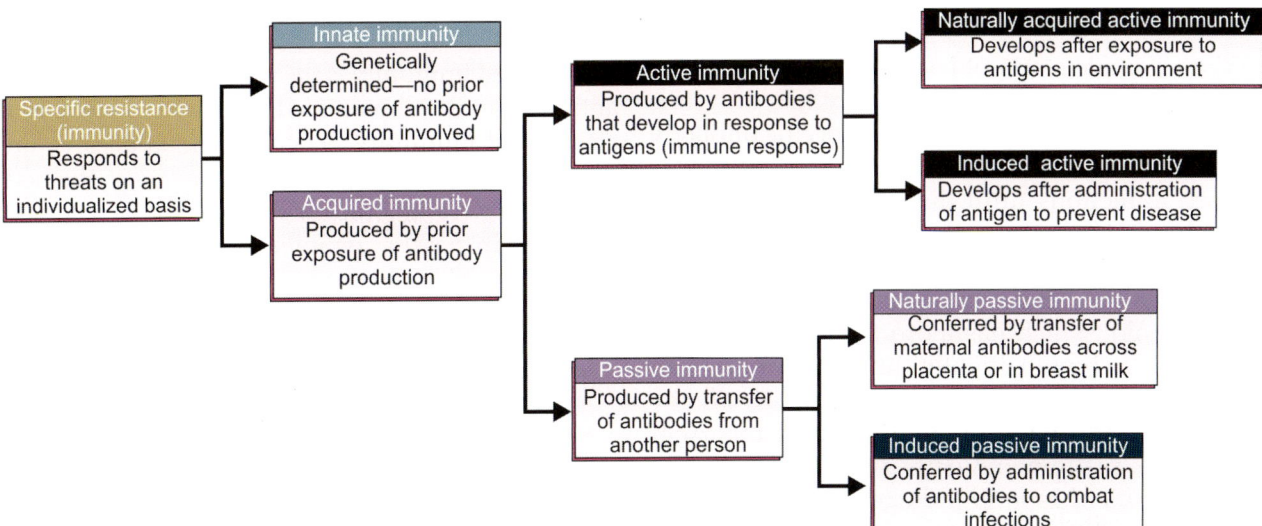

Fig. 10.19: Types of immunity *(Martini et al, 2008)*

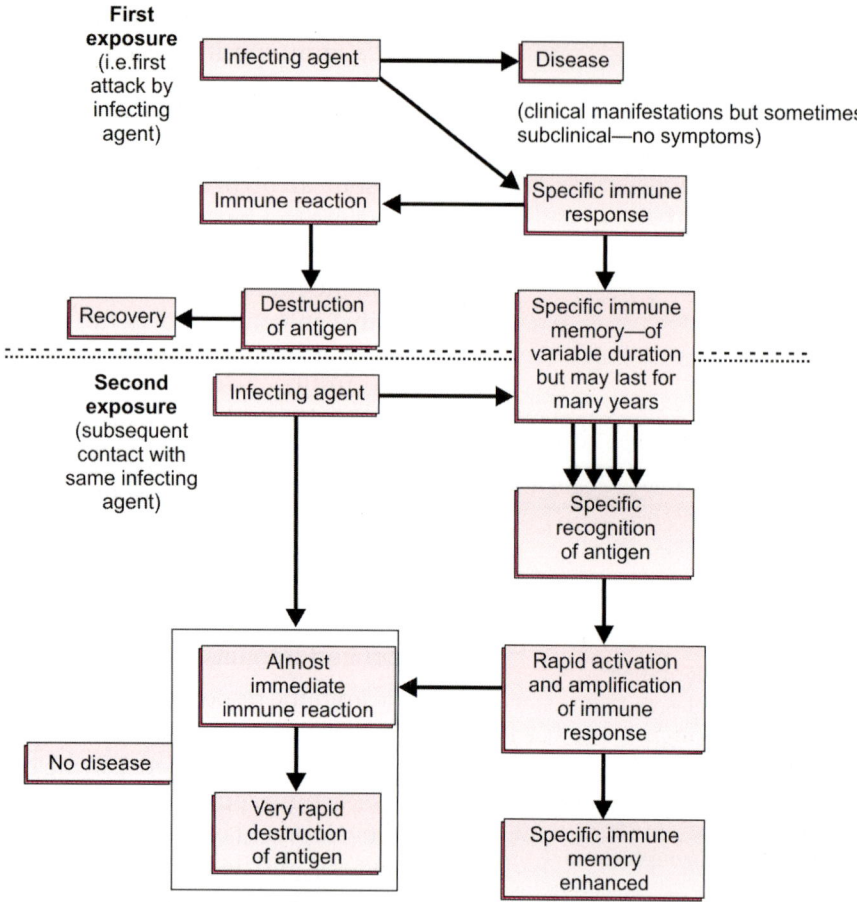

Fig. 10.20: The sequence of events in an infection

2. A secondary response results when a repeat exposure to the same antigen occurs. Even years later, the memory cells stimulate production of large numbers of the matching antibodies or T cells very quickly.

When a single strain of bacteria or virus causes a disease, the affected person usually has only one episode of the disease because the specific antibody is retained in the memory. Young children are subject to many infections until they establish a pool of antibodies. As one ages, the number of infections declines. However, when there are many strains of a bacteria or virus causing a disease, for example, the common cold, which has more than 100 causative organisms, each with slightly different antigens, an individual never develops antibodies to all the organisms, and therefore, he or she has recurrent colds. The influenza virus, which affects the respiratory tract, has several antigenic forms, e.g. type A and type B. These viruses have various strains that mutate or change slightly over time. For this reason,

a new influenza vaccine is manufactured each year, its composition based on the current antigenic forms of the virus most likely to cause an epidemic of the infection.

Acquired immunity is the resistance to infection by antibody- and cell-mediated immunity. One way of classifying immunity is active versus passive and natural versus artificial. In *active immunity*, the body makes its own antibodies or T cells against a pathogen, whereas in *passive immunity*, the body acquires antibodies or T cells produced by another person or an animal. Either type of immunity can occur naturally or, for treatment and prevention purposes, it can be induced artificially. Thus we can recognize four classes of immunity under this scheme.

So immunity is acquired in four ways (Fig. 10.19, Table 10.2).

Active immunity develops when the person's own body develops antibodies or T cells in response to a

Table 10.2: Types of acquired immunity

Type	Mechanism	Memory	Example
Natural active	Antibodies are formed in the body in response to exposure to an antigen. Sometimes providing permanent immunity (measles, chickenpox, yellow fever). Long-lasting (years to lifetime).	Yes	Person has chickenpox once
Artifical active	Vaccine (live or attenuated organisms) is injected into person to stimulate the production of specific anti-bodies. May require booster injections. Long-lasting (years to lifetime).	Yes	Person has measles vaccine and gains immunity
Natural passive	Antibodies are acquired from a source outside the body. Antibodies from an immune pregnant woman pass to the fetus through the placenta or to the baby in milk during breastfeeding. The newborn baby receives temporary (several weeks or months) immunity against diseases to which the mother has active immunity. May be effective for several months.	No	Placental passage during pregnancy or ingestion of breast milk
Artifical passive	Immune serum from immunized animal or human beings is injected into exposed individual, who receives specific antibodies (diphtheria, tetanus). Effective for weeks to months.	No	Gammaglobulin if recent exposure to microbe

specific antigen introduced into the body. This process takes a few weeks, but the result usually lasts for years because memory B and T cells are retained in the body.

- *Active natural immunity* may be acquired by direct exposure to an antigen, for example, when a person has an infection and then develops antibodies. Active natural immunity signifies the production of one's own antibodies or T cells as a result of **vaccination** against diseases such as smallpox, tetanus, or influenza. A **vaccine** consists of either dead or *attenuated* (weakened) pathogens which can stimulate an immune response but normally cause little or no discomfort or disease. In some cases, periodic "booster shots" are given to restimulate immune memory and maintain a high level of protection. Vaccination has eliminated smallpox worldwide and greatly reduced the incidence of life-threatening childhood diseases, but many people continue to die from influenza and other diseases that could be prevented by vaccination (Table 10.3).

- *Active artificial immunity* develops when a specific antigen is purposefully introduced into the body, stimulating the production of antibodies. For example, a vaccine is a solution containing dead or weakened (attenuated) organisms that stimulate the immune system to produce antibodies but do not result in the disease itself. Work continues on the development of vaccines utilizing antigenic fragments of microbes or genetically altered forms. A long list of vaccines is available including polio, diphtheria, measles, and chickenpox. Infants begin a regular schedule of immunizations/vaccines shortly after birth to reduce the risk of serious infections and in hopes of eradicating some infectious diseases.

The occurrence of many infectious diseases, such as polio and measles, has declined where vaccines have been well utilized. Believing smallpox (variola) had been eradicated in many countries by the mid-1950s, the U.S. discontinued the smallpox vaccine in 1972. The World Health Organization (WHO) worked toward worldwide eradication and the last case of smallpox was recorded in 1977. Polio vaccination was implemented in 1954, and cases are a rare occurrence today. Unfortunately, not all individuals agree with immunization programs, therefore, infectious diseases persist. The search continues for additional vaccines against AIDS and malaria, and so forth. Research is also continuing on genetic vaccines, where only a strand of bacterial DNA would form the vaccine, thus reducing the risks from injection of the microorganism.

A toxoid is an altered or weakened bacterial toxin that acts as an antigen in a similar manner.

A booster is an additional immunization, given perhaps 5 or 10 years after initial immunization, that "reminds" the immune system of the antigen and promotes a better secondary response.

Table 10.3: Common immunization

Immunization target	Type of immunity provided	Vaccine type	Remarks
Viruses			
Polyviruses	Active	Live, attenuated	Oral
	Active	Killed	Booster every 2–3 years
Rubella	Active	Live, attenuated	
	Passive	Human antibodies (pooled)	
Mumps	Active	Live, attenuated	
Measles (rubeola)	Active	Live, attenuated	May need second booster
Hepatitis A	Passive	Human antibodies (pooled)	
Hepatitis B	Active	Killed	May need periodic boosters
	Passive	Human antibodies (pooled)	
Smallpox	Active	Live, related virus	Boosters every 3–5 years (no longer required as disease appears to have been eliminated)
Yellow fever	Active	Live, attenuated	Booster every 10 years
Herpes zoster	Passive	Human antibodies (pooled)	
Rabies	Passive	Human antibodies (pooled)	
Bacteria			
Typhoid	Active	Killed	Booster every 2, 3 or 5 years, depending on vaccine type
Tuberculosis	Active	Live, attenuated	
Tetanus	Active	Toxins only	Booster every 5–10 years
	Passive	Human antibodies (pooled)	
Diphtheria	Active	Toxins only	Boosters every 10 years
Streptococcal pneumonia	Active	Bacteria and cell-wall components	
Botulism	Passive	Horse antibodies	
Rickettsia: Typhus	Active	Killed	Boosters yearly
Haemophilus influenzae B (HiB)	Active	Killed	May need periodic boosters
Other toxins			
Snake bite	Passive	Horse antibodies	
Spider bite	Passive	Horse antibodies	
Venomous fish	Passive	Horse antibodies	
Spine	Passive	Horse antibodies	

An example of the commonly used vaccine is the DPT (diphtheria/pertussis/tetanus) vaccine. This vaccine contains antigenic proteins from the bacteria that cause diphtheria, whooping cough, and tetanus. It is administered at several intervals during the first five years of life and provides protection against infection from these bacteria. Some vaccines will impart lifelong immunity, while others must be periodically followed with a "booster dose" to ensure continued protection.

An example of the clinical use of both active and passive immunities is the regimen used for the prevention of tetanus.

Most people from the developed countries have received some form of tetanus vaccination during their life. These people typically have some antibodies to tetanus and often need nothing more than a tetanus booster. However, some people have never received any sort of tetanus vaccination. When they seek treatment for a tetanus-prone wound, they must receive prophylaxis for tetanus in addition to care for their wound. This is best achieved by providing both passive and active immunities. To provide immediate protection, the patient is administered antibodies specific for tetanus (tetanus immune globulin). The tetanus immune globulin provides passive immunity until the body's immune system can respond to the vaccination and develops antibodies specific for tetanus. This should be followed by periodic tetanus boosters until the patient's immunization program is complete.

Passive immunity occurs when antibodies are transferred from one person to another. These are effective immediately but offer only temporary protection because memory has not been established in the recipient, and the antibodies are gradually removed from the circulation. There are also two forms of passive immunity:

- *Passive natural immunity* is a temporary immunity that results from acquiring antibodies produced by another individual. The only natural way for this to happen is for a fetus to acquire antibodies from the mother through the placenta before birth or for a baby to acquire it through the colostrum or breast milk after birth.
- *Passive artificial immunity* is a temporary immunity that results from the injection of an *immune serum* obtained from another individual or from animals (such as horses) that produced antibodies against a certain pathogen. The serum containing the antibodies is called the immune serum. An example is the administration of the rabies antiserum or snake antivenom. Passive immunity is used against botulism, diphtheria, whooping cough, rabies, tetanus, and rattle-snake venom. Sometimes immunoglobulins are administered to an individual who has been immunized in order to reduce the effects of the infection (e.g. hepatitis B). Artificial passive immunity is particularly useful when a

person has been exposed to a dangerous disease and must be immunized as quickly as possible. Immune serum is used for emergency treatment of snakebites, botulism, tetanus, rabies, and other diseases. Although the protection of artificial passive immunity is immediate upon injection, it lasts only a few weeks.

FUNCTIONS OF THE IMMUNE SYSTEM

The purpose of the immune response is to inactivate or destroy pathogens, abnormal cells, and foreign molecules (such as toxins) (Table 10.4). It is based on the activation of lymphocytes by specific antigens through the process of antigen recognition. Figure 10.21 presents an overview of the immune response. When an antigen triggers an immune response, it usually activates T cells first and then B cells. T cells are typically activated by phagocytes that have engulfed the antigen (sometimes T cells are activated by abnormal body cells). Once activated, the T cells both attack the antigen and stimulate the activation of B cells. The activated B cells mature into cells that produce antibodies. The circulating antibodies bind to and attack the antigen.

The functions of the immune system is illustrated in Table 10.4.

COMPONENTS OF THE IMMUNE SYSTEM

The immune system consists of the lymphoid structures, the immune cells, and the tissues concerned with immune cell development (Box 10.2). Many chemical mediators in the body have essential functional

Table 10.4: Functions of the immune system

Function	Humoral	Cellular
Processing of antigen	T-helper cells and macrophages	Macrophages plus antigens of major histocompatibility complex (MHC)
Cellular recognition of antigen	Receptors on B lymphocytes are sensitive to specific chemical configurations	T lymphocytes with receptors to specific subsets of MIC antigens
Cellular response to presentation of antigen	Specific colonies of B lymphocytes multiply and produce plasma cells and memory cells	Specific colonies of T lymphocytes multiply and produce effector T cells and memory T cells
Cellular action aganist antigen	Plasma cells produce specific immunoglobulin (antibodies); memory cells become plasma cells, with later antigen contact	Effector T cells produce cytokines; memory T cells become effector T cells, with later antigen contact
Eradication of antigen	Reaction with specific antibody is facilitated by non-specific branch of the immune system; antigen is removed by cells of a nonspecific branch	Destruction of antigen by cytokines and elements of the immune system.

Box 10.2: Major components of the immune system and their functions

Antigen	Foreign substance or component of cell that stimulates immune response
Antibody	Specific protein produced in humoral response to bind with antigen
Autoantibody	Antibodies against self antigen; attacks body's own tissues
Thymus	Gland located in the mediastinum, large in children, decreasing size in adults. Site of maturation and proliferation of T lymphocytes
Lymphatic tissue	Contains many lymphocytes, filters body fluids, removes foreign matter, immune response
Bone marrow	Source of stem cells, leucocytes, and maturation of B lymphocytes
Cells Neutrophils	White blood cells for phagocytosis; nonspecific defense; active in inflammatory process
Basophils	White blood cells: Bind IgE, release histamine in anaphylaxis
Eosinophils	White blood cells: Participation in allergic responses
Monocytes	White blood cells: Migrate from blood into tissues to become macrophages
Macrophages	Phagocytosis; process and present antigens to lymphocytes for the immune response
Mast cells	Release chemical mediators such as histamine in connective tissue
B lymphocytes	Humoral immunity-activated cell becomes an antibody-producing plasma cell or a B memory cell
Plasma cells	Develop from B lymphocytes and secrete specific antibodies
T lymphocytes	White blood cells: Cell-mediated immunity
Cytotoxic or killer T cells	Destroy antigens, cancer cells, virus-infected cells
Memory T cells	Remember antigen and quckley stimulate immune response on re-exposure
Helper T cells	Activate B and T cells; control or limit specific immune response
NK lymphocytes	Natural killer cells destroy foreign cells, virus-infected cells, and cancer cells
Chemical mediators complement	Group of inactive proteins in the circulation that, when activated, stimulate the release of other chemical mediators, promoting inflammation, chemotaxis, and phagocytosis
Histamine	Released from mast cells and basophils, particulary in allergic reactions. Cause vasodilation and increased vascular permeability or edema, also contraction of bronchiolar smooth muscle, and pruritus
Kinins (e.g. brandykinin)	Cause vasodilation, increased permeability (edema), and pain
Prostaglandins	Group of lipids with varying effects. Some cause inflammation, vasodilation and increased permeability, and pain
Leukotrienes	Group of lipids, derived from mast cells and basophils, which cause contraction of bronchiolar smooth muscle and have a role in development of inflammation
Cytokines (messengers)	Includes lymphokines, monokines, interferons, and interleukins; produced by macrophages and activated T lymphocytes; stimulate activation and proliferation of B and T cells, communication between cells; involved in inflammation, fever, and leukocytosis
Tumor necrosis factor (TNF)	A cytokine active in the inflammatory and immune responses; stimulates fever, chemotaxis, mediator of tissue wasting, stimulates T cells, mediator in septic shock (decreasing BP), stimulates necrosis in some tumors
Chemotactic factors	Attract phagocytes to area of inflammation

roles as well. The lymphoid structures, including the lymph nodes, the spleen and tonsils, the intestinal lymphoid tissue, and the lymphatic circulation which has been discussed before, form the basic structure within which the immune response can function.

The immune cells, or lymphocytes, as well as macrophages provide the specific mechanism for the identification and removal of the foreign material. All cells originate in bone marrow, and the bone marrow and thymus have roles in the maturation of the cells.

The blood and circulatory system provide a major transportation and communication network for the immune system.

Antigens

An antigen is a protein or polysaccharide molecule that, when introduced into the body as a foreign substance, causes the production of specific antibodies, the proliferation of specific T cells, or both. Almost any protein is capable of acting as an antigen.

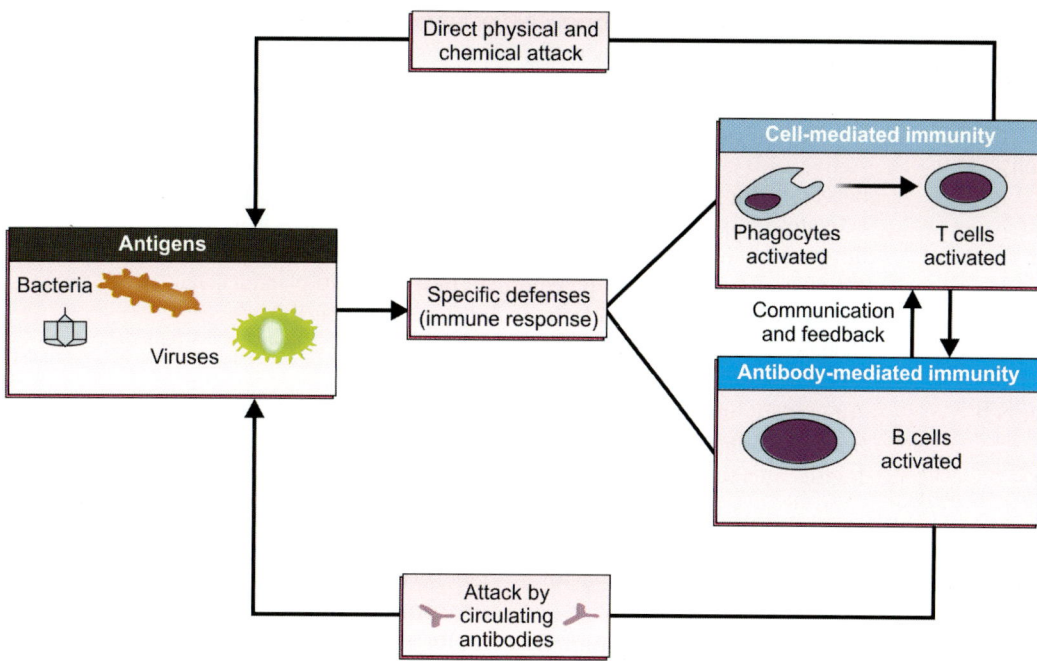

Fig. 10.21: An overview of the immune response *(Martini et al, 2008)*

Incompatible blood cells, proteins on the surfaces of transplanted tissues, pollen, dust, animal dander (flaking skin), animal hair, some components of food, bacteria and toxins are common examples of potential antigens.

Certain small substances with very low molecular weights can be antigenic. Such substances, called Haptens, are reactive only when they are combined with a much larger carrier molecule, such as protein. The antibiotic penicillin is an example of a hapten. In some patients who receive penicillin for the first time, it combines with a protein carrier to cause the formation of antibodies against penicillin. Subsequent doses of penicillin will cause the antibodies to react with the small penicillin molecule, producing a severe immune response (an allergy) to the penicillin.

Cells

The primary cell in the immune response is the lymphocyte, one of the leukocytes or white blood cells produced by the bone marrow (Box 10.3). Mature lymphocytes are termed immune-competent cells—cells that have the special function of recognizing and reacting with antigens in the body. The two groups of lymphocytes, T and B lymphocytes, determine which type of immunity will be initiated, either cell-mediated immunity or humoral immunity (Figs 10.22 to 10.24).

- *T lymphocytes (T cells)* arise from stem cells (incompletely differentiated cells held in reserve in the body) in the bone marrow and then travel to the thymus for further differentiation and development of cell membrane receptors. Cell-mediated immunity develops when T lymphocytes with protein receptors on the cell surface recognize antigens on the surface of target cells and directly destroy the invading antigens. These specially programmed T cells then reproduce, creating an 'army' to battle the invader, and they also activate other T and B lymphocytes. T cells are primarily effective against virus-infected cells, fungal and protozoal infections, cancer cells, and foreign cells such as transplanted tissue. There are a number of subgroups of T cells, marked by differ-ent surface receptor molecules, each of which has specialized function in the immune response.

- The cytotoxic CD8 positive T-killer cells destroy the target cell by binding to the antigen and releasing damaging enzymes or chemicals, such as monokines and lymphokines, which may destroy foreign cell membranes or cause an inflammatory response, attract macrophages to the site, stimulate the proliferation of more lymphocytes, and stimulate hematopoiesis. Phagocytic cells then clean up the debris. The helper CD4 positive T cell facilitates the immune response. A sub-group, the memory T cells,

Box 10.3: Principal cells of immune system

Type of cell	Major functions
B cell	Differentiates into antibody-secreting plasma cells when stimulated by antigen
T cell	
• Helper T cell	Activates B cells after B cells encounter specific antigens by releasing B cell growth factor; necessary for appropriate responses of cytotoxic T cells and suppressor T cells to antigens; activates lymphokines that activate macrophages.
• Suppressor T cell	Suppresses autoimmune responses, excessive antibody production; regulates activities of cytotoxic T cells; inhibits development of B cells into plasma cells.
• Cytotoxic T cell	Attacks-infected cells and tumor cells; is antigen-specific
• Delayed hyper-sensitivity T cell	Releases lymphokines, which assist in macrophage activity
Natural killer cell	Attacks any intracellular foreign microorganism; not antigen specific
Plasma cell	Secretes antibodies that mark foreign substances for destruction
Macrophage	Ingests microorganisms, presents antigens to T cells to initiate specific immune response

remains in the lymph nodes for years, ready to activate the response again, if the same invader returns.

Two subgroups of T cells have gained prominence as markers in patients with acquired immuno-deficiency syndrome (AIDS) (Figs 10.23 and 24). T-helper cells have "CD4" molecules as receptors on the cell membrane and the killer T cells have "CD8" molecules. These receptors are important in T cell activation. While the CD8+ cells are primarily cytotoxic, CD4+ T cells regulate all the cells in the immune system, the B and T lymphocytes,

macrophages, and natural killer (NK) cells, by secreting the "messenger" cytokines. The human immunodeficiency virus (HIV) destroys the CD4 cells, thus crippling the entire immune system. The ratio of the CD4 to CD8 T cells (normal is 2:1) is closely monitored in AIDS patients as a reflection of the progress of the infection.

• The B lymphocytes or B cells are responsible for humoral immunity through the production of antibodies or immunoglobulins. B cells are thought to mature in the bone marrow and then proceed to the spleen and lymphoid tissue (Box 10.4).

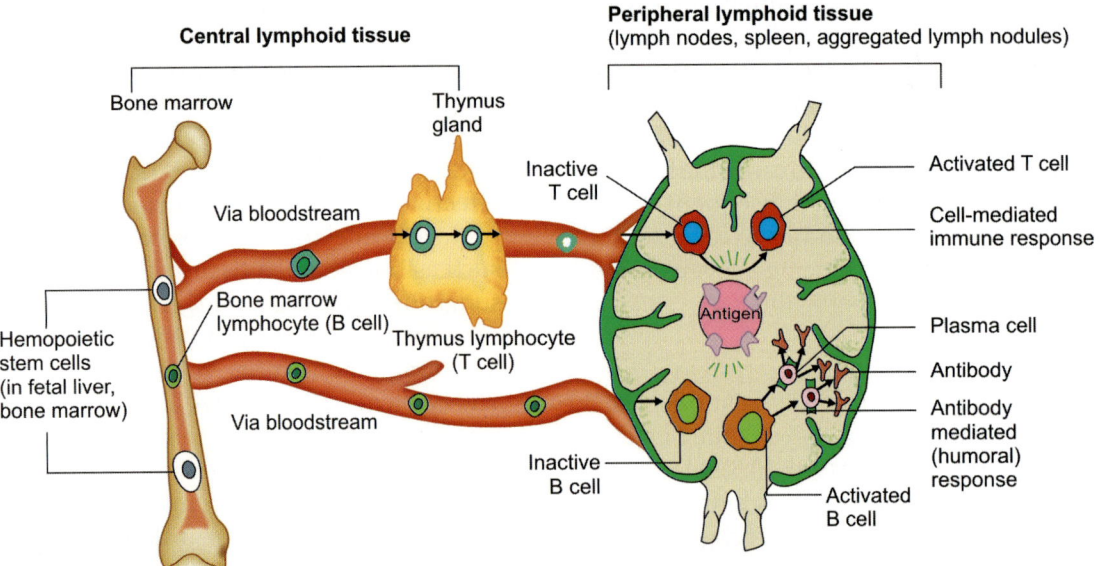

Fig. 10.22: The development of T and B cells from hemopoietic stem cells in the fetal liver and postnatal bone marrow. Some stem cells mature in the bone marrow into B cells, which become plasma cells. T cells mature only after the precursor stem cells migrate to the thymus gland via the bloodstream. T and B cells are activated when they come in contact with a specific antigen in peripheral lymphoid tissue *(Wynsberghe et al, 1995)*

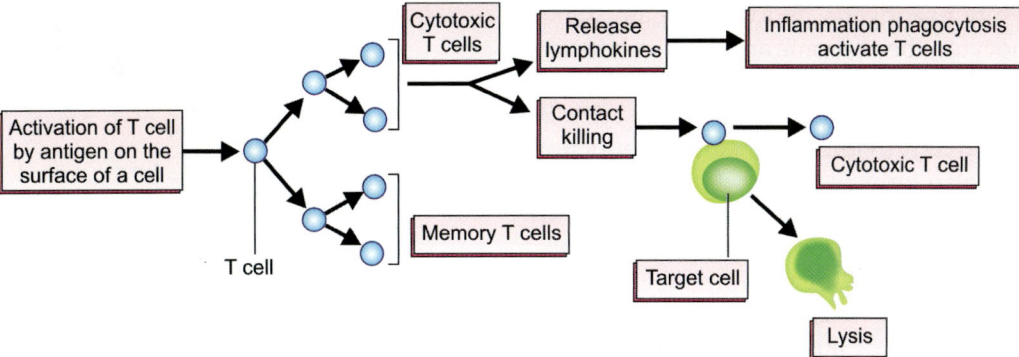

Fig. 10.23: Stimulation and effects of T cells. When activated, T cells form cytotoxic T cells and memory cells. The cytotoxic T cells cause lysis of target cells or release lymphokines that promote the destruction of the antigen. The memory T cells are responsible for the secondary response *(Seeley et al, 1996)*

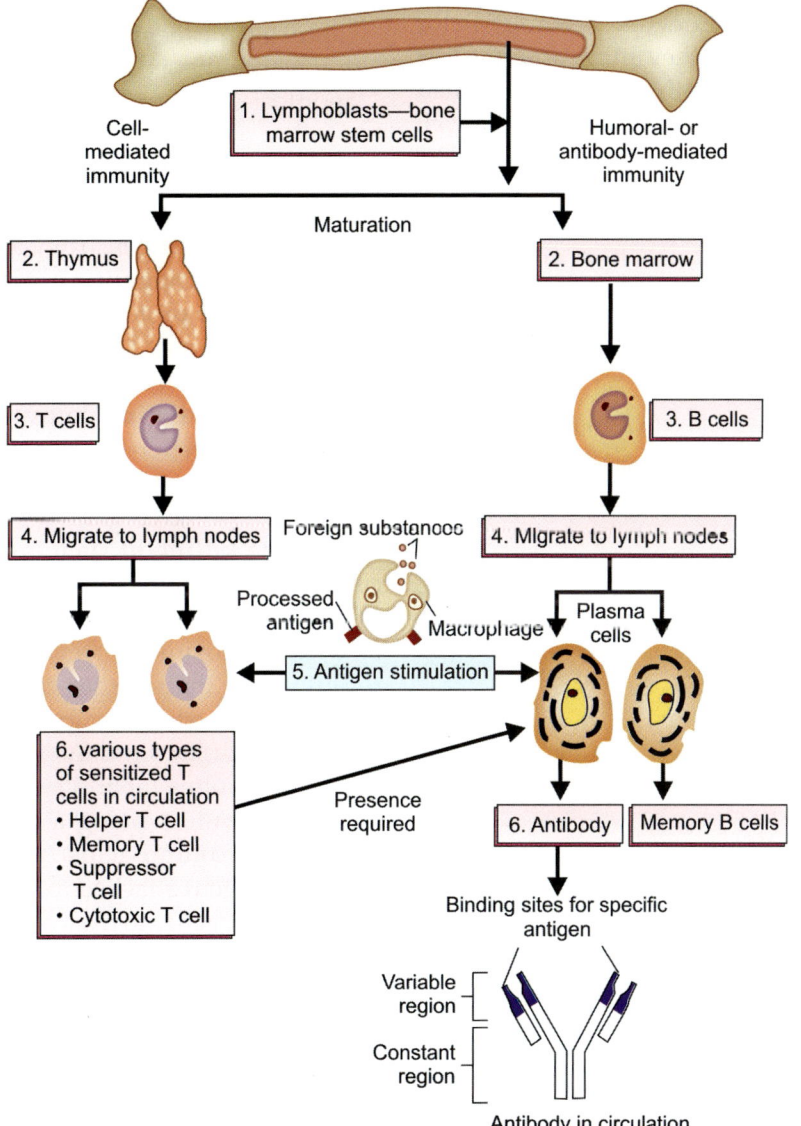

Fig. 10.24: Development of cellular and humoral immunities *(Gould, 2006)*

After exposure to antigens, and with the assistance of T lymphocytes, they become antibody producing plasma cells. B lymphocytes act primarily against bacteria and viruses that are outside body cells. B-memory cells that provide for repeated production of antibodies also form.

- *Natural killer (NK) cells* are large lymphocytes with a nonspecific role, produced in red bone marrow. They account for 1 to 3% of all lymphocytes. They kill certain tumor and virus-infected cells. NK cells are classified as part of innate immunity, because they do not exhibit specity memory. Instead, NK cells recognize a general class of cells such as tumor cells, rather than a specific type of tumor cell. The natural killer (NK) cells are lymphocytes distinct from the T and B lymphocytes. Without prior exposure and sensitization, they attack and lyse *host cells* (cells of one's own body) that have either turned cancerous or become infected with viruses, as well as bacteria and cells of transplanted tissues. The continual "patrolling" of the body by NK cells "on the lookout" for abnormal cells is called *immunological surveillance.* When an NK cell recognizes an abnormal cell, it secretes proteins called **performs,** which bind to the enemy cell surface and make holes in its membrane. This has

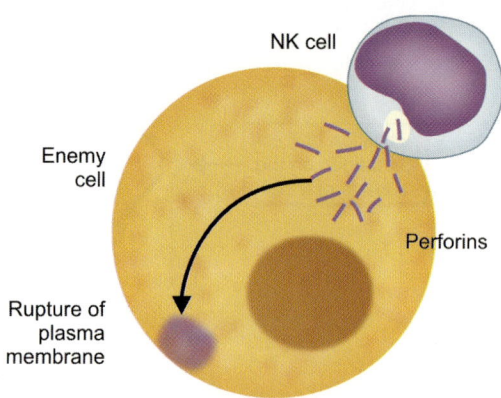

Fig. 10.25: The action of perforin *(Saladin, 2003)*

generally been thought to destroy host cells by rupturing the membrane (Fig. 10.25), although there is a newer theory that perforin induces target cell apoptosis.

Antibodies (Immunoglobulins)

Antibodies are proteins produced by B cells in response to an antigen. They are specialized to react with antigens, triggering a complex process, called immunity, that protects the body by destroying the invader. In contrast to phagocytosis, which provides an immediate defense against infections, antibodies contribute an active immunity that provides relatively long-term protection against reinfection by the same microorganism or chronic infections. **Antibodies cannot kill foreign organisms on their own, but they initiate the killing of such organisms by activating complement, phagocytes, and natural killer T cells** (Fig. 10.26). Antibodies can also combine with viruses or bacterial toxins to prevent them from bindig to receptors on their target cells. Because antibodies belong to the globulin group of proteins and are involved with the immune response, they are called immunoglobulins (abbreviated as Ig). Antibodies or immunoglobulins being a protein, have a unique sequence of amino acids (variable portion, which binds to antigen) attached to a common base (constant region that attaches to macrophages). Antibodies bind to the specific matching antigen, destroying it. This specificity of antigen for antibody, similar to a key opening a lock, is a significant factor in the development of immunity to various diseases. Antibodies are found in the general circulation, forming the globulin portion of the plasma proteins, as well as in lymphoid structures. Imunoglobulins are

---

Box 10.4: Functions of the humoral immune system*

1. First encounter with antigen (primary response)
   a. Latent period
      - Antigen is processed.
      - B lymphocyte clone is selected.
      - Differentiation and proliferation.
      - Plasma cells produce specific immunoglobulin.
   b. Specific immunoglobulin (IgM) level increases first in serum followed by IgG.
   c. IgM levels later fall to zero.
   d. IgG levels fall; however, some stay the same.
2. Second encounter with antigen (secondary response)
   a. Latent period is short
      - Antigen is processed
      - Memory cells are selected; become plasma cells
      - Plasma cells produce specific immunoglobulins
   b. IgM levels increase first
   c. IgG levels increase to 50 times the level found in the primary response
   d. IgM levels fall later
   e. IgG levels fall alter, but a significant serum level is usually maintained.

* Modified from Thomson NC, Kirkwood EM, Lever RS. In Thomson et al, 1990

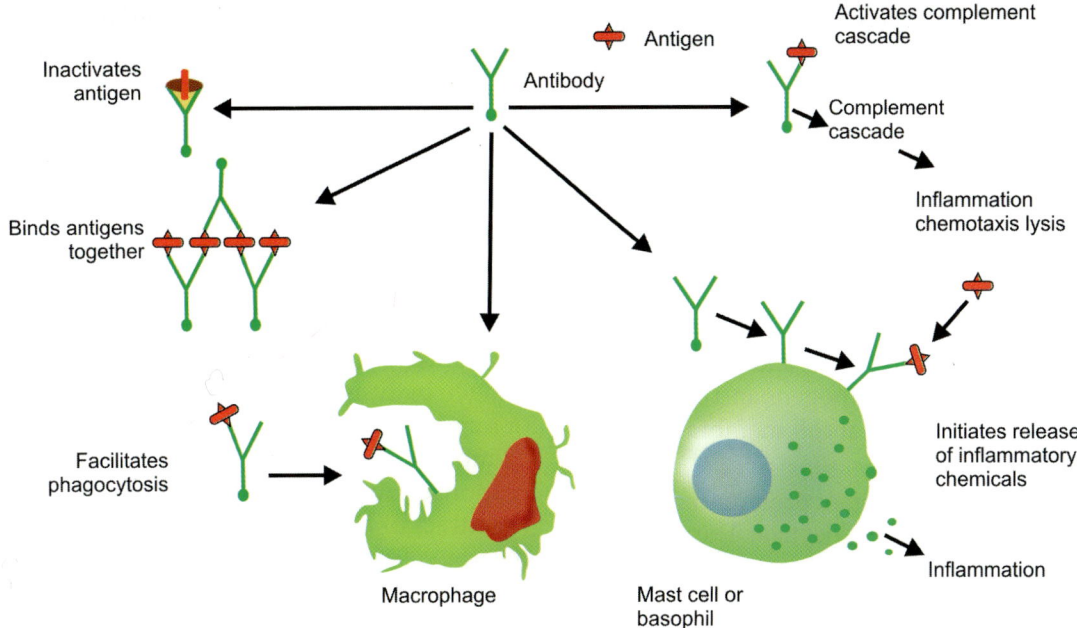

Fig. 10.26: Effects of antibodies. Antibodies directly affect antigens by inactivating the antigens or binding the antigens together. Antibodies indirectly affect antigens by activating other mechanisms through the constant region of the antibody. Indirect mechanisms include increased phagocytosis resulting from antibody attachment to macrophages. Increased inflammation resulting from the release of inflammatory chemicals from mast cells or basophils, and activation of complement *(Seeley et al, 1996)*

abundant in the body, making up about 20% of the total weight of plasma proteins. Immunoglobulins are divided into five classes, each of which has a special structure and function (Table 10.5).

The function of the antibodies can be listed as follows:

The function of antibodies is to eliminate antigens. The formation of an antigen–antibody complex may cause their elimination in several ways:

1. *Neutralization:* Antibodies can bind to viruses or bacterial toxins, which make them incapable of attaching to a cell. This mechanism is called neutralization.

2. *Agglutination and precipitation:* When a large number of antigens are close together, one antibody molecule can bind to antigenic sites on two different antigens. In this way, antibodies can tie antigens together and create large complexes. When the antigen is a soluble molecule (such as a bacterial toxin), the complex may then be too large to stay in solution. The resulting insoluble complex settles out of body fluids in a process called precipitation. The formation of large complexes is called agglutination. The clumping

Table 10.5: Immunoglobulins and their functions*

IgG	Most common antibody in the blood; produced in both primary and secondary immune responses; activates complement; includes antibacterial, antiviral and antitoxin antibodies. Crosses placenta, creates passive immunity in newborn. Four subclasses: IgGl, IgG2, IgG3, IgG4. Can bind to mast cells.
IgM	Bound to B lymphocytes in circulation and is usually the first immunoglobulin produced; Confined to intravascular space, activates complement; forms natural antibodies; is involved in blood ABO type incompatibility reaction.
IgA	Found in secretions such as tears, saliva and nasal mucus, in mucous membranes, and in colostrums to provide protection for newborn child.
IgE	Increased in parasitic and atopic diseases. Binds to mast cells in skin and mucous membranes; when linked to allergen, causes release of histamine and other chemicals, resulting in inflammation. Key antibody in pathogenesis of type I hypersensitivity reactions
IgD	Attached to B cells; activates B cells

* *Modified from Thomson NC, Kirkwood EM, Lever RS. In: Thomson NC, et al (eds). Handbook of Clinical Allergy. Oxford, Blackwell Scientific, 1990.*

of red blood cells that occurs when incompatible blood types are mixed in an agglutination reaction.

3. *Activation of complement:* Upon binding to an antigen, portions of the antibody molecule change shape, and expose areas of the constant segments that bind complement proteins. The bound complement molecules then activate the complement system, which destroys the antigen.

4. *Attraction of phagocytes:* Antigens covered with antibodies attract eosinophils, and macrophages—cells that phagocytize pathogens and destroy cells with foreign or abnormal cell membranes.

5. *Enhancement of phagocytosis:* A coating of antibodies and complement proteins makes some pathogens easier to phagocytize. The antibodies involved are called opsonins and the effect is known as opsonization.

6. *Stimulation of inflammation:* Antibodies may promote inflammation by stimulating basophils and mast cells. This action can help mobilize nonspecific defenses and slow the spread of the infection to other tissues.

Complement System

Plasma contains 11 special complement proteins that constitute the complement system. The term complement refers to the fact that this system complements the actions of antibodies.

The complement system primarily deals with organisms that have invaded the bloodstream. It is also actively involved in the acute inflammatory response. The complement system is frequently activated during an immune reaction with IgG or IgM. This system involves a group of inactive proteins circulating in the blood. When an antigen–antibody complex binds to the first complement component, Cl, a sequence of activating steps occurs (similar to a blood clotting cascade).

Eventually, this results in the destruction of the antigen by lysis when the cell membrane is damaged, or fragment may attach to a marking it for phagocytosis. Complement activation also initiates an inflammatory response. So complement activation is known to: (1) attract phagocytes, (2) stimulate phagocytosis, (3) destroy cell membrane, and (4) promote inflammation.

Chemical Mediators

A number of chemical mediators such as histamine or interleukins may be involved in an immune reaction, depending on the particular circumstances. These chemicals have a variety of function, such as signaling a cellular response or causing cellular damage (Table 10.6).

Interferons

These are small proteins released by activated lymphocytes, macrophages, and tissue cells. Normal cells exposed to interferon molecules respond by

Table 10.6: Chemical mediators in the inflammatory response

Chemical	Source	Major action
Histamine	Mast cell granules	Immediate vasodilation increased capillary permeability to form exudates.
Chemotactic factors	Mast cell granules	For example, attract neutrophils to site.
Platelet activating factors (PAF)	Cell membranes of platelets	Activate neutrophils Platelet aggregation.
Cytokines (interleukin, lymphokines), leukotrienes, interferons.	T lymphocytes Macrophages Synthesis from arachidonic acid in mast cells.	Increase plasma proteins, ESR. Induce fever, chemotaxis, leukocytosis. Later response: • Vasodilation • Increased capillary permeability, and • Chemotaxis.
Prostaglandins (PGs)	Synthesis from arachidonic acid in mast cells.	Vasodilation, increased capillary permeability, pain, fever, potentiate histamine effect.
Kinins (e.g. bradykinin)	Activation of plasma proteins (kinogen).	Vasodilation, increased capillary permeability, pain, chemotaxis.
Complement system	Activation of plasma protein cascade	Vasodilation, increased capillary permeability, chemotaxis, increased histamine release.

producing antiviral proteins that interfere with viral replication inside the cell. In addition to slowing the spread of viral infections, interferons stimulate the activities of macrophages and NK cells. Interferons are examples of cytokines which are chemical messengers that are released by tissue cells and coordinate local activities. Most cytokines act within one tissue, but those released by cellular defenders also act as hormones; they affect the activities of cells and tissues throughout the body.

PROPERTIES OF IMMUNITY

Immunity has four general properties:

1. *Specificity:* A specific defense is activated by a specific antigen, and the immune response targets only that particular antigen. This process is known as antigen recognition. *Specificity* occurs because the cell membrane of each T cell and B cell has receptors that will bind only one specific antigen and ignore all other antigens. Each lymphocyte will inactivate or destroy that specific antigen only, without affecting other antigens or normal tissues.

2. *Versatility:* In the course of a normal lifetime, an individual encounters an enormous number of antigens—perhaps tens of thousands. Your immune system cannot anticipate which antigens it will encounter, so it must be ready to confront any antigen at any time. The immune system achieves versatility by producing millions of different lymphocyte populations, each with different antigen receptors, and through variability in the structure of synthesized antibodies. In this way, the immune system can produce appropriate and specific responses to each antigen when exposure does occur.

3. *Memory:* The immune system remembers antigens that it encounters. As a result of immunologic memory, the immune response to a second exposure to an antigen is stronger and lasts longer than the response to the first exposure. During the initial response to an antigen, lymphocytes sensitive to its presence undergo repeated cell divisions. Two kinds of cells are produced: some that attack the antigen and others that remain inactive unless they are exposed to the same antigen at a later date. These latter cells— memory cells— enable the immune system to remember previously encountered antigens and launch a faster, stronger response, if one of them ever appears again.

4. *Tolerance:* Although the immune response targets foreign cells and compounds, it generally ignore normal tissues and their antigens. Tolerance is said to exist when the immune system does not respond to such antigens. Any B cells or T cells undergoing differentiation (in the bone marrow and thymus respectively) that react to normal body antigens are destroyed. As a result, normal B and T cells will ignore normal (or self) antigens and will attack foreign (or nonself) antigens.

IMMUNE RESPONSES

The two types of lymphocytes (B and T) display different responses to antigens:

- *The antibody-mediated (humoral) response:* The humoral (antibody-mediated) immunity, named for the fluids or "humors" of the body, is an indirect attack that employs antibodies. Antibodies occur in the body fluids and on the plasma membranes of some lymphocytes. Circulating antibodies bind to bacteria, toxins, and extracellular viruses, tagging them for destruction by mechanisms described later. You will find cellular and humoral immunity summarized and compared in Table 10.7 following discussion of the details of the two processes.

- *The cell-mediated response:* The cell-mediated immunity is based on the action of lymphocytes that directly attack diseased or "suspicious" cells, including those of transplanted tissues, cells infected with viruses or parasites, and cancer cells. Lymphocytes lyse these cells or release chemicals that enhance other defenses such as inflammation (Table 10.7).

1. Humoral (Antibody-mediated) Response

The body has millions of populations of B cells. B cell carries its own particular antibody molecules in its cell membrane. If corresponding antigens appear in the intestinal fluid, they will be bound by those antibiodies.

Humoral (antibody-mediated) immunity, named for the fluids or "humors" of the body, is an indirect attack that employs antibodies. Antibodies occur in the body fluids and on the plasma membranes of some lymphocytes. Circulating antibodies bind to bacteria, toxins, and extracellular viruses, tagging them for destruction by mechanisms described later. You will

Table 10.7: Some comparisons between humoral and cellular immunities

	Cellular immunity	Humoral immunity
Pathogens	Transplanted tissues and organs, cancer cells, infected cells,	Bacteria, toxins, mismatched RBCs, extracellular viruses
Effector cells	Cytotoxic T cells	Plasma cells (develop from B cells)
Other cells involved in attack	Helper T cells, suppressor T cells	Helper T cells
Antigen preseting cells	B cells, macrophages, nearly all cells.	B cells
Chemical agents of attack	Performs, lymphokines, tumor necrosis factor	Antibodies, complement

find cellular and humoral immunities summarized and compared in Table 10.7 following discussion of the details of the two processes.

When B cells come in contact with a specific antigen for the first time, they respond by first dividing and then developing into **plasma cells,** which produce specific soluble **antibodies** and secrete them into the blood and lymph. The reaction is called the primary immune response (Fig. 10.27).

The plasma cells are larger than B cells and contain an abundance of rough endoplasmic reticulum. Plasma cells develop mainly in the germinal centers of the lymphatic follicles of the lymph nodes. About 10% of the plasma cells remain in the lymph node, but the rest leave the lymph nodes, take up residence in the bone marrow and elsewhere, and there produce antibodies until they die. A plasma cell secretes antibodies at the remarkable rate of 2,000 molecules per second over a lifespan of 4 to 5 days. These antibodies travel throughout the body in the blood and other body fluids. The first time you are exposed to a particular antigen, your plasma cells produce mainly an antibody class called IgM. In later exposures to the same antigen, they produce mainly IgG.

Antibodies are not capable of independent movement. Instead they are carried by the blood and lymph to the site of an infection or injury, where they bind to specific antigen that caused the antibodies production. Because such body fluids were once referred to as humors, this type of immunity involving B cells in the production of antibodies is also called humoral immunity, is most active against extracellular pathogens such as bacteria, viruses, toxins, and other soluble foreign proteins.

B cell activation and maturation into antibody-secreting plasma cells occur following the binding of antigen to the B cell's surface receptor. The helper T cells amplify this process by secreting chemical signals called cytokines. The types of cytokines important for the production of plasma cells are called interleukins because they transmit messages between (inter) white blood cells (leukocytes).

Not all activated B cells develop immediately into antibody-secreting plasma cells. Some retain their previous appearance as smaller, inactivated cells, instead of circulating for a short time in the blood or lymph, they remain in lymphoid tissue for a long time. Such activated but apparently inactive B cells are called **B memory cells** because they have the ability to remember the sensitizing antigen and react to it the next time it appears. Such a secondary immune response occurs at the second and subsequent exposures to the same antigen that produced the primary immune response.

A secondary response starts faster and releases many more antibodies than a primary response does. For this reason, a second tissue or organ transplant from a single donor is usually rejected much faster than the first transplant. Memory cells are capable of multiplying during a secondary response, which makes them even more effective against a recurring antigen. If a totally new antigen is introduced, the primary immune response is elicited all over again, indicating that lymphocytes have an antigen-specific memory, reacting appropriately to each exposure to an antigen.

2. Cell-mediated Response

Cellular (cell-mediated) immunity is based on the action of lymphocytes that directly attack diseased or "suspicious" cells, including those of transplanted tissues, cells infected with viruses or parasites, and cancer cells. Lymphocytes lyse these cells or release chemicals that enhance other defenses such as inflammation.

T cells also respond to specific antigens, but they do not produce antibodies as B cells do.

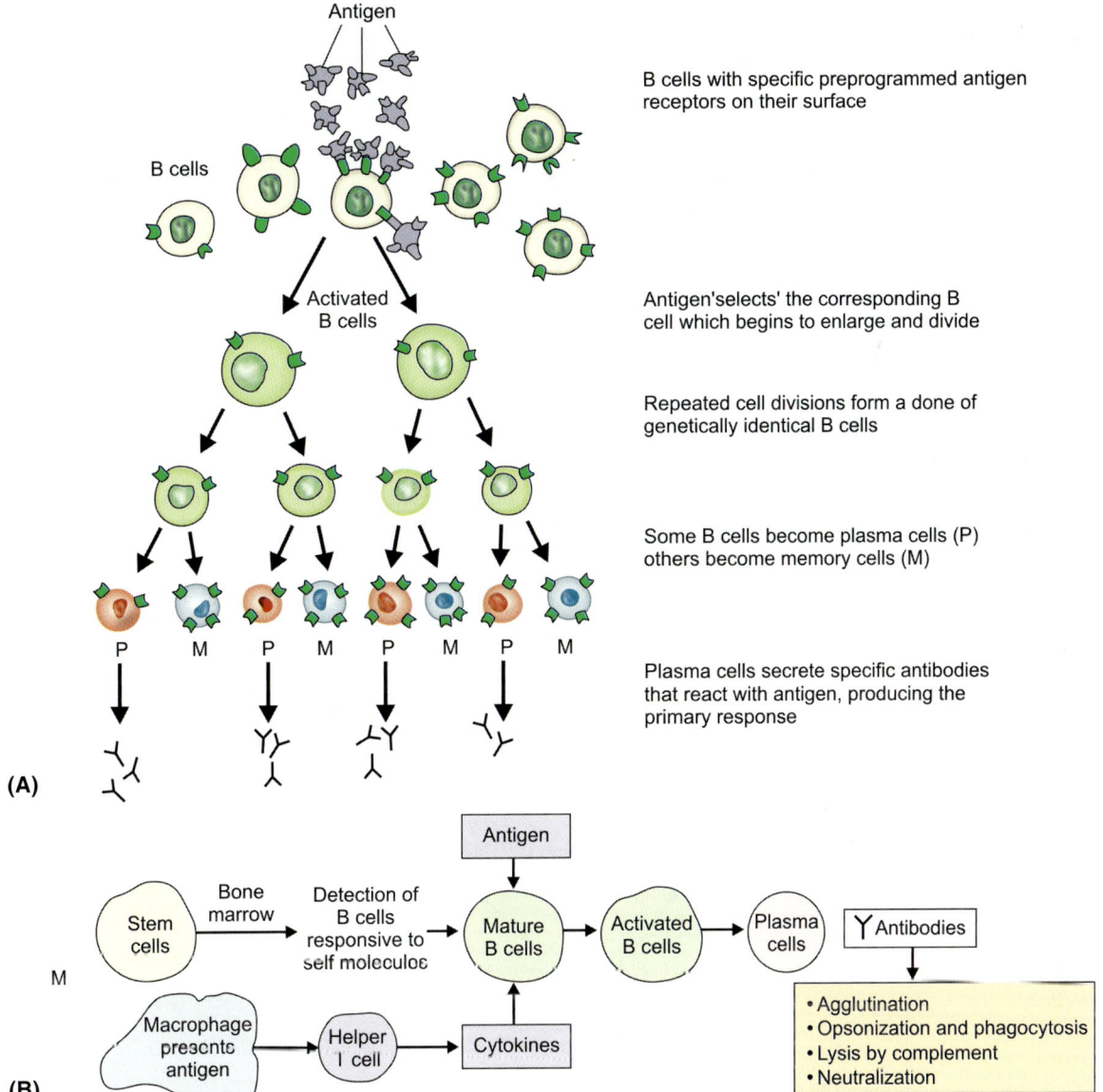

Antigen

B cells

B cells with specific preprogrammed antigen receptors on their surface

Activated B cells

Antigen 'selects' the corresponding B cell which begins to enlarge and divide

Repeated cell divisions form a done of genetically identical B cells

Some B cells become plasma cells (P) others become memory cells (M)

P M P M P M P M

Plasma cells secrete specific antibodies that react with antigen, producing the primary response

(A)

Antigen

Stem cells → Bone marrow → Detection of B cells responsive to self molecules → Mature B cells → Activated B cells → Plasma cells → Y Antibodies

M

Macrophage presents antigen → Helper T cell → Cytokines

• Agglutination
• Opsonization and phagocytosis
• Lysis by complement
• Neutralization

(B)

Fig. 10.27: Antibody-mediated (humoral) immunity. **(A)** Colonal selection and proliferation of B cells in antibody-mediated (humoral) immunity. **(B)** Summary of antibody-mediated (humoral) immunity *(Wynsberghe et al, 1995)*

T cells give protection by:

1. Producing chemicals that destroy antigens, if the antigen is an infecting virus.
2. Inducing macrophages or other host cells to destroy the antigen.
3. Stimulating cytotoxic T cells to destroy infected host cells or
4. Regulating the immune response to make certain that the system does not overact to the point where it damages the body. The protective method of T cells is called cell-mediated immunity

because it involves direct contact between T cells and antigen (Fig. 10.28).

Cell-mediated immunity operates against intracellular pathogens such as multicellular parasites and fugi, and also against cancer cells and tissue transplants. It is active against any cells that contain an infecting bacterium or virus. Some intracellular parasites are not attacked by the soluble antibodies prominent in antibody-mediated immunity because the antibodies are unable to cross the host-cell membranes to reach the parasites.

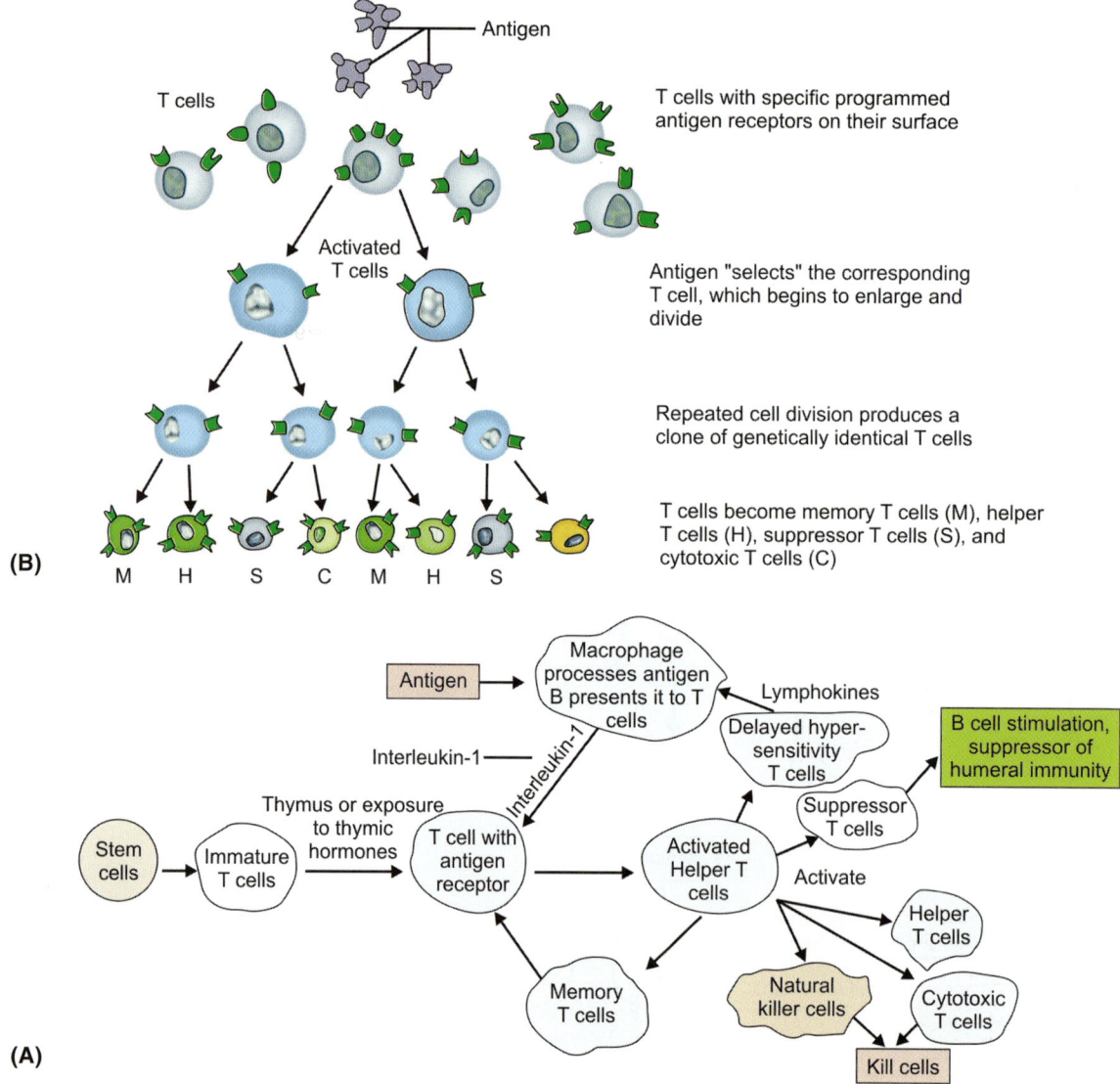

Fig. 10.28: Cell-mediated immunity. **(A)** Colonal selection and proliferation of T cell in cell-mediated immunity. **(B)** Summary of cell in cell-mediated immunity *(Wynsberghe et al, 1995)*

How T Lymphocytes Help Fight Cancer Cells?

One of the problems in treating cancer is the fact that chemotherapy, while possibly destroying cancer cells and prolonging the life of the patient, usually damages the immune system and a damaged immune system has little or no chance to destroy cancer cells effectively and permanently. Now researchers at the Ludwig Institute for Cancer Research in Brussels have proven that most tumor cells display antigens that can stimulate antigen receptors on cytotoxic T cells, causing the T cells to destroy the tumor cells. According to the concept of immune surveillance, the immune system detects tumor cells and destroys them before a tumor can form. T cells, NK cells and macrophages are involved in the destruction of tumor cells.

Immune surveillance may exist for some forms of cancer caused by viruses. However, the immune response appears to be directed more against the viruses rather than against tumor in general. Only a few cancers are known to be caused by viruses in humans. For most tumors, the response of the immune system may be ineffective and too late.

Cancer researchers are looking for ways to use tumor-cell antigens to trigger T cells in the body's immune system in the most efficient way. The production of antigens within tumor cells takes place in several steps. T cells that have appropriate antigen receptors can then attack the cell. In this way, cancer tumor cells can be destroyed by a cellular mechanism without injuring nearby tissue or harming the immune system.

In a related procedure, scientists have removed cancer cells from patients suffering from B cell lymphoma and treated the cells with a vaccine that makes them more stimulating to the immune system. The vaccinated cells are then reinjected under the patient's skin, increasing the activity of the immune system. If this technique is successful with a large group of patients, researchers intend to use it for other diseases, including diabetes, sclerosis, and rheumatoid arthritis.

An effective approach to treat cancer would be to destroy only cells displaying tumor antigens. The use of monoclonal antibodies, administering cytokines, and injecting tumor-specific cytotoxic T cells that have been isolated and stimulated outside of the body are examples. To date, such attempts have had only limited success and often produce undesirable side effects.

III. UPSETS OF THE IMMUNE RESPONSE

The complicated and delicately balanced immune mechanisms clearly have been developed to protect against antigens, particularly infections. When these immune reactions are upset, the protective mechanism can itself be a source of disease states. There are three main categories of disease states:
A. Autoimmune diseases
B. Immune-deficiency states (suppression of the immune response)
C. Hypersensitivity states

A. AUTOIMMUNE DISEASES

Early in embryonic development, lymphocytes with receptors for antigen determinants on self molecules are either eliminated or suppressed. This allows the immune system (Fig. 10.29) to respond only to foreign (non-self) antigens and to show tolerance for its own (self) antigens.

When tolerance to self antigens breaks down, however, the body forms antibodies to its own antigens, resulting in autoimmunity "protection against one's self" and autoimmune disease results. In other words, the immune system reacts either too vigorously or directs its attack against the wrong targets (Fig. 10.30).

Autoimmune diseases are failures of self-tolerance—the immune system fails to distinguish self-antigens from foreign antigens and produces **autoantibodies** that attack the body's own tissues. There are some reasons why self-tolerance may fail, among these reasons:

1. *Cross-reactivity:* The formation of cross-reacting antibodies against foreign antigens that also attack the patient's own antigens. Some antibodies against foreign antigens react to similar

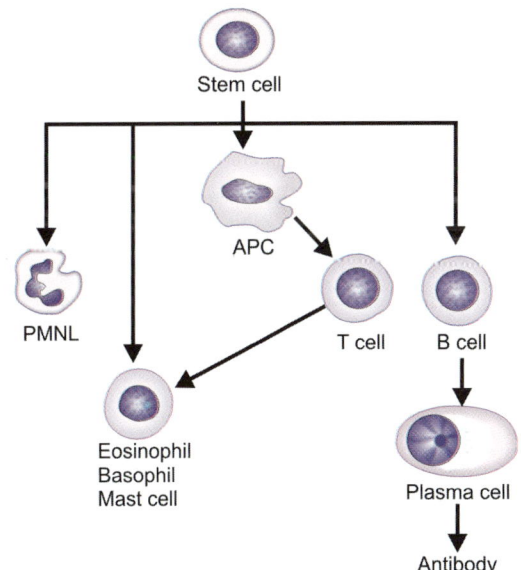

Fig. 10.29: Components of immune response; all are leukocytes. APC = antigen-presenting cell, PMNL = polymorphonuclear leukocyte *(Scully and Cawson, 2005)*

self-antigens. In rheumatic fever, for example, a *Streptococcus* infection stimulates production of antibodies that react not only against the bacteria

A. AUTOIMMUNE DISEASES

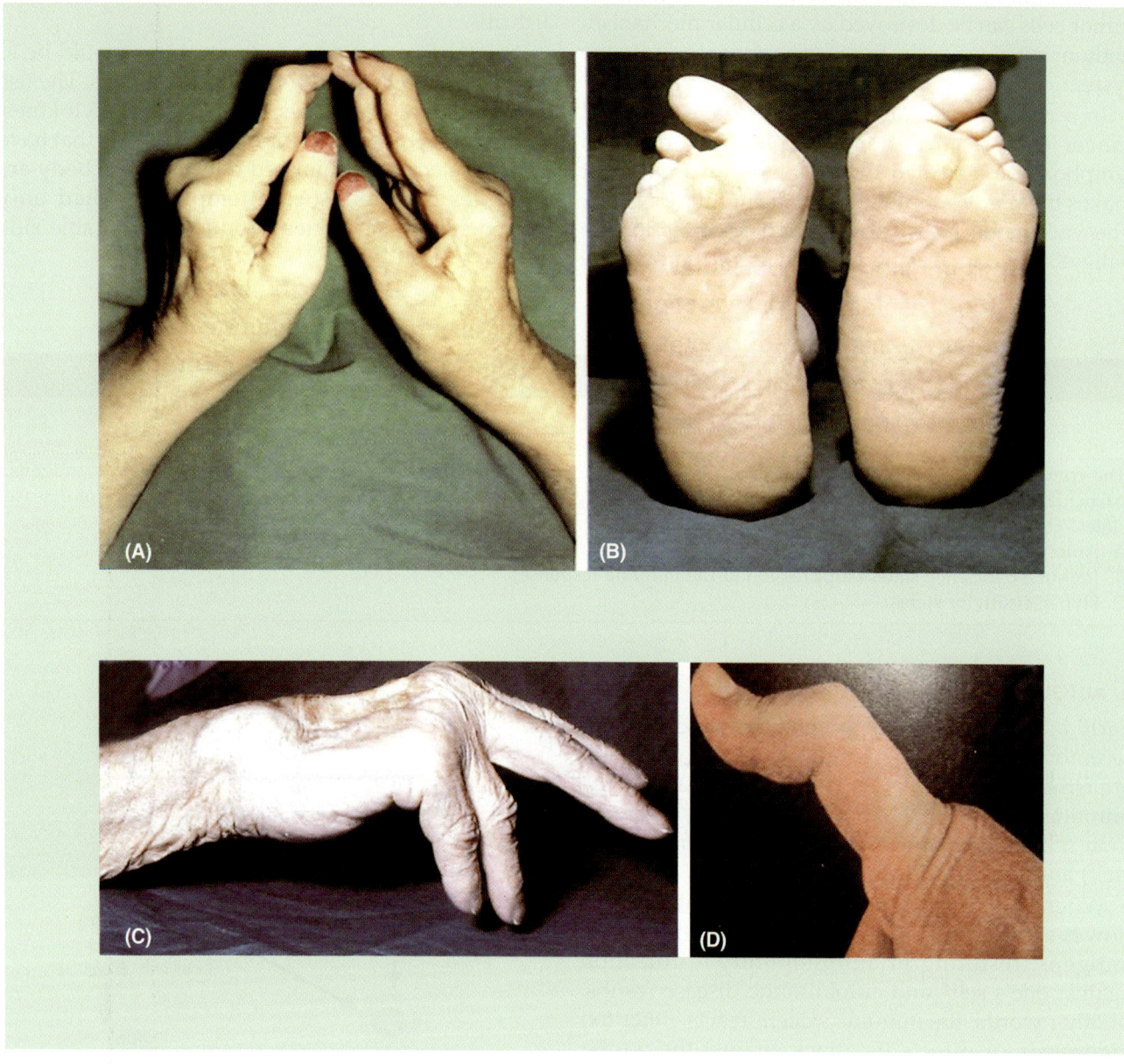

Plate XIII: **(A)** Rheumatoid arthritis. Swan-neck deformity of the proximal interphalangeal (PIP) and flexion of the distal interphalangeal (DIP) affecting both hands. **(B)** Metatarsophalangeal (MTP) involved of both feet. Note the calluses overlying the affected joints (Norman and Bramley, 1990). **(C)** Rheumatoid arthritis. A extensor tendon rupture affecting the ring and little fingers, and associated with arthritis of the wrist and dorsal tendosynovitis (note the swelling on the back of the wrist). **(D)** Boutonniere deformity. This common deformity in advanced rheumatoid arthritis results from the rupture of the central slip of the extensor tendon over the proximal interphalangeal joint. The lateral slips of the extensor tendon mechanism are displaced to the sides and maintain the deformity *(Forbes and Jackson, 2003)*

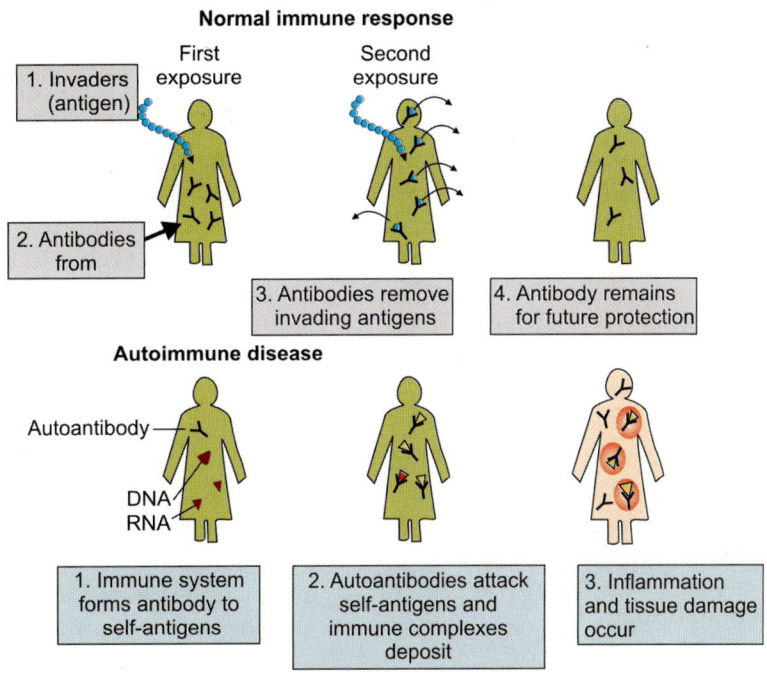

Fig. 10.30: The autoimmune response *(Gould, 1996)*

but also against antigens of the heart tissue. It often results in scarring and stenosis (narrowing) of the mitral and aortic valves.

2. *Change in the structure of self-antigens:* Alternation of the patient's own (self) antigens that causes them to become antigenic and provoke an immune reaction (Fig. 10.31). Viruses and drugs may change the structure of self-antigens and cause the immune system to perceive them as foreign.

An immune reaction is generated against the altered antigen, which may injure the antigenically similar self-antigen as well. One theory of the cause of type I diabetes mellitus is that a viral infection alters the antigens of B cells of the pancreatic islets, which leads to an autoimmune attack on the cells.

3. *Defective regulation of the immune response by regulator T lymphocytes:* Defective regulation of the immune system by helper-suppressor T lymphocytes may lead to autoimmune disease by permitting lymphocytes directed against self-antigens to become activated and to attack one's own cells and tissues. When lymphocytes are programmed to respond to specific antigens (develop immune competence) in the thymus and bone marrow as the immune system is developing, some lymphocytes are inadvertently programmed

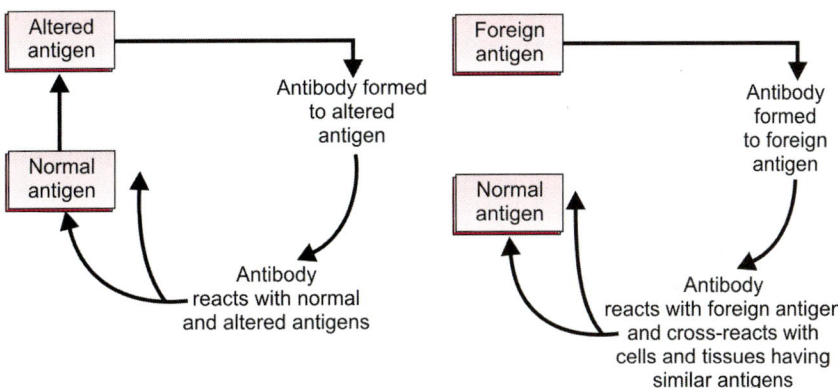

Fig. 10.31: Two mechanisms postulated to cause autoantibody formation *(Leonard and Crowley, 2004)*

to respond to self-antigens. These cell populations are either destroyed, inactivated, or suppressed so that they do not function. As a result, a normally functioning immune system does not attack self-antigens. Not all self-antigen-reacting lymphocytes are destroyed, however. Some are only suppressed and their "attack" functions are held in check by suppressor T-lymphocytes. If the regulator function of suppressor T cells is impaired, lymphocytes programmed to recognize self-antigens are freed from suppressor T cell restraint. They become activated and attack one's own cells and tissues. On the other hand, hyperactivity of helper T cells may stimulate the immune system excessively, which may also activate previously suppressed self-reactive lymphocytes and induce autoimmune disease.

Autoimmune Disease Manifestations and Mechanisms of Tissue Injury

The manifestations of autoimmune disease depend on which cells or tissue components are targeted for attack by the immune system. The mechanisms of tissue injury are those described in connection with immune-mediated hypersensitivity reactions and may include humoral mechanisms, or a combination of both.

Autoantibody-associated tissue injury results when antibody becomes attached to the cell membrane of the target cells, activating complement and causing complement-mediated destruction of the target, usually assisted by activated macrophages and killer lymphocytes (Type II reaction). Alternatively, antigen and antibody may combine to form immune complex that are deposited in the tissues and induce a similar type of complement-mediated tissue injury (Type III reaction). Cell-mediated destruction of target tissues is caused by sensitized T lymphocytes that secrete lymphokines, which generate a destructive inflammatory reaction in the target tissues or organ (Type IV reaction).

Not all autoantibodies destroy target tissue. Sometimes they derange the function of the target but do not destroy it. The thyroid gland, for example, may be attacked by two different types of autoantibodies. One type destroys thyroid cells and impairs thyroid function, causing hypothyroidism. Another type stimulates the thyroid cells and makes them hyperfunction, causing hyperthyroidism.

Examples of autoimmune disease are: In T cell disorders, cell-mediated immunity is principally affected but antibody production may also be impaired. Autoimmune disease operates through the same mechanisms as hypersensitivity reactions except that the reaction is stimulated by self-antigen. Examples of autoimmune diseases include thrombocytopenia, lupus erythematosus, rheumatoid arthritis, rheumatic fever, diabetes mellitus (type I), and myasthenia gravis (Table 10.8).

a. *Myasthenia gravis*, in which a person makes antibodies against the acetylcholine receptors on skeletal muscles. The receptors cease to function properly, causing among other things difficult breathing that may lead to death. Entitled "neuromotor deficits". The disease usually can be ameliorated for several hours by administering neostigmine or some other anticholinestrase drug. This allows larger than normal amounts of acetylcholine to accumulate in the synaptic space. Within minutes, some of these paralyzed people can begin to function almost normally, that is, until a new dose of neostigmine is required a few hours later. Myasthenia gravis will be discussed in Chapter 12.

b. *Primary thyrotoxicosis* (Graves' disease), where excessive amounts of thyroid hormone are produced. LATS (long acting thyroid stimulator), an IgM autoantibody, combined with antigen on the thyroid cell surface and produces changes mimicking those produced by TSH (thyroid stimulating hormone)—physiologically manufactured by the pituitary. Graves' disease was discussed in Chapter 9 entitled "Thyroid and Parathyroid glands".

c. One type of **glomerulonephritis** in which the person becomes immunized against the basement membranes of glomeruli.

d. *Lupus erythematosus*, in which the person becomes immunized against many different body tissues at the same time, a disease that causes extensive damage and often rapid death.

e. *Rheumatic fever*, in which the body becomes immunized against tissues in the joints and heart, especially the heart valves, after exposure to a specific type of streptococcal toxin that has an epitope in its molecular structure similar to the structure of some of the body's own self-antigen.

f. *Rheumatoid arthritis*, in rheumatoid arthritis (used to be called rheumatism) certain cells of the immune system (T cells) attack the joint cartilage. Rheumatoid arthritis will be discussed here.

Table 10.8: Some autoimmune diseases

Disease	Specificity of autoantibodies against	Result
Addison's disease	Adrenal gland	Weakness, skin pigmentation changes, weight loss, electrolyte imbalance
Autoimmune hemolytic anemia	Erythrocyte antigens	Hemolysis, anemia
Goodpasture's syndrome	Basement membrane (kidney, lung)	Pulmonary hemorrhage, kidney failure
Hashimoto's thyroiditis	Thyroid antigens	Goiter, abnormal changes in thyroid gland
Idiopathic thrombo-cytopenic purpura	Platelets	Hemorrhages in skin and mucous membranes
Diabetes (type I)	T cells	Beta cells in pancreas destroyed
Multiple sclerosis	Macrophages, T cells	Myelin progressively destroyed
Myasthenia gravis	Acetylcholine receptors on skeletal muscle cells	Progressive neuromuscular weakness, breathing difficulty
Pernicious anemia	Intrinsic factor	vit.B_{12} absorption from intestine prevented, severe anemia
Rheumatoid arthritis	Immunoglobulin	Inflammation and deterioration of joints and connective tissue
Systemic lupus erythmatosus	DNA, nuclear antigens	Facial rash, lesions of blood vessels, heart and kidneys.

RHEUMATOID ARTHRITIS

- Rheumatoid arthritis is a chronic polyarthritis characterized by bilateral symmetrical joint involvement, radiological erosions, and positive tests for rheumatoid factor.
- Rheumatoid arthritis begins when the body produces antibodies to fight an infection. Failing to recognize the body's own tissues, a misguided antibody known as *rheumatoid factor* also attacks the synovial membranes. Inflammatory cells accumulate in the synovial fluid and produce enzymes that degrade the articular cartilage. The synovial membrane thickens and adheres to the articular cartilage, fluid accumulates in the joint capsule, and the capsule is invaded by fibrous connective tissue. As articular cartilage degenerates, the joint begins to ossify, and sometimes the bones become solidly fused and immobilized, a condition called *ankylosis*.

Rheumatoid arthritis is a chronic systemic inflammatory disorder that may affect many tissues and organs, but principally attacks synovial joints (Fig. 10.32). Genetic predisposition with familial predisposition and viral infections are among the proposed causes of rheumatoid arthritis. As with some other autoimmune diseases, there is a genetic susceptibility to rheumatoid arthritis that is related to the individual's HLA antigens. About half of the persons with rheumatoid arthritis have the HLA antigen designated HLA-DR4, which is present in only about 20% of control subjects, and this is considered a highly significant difference. About 1% of the world's population is afflicted by rheumatoid arthritis, women three times more often than men. Onset is most frequent between the ages of 40 and 50, and the incidence increases with aging. When it occurs in child, it is usually severe.

Rheumatoid arthritis is considered as a multiorgan chronic autoimmune disease. The disease often commences rather insidiously with symmetrical involvement of the small joints such as the fingers,

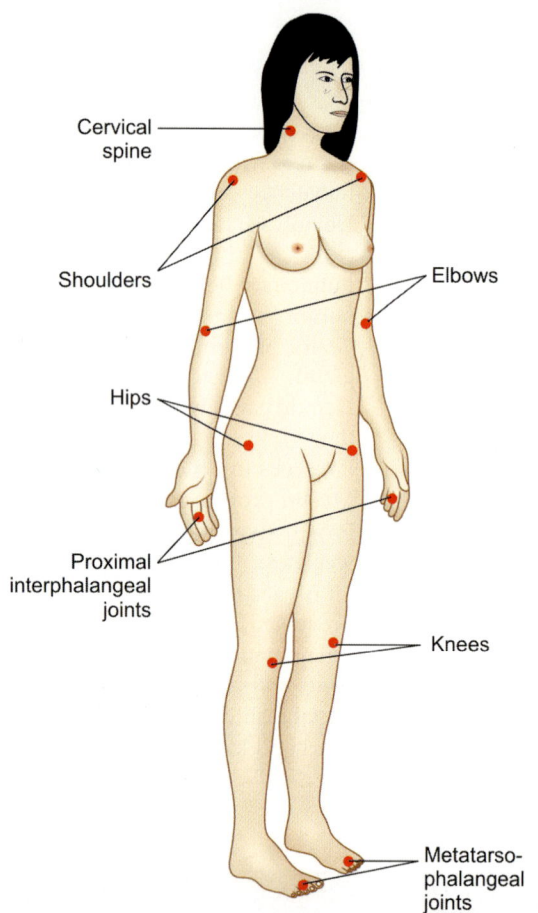

Fig. 10.32: Joints commonly affected by rheumatoid arthritis *(Forbes & Jackson, 2003)*

individual's own gamma globulin. Immune complexes composed of gamma globulin and autoantibody form within the joints which activate complement and attract inflammatory cells that damage the joints. The lymphocytes and macrophages (activated monocytes) in the synovial tissues also contribute to joint damage by secreting various injurious cytokines, including tumor necrosis factor and interferon.

Much of the joint damage characteristic of rheumatoid arthritis appears to be caused by tumor necrosis factor, which is very destructive cytokine. Because of the systemic nature of the disease and the presence of autoantibodies, rheumatoid arthritis is often classified as one of the autoimmune diseases.

Although any organ can be involved, rheumatoid arthritis most frequently involves the synovium of joints, eventually leading to the destruction of involved joints and resulting in severe disabilities and deformities. The involved synovium contains T and B cell lymphocytes, plasma cells, macrophages and synovial fibroblasts. It is now believed that a great interplay of all of these cells results in joint degradation (Fig. 10.33).

Increased osteoclastic activity is thought to be due to receptor activation of T cells. The T cells stimulate the synovial fibroblasts to secrete cytokines that promote inflammation. Additionally, the synovial fibroblasts secrete enzymes that degrade the cartilage. B cells secrete rheumatoid factor and other autoantibodies, which can be detected in the serum. In addition to the inflamed synovium, the subchondral bone can also become chronically inflamed.

followed by inflammation and destruction of additional joints (e.g. wrists, elbows, knees, upper cervical vertebrae, and temporomandibular joints). The process produces an inflammatory response of the synovium (synovitis) secondary to hyperplasia of synovial cells, excess synovial fluid, and the development of pannus in the synovium.

The pathology of the disease process often leads to the destruction of the articular cartilage and ankylosis of joints. The inflammatory process has other effects on the body, e.g. rheumatoid or subcutaneous nodules may form on the extensor surfaces of the ulna, on the pericardium, pleura, heart valves, or sclera.

PATHOPHYSIOLOGY

The blood and synovial tissues of patients with rheumatoid arthritis often contain a substance called rheumatoid factor, which is an autoantibody produced by B lymphocytes that is directed against the

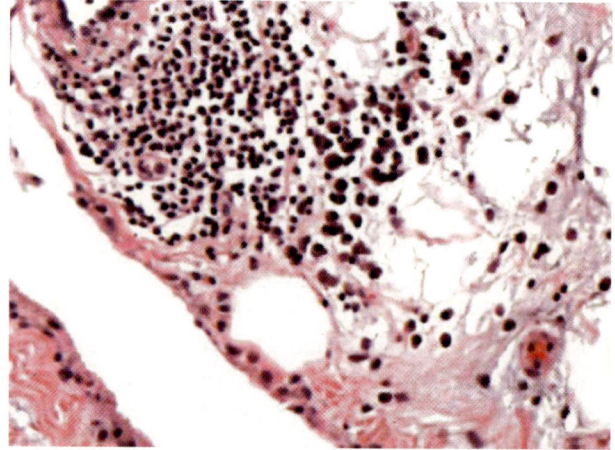

Fig. 10.33: Typical inflammatory infiltrate in rheumatoid arthritis consists of lymphocytes and plasma cells *(H and E, 4000x)*

The barrage of inflammatory cells and release of cytokines, interleukins (ILs), metalloproteases, and antigens lead to the histologic findings of synovial hyperplasia, inflammation, germinal center formation, increased osteoclasts, and cartilage destruction and bone resorption. The joints in the head and neck will become edematous with a plasma cell and lymphocytic infiltrate in the synovium and underlying articular architecture.

The capsular tissue will form a pannus also with lymphocytes. As the bone resorbs, the articular surface of the condyle will be destroyed. The inflammation can extend into the surrounding periarticular tissue, leading to further joint instability. Twenty-five percent of seropositive patients develop necrotizing granulomatous nodules (rheumatoid nodules). The nodule contains a fibrinoid center with peripheral palisading histiocytes, giant cells, and lymphocytes (Fig. 10.34). These typically occur in the soft tissue, but occasionally can be seen in bone and cartilage (trachea, larynx, ear).

SIGNS AND SYMPTOMS

i. Joints (other than the temporomandibular joint)
ii. Rheumatoid arthritis involving the temporomandibular joint
iii. Non-articular manifestations of rheumatoid arthritis

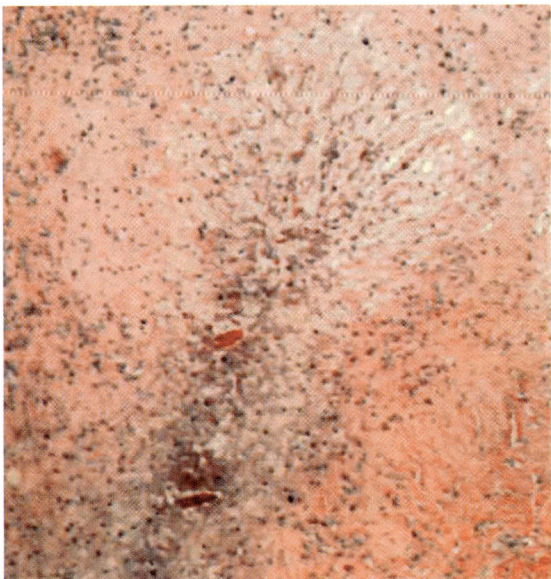

Fig. 10.34: Rheumatoid nodule composed of histiocytes, giant cells, and lymphocytes surrounding a fibrin center *(H and E, 200x)*

I. Joints (Other than the temporomandibular joint)

Rheumatoid arthritis is insidious at onset, often becoming manifest as mild general aching and stiffness. Inflammation may be apparent first in the fingers, feet, or wrists, (Plate XIII, Figs 10.35 to 10.37). It affects joints in a symmetrical (bilateral) fashion, and usually more than one pair of joints are involved. The joints appear red, warm, swollen and often are very sensitive to touch as well as painful. Joint stiffness occurs following rest, which then eases with mild activity as circulation through the joint improves. The stiffness of rheumatoid arthritis is a morning stiffness rather than an immobility stiffness and the duration of the morning stiffness provides a useful index of

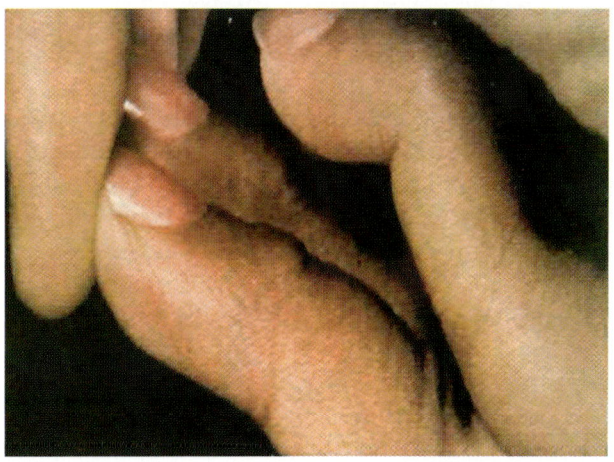

Fig. 10.35: Swan-neck deformity is common in advanced rheumatoid arthritis. It is brought about by disruption of the volar plate of the proximal interphalangeal joint, sometimes with associated rupture of the insertion of the flexor sublimis

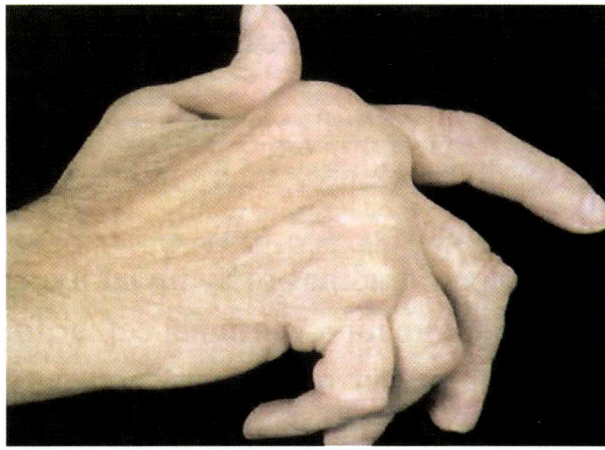

Fig. 10.36: Rheumatoid arthritis destroys articular cartilage and produces crippling deformities *(Wynsberghe et al, 1995)*

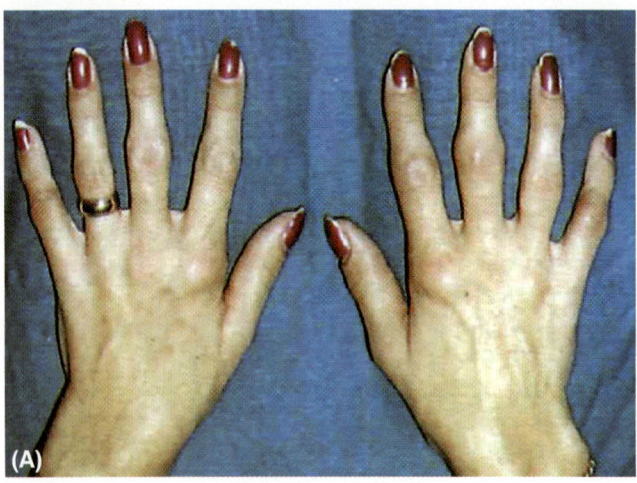 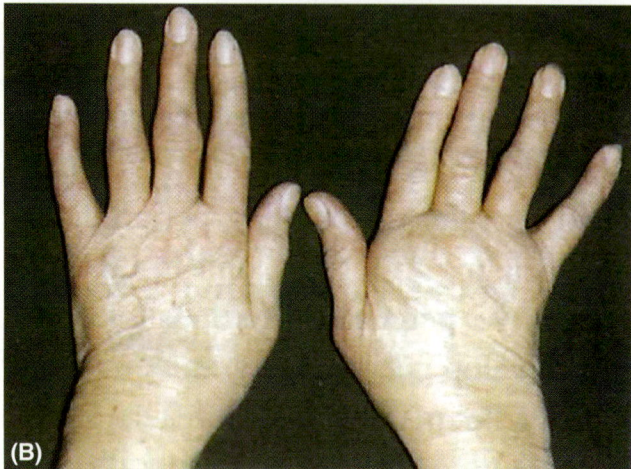

Fig. 10.37: Rheumatoid arthritis. **(A)** Note the spinding of the proximal interphalangeal (PIP) and the swelling of the second metacarpophalangeal (MCP), the wrists, toes are involved. **(B)** Ulnar deviation of the right (dominant) hand. Note also the PIP swelling *(Norman and Bramley, 1990)*

the degree of inflammation in the joints but typically it lasts for more than an hour. Tenderness reflects the synovial inflammation. It is of mild to intermediate degree, but is not of severity seen in patients with gout, septic arthritis or rheumatic fever. The nature of the swelling is soft and "boggy" and there is often an effusion present.

Radiologic Features

X-rays of the hands and feet are generally performed in people with a polyarthritis. Other medical imaging techniques as magnetic resonance imaging and ultrasound are also used in rheumatoid arthritis. The radiographic abnormalities of the bone, joint and soft tissue in RA are well known. Changes are distributed symmetrically and consist of soft tissue swelling, regional osteoporosis, diffuse loss of joint space, marginal and central erosions, and fibrous ankylosis. The synovium of bursae and tendon sheaths is also affected.

The radiologic features can conveniently be divided into early and late changes as follows.

Early changes: These include juxta-articular osteoporosis with erosions. These are usually peri-articular and the transition between marked bone loss in juxta-articular osteoporosis and the earliest change of erosion is often difficult to ascertain, the articular cortical bone plate being so thinned as to difficult to delineate. Erosions once established, range from minute irregularities in the bone surface to larger "cortical bites" often measuring a few millimeter across.

Late changes: Loss of joint space is due to destruction of the articular cartilage by synovial pannus. Confluence of erosions may eventually lead to changes in the normal morphology of the articular surface. Severe joint destruction or changes in peri-articular tissues may lead to alternation of the axial alignment of one bone on another (Figs 10.38 to 10.40). The term "subluxation" is used when some degree of articular contact is retained (Figs 10.41 and 10.42).

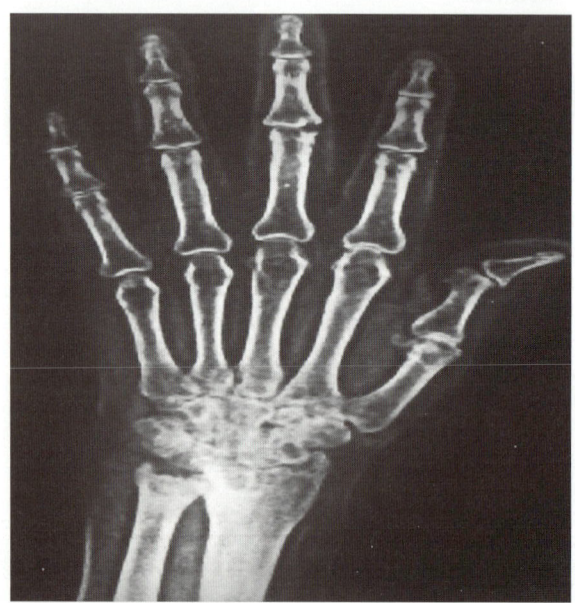

Fig. 10.38: Advanced rheumatoid arthritis. All the typical changes are seen: soft tissue swelling specially around the wrist, bone erosions, joint space narrowing particularly in the radiocarpal joint

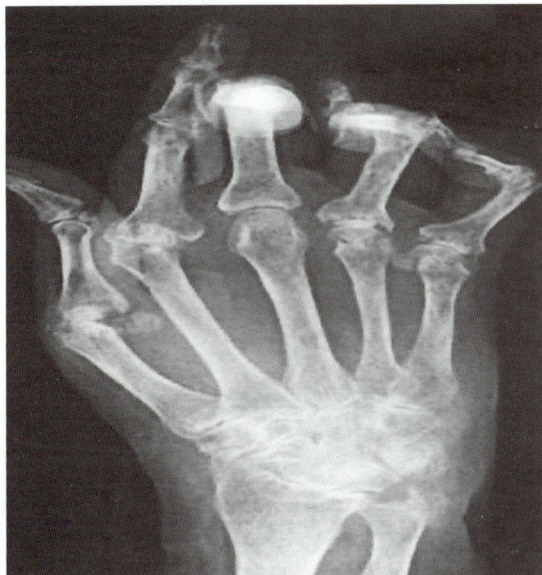

Fig. 10.39: Radiograph illustrating destruction of articular surfaces involving the interphalangeal and metacarpophalangeal joints *(Scutellari and Orzincolo, 1998)*

Total loss of contact between joint surfaces is usually described by the more orthopedic term "dislocation". Ankylosis may develop. The humerous head and glenoid fossa may show severe destruction (Fig. 10.43). Subluxation of the cervical vertebrae (Figs 10.44 and 10.45) and necrosis of the thoracic spine may occur.

Diagnosis: The diagnosis is not difficult in patients with typical clinical and radiologic features.

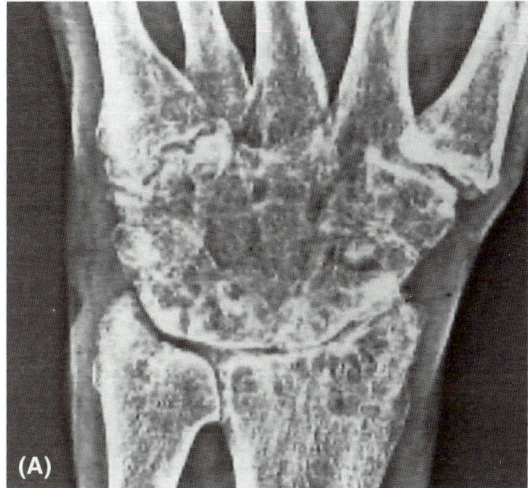

(A)

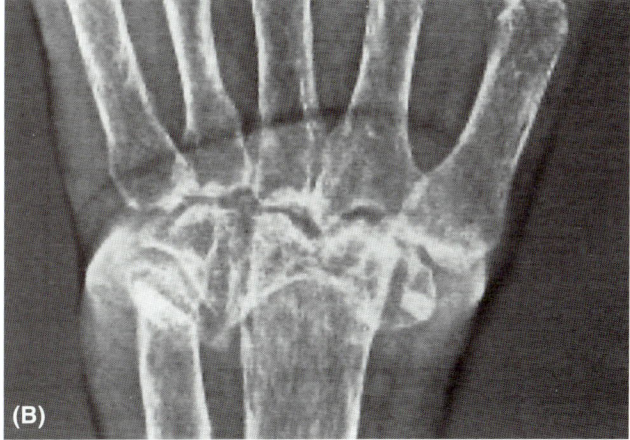

(B)

Fig. 10.41: Xenoradiography of the wrist. **(A)** Bone ankylosis of all the carpal bones. **(B)** Destruction and lysis of the proximal carpal bones and radiocarpal subluxation *(Scutellari and Orzincolo, 1998)*

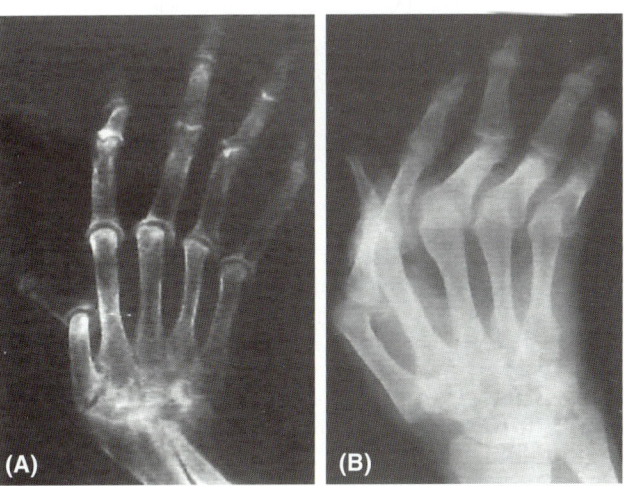

(A) (B)

Fig. 10.40: Malalignment and subluxation in the late stage of RA, with bone resorption of proximal carpal bones and distal ulna **(A)**, En boutonniere hand deformity **(B)**

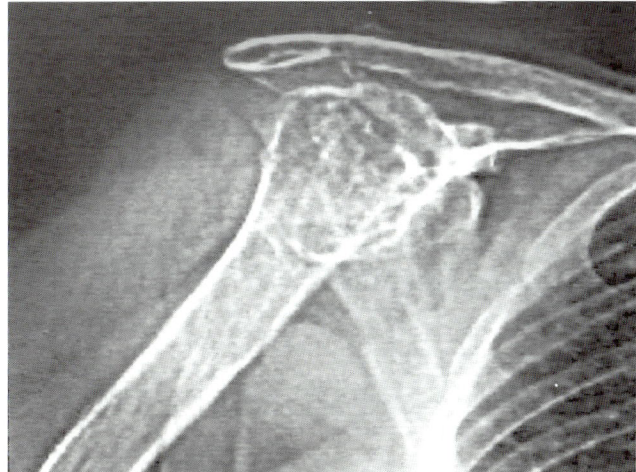

Fig. 10.42: Bone resorption of the humeral head and glenoid fossa of the right shoulder *(Scutellari and Orzincolo, 1998)*

Glenoid fossa of scapula

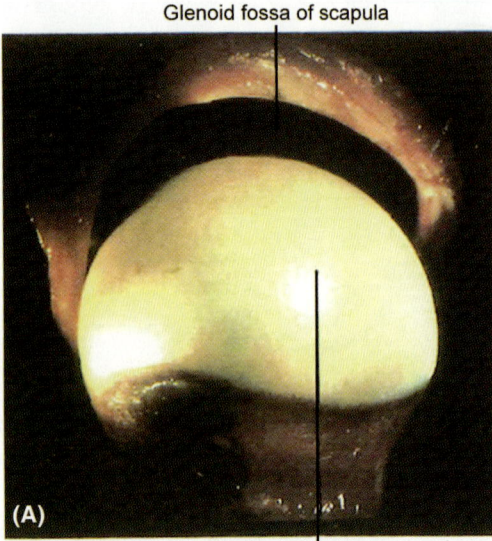

(A)

Head of humerus

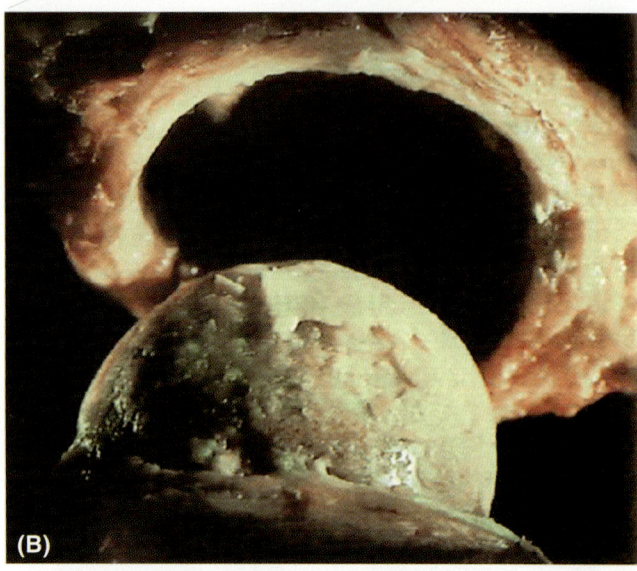

(B)

Fig. 10.43: (A) The head of a healthy humerus. **(B)** The diseased joint of a person with rheumatoid arthritis. The articular cartilage has been removed *(Donna et al, 1995)*

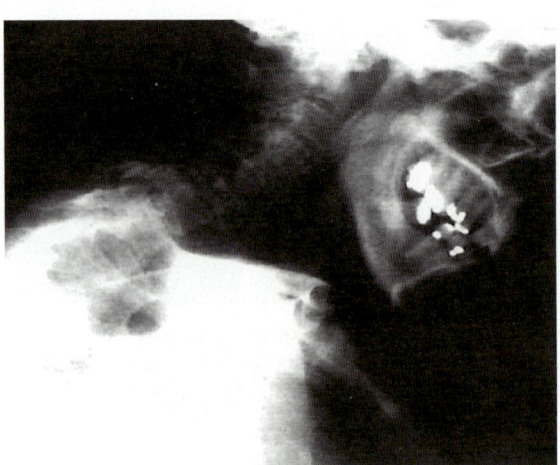

Fig. 10.44: Rheumatoid arthritis. Severe cervical subluxation marked at C6/7 level *(Norman and Bramley, 1990)*

The following diagnostic criteria have been proposed in atypical cases (Arnett et al, 1988):
1. Morning stiffness.
2. Soft tissue swelling of three or more joints observed by a physician.
3. Swelling of the proximal interphalangeal, metacarpophalangeal or wrist joints.
4. Symmetric arthritis.
5. Rheumatoid nodules.
6. Presence of rheumatoid factor.
7. Typical radiographic findings, i.e. erosions with or without periarticular osteopenia in the hand and wrist joitns.

Criteria 1 through 4 must have been present for at least 6 weeks. RA is defined by the presence of four or more criteria.

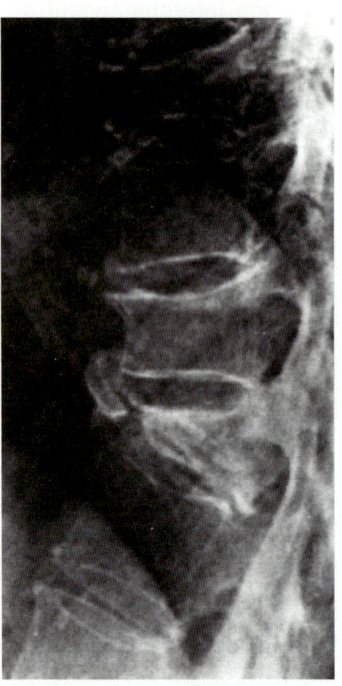

Fig. 10.45: Osteonecrosis of a distal vertebral body of the thoracic spine after long-term corticosteroid therapy, note anterior wedging of the body, crush fracture, and intraosseous vacuum phenomenon *(Scutellari and Orzincolo, 1998)*

II. Rheumatoid Arthritis Involving the Temporomandibular Joint

Incidence

Involvement of the temporomandibular joint in rheumatoid arthritis varies widely among references.

Clinical TMJ involvement is found in 4–80% of RA patients (Ogus, 1975; Raustia AM, Pyhtinen, 1991; Yoshida et al, 1998; Yamakawa et al, 2002; Gynther et al, 1997), so wide a range might be due to different examinations performed, patients selection, and the use of different criteria for classifying joint involvement. Temporomandibular joint involvement is frequently overlooked by rheumatologists or by the patients themselves, for the following reasons:

1. Compared with other joints like the hands and knees where frequent motion or weight-bearing is unavoidable in daily life, the joints of the stomatognathic system are less of a problem for RA patients. They can subjectively reduce its motion by talking less or by avoiding chewing hard food. This explains treatment is focused on other joints for upper extremity function or weight-bearing (Syrjianen, 1985; Goupille et al, 1990).

2. The joints involved with R A are usually swollen, such swelling is not evident in the temporomandibular joint. The TMJ is structurally different from other joints. It has special retrodiscal tissue that is rich in blood vessels, which may act as a highly efficient drainage system for joint exudates (Okeson, 1993).

3. The mandibular function is not significantly restricted despite severe TMJ destruction. This might be due to the presence of specialized articular disk structure, which divides the TMJ into two distinct cavities, the upper and lower one which allows a certain range of mouth opening. This may also constitute an important cause for reduced self-awareness of TMJ problems among RA patients.

About 50–60% of patients show some manifestations during the course of their disease (Breslow, 1975; Hampf et al, 1985). Some texts reported that temporomandibular joint involvement is typically a late sequela of RA, although rarely it is the first presenting sign. However, involvement of temporomandibular joint is more frequent in patients with > 5 years duration of RA (Ogus, 1975). When the TMJ is affected, it is usually bilateral. However, it is curious that even in patients with severe and widespread joint disease, handicapping involvement of the temporomandibular joint is only rarely observed (Toller, 1974; Norman, 1982).

Roentgenographic examination

There is no radiological criterion that is pathognomonic for generalized osteoarthritis or rheumatoid arthritis. The following features can be observed in rheumatoid arthritic temporomandibular joint:

- Reduced joint space
- Marginal erosion of the articular cortical surfaces.
- Bone destruction may be severe and may lead to complete condylar loss.
- Devastating effects on jaw relationship and function, e.g. open bite deformity.
- In some cases, there may be outgrowths (osteophytes)
- Fibrous ankylosis with limited mouth opening.

Clinical Feature

The most common symptoms are morning stiffness, decreased range of motion, crepitus, swelling and pain (Figs 10.46 and 10.47). Progressive trismus is less common in adult rheumatoid arthritis. Malocclusion and open bite deformity (Figs 10.48 to 10.50) may develop due to condylar damaged. Daily activities become difficult, including food preparation, and oral hygiene. With each exacerbation and as the joint damage progresses, the functions of the affected joints become further impaired.

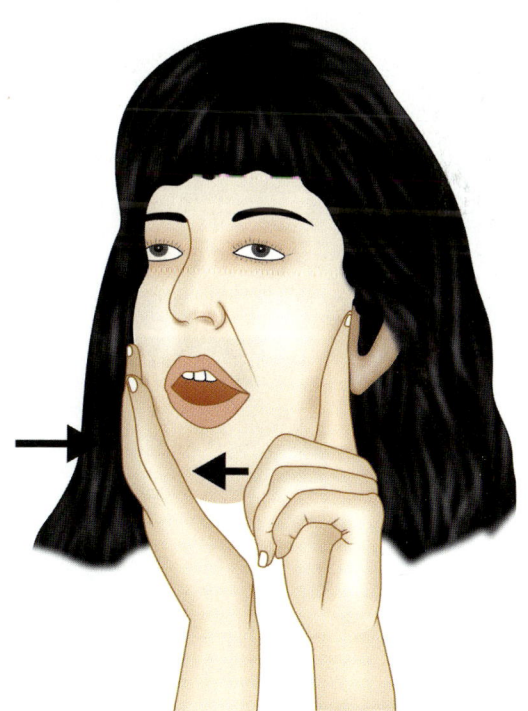

Fig. 10.46: Pre-auricular pain and deviation of the mid-mandibular incisor line on attempt to open the mouth due to rheumatoid arthritis involving the right TMJ

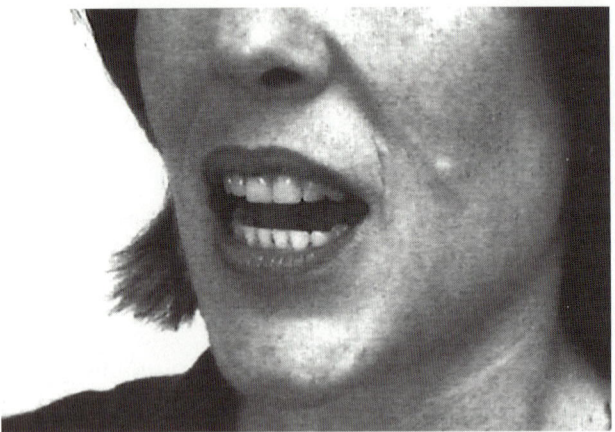

Fig. 10.47: Myofibrotic contracture has caused permanent restriction in mandibular opening due to bilateral involvement of the TMJ by rheumatoid arthritis

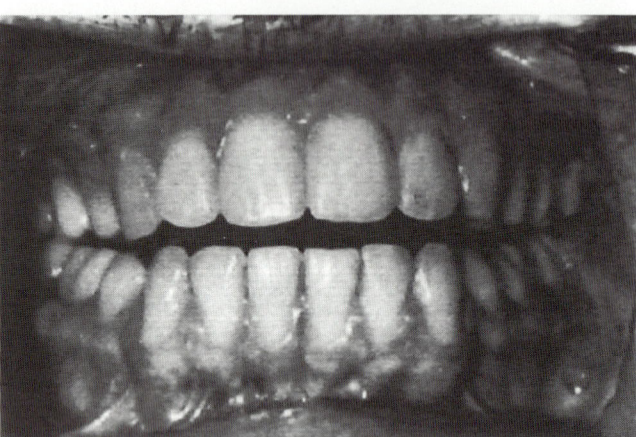

Fig. 10.48: Malocclusion "open bite" from severe condylar bone loss due to rheumatoid arthritis

Diagnostic imaging includes plain radiography (transcranial view of both the right and left sides with the mouth closed and open), tomography, arthrography, CT, and MRI.

The rheumatoid process may result in progressive destruction of the articular eminence and subarticular bone of the condyle (Figs 10.51 to 10.57). Although not specific to RA, erosion and cysts-like bone resorption of the mandibular condyle commonly occur. The meniscus may be subject to gradually increasing damage until it becomes perforated and eventually destroyed. Radiographs reflect these pathological processes and may show progressive resorption of the condyle. The severity of these

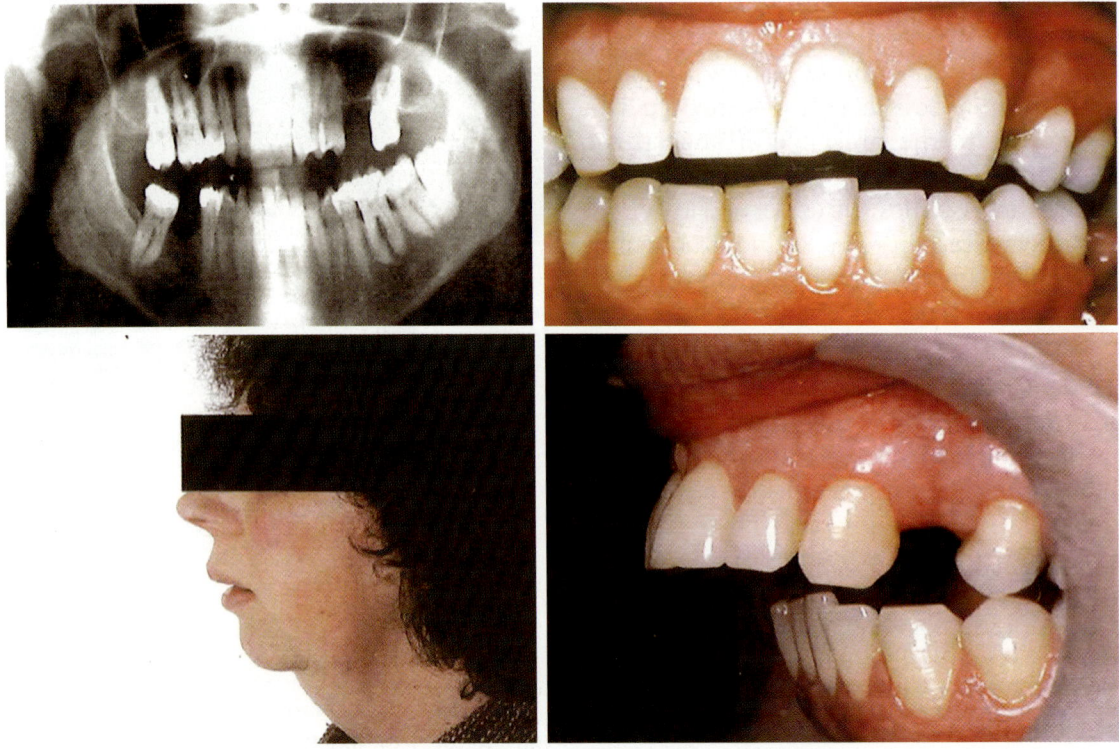

Fig. 10.49: Rheumatoid arthritis. Onset, in this patient, occurred in the late 20s, progressing to anterior open bite and retrognathia, due to bilateral condylar destruction, by the mid-30s *(Norman and Bramley, 1990)*

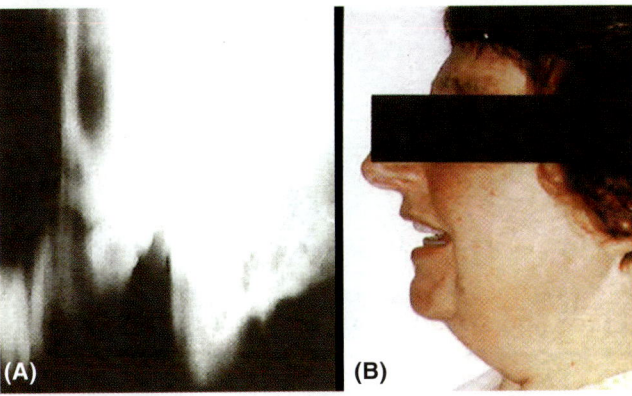

Fig. 10.50: Rheumatoid arthritis. **(A)** Late onset, **(B)** After 10 years steroid therapy, anterior open bite, destruction of the condyle and formation of the neoarthrosis *(Norman and Bramley, 1990)*

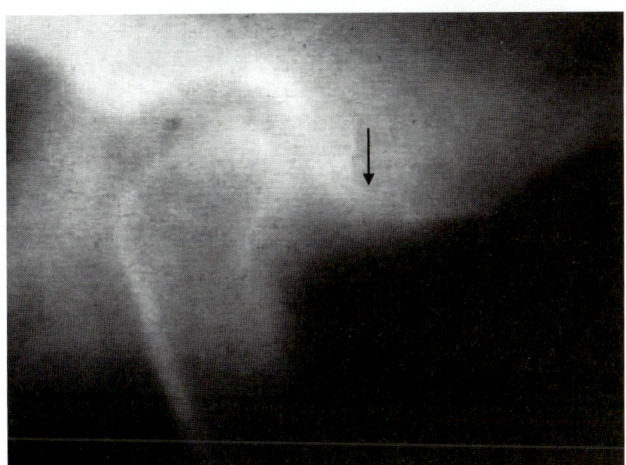

Fig. 10.51: Rheumatoid arthritis TMJ showing loss of cortical bone covering the summit of the articular eminence

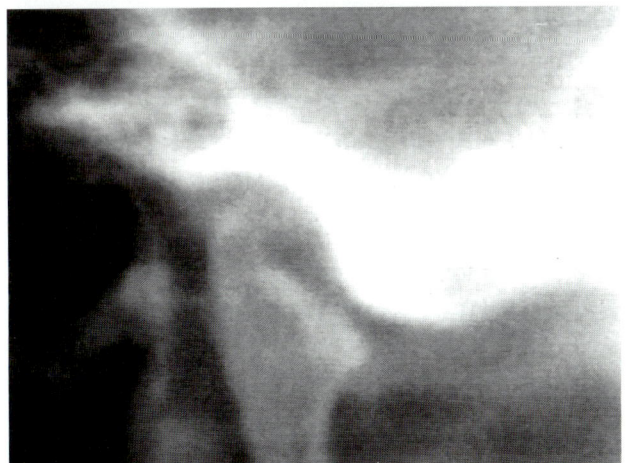

Fig. 10.52: A lateral tomogram of a temporomandibular joint affected by rheumatoid arthritis. Showing sclerosis of the anterosuperior condylar surface and subcortical bone resorption

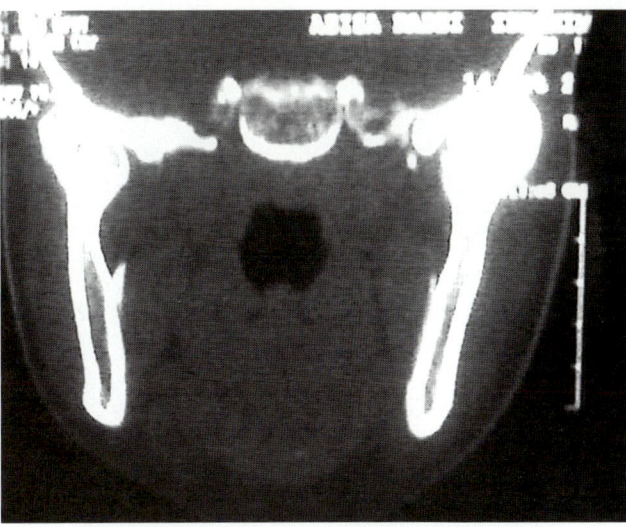

Fig. 10.53: When rheumatoid arthritis involves the temporo-mandibular joint, the roentgenographic picture reveals loss of joint space, subcortical bone resorption of the mandibular condyles, loss of integrity of the articular surfaces of the condyles, glenoid fossa and articular eminence

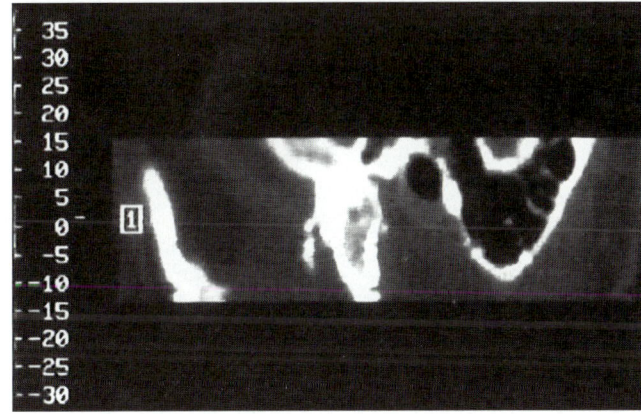

Fig. 10.54: Sagittal reformation of 1.5 mm thick axial CT sections obtained at 0.1 mm intervals through the joint. This patient has severe limitation of opening on the left. CT demonstrates severe osteoarthritis changes without bony ankylosis seen. Fibrous ankylosis cannot be excluded

changes, with reduction of the condyle to a mere remnant, is not as common in adult rheumatoid arthritis as in the juvenile-onset disease. Adults presented with severely resorbed condyles usually have a history of juvenile inflammatory arthritis, and hypoplastic changes are commonly present in these patients. In severe cases, erosion of the condylar head and fibrosis can lead to mandibular micrognathia and anterior open bite.

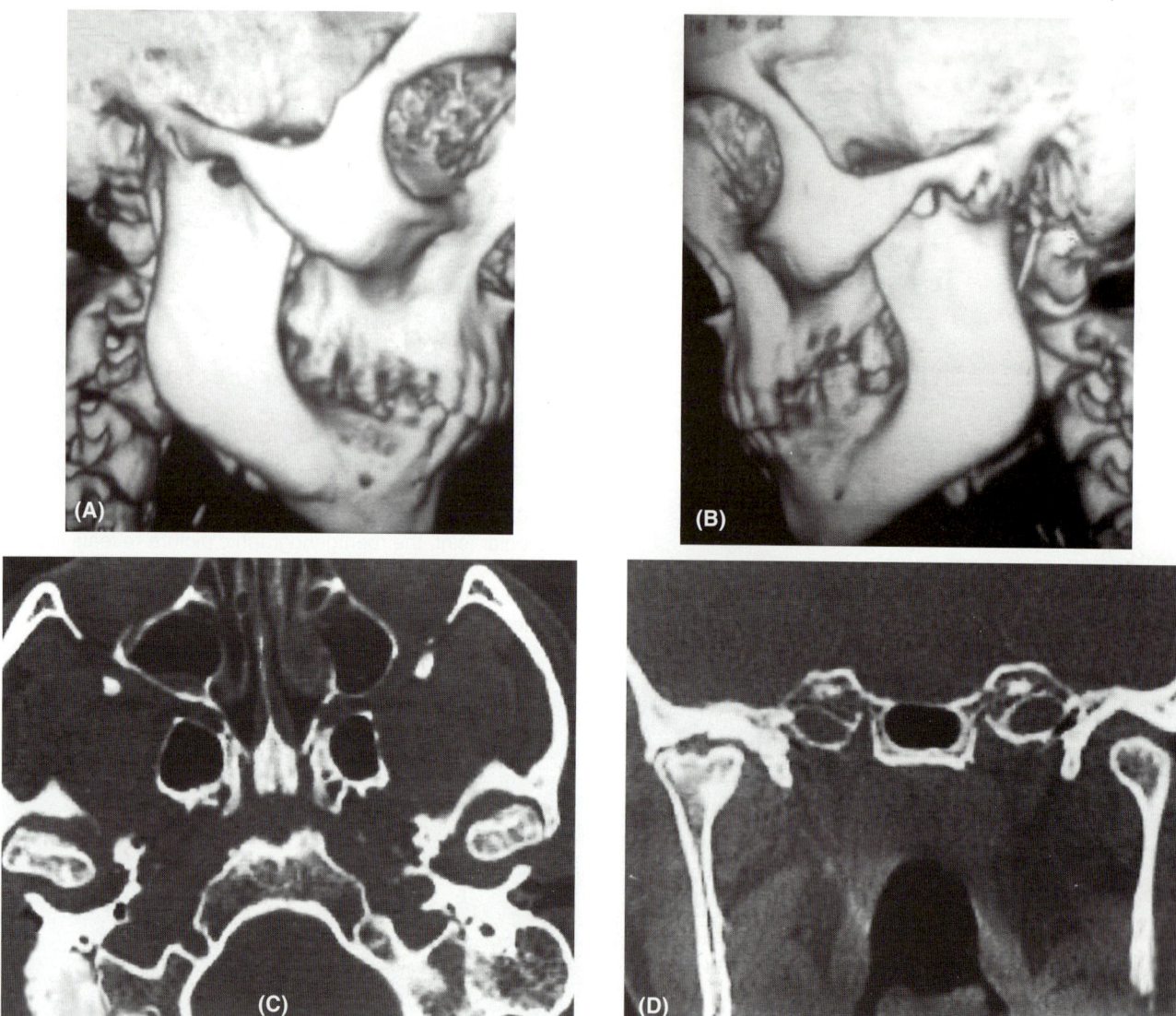

Fig. 10.55: (A and B) Three-dimensional CT showing erosion of the mandibular condyles. **(C and D)** CT of the TMJ coronal and axial sections. Erosion and asymmetric condyle remodeling, with flattening and sclerosis *(Scutellari and Orzincolo, 1998)*

III. Non-articular Manifestations of Rheumatoid Arthritis

RA often affects the soft tissue, resulting in vasculitis, rheumatoid nodule, lymphadenopathy, Sjogren's syndrome, keratoconjunctivitis, iritis, scleritis, neuropathy secondary to small vessel angiitis or compression, myositis and amyloidosis.

Systemic signs are obvious during exacerbations and are thought to arise from the circulating immune factors. They include fatigue, anorexia, mild fever, generalized lymphadenopathy, and generalized aching. Although the bone findings of RA are not unique to the head and neck, the clinical manifestations can be quite dramatic.

Soft tissue surrounding joints: Subcutaneous nodules are firm, intradermal and generally occur over pressure points, typically the elbows, the finger joints and Achilles tendon (Figs 10.58 to 10.60). They occur on the sacrum and occiput in bed-bound patients. They may ulcerate and become infected, but usually resolve when the disease comes under control. The nodules can be removed surgically or injected with corticosteroids, if causing as problem. They tend to occur. Histologically, there is a necrotic center surrounded by rows of activated macrophages. This resembles synovitis without a synovial space.

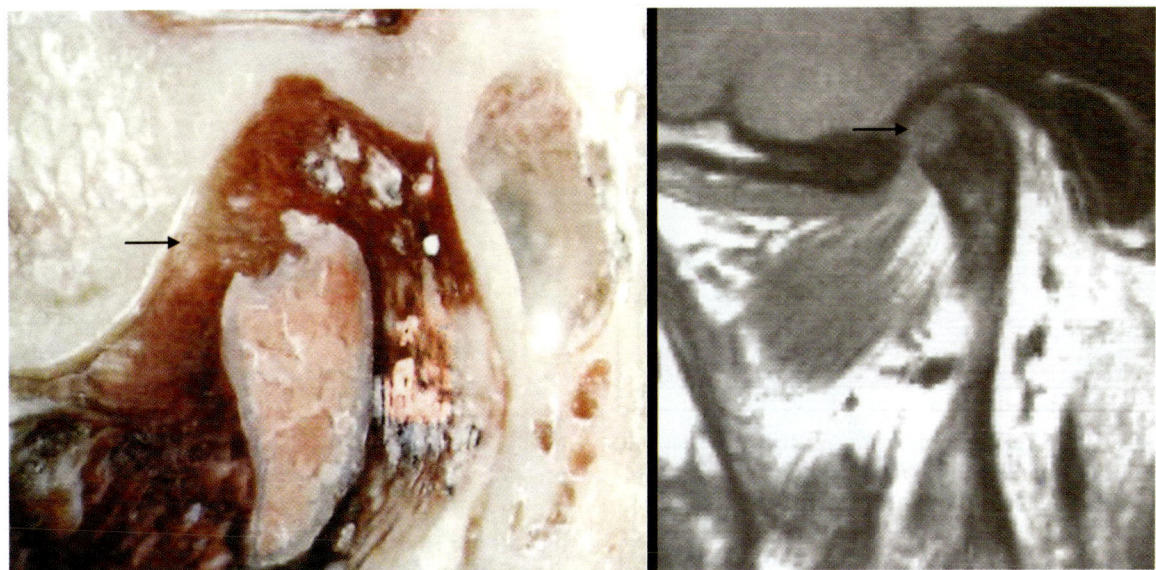

Fig. 10.56: Rheumatoid arthritis. An MRI shows completely destroyed disk, replaced by fibrous or vascular pannus and cortical punched-out erosion (arrow) with sclerosis in condyle

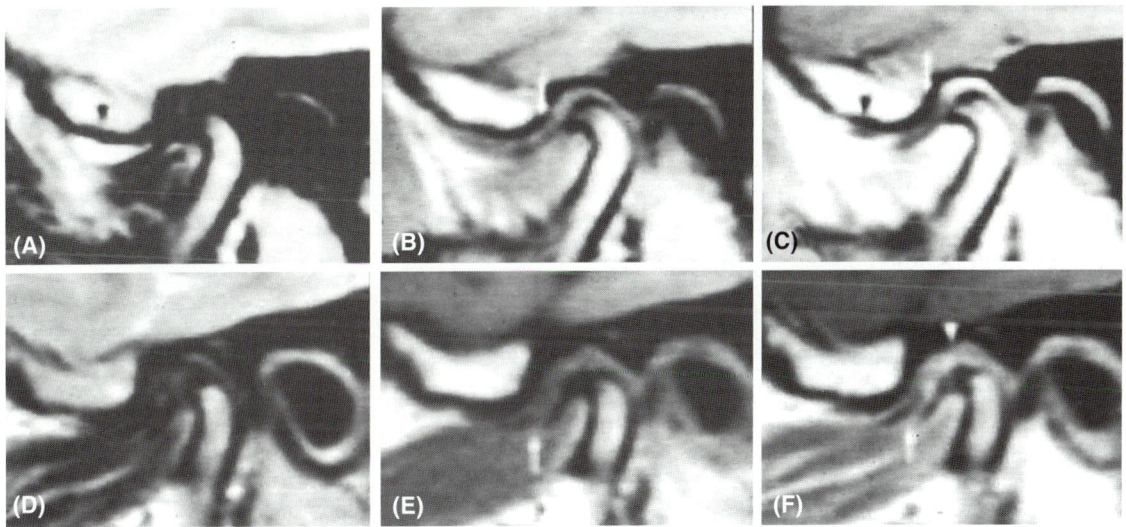

Fig. 10.57: Rheumatoid arthritis and disk displacement of right **(A, B, C)** and left **(D, E, F)** joints. T2-weighed MRI shows joint effusion in upper compartment of anterior recess (arrowhead). **B, C,** T1-weighed pre-Gd, **(B)** and T1-weighed post-Gd, **(C)** MRI shows anteriorly displaced disk (arrow) and contrast enhancement in peripheral rim of joint effusion (arrowhead) and in posterior attachment, consistent with thickened synovium. Secondary osteoarthritis **(D)** T2-weighed MRI shows no effusion. **(E, F)** T1-weighed pre-Gd, **(E)** and T1-weighed post-Gd, **(F)** MRI shows anteriorly placed disk (arrow) and slight contrast enhancement around disk and in joint space (arrowhead), consistent with thickened synovium

Tenosynovitis of affected flexor tendons in the hand can cause a trigger finger. Swelling of the extensor tendon sheath over the dorsum of the wrist is common. Muscle wasting around joints is common. Muscle enzyme concentrations are normal; myositis is extremely rare. Corticosteroid-induced myopathy may occur.

Lungs: Peripheral, intrapulmonary nodules are usually asymptomatic but may cavitate. Other manifestations are: serositis causing pleural effusion,

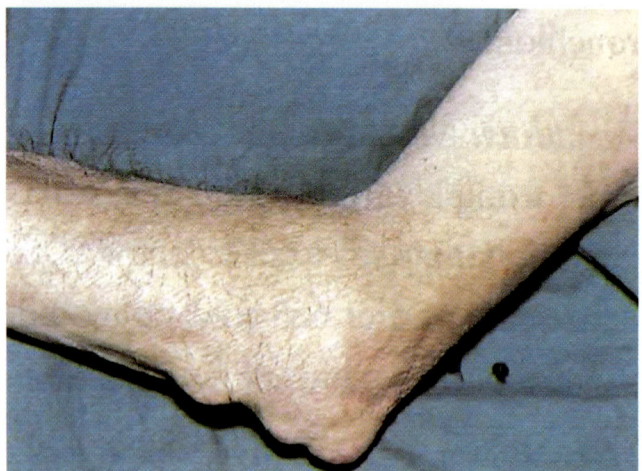

Fig. 10.58: Rheumatoid nodules are formed in the under-surface of the feet

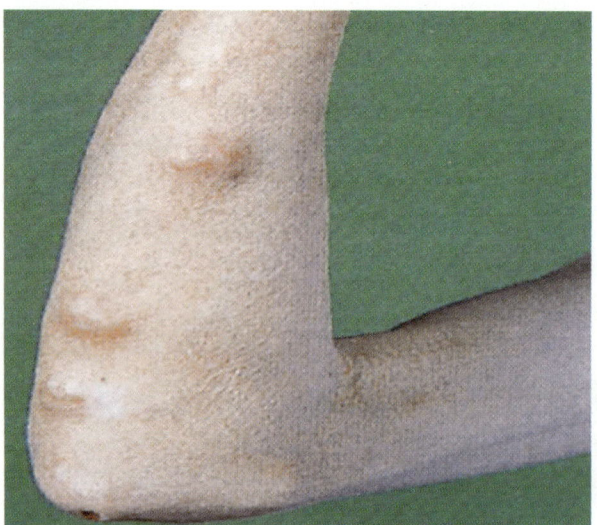

Fig. 10.59: Rheumatoid nodules. The upper forearm and elbow are the most common sites for skin nodules in rheumatoid arthritis. These nodules result from vasculitis, and they may ulcerate or become necrotic, as has occurred at the elbow in this patient. Such nodules are often painless and cause no symptoms, but surgery is occasionally indicated for cosmetic reasons *(Forbes and Jackson, 2003)*

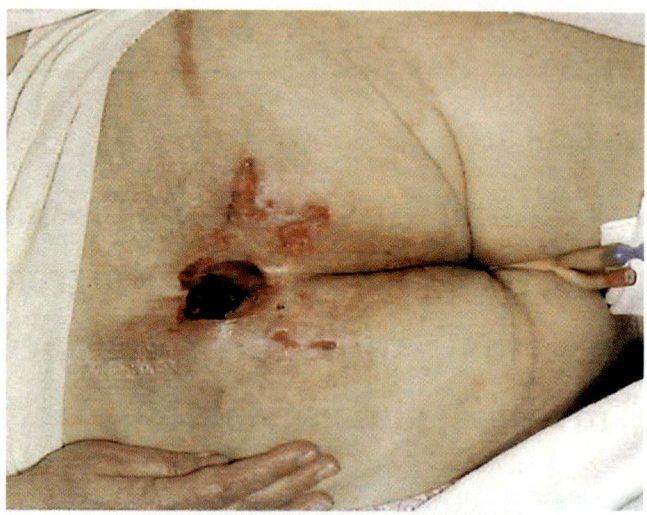

Fig. 10.60: Rheumatoid arthritis. Extensive sacral ulceration associated with rheumatoid arthritis, possibly due to rupture of rheumatoid nodules *(Norman and Bramley, 1990)*

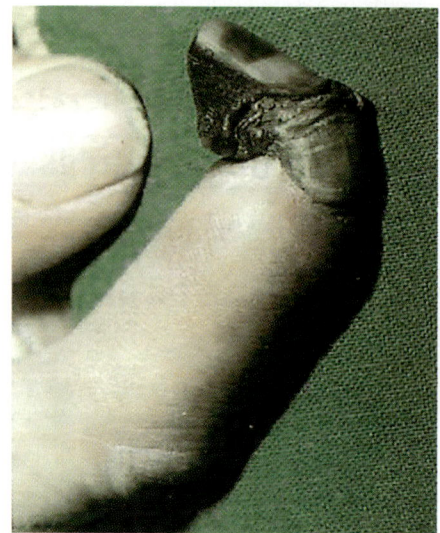

Fig. 10.61: Rheumatoid arthritis. Showing severe digital arthritis associated with gangrene (the finger ends ultimately separated, leaving healing stumps) *(Norman and Bramley, 1990)*

pleural nodules, fibrosing alveolitis, obstructive bronchiolitis.

Vasculitis: Vasculitis is caused by immune complex deposition in arterial walls. Smoking is a risk factor. Other manifestations are: nail-fold infarcts due to cutaneous vasculitis (Fig. 10.61), widespread cutaneous vasculitis with necrosis of the skin, mononeuritis multiplex, bowel infarction due to necrotizing arteritis of the mesenteric vessels.

The larynx: The larynx contains two symmetric joints, the cricoarytenoid and the cricothyroid joints. The cricoarytenoid joints contribute to the movement of the true vocal cords, so when cri-coarytenoid arthritis occurs, the patient may experience hoarseness, fullness in the throat, dyspnea, dysphagia, and stridor. It is estimated that 26 to 78% of patients with RA will have some laryngeal involvement, but only a quarter of these patients will have symptoms.

The heart and peripheral vessels: Clinical pericarditis is rare. In strongly seropositive RA, echocardiogram or postmortum studies, however, show that 30–40 of patients have pericardial involvement. Endocarditis and myocardial disease are rarely seen.

The nervous system: Neuropathies, either mononeuritis multiplex or a sensory loss in a glove and stocking pattern, are due to vasculitis of the vasa nervosum. Compression neuropathies such as carpal or tarsal tunnel syndrome are due to local synovial hypertrophy. Atlantoaxial subluxation can cause serious neurological abnormalities.

The eyes: Scleritis and episcleritis occur in severe, seropositive disease and produce painful red lesions in the eye (Fig. 10.62). Scleritis may lead to perforation of the eye and requires active treatment with local and systemic corticosteroids.

The kidneys: Amyloidosis causes the nephritic syndrome and renal failure. Presentation is with proteinuria. It occurs rarely in severe, long-standing rheumatoid disease and is due to the deposition of highly stable amyloid A protein (SAP) in the intercellular matrix of a variety of organs. SAP is an acute-phase reactant, produced normally in the liver. It is rare and proteinuria in RA is more commonly due to disease-modifying antirheumatic drugs (DMARDs).

The spleen, lymph nodes, and blood: Felty's syndrome is splenomegaly and neutropenia in a patient with RA. Leg ulcers or sepsis are complications. HLA-DRW4 is found in 95% of patients, compared with 70% of patients with RA alone. The

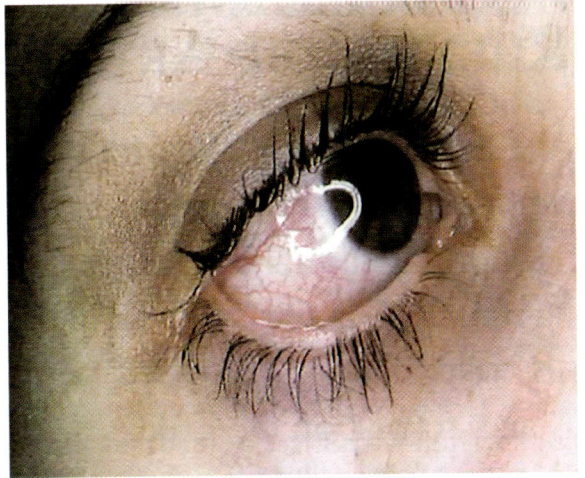

Fig. 10.62: Scleritis. Note the diffuse, mainly fine-vessel injection of the sclera *(Norman and Bramley, 1990)*

Criteria for the diagnosis of rheumatoid arthritis (American College of Rheumatology, 1987 revision):
- Morning stiffness ≥ 1 hour
- Arthitis of three or major joints
- Arthitis of hand joint and wrists
- Symmetrical arthritis
- Subcutaneous nodules
- A positive serum rheumatoid factor
- Tpical radiological changes (erosion and/or periarticular osteopenia)

Four or more criteria are necessary for diagonsis.

lymph nodes may be palpable, usually in the distribution of affected joints. There may be peripheral lymphedema of the arm or leg.

Anemia is almost universal and is usually the normochromic normocytic anemia of chronic disease.

The American Rheumatism Association has established criteria for diagnosis based on the manifestations and length of time they persist, for example, swelling of three joints for a minimum of 6 weeks. The severity of the condition varies from mild to severe, reflecting the number of joints affected, the degree of inflammation, and the rapidity of the progression.

PROGRESSION OF RHEUMATOID ARTHRITIS

In the affected joints, the first step in the development of rheumatoid arthritis is an abnormal immune response, causing inflammation of the synovial membrane with vasodilation, increased permeability, and formation of exudates, causing the typical red, swollen, and painful joint. This synovitis appears to result from the immune abnormality. Rheumatoid factor, an antibody against immunoglobulin G, as well as other immunologic factors, is present in the blood in the majority of patients with RH arthritis. RF is also present in synovial fluid. After the first period of acute inflammation, the joint may appear to recover completely. As the pathologic process continues, the following manifestations are observed:

1. *Synovitis:* Inflammation recurs, synovial cells proliferate.
2. *Pannus formation:* Granulation tissue from the synovium spreads over the articular cartilage. This granulation tissue, called pannus, releases enzymes and inflammatory mediators, destroying the cartilage.
3. *Cartilage erosion:* Cartilage is eroded by enzymes from the pannus, and in addition, nutrients that

Typcial presentation of rheumatoid arthritis

- **Palindromic:** Monoarticular attacks lasting 24–48 hours; 50% progress to other types of RA.
- **Transient:** A self-limiting disease, lasting less than 12 months and leaving no permanent joint damage. Usually seronegative for IgM rheumatoid factor. Some of these may be undetected postviral arthritis.
- **Remitting:** There is a period of several years during which the arthritis is active but then remits, leaving minimal damage.
- **Chronic, persistent:** The most typical form, it may be seropositive or seronegative for IgM rheumatoid factor. The disease follows a relapsing and remitting course over many years. Seropositive patients tend to develop greater joint damage and long-term disability. They warrant earlier and more aggressive treatment with disease-modifying agents.
- **Rapid progressive:** The disease progresses remorselessly over a few years and leads rapidly to severe joint damage and disability. It is usually seropositive, has a high incidence of systemic complications and is difficult to treat.

are normally supplied by the synovial fluid to the cartilage are cut off by the pannus. Erosion of the cartilage creates an unstable joint.

4. *Fibrosis:* In time, the pannus between the bone ends becomes fibrotic, limiting movement. This calcifies and the joint space is obliterated.

5. *Ankylosis:* Joint fixation and deformity develop.

During each exacerbation or acute period, inflammation and further damage occur in joints previously affected, and additional joints become affected by synovitis. During this process, other changes frequently occur around the joint:

- Atrophy of muscles— the acute inflammation leads to disuse atrophy of the muscles and stretching of the tendons and ligaments, thus decreasing the supportive structures in the unstable joint.
- The alignment of the bones in the joint shifts, depending on how much cartilage has been eroded and the balance achieved between muscles. Mobility is greatly impaired as the various joints become damaged and deformed. Walking becomes very difficult when the knees or ankles are affected.
- Inflammation and pain may cause muscle spasm, further drawing the bones out of normal alignment.
- Contractures and deformity with subluxation develop. Various contractures and deformities, such as ulnar deviation, swan neck deformity, or boutonniere, may occur in the hands depending on the degree of flexion and hyperextension in the joints.

LABORATORY FEATURES

Laboratory investigations contribute to the diagnosis and assessment of the degree of inflammatory activity, although clinical features remain the most important clues in diagnosis and management.

1. Blood Count

- Anemia tends to occur in active disease and has the features of iron-deficiency anemia but with a normal or low iron-binding capacity. Pernicious anemia is significantly more common in rheumatoid arthritis patients than in the general population.
- A raised erythrocyte sedimentation rate (ESR) provides a reasonable index of disease activity although, very high ESR level should raise the question of an associated connective tissue disorder such as systemic lupus erythematosus (SLE), malignancy, or septic arthritis.

2. Serology

- About 80% of patients with clinical rheumatoid arthritis have a positive rheumatoid factor test. Rheumatoid factors are circulating autoantibodies, which have the Fc portion of IgG as their antigen. The nature of the antigen means that they self-aggregate into immune complexes and thus activate complement and stimulate inflammation, causing chronic synovitis.

Transient production of rheumatoid factors is an essential part of the body's normal mechanism for removing immune complexes, but in RA they show a much higher affinity and their production is per-sistent and occurs in the joints. They may be of any immunoglobulin class (IgM, IgG, or IgA), but the most common tests employed clinically detect IgM rheuma-toid factor. Around 70% of patients with polyarticular RA have IgM rheumatoid factor in serum.

The term seronegative RA is used for patients in whom the standard tests for IgM rheumatoid factor are persistently negative. They tend to have a more limited pattern of synovitis.

Seronegative arthritis may become seropositive with time or remain seronegative. The titre of rheumatoid factor correlates to some degree with prognosis in rheumatoid arthritis and with systemic features. High-titre disease tends to be more destructive and more likely to be associated with systemic features, including nodules. IgM rheumatoid factor is neither diagnostic of RA, and proteinuria nor does its absence rule the disease out; but it is useful predictor of prognosis. A persistently high titre in early disease implies more persistently active synovitis, more joint damage and greater disability eventually, and justifies earlier use of DMARDs.

- The histocompatibility antigens HLA-A DW4 and HLA DRW4 are present in 50% of patients, a finding that have been helpful in ascribing a genetic influence in the etiology of rheumatoid arthritis.

3. Aspiration of the Joint

The synovial fluid in rheumatoid arthritis shows all the features of a non-specific inflammatory exudates; it is turbid, yellow/green, of low viscosity, clot-positive and has up to 30,000 WBC/mm^3. Marked turbidity and a high WBC count should raise the question of septic arthritis.

1. *Disease-modifying Antirheumatic Drugs* (DMARDs)

Failure of satisfactory suppression of the inflammatory process with NSAIDs combined with corticosteroids may indicate the use of disease-modifying antirheumatic drugs (DMARDs) which are remission-inducing agents.

DMARDs, which mainly act through cytokines inhibition, reduce inflammation, as reflected by a reduction of joint swelling, a fall in the plasma acute phase reactants and slowing of the development of joint erosions and irreversible damage. Their beneficial effect is not immediate (hence slow-acting agents) and may be parual or transient. The problem with all DMARDs is their effect is often only partial, achieving between 20 and 50% improvement.

Complications of rheumatoid arthritis

Complications of the condition
Ruptured tendon
Ruptured joints
Joint infection
Spinal cord compression (atlantoaxial or upper cervical spine)
Amyloidosis (rare)
Side effects of therapy
Dyspepsia
Gastrointestinal bleeding
Perforation
Anemia
Renal impairment
Bone marrow hypoplasia

Treatment

Management of rheumatoid arthritis

- Establish the diagonsis clinically.
- Use NSAIDs and analgescis to control symptoms.
- Try to induce remission with i.m. depot methylprednisolone 80–120 mg, if synovitis persists beyond 6 weeks.
- If synovitis recurs, refer to a rheumatologist to start sulfasalazine or methotrexate. Give a second dose of i.m. depot methylprednisolone.
- Refer for physiotherapy and general advice through a specialist team.
- If there is no significant improvement in 6–12 weeks as measured by less pain, less morning stiffness and reduced acute-phase response, consider a combination of methotrxate and sulfasalazine.
- If no better, consider an alternative agent, such as gold, D-penicillamine or leflunamide.
- If still no better, consider anti-TNF-α therapy.
- If still no better, surgery is considered where total joint replacement is performed.

Nonetheless there is good evidence that DMARDs control symptoms and signs of joint inflammation and their withdrawal leads to a flare.

These disease-modifying antirheumatic drugs (DMARDs)include gold salts, penicillamine, sulfasalazine, methotrexate, and antimalarials (hydroxychloroquine), gold (sodium aurothiomalate) and leflunamide. These agents have proven useful in some cases. These drugs are slow-acting, powerful, anti-inflammatory agents with potentially serious toxic effects, and careful monitoring of each of these drugs is, therefore, mandatory. It is important to ensure regular checks of urine and blood during gold therapy, of urine with penicillamine, and regular ophthalmic checks when using antimalarials.

2. *Tumor Necrosis Factor (TNF-α) Blockers*

The recent availability of agents that block TNF-α is beginning to alter the traditional use of DMARDs. Infliximab is a monocolonal antibody against TNF-α and is given intravenously. Infliximab is coprescribed with methotrexate to prevent loss of efficacy because of antibody formation. Both products slow or halt erosion formation in up to 70% of patients with RA and produce healing in a few.

3. *Anti-inflammatory Analgesics*

Anti-inflammatory analgesics are to control pain. Most patients with RA are unable to cope without an NASID to relieve night pain and morning stiffness. NSAIDs do not reduce the underlying inflammatory process. They all act on the cyclo-oxygenase (COX) pathway, but newer drugs are more specific for blocking the COX-2 enzyme. The individual response to NSAIDs varies greatly. It is desirable, therefore, to try several different drugs for a particular patient in order to find the best. Each compound should be given for at least a week.

4. Glucocorticoids

They are powerful disease-controlling drugs, but are avoided in the long term because side effects are inevitable. In more severe cases, glucocorticoids may be prescribed, and administered either orally or as intra-articular injections (Fig. 10.63). Predisolone (or prednisone) 40–120 mg i.m. is the corticosteroid of choice. Patients like the effects of glucocorticoids because the drug promotes a feeling of well-being and improves the appetite. However, there are a number of potential complications with long-term use of these drugs, so they should be used only during acute episodes or taken on alternate days at the lowest effective dose.

5. Physiotherapy

Patients with RA need constant advice and support from physiotherapists and nurse specialists, especially while they are learning to adjust. A combination of rest for active arthritis and excercises to maintain joint range and muscle power is essential. Physiotherapy is carried out to maintain mobility and strengthen the weak muscles.

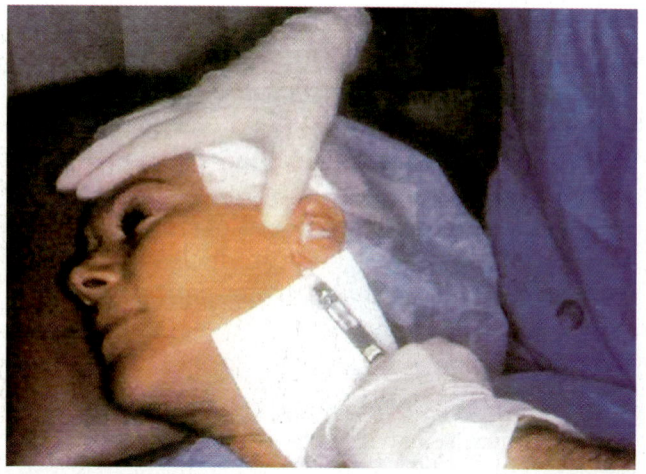

Fig. 10.63: Intra-articular injection of corticosteroid "Debrofos"

> **Problems associated with the use of corticosteroids**
> - Patients are increasingly anxious about the use of corticosteroids because of adverse publicity about their potential side effects. This must be discussed frankly and the risks of not treating them be described and balanced against the risks of the drug itself.
> - Patients must be warned to avoid sugars and saturated fats and to eat less because of the risk of weight gain.
> - The skin becomes thin and easily damaged.
> - Monitor for diabetes and hypertension
> - Ctataract formation may be accelerated.
> - Osteoporosis develops within 6 months on doses above 7.5 mg daily, and hormone replacement therapy and/or calcium and vitamin D and bisphosphonate are used.

The general management of the disease naturally includes:
- Exercise in a hydrotherapy pool is popular and effective.
- During acute episodes, the involved joints may require splinting to prevent excessive movement and to maintain alignment.
- Appropriate body poisitioning and body mechanics when walking or moving also help to maintain function.
- Assistive devices such as wrist support or padded handles with straps are available to help the patient cope with daily activities and to reduce contractures.

When the temporomandibular joints are involved by RA, the following physiotherapeutic management is advised.

a. Muscular excercises (Fig. 10.64).

b. Disengagement of occlusion, i.e. "separation of teeth" by the costrucion of a maxillary or mandibular bite planes to nullify occlusal abnormalities, help decompression of the edemetous retrodiscal tissues and synovial membrane and assists in alleviating the preauricular pain (Fig. 10.65).

c. The use of heat and cold modalities can be very effective when they are used correctly.

These measurements usually lead to improvement of jaw function (Fig. 10.66).

6. Surgical Intervention

Surgery should be considered carefully in the long-term approach to patient management. Its main objectives are prophylactic, to prevent joint

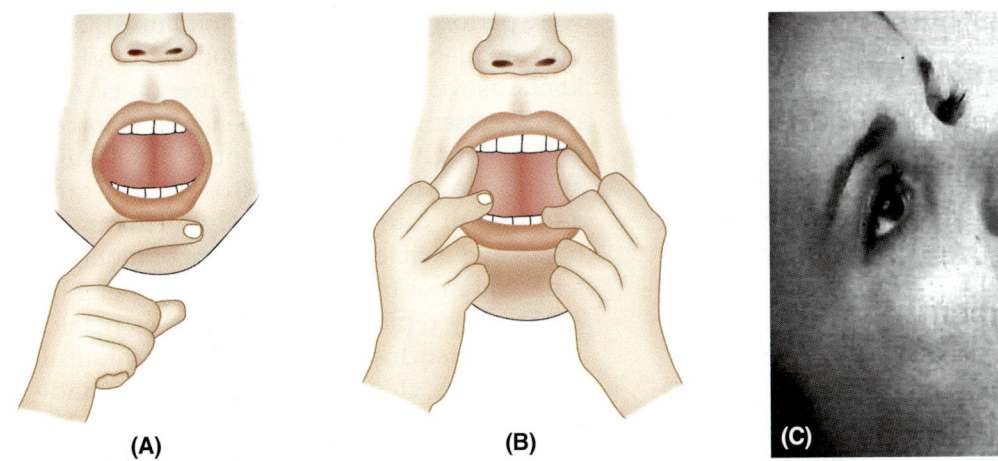
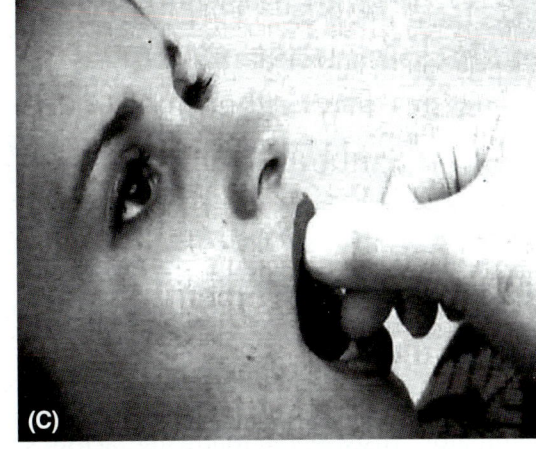

(A)　　　　**(B)**　　　**(C)**

Fig. 10.64: (A) Heavy downward pressure is applied to the symphysis menti region as an isotonic exercise to strengthen the jaw muscles. Gentle but steady pressure is placed on the premolar teeth **(B)** or lower incisors **(C)** for approximately 10 to 15 seconds to activate the muscles of mastication

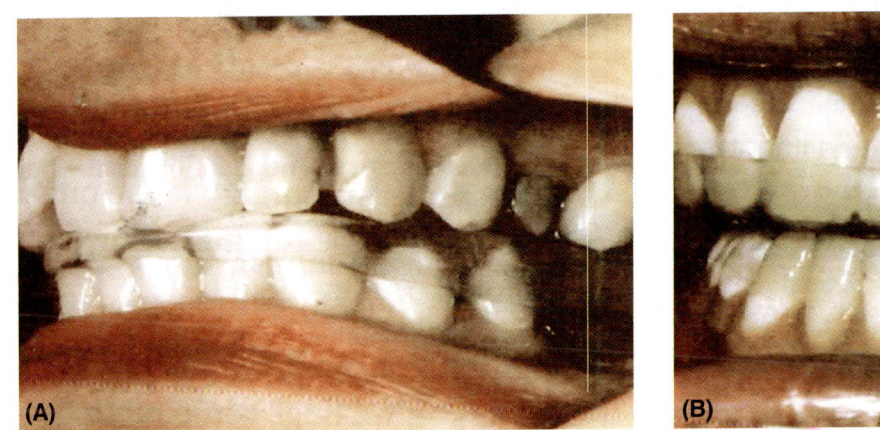
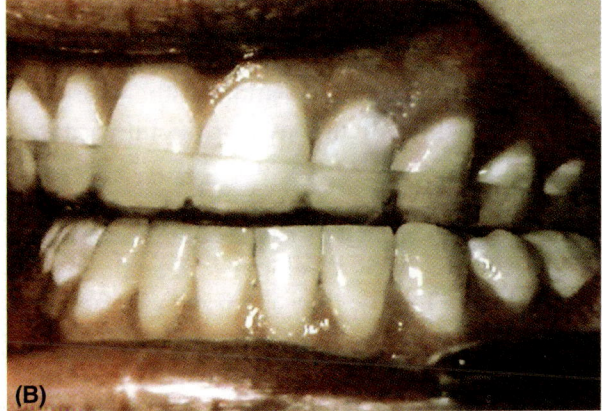

(A)　　　　　　　　　　**(B)**

Fig. 10.65: The occlusion is disengaged by wearing either a mandibular **(A)** or a maxillary **(B)** stabilization splint. Disengaged occlusion "separation of teeth" leads to decompression of the edematous retrodiscal tissues and synovial membrane, assists in alleviating the preauricular pain

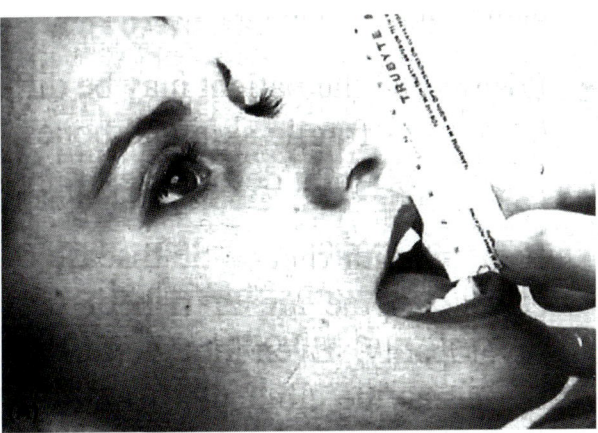
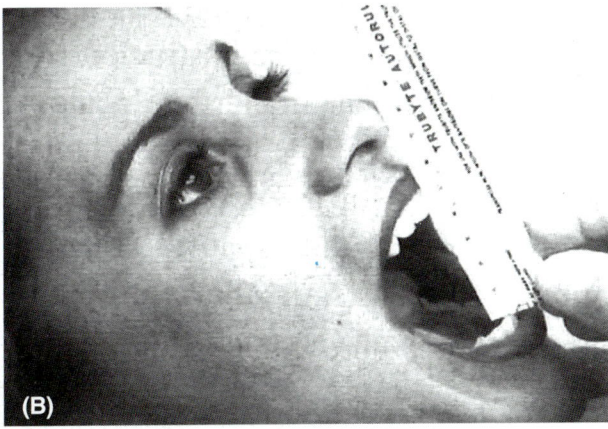

(B)

Fig. 10.66: Measuring the range of mouth opening. **(A)** The patient is asked to open the mouth until pain is felt. At this position, the distance between the incisal edges of the anterior teeth is measured. This measurement is called the maximum comfortable mouth opening. **(B)** Following muscular exercises, the range of comfortable opening is increased

destruction and deformity, and reconstructive, to rest one function.

Single-joint disease can be treated by surgical synovectomy to reduce the bulk of inflamed tissue and prevent damage. Excision arthroplasties of the metatarsal heads reduce metatarsal pain and relieve pressure points. The major surgical advance has been the development of total replacement arthroplasty of the hip, knee, finger, joints, elbows and shoulders. Such procedures need careful planning and preparation, and the expected outcomes and risks should be explained to the patient.

When considering surgery in the presence of rheumatoid disease, the following factors should be considered:

- The effects on coagulation of drug therapy involving corticosteroids, antibiotic cover, and NSAIDs. The adult patient with severe secondary osteoarthritis, whose rheumatoid disease started in childhood and who is maintained on NSAIDs and steroids, may pose a formidable surgical and anesthetic problem.
- Positioning the patient may be difficult because of fragile skin and bones, and because of joint deformities.
- Patients with rheumatic disease of the cervical spine are at risk of cervical myelopathy. Even though the cervical spine may be clinically trouble free, it is wise to place these patients in a soft collar pre-operatively, if only to remined medical and non-medical personnel handling the patients that the neck is vulnerable.

The following surgical approaches are indicated:

a. *Synovectomy* to remove the pannus and reduce contractures. In the active stage of the disease, synovectomy may limit the extent of the destruction, but surgeons are relatively invited to see the patient at this stage and more commonly the disease process is more advanced. It appears that of all small joints, the TMJs have less synovial tissue than those of the hands and feet and symptoms are, therefore, less marked.

b. *Joint prosthesis (arthroplasty):* Surgery can supply joint replacement and much more normal appearance and function. Arthroplasty, a treatment of last resort, is the replacement of a diseased joint with an artificial device called a *prosthesis.* Joint prostheses are now the most common orthopedic procedure for the elderly (Figs 10.67 and 10.68). The first knee replacements were performed in the 1970s. Joint prostheses are now available for finger, shoulder, and elbow joints, as well as for hip and knee joints. Arthroplasty presents ongoing challenges for biomedical engineering. An effective prosthesis must be strong, non-toxic, and corrosion resistant. In addition, it must bond firmly to the patient's bones and enable a normal range of motion with a minimum of friction. The heads of long bones are usually replaced with prostheses made of a metal alloy such as cobalt-chrome, titanium alloy, or stainless steel. Joint sockets are made of polyethylene. Prostheses are bonded to the patient's bone with screws or bone cement. About 80 to 90% of hip replacements and at least 60% of ankle replacements are still functional 2 to 10 years later. The most common form of failure is detachment of the prosthesis from the bone. This problem has been reduced by using *porous-coated prostheses,* which become infiltrated by the patient's own bone and create a firmer bond. A prosthesis is not as strong as a natural joint, however, and is not an option for many young, active patients.

Arthroplasty has been greatly improved by *computer-assisted design and manufacture (CAD/CAM).* A computer scans X-rays from the patient and presents several design possibilities for review. Once a design is selected, the computer generates a program to operate the machinery that produces the prosthesis. CAD/CAM has reduced the waiting period for a prosthesis from about 12 weeks to about 2 weeks and has lowered the cost dramatically.

Concerning temporomandibular joint involvement, in **jeuvenile rheumatoid arthritis** where there is progressive destruction, fibrous ankylosis may follow, and in addition the mandibular condyles may be completely destroyed resulting in an increasing anterior open bite and retrognathia (Fig. 10.49). The totally destroyed joints in the growing child may need to be replaced with a bilateral costochondral graft, although obviously not in the presence of active disease. Later a mandibular advancement and genioplasty will be carried out. Although pain, effusion and restricted movement may initiate the referral, it is progressive retrognathia and micrognathia which become a concern to the mother and child. With the active disease controlled, an assessment should be made by rheumatologist, surgeon and orthodontist, and a long-term treatment plan drawn up.

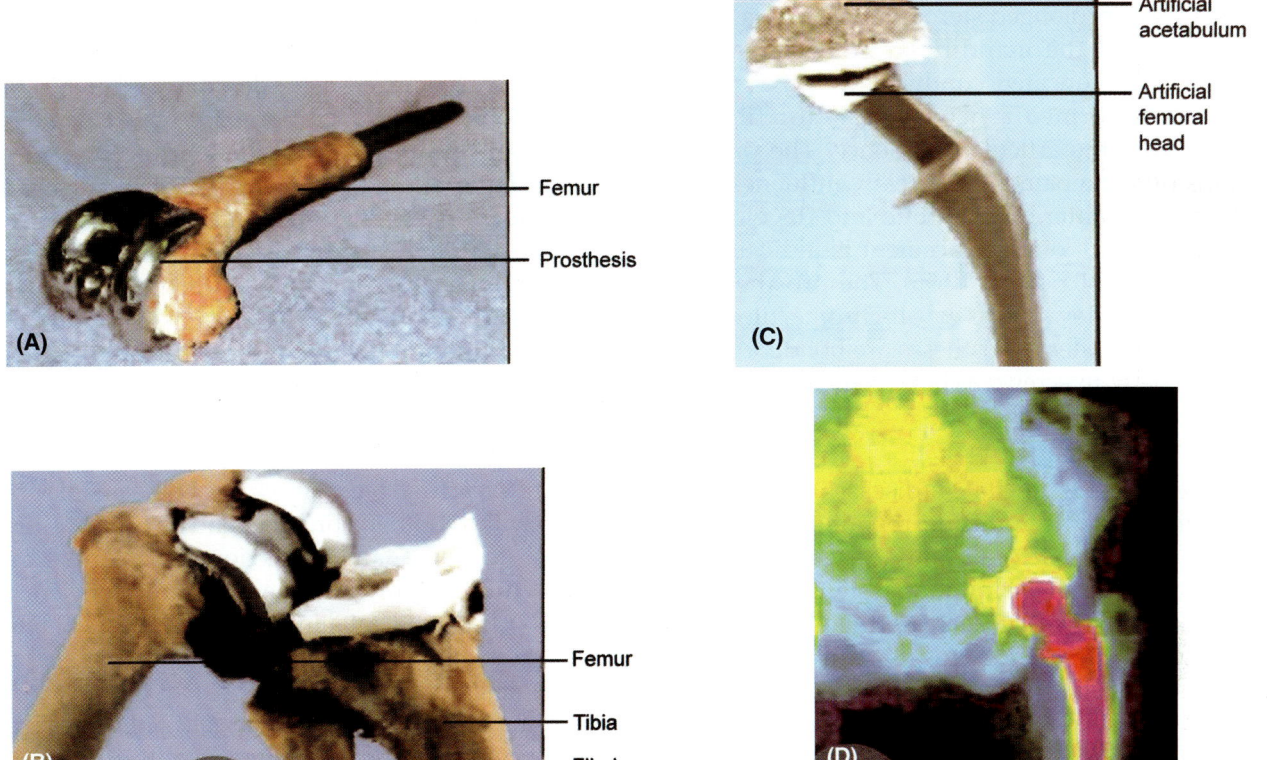

Fig. 10.67: Joint prosthesis. **(A)** An artificial femoral head inserted into the femur. **(B)** An artificial knee joint bonded to a natural femur and tibia. **(C)** A porous coated hip prosthesis. The cap-like portion replaces the acetabulum of the os coxae, and the ball and shaft shown below are bonded to the proximal end of the femur. **(D)** X-ray of a patient with a total hip replacement *(Saladin, 2003)*

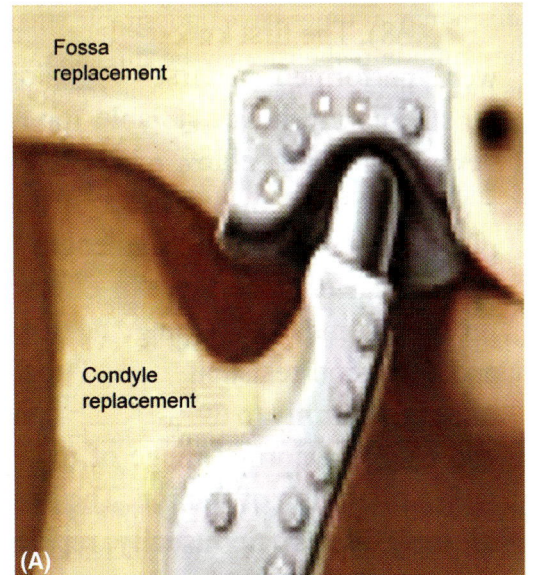

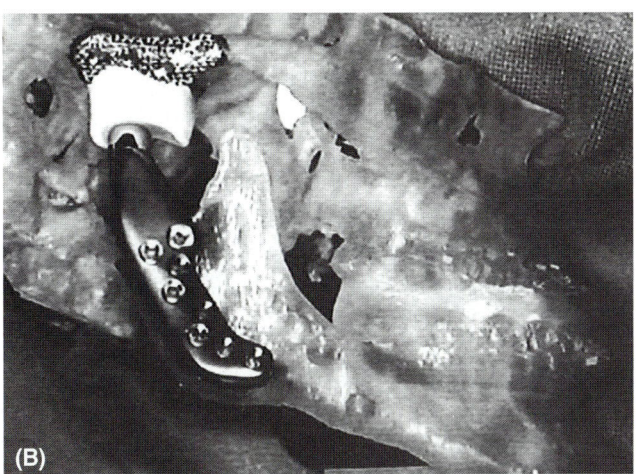

Fig. 10.68: Total temporomandibular joint replacement

In the adult patient with late onset rheumatoid disease and a history of prolonged steroid therapy, it is quite common to find the mandibular condyle totally destroyed. The truncated condylar neck may have subluxated or formed a neoarthrosis (or fibrous ankylosis) with the articular eminence. The patient complains of some pain but is greatly influenced by the progressive anterior open bite and developing retrognathia. Total joint replacement is indicated in such cases (Figs 10.54 and 10.56). The prosthesis is made of a metal alloy such as cobalt-chrome, titanium alloy, or stainless steel. Prostheses are bonded to the patient's bone with screws or bone cement.

B. IMMUNE DEFICIENCY STATES

Immunodeficiencies are states (diseases) that result from a defect in the immune response, or from improper response of the immune system. It is a failure of some part of the immune system to function properly. Conditions that decrease the effectiveness of the immune system, or destroy its ability to respond to antigens altogether are called immunodeficiency. Immunodeficiency diseases may result from a complete absence of B or T cells or a decrease in their number or activity. If B cells are few in number or absent, the person will be vulnerable to bacterial infections (but not viral infections, if T cells are normal). If T cells are absent or low in number, the person is particularly vulnerable to viral infections, parasites, and tumor cells.

Categorization of Immunodeficiency

1. *Congenital immunodeficiency states:* Usually involve failure of the fetus to form adequate number of B cells, T cells, or both.
2. *Acquired immune deficiency:* Acquired immuno-deficiency can result from many different causes. For example, inadequate protein diet inhibits protein synthesis and, therefore, antibody levels decrease. The immune system can be depressed as a result of stress, drugs (e.g. to protect graft rejection), or illness. Diseases such as leukemia cause an overproduction of lymphocytes that do not function properly.
   Acquired immunodeficiency syndrome (AIDS), is a non-hereditary disease contracted after birth. It is a life-threatening disease caused by the human immunodeficiency virus (HIV). Acquired immune deficiency syndrome (AIDS) is a disease in which the number of the helper T cells is decreased, making the affected person vulnerable to infections. AIDS is the terminal stage of infection with the human immunodeficiency virus (HIV), which is recognized as undergoing a number of mutations. AIDS-related complex, which includes cervical lymphadenopathy, oropharyngeal candidiasis, and hairy leukoplakia is precursor to full-blown AIDS. Infections characteristic of AIDS are pneumocystis carini pneumonia and disseminated myobacterial infection. Kaposi's sarcoma is the tumor most often associated with the condition. AIDs is presented as a group of conditions that involve a severely depressed immune response resulting from infection with the human immunodeficiency virus (HIV).

3. *Severe combined immunodeficiency:* Some people are born without either B or T cells and have practically no protection against infection. This condition, known as severe combined immunodeficiency (SCID), is usually fatal in the first few years of life. Children with SCID are sometimes helped by transplants of bone marrow or fetal thymus, but in some cases the transplanted cells fail to survive and multiply or transplanted T cells attack the patient's tissues. Unless the person suffering from SCID is kept in a sterile environment or is provided with a compatible bone marrow transplant, death from infection results.

Cell-mediated and humoral immune responses protect against potentially harmful microorganisms and other foreign substances. The same immunologic mechanism may at times have undesirable effects:

1. The immune response may be directed against the individual's own cells or tissue components, leading to autoimmune diseases.
2. The immune response is responsible for the rejection of transplanted organs.
3. The immune response may lead to Rh hemolytic disease in newborn infants.

Also, the undesirable immunologic effect may develop as a result of some diseases or some administrated drugs.

Diseases which Suppress the Immune Response

1. *Autoimmune disease,* e.g. rheumatoid arthritis, carries a minor increased risk of infection.
2. *Chronic renal failure:* Moderately increased risk.
3. *Deficiency states:* Anemia carries minor increased risk.

B. IMMUNE DEFICIENCY STATES

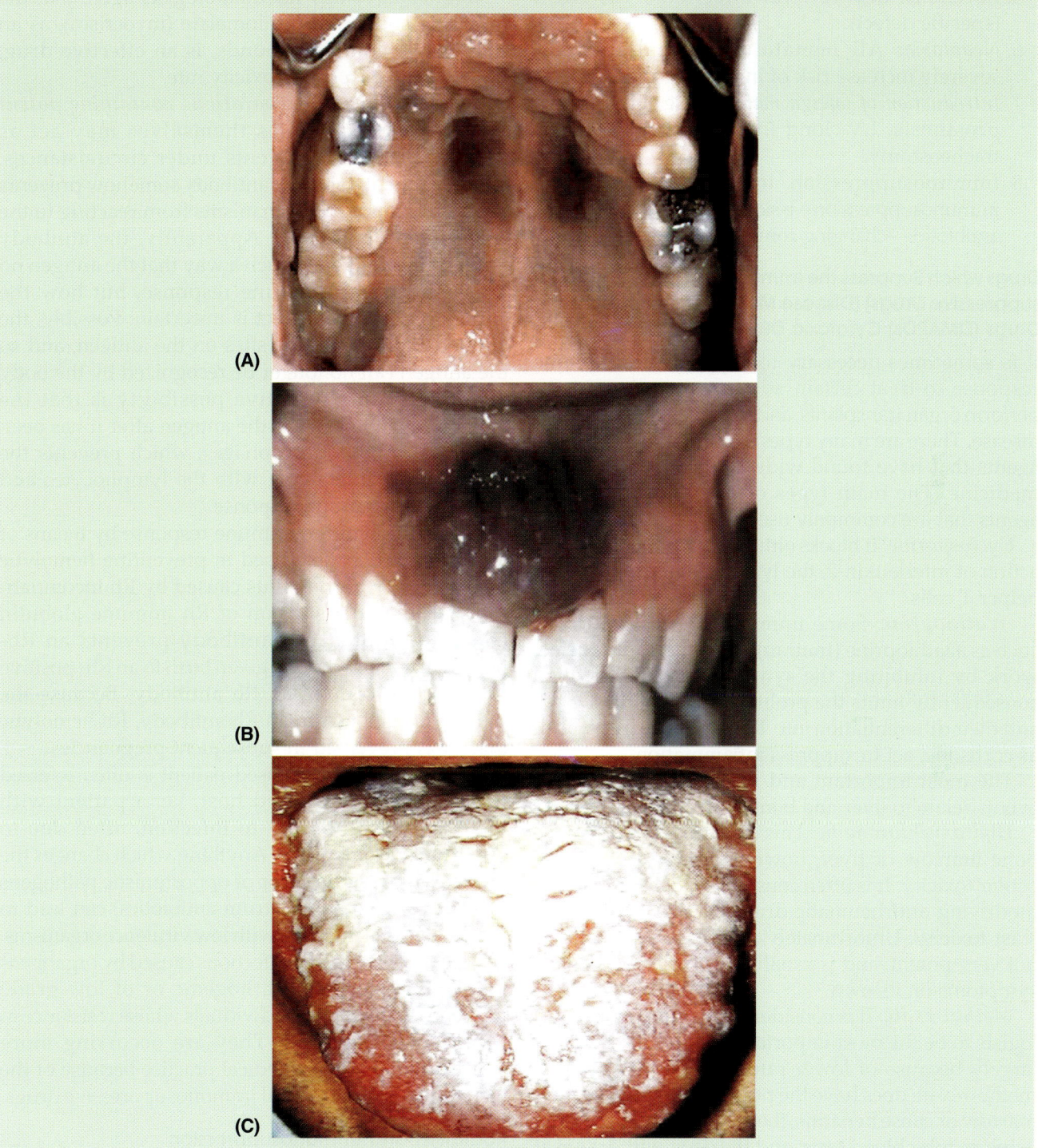

(A)

(B)

(C)

Plate XIV: Kaposi's sarcoma. **(A)** Bilateral areas of brownish discoloration of the midline of the hard palate. Also note the brown exophytic mass palatal to the maxillary third molar. **(B)** Hemorrhagic and exophytic mass of the anterior maxillary gingiva (*About Table, 2006*). **(C)** Extensive oral infection with *Candida albicans* in a patient with HIV infection. Note the great changes in the tongue and the angular chelitis

4. *Diabetes mellitus* is common and carries a moderate increases risk of infection.
5. *Infections:* Severe viral infections, TB, AIDS (specific defect).
6. *Neoplasia:* All hematological malignances severely increase risk of infection.
7. *Introduction of foreign material,* e.g. heart valve prosthesis, I.V. long lines in intensive care, tracheostomy.
8. Immunosuppression in transplant surgery, immunosuppression—a side effect of tumor therapy, antibiotics—changing commensal populations.

Drugs which Suppress the Immune Response (Immuno-suppressive Drugs) (Disease Modifying Anti-rheumatic Drugs (DMARDs) Cytotoxic Durgs)

It is sometimes necessary to suppress the immune response to treat certain autoimmune diseases, to perform organ transplants, and to prevent Rh hemolytic disease. There are many types of immu-nosuppressive agents that have found wide application in clinical medicine. The main types of immunosuppressive agents that are commonly used by physician are:

Cyclosporine: It blocks either the production or the action of interleukin-2, the lymphokine produced by helper T cells.

Azathioprine: Some immunosuppressive drugs such as azathioprine (Imuran) and 6-mercaptopurine, work by inhibiting the synthesis of DNA, which consequently limits the proliferation of lymphocytes and their differentiation into T cells. Other drugs, such as cortisone, act to suppress inflammation.

The most important and most common adverse events relate to liver and bone marrow toxicity.

Hydroxychloroquine: This drug does not affect the bone marrow or liver, however, may rarely cause ocular toxicity. It is often considered to be the disease modifying antirheumatic drug (DMARDs) with the least toxicity. Unfortunately, hydroxychloroquine is not very potent, and is usually insufficient to control symptoms on its own.

Methotrexate: It is considered by many rheumato-logists to be the most important and useful DMARD, largely because of lower rate of toxicity. Although methotrexate does have the potential to suppess bone marrow or cause hepatitis, these effects can monitored using regular blood tests, and the drug withdrawn at an early stage.

Corticosteroids: They suppress the inflammatory response and impair phagocytosis. They also inhibit protein synthesis, thereby suppressing the growth and division of lymphocytes and inhibiting antibody formation by plasma cells.

Gold compounds: Rheumatologists agree that the injectable sodium aurothiomalate (myocrisin), as an example of gold compounds, is an effective drug, however, it has a great toxicity rate.

Gamma globulin preparations containing potent antibodies: Antibodies themselves may act as immunosuppressive agents under circumstances. Given a patient a specific antibody somehow prevents the body's immune mechanisms from reacting to the corresponding antigen. Apparently, the antibody binds to the antigen in such a way that the antigen no longer incites an immune response, but how the antibody exerts this effect is uncertain. Possibly, the antibody covers specific sites on the antigen, and so the antigen can no longer be recognized by the body as foreign. An alternative possibility is that the antibody combines with the antigen after it has been processed by the macrophages, which prevents the antigen from interacting with the lymphocytes and inducing an immune response.

Suppression of the immune response by means of an antibody is widely used in preventing hemolytic disease of newborn infants caused by Rh incompatibility. The administration of Rh immune globulin containing potent Rh antibody prevents an Rh-negative mother who has given birth to an Rh- positive infant from forming an Rh antibody. Because the mother does not form an Rh antibody, Rh hemolytic disease is prevented in subsequent pregnancies.

An immunocompromised patient is often referred to immunocompromised host, i.e. a patient with increased susceptibility to infection, often due to opportunistic organisms. Anything which changes the host environment in favor of opportunistic pathogens (e.g. surgery, broad spectrum antibiotics) can lead to potentially fatal infection with low virulence organisms. The term opportunistic infections caused by organisms which are often non-pathogenic or of low grade virulence, occurring in individuals whose resistance to infection is impaired. They are occurring more frequently in modern medical practice because of the increasing use of powerful immunosuppressive drugs.

Radiation and Immunosuppression

Radiation destroy normal cells. It exerts its immunosuppressive effects by destroying lymphoid tissue, which plays a key role in both cell-mediated and humoral immunities.

ACQUIRED IMMUNODEFICIENCY SYNDROME (AIDS)
HUMAN IMMUNODEFICIENCY VIRUS (HIV)

AIDS, an immunodeficiency disease, is caused by a retrovirus, the human immunodeficiency virus (HIV) that targets primarily helper T cells. As the number of T cells falls, the normal immune response breaks down.

Introduction

- Immunocompromised patients are a group of individuals who present special problems because of defect in, or suppression of their immune system. The condition with the highest profile among these is AIDS.

- All human immunodeficiency virus (HIV) -infected individuals develop oral alterations during the course of HIV disease. They range from asymptomatic and subtle changes of the oral mucosa that are secondary to a decreased salivary flow or candidiasis to rapidly destructive lesions, such as necrotizing stomatitis, necrotizing ulcerative periodontitis, and cancers. It is important to realize that none of these lesions is specific for HIV disease, and all can be found in other immune-suppressed individuals. Thus oral lesions found in HIV-infected patients may be important markers for disease progression.

- All dentists need to be able to screen for abnormalities in the oral cavity. Similarly, dentists need to refer those patients with lesions beyond their expertise to more experienced providers. Treatment of certain oral lesions can be handled in a dental office on an outpatient basis. Ideally dental care providers should feel confident in treating common lesions, such as oral candidiasis, oral hairy leukoplakia, some HIV-related periodontal conditions, and minor apthous ulcerations, and provide symptomatic pain relief.

- As with all other patients, the main concerns for dentists treating HIV- infected individuals are increased bleeding tendencies, postoperative infections, drug interactions, and adverse reactions.

Acquired immunodeficiency diseases are non-hereditary diseases contracted after birth. The best-known example is **acquired immunodeficiency syndrome (AIDS),** a group of conditions that involve a severely depressed immune response resulting from infection with the **human immunodeficiency virus (HIV)** (Box 10.5).

On June 5, 1981, when the Centers for Disease Control (CDC) reported five cases of pneumocystis carinii pneumonia in young homosexual men in Los Angeles, few suspected that it heralded a pandemic of acquired deficiency syndrome (AIDS). The human immunodeficiency virus (HIV) was first isolated from a patient with AIDS in 1983. Twenty-five years since the first report, more than 67 million persons have been infected with HIV, and more than 25 million have died of AIDS.

INCIDENCE

The rise of AIDS in Central Africa is in no way coincidental to the massive smallpox vaccination in Africa in the late 1960s and 1970s. One possibility is iatrogenic infection through contaminated needles employed in the vaccination campaigns because of unavailability of disposable needles (Siebert C Times August 1994, Van de Perre P et al, 1984). In Central and West Africa, (Zaire, Uganda, Rwanda, Burundi, Senegal) HIV was transmitted through promiscuity and contact with prostitutes (426–429) (Van de Perre P et al, 1984, Piot et al, 1984, Clumeck et al, 1984, Clumeck et al, 1985).

HIV spread to Haiti and then the United States via tourist/immigrant contacts with prostitutes. AIDS first appeared in the United States among homosexuals and Haitian immigrants in two major cities with large homosexual populations: namely New York City and San Francisco (430. Center for Disease Control, 1982).

It was initially termed the "gay-related immune deficiency syndrome." The San Francisco Chronicle newspaper published the "seven deadly symptoms" associated with the disease:

i. Persistent fever for more than four or five days

ii. Unexplained weight loss of 10 to 20 pounds in a few months

iii. General aches and pains similar to an acute viral syndrome for over 10 days

iv. Sore or swollen lymph glands for over a week

v. Appearance of blue or purplish skin spots (KS)

vi. Persistent or worsening herpes sores for over five weeks

Box 10.5

The human immune deficiency virus (HIV) infects and destroys CD4-T lymphocytes, macrophages are also affected.

Infection
CD4> 500×10^6. Asymptomatic or a short febrile illness. Although the patient's cells contain HIV, tests for antibodies may be negative for up to several months.

Latent period
CD4—$200–500 \times 10^6$. Virus present in lymphocytes: may be persistent lymph node enlargement and fever.

AIDS
CD4 < 200×10^6
Infections and tumors

Infection
• Opportunistic
• Others

Tumors
• Kaposi's sarcoma
• Lymphomas

The whole range of opportunistic infection, including virus infection (e.g. herpes simplex virus) occurs. The diagram shows the more common AIDS-associated diseases and sites.

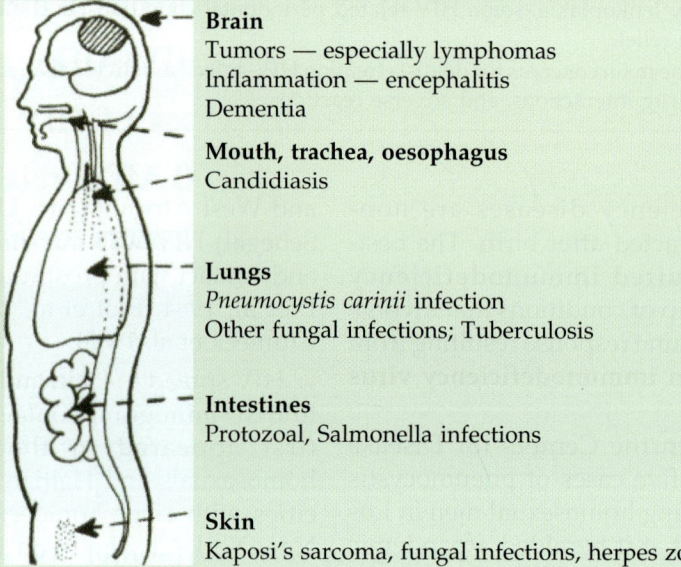

Brain
Tumors — especially lymphomas
Inflammation — encephalitis
Dementia

Mouth, trachea, oesophagus
Candidiasis

Lungs
Pneumocystis carinii infection
Other fungal infections; Tuberculosis

Intestines
Protozoal, Salmonella infections

Skin
Kaposi's sarcoma, fungal infections, herpes zoster

Blood changes
Antibodies: Specific antibodies appear up to six months after infection and form the basis of the diagnostic test for HIV. The antibody titre may fall greatly late in the disease.
Immunoglobulins: They are usually elevated in the early stage. CD4 lymphocytes may be severely reduced, producing a lymphopenia.

vii. Loss of sensorimotor ability or defects in mental or neurological function (Levy, 2006).

These are the characteristic features of HIV infection. During that era, promiscuity among segments of the homosexual community reached gargantuan proportions, with possible pro annum sexual contacts numbering in the hundreds (Maraior et al, 1982).

The circle of vulnerability has widened to include intravenous drug abusers, hemophiliacs, and other recipients of infected blood and blood products. In the United States, the incidence of new cases and related deaths continued to increase until the mid-1990, when the use of HAART became widespread. As of 2003, more than 1 million persons in the United States are living with HIV/AIDS; approximately 40,000 new cases of HIV infection and 16,000 to 17,000 AIDS-related deaths occur annually [Centers for Disease Control and Prevention (CDC), 2007].

Transmission is greatest among the male-to-male sexual contact group [Centers for Disease Control and Prevention (CDC), 2007]. Globally, an estimated 38 million people (range 35–42 million) are living with HIV/AIDS. The devastating impact of this disease, with respect to suffering, mortality, disruption to families, local economies, and infrastructure is greatest in Sub-Saharan and South Africa, where 25 million (range 23.1–27.9 million) are living with HIV/AIDS (4UNAIDS, 2004).

PATHOLOGY

The primary target cell of HIV is the CD4+ helper T lymphocyte. The DNA of HIV is incorporated into the DNA of the lymphocyte and is present for the life of the cell. In most viral infections, host antibodies that are protective against the organism usually are formed. In people with HIV infection, antibodies are developed but are not protective. Like other viruses, HIV can only be replicated by a living host cell. It invades helper T (CD4) cells, dendritic cells, and macrophages. HIV adheres to a target cell by means of one of its envelope glycoproteins.

Table 10.9 summarizes the criteria for HIV infection, the CD4 lymphocyte categories that are used to guide clinical and therapeutic management of HIV-infected individuals, and the clinical categories for HIV/AIDS.

By destroying TH cells by HIV, the humoral immunity and cellular immunity are abolished (Fig. 10.69). The viruses may remain silent, cause cell death, or produce syncytial fusion of the cells, which disrupts their normal functions. A subsequent decrease in T-helper cell numbers occurs, with a resultant loss in immune function. The normal response to viruses, fungi and encapsulated bacteria is diminished.

Normally, the TH count is 600 to 1,200 cells/μL of blood, but a criterion of AIDS is a TH count less than 200 cells/μL. With such severe depletion of TH cells, a person succumbs to opportunistic infections with *Toxoplasma* (a protozoan previously known mainly for causing birth defects), *Pneumocystis* (a group of

Table 10.9: CD4 + lymphocytes categories: Used to guide clinical and therapeutic actions in the management of HIV-infected adolescents and adults

Category 1: Greater or equal to 500 cells/mL	Equal stage, opportunistic infections rare.
Category 2: Between 200–499 cell/mL	Intermediate stage, early signs of HIV infection
Category 3: Less than 200 cells/mL	Advanced stage, opportunistic infections occur in this range.

respiratory fungi), herpes simplex virus, cytomegalovirus (which can cause blindness), or tuberculosis bacteria. White patches may appear in the mouth, caused by *Candida* (thrush) or Epstein-Barr virus (leukoplakia). A form of cancer called Kaposi sarcoma, common in AIDS patients, originates in the endothelial cells of the blood vessels and causes bruise like purple lesions visible in the skin.

Like other viruses, HIV can only be replicated by a living host cell. It invades helper T (CD4) cells, dendritic cells, and macrophages. HIV adheres to a target cell by means of one of its envelope glycoproteins and "tricks" the target cell. By destroying TH

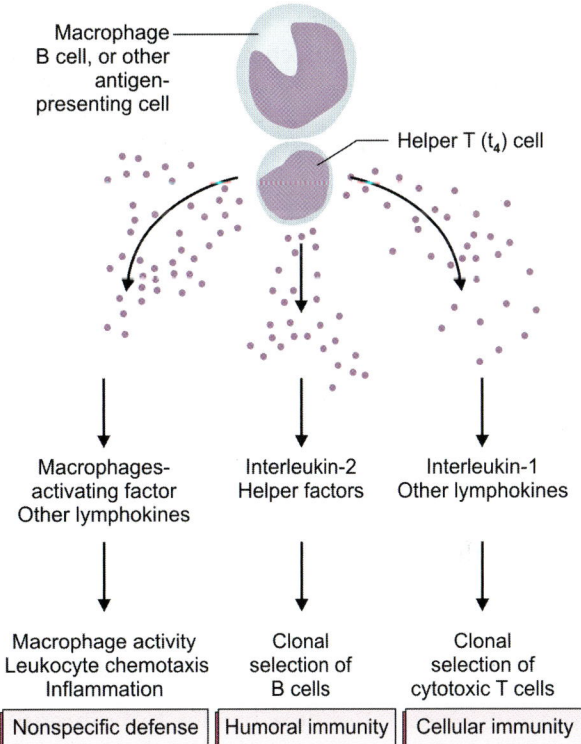

Fig. 10.69: The role of helper T cells in defense and immunity *(Saladin, 2003)*

cells, HIV strikes nonspecific defense, humoral immunity, and cellular immunity.

The incubation period—from the time of infection to the time of the first symptoms—can range from a few months to 12 years. Flu-like episodes of chills and fever occur as HIV attacks TH cells. At first, antibodies against HIV are produced and the TH count returns nearly to normal. As the virus destroys more and more cells, however, the signs and symptoms become more pronounced: night sweats, fatigue, headache, extreme weight loss, and lymphadenitis.

On introduction of HIV an indefinite percentage of those infected will have an acute self-limited viral syndrome. This is followed by an asymptomatic stage, which averages 8–10 years. The length of asymptomatic period is variable and may be affected by the nature of the virus, the host immune reaction or external factors that may delay or accelerate the process. Almost inevitably, the final symptomatic stage develops.

Patients with full-blown AIDS show no response to standard skin tests for delayed hypersensitivity. Slurred speech, loss of motor and cognitive functions, and dementia may occur as HIV invades the brain by way of infected macrophages and induces them to release toxins that destroy neurons and astrocytes. Death from cancer or infection is inevitable, usually within a few months but sometimes as long as 8 years after diagnosis. Some people, however, have been diagnosed as HIV-positive and yet have survived for 10 years or longer without developing AIDS.

In general, the universal precautions used for bacterial, mycotic, and other viral processes will protect the dentist, office staff, and other patients from the spread of the virus that causes AIDS. It is also important that patients with depressed immune function be afforded extra care to prevent the spread of infection to them. Thus all patients infected with HIV who have CD4+ T lymphocyte counts of less than 200/uL or category B or C HIV infection should be treated by doctors and staff free of clinically evident infectious diseases. These patients should not be put in a circumstance in which they are forced to be closely exposed to patients with clinically apparent symptoms of a communicable disease.

About 1% of HIV's genes mutate every year. This rapid rate of mutation is a barrier to both natural immunity and development of a vaccine. Even when immune cells do become sensitized to HIV, the virus soon mutates and produces new surface antigens that escape recognition. The high mutation rate also would quickly make today's vaccine ineffective against tomorrow's strain of the virus. Another obstacle to treatment and prevention is the lack of animal models for vaccine and drug research and development. Most animals are not susceptible to HIV. The chimpanzee is an exception, but chimpanzees are difficult to maintain, and there are economic barriers and ethical controversies surrounding their use.

The AIDS epidemic has triggered an effort of unprecedented intensity to find a vaccine or cure. HIV is a difficult pathogen to attack. Since it "hides" within host cells, it usually escapes recognition by the immune system. In the brain, it is protected by the blood-brain barrier.

MODE OF TRANSMISSION

The mode of transmission for those visiting from other planet, is:

1. Traumatic.
2. Vaginal sex (semen, vaginal secretions).
3. As a recipient of contaminated blood or blood products.
4. Mother to fetus transmission (milk).
5. IV drug abusers.

In infected individuals, the virus can be found in most bodily fluids. HIV can be recovered from serum, blood, saliva, semen, tears, urine, breast milk, ear secretions, and vaginal secretions. The most frequent routes of transmission are sexual contact (vaginal, anal, or oral), parenteral exposure to blood, or transmission from mother to fetus during the perinatal period. Infection also has been documented to be caused by artificial insemination, breastfeeding from infected mothers, and organ transplantation.

Homosexuals: Because of its relative inability to survive outside the host organism, HIV (the cause of acquired immunodeficiency syndrome [AIDS]), acts in a fashion similar to other sexually transmitted infectious disease agents. That is, transfer of the virions from one individual to another requires direct contact between virusladen blood or secretions from the infected host organism and a mucosal surface or epithelial wound of the potential host. Evidence has shown that the HIV loses its infectivity once desiccated.

Worldwide, about 75% of HIV infections are acquired through heterosexual, predominantly vaginal intercourse. In the United States, most cases occur in men who have sex with other men, but adolescents are the fastest rising group of AIDS patients because of the increasing exchange of unprotected sexual intercourse.

Homosexual men with a history of syphilis or genital herpetic infection have a threefold to eightfold increased risk of being HIV-positive. This statistic may suggest that genital ulceration may act as a portal of entry for the HIV.

Recipient of contaminated blood or blood products: Recipients of blood products are included in the high-risk groups. Transfusion recipients who were at risk prior to screening of blood products now have a minimal risk. Many hemophiliacs became infected with HIV through blood transfusions before preventive measures were implemented in 1984, but all donated blood is now tested for HIV and the risk of infection is less than 1%. Now HIV cannot be contracted by donating blood.

Casual contact: AIDS is not known to be transmitted through casual contact— for example, to family members, friends, coworkers, classmates, or medical personnel in charge of AIDS patients. It is not transmitted by kissing. Despite some speculation and fear, it has not been found to be transmitted by mosquitoes or other blood-sucking arthropods.

Saliva: Researches have debated the infectiousness of oral fluids. HIV has been found to be present in oral fluids, but saliva appears to reduce the ability of HIV to infect its target cells, lymphocytes. Reports of transmission by oral fluids are rare, and it appears this is not a significant source for the transmission of aids. In spite of this, reports have documented the transmission of AIDS during breastfeeding from the oral fluids of postpartum infected infants to their previously non-infected mothers. In addition, rare examples have been documented reporting the transmission of HIV infection by contamination of the oral fluids during cunnilingus or repeated passionate kissing. However, some reports point out that oral fluids can be infectious and are not completely protective against oral introduction of HIV. Although saliva is known to contain a number of anti-HIV inhibitory factors, the presence of aphthae, erosions ulcerations, and hemorrhagic inflammatory pathosis (gingivitis, periodontitis) may predispose an individual to oral transmission. **In summary, the best precaution against infection is avoidance of all body fluids of infected patients.**

In addition, extremely few people carrying the HIV secretes the virus in their saliva, and those who do tend to secrete extremely small amounts.

No epidemiologic evidence supports the possibility of HIV infection by saliva alone. Even the blood of patients who are HIV-positive has low concentrations of infectious particles (106 particles/mL as compared with 1013 particles/mL in hepatitis patients). This probably explains why professionals who are not in any of the known high-risk groups for HIV positivity have an extremely low probability of contracting it, even when exposed to the blood and secretions of large numbers of patients who are HIV-positive during the performance of surgery or if accidentally autoinoculated with contaminated blood or secretions. Nevertheless, until the transmission of HIV becomes fully understood, prudent surgeons will take steps to prevent the spread of infection from the HIV-carrying patient to themselves and their assistants through the use of universal precautions, including barrier techniques. Since the initial years of the epidemic, blood screening methods have improved dramatically and reduced the risk for HIV infection to as low as one in two million blood donations.

Infected mothers: HIV is transmitted through blood, semen, vaginal secretions, and breast milk. It can be transmitted from mother to fetus through the placenta or from mother to infant during childbirth or nursing. HIV occurs in saliva and tears, but is not believed to be transmitted by those fluids.

Infected mothers create a huge increase in HIV positive children. Antenatal testing for HIV is crucial as is avoiding breastfeeding. Zidovudine (AZT) therapy and delivery by caesarean section dramatically decrease vertical transmission.

The risk of transmission from infected mothers to newborns has been reduced from 25–30% to 2% (95% reduction) because of widespread prenatal HIV testing, prophylactic use of antivirals, elective cesarean section performed before onset of labour and avoidness of breastfeeding.

Signs and Symptoms

Primary HIV infection may be entirely asymptomatic, but more than half of infected patients present with fever, malaise, myalgias, diarrhea, pharyngitis, macular erythematous rash, lymphadenopathy, splenomegaly, and/or weight loss. The acute illness occurs three to six weeks after primary exposure and may last up to two weeks; milder symptoms may persist for months. Clinical manifestations commonly involve the head and neck. Mucosal ulcerations can accompany acute HIV seroconversion; they are probably the direct result of HIV infection (chancre of HIV). These lesions are multiple, painful, small (0.3–1.5 cm) discreet ulcers, which have been reported on the palate, esophagus, anus, and penis and relate to sexual activity (Rabeneck L, 1990).

Opportunistic infections are rare for early stage patients with CD4 counts greater than 500 cells/mm^3 (Table 10.9). Intermediate stage patients with CD4 counts between 500 and 200 cells/mm^3 may manifest some early signs of HIV infection. AIDS (advanced stage infection) is diagnosed with counts less than 200 cells/ mm^3. Opportunistic infections occur in this CD4 count range, especially with counts below 50 cells/ mm^3. OC, oral hairy leukoplakia (OHL), KS, non-Hodgkin's lymphoma (NHL), and necrotizing ulcerative gingivitis/periodontitis are strongly associated with HIV; these conditions may be present in up to 50% of seropositive patients and up to 80% of AIDS patients. Painful HSV lesions may be present, and reactivation of herpes zoster may be seen.

Oral Manifestations of HIV Infection and AIDS

Oral lesions occur commonly in HIV-seropositive patients. The underlying severe immunodeficiency leads to a number of oral manifestations which, although not pathognomonic, should raise the possibility of HIV infection, i.e. in general, they are not specific to HIV infection and simply reflect the immunocompromised state. Thus many of the oral lesions occur in patients who are immunocompromised for others reasons. The current classification of these lesions is based on the strength of association with HIV infection (Box 10.6). Three groups are recognized:

1. Group *I* lesions strongly associated with HIV infection.
2. Group *II* lesions less commonly associated with HIV,
3. Group *III* lesions seen in HIV infections.

Group I Strongly Associated with HIV

- *Candidiasis:* Seen in 60% of HIV patients as early manifestation. Erythematous (early), hyperplastic, pseudomembranous (late), and angular cheilitis in young people (most common feature of HIV).

Box 10.6: Lesions associated with HIV infection

Group I: Lesions strongly associated with HIV infections
1. Candidiasis:
   a. Erythematous
   b. Psuedomembranous
   c. Angular cheilitis
   d. Median rhomboid glossitis.
2. Hairy leukoplakia
3. Kaposi's sarcoma
4. Non-Hodgkin's lymphoma
5. Periodontal diseases:
   a. Linear gingival erythema.
   b. Acute necrotizing ulcerative gingivitis.
   c. Acute necrotizing ulcerative periodontitis.

Group II: Lesions less commonly associated with HIV infection
1. Atypical ulceration
2. HIV-associated salivary gland disease (HIV-SGD):
   a. Xerostomia and/or
   b. Swelling of the major salivary glands.
3. Necrotizing ulcerative stomatitis
4. Thrombocytopenic purpura
5. Viral infections:
   a. Cytomegalovirus
   b. Herpes simplex virus
   c. Human papillomavirus
   d. Varicella zoster

Group III: Lesions seen in HIV infection
1. Bacterial infections
2. Drug reactions
3. Gungal infections
4. Neurological disturbances:
   a. Facial nerve palsy.
   b. Trigeminal neuropathy.

- *Hairy leukoplakia:* Bilateral, white, non-removable corrugated lesions of the tongue, unaffected by antifungals but usually resolves with acyclovir or valacyclovir. It is a predictor of bad prognosis and possible development of lymphoma.
- *HIV gingivitis:* Unusually severe gingivitis for the general state of the mouth. Often characterized by linear gingival erythema, intense red band along gingival margin.
- *Acute ulcerative gingivitis:* Occurs in young, otherwise healthy mouths.
- *HIV periodontitis:* With severe localized destruction of the periodontal membrane.

- *Kaposi's sarcoma:* Commonest malignancy among HIV patients. Radiotherapy is effective. One or more erythematous/purplish macules or swelling, frequently on the palate. 50% occur intra- or periorally.
- *Non-Hodgkin's lymphoma:* Similar to the above.

Group II Less Strongly associated with HIV

- Atypical oropharyngeal ulceration.
- Idiopathic thrombocytopenic purpura.
- HIV associated salivary glands disease HIV children greater than adult. Similar to Sjogren syndrome.
- Wide range of common viral infections.

Group III Possible association with HIV

- Wide range of rare bacterial and fungal infections.
- Cat scratch disease.
- Drug reactions.
- Neurological abnormalities (facial nerve palsy, trigeminal neuropathy).
- Osteomyelitis/sinusitis/submandibular cellulitis.
- Squamous carcinoma.
- Clearly, the conditions in group III are likely to be seen in patients who are HIV –ve at least as often as in patients who are HIV +ve.
- Persistent generalized lymphadenopathy, otherwise inexplicable lymphadenopathy greater than 1 cm persisting for 3 months, at two or more extrainguinal sites. Cervical nodes particularly commonly affected may be prodromal or a manifestation of AIDS.

Erythematous and Pseudomembranous Candidiasis

Most common oral fungal infections seen in association with HIV infection. Various studies report the frequency of oral candidiasis ranging from 7 to 90%. Erythematous candidiasis generally occurs early in the disease process, whereas pseudomembranous candidiasis is a later manifestation, occurring when the patient is severely immunosuppressed. Both forms are highly predictive of the development of AIDS (Figs 10.70 to 10.73).

Hairy Leukoplakia

Usually asymptomatic. Characterized by bilateral vertically corrugated white patches on the lateral margins of the tongue. May affect the ventral surface, where it assumes a more homogenous appearance. Rarely may involve other parts of the oral mucosa (buccal mucosa and palate) although when it affects these unusual sites it also always present on the lateral margin

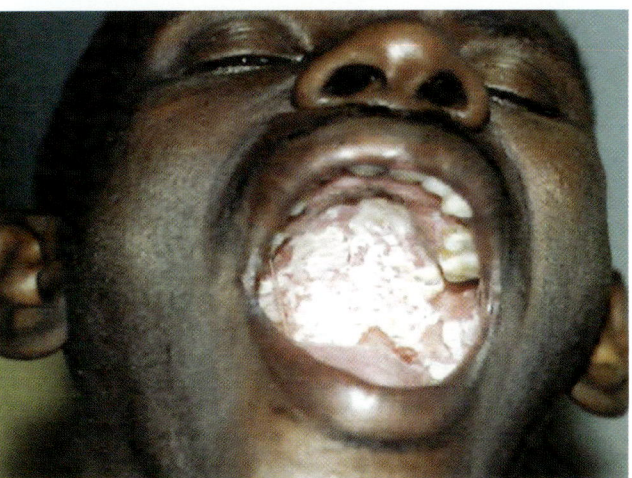

Fig. 10.70: Oral candidiasis: Removable whitish plaques on the palate are seen in this HIV patient with pseudo membranous candidiasis *(Neville et al, 2002)*

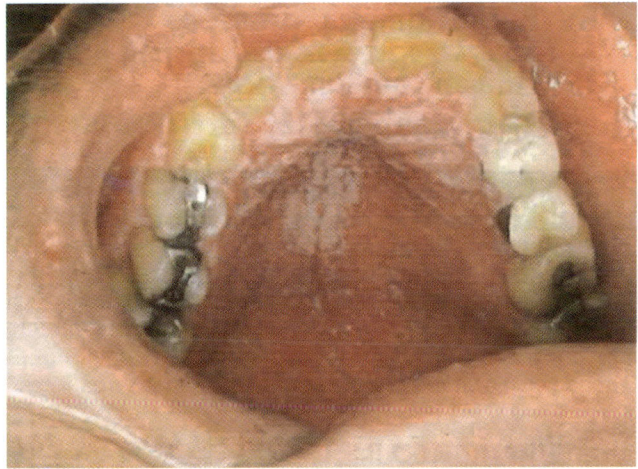

Fig. 10.71: Chronic oral florid candidiasis in patient with AIDS related complex *(from Silverman, S, jr; JADA, 1986)*

of the tongue. Originally considered to be pathognomonic of HIV infection. Although as the lesion has been described in other immunosuppressed patient groups (e.g. organ transplant recepient's, patients receiving chemotherapy for acute leukemia) it is now simply regarded as a marker of underlying immunodeficiency (Figs 10.74 to 10.76).

Histopathology: OHL is composed of hyperplastic, hyperparakeratotic squamous epithelium with "hair-like" keratin projections forming an irregular ridged surface.

Kaposi's Sarcoma

Before the advent of AIDS and HIV infection, Kaposi's sarcoma (KS) was seen mainly among elderly Jewish

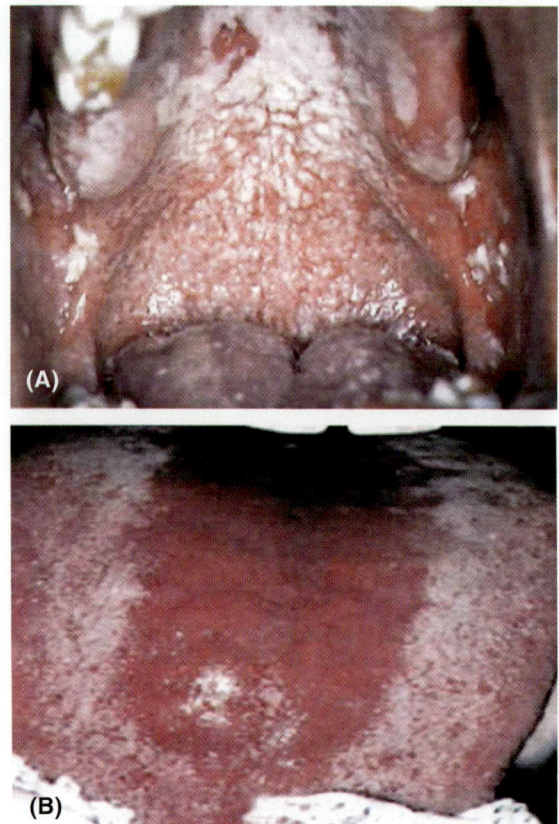

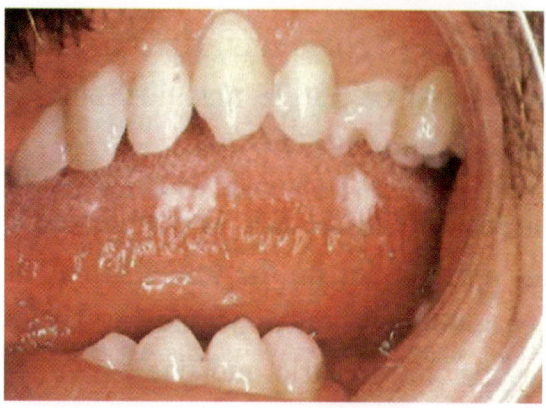

Fig. 10.74: Limited hairy leukoplakia in AIDS patient

Fig. 10.72: Candidiasis. **(A)** Diffuse white alteration of the palate bilateral buccal mucosa, and dorsal tongue. The surface material can be rubbed off, and smear revealed numerous fungal organisms. **(B)** Large central zone of erythema and papillary atrophy of the dorsal surface of the tongue. Cytopathologic smear revealed numerous fungal organisms

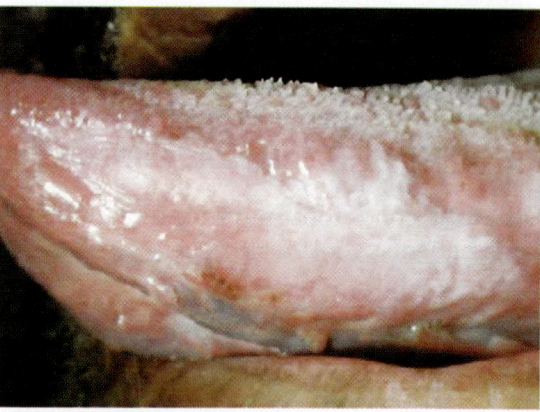

Fig. 10.75: Hairy leukoplakia corrugated appearance of lesions on lateral tongue border. *(Source: courtesy of Dr. Marie Ramer DDS, Mount Sinai, New York, USA)*

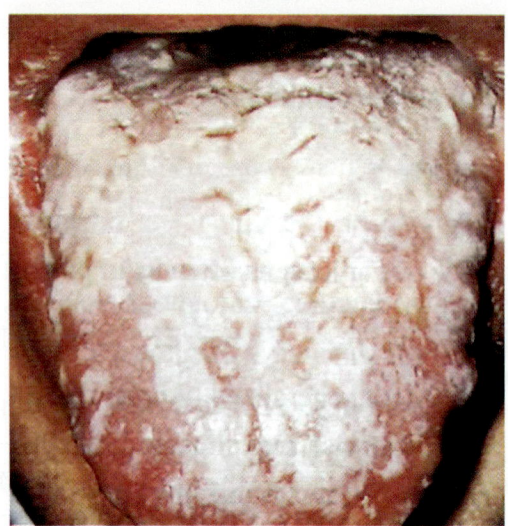

Fig. 10.73: Extensive oral infection with *Candida albicans* in a patient with HIV infection. Note the great changes in the tongue and the angular cheilitis

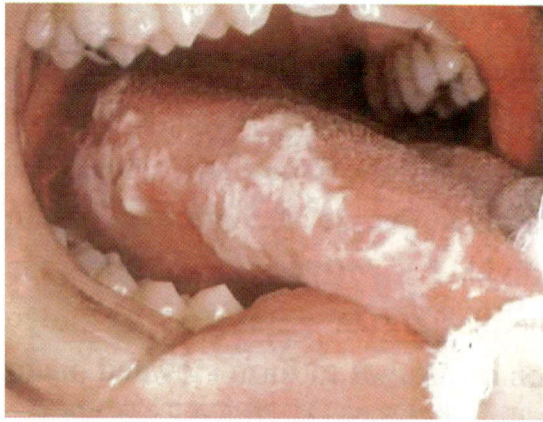

Fig. 10.76: Extensive hairy leukoplakia in AIDS patient. Hairy Leukoplakia usually indicates infectivity by the AIDS related virus and risk of immunosuppression *(from Silverman, S, jr; JADA, 1986)*

males of eastern European or Mediterranean descent, and an endemic form was recognized in southern Africa. AIDS associated KS is seen almost exclusively in male homosexuals and is rare among other risk categories for HIV infection.

KS is a multicentric, angioproliferative disorder characterized by proliferating spindle cells, inflammation, and neoangiogenesis (Feller L et al, 2007). Presents as red or purple maculopapular lesions (Figs 10.77 to 10.79).

Clinically, classic KS is manifested as soft red nodules on the lower limbs, and less commonly, on upper limbs. Lesions may be multicentric and coalescent, but rarely exceed 2 cm in size. Classic KS may uncommonly affect the head and neck; 8% involve facial skin or eyelids, nose, and ears and only 2% affect the mucosa (conjunctiva, palate, tongue, gingiva and tonsil) (Gnepp DR et al, 1984;. Bottler et al, 2007; Venizelos et al, 2008).By contrast, HIV-KS commonly affects cutaneous head and neck sites (32%) and oral and perioral tissues including mucosal surfaces [palate, gingiva, buccal mucosa, dorsal tongue, larynx, trachea, paranasal sinuses (19%)] (Feller L et al, 2007; Gnepp DR et al, 1984, 1997; Parikh and Freeman, 1992). Actually Kaposi's sarcoma may involve skin anywhere in the body (Fig. 10.80), caused by infection with human herpes virus (HHV).

KS evolves through three stages: patch, plaque, and nodular. The patch stage, which is the earliest stage, is characterized by single or multiple, flat, bruise-like, blue, purple, red macules. Multiple individual lesions may become confluent. The plaque stage represents the progression of patches to form elevated plaques. The nodular stage is characterized by raised, spongy

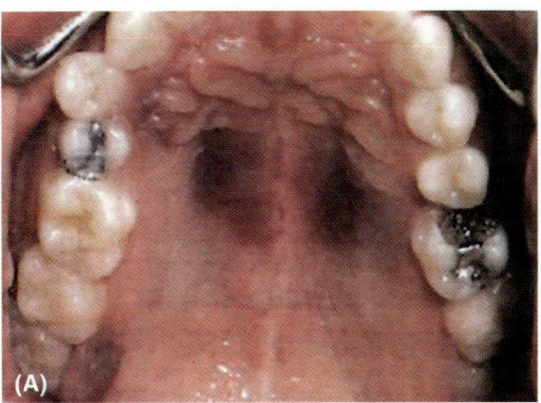

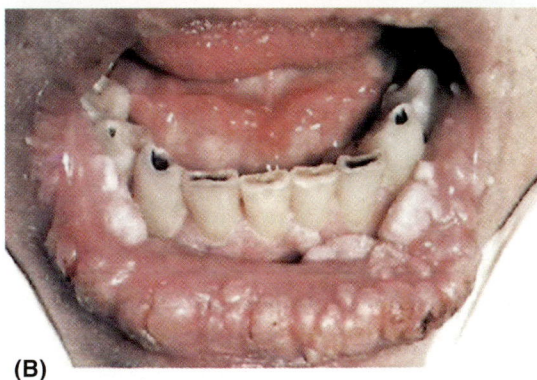

(B)

Fig. 10.78: Kaposi's sarcoma. **(A)** Bilateral areas of brownish discoloration of the midline of the hard palate. Also note the brown exophytic mass palatal to the maxillary third molar. **(B)** Hemorrhagic and exophytic mass of the anterior maxillary gingiva *(AbouTable, 2006)*

lesions and exophytic masses, which can become fixed as they invade underlying tissue. Refer to Chapter 15, "K" Kaposi's Sarcoma, page 449.

Treatment choices are based on symptoms, location and extent of the lesion, and the general medical condition of the patient. KS is usually very responsive

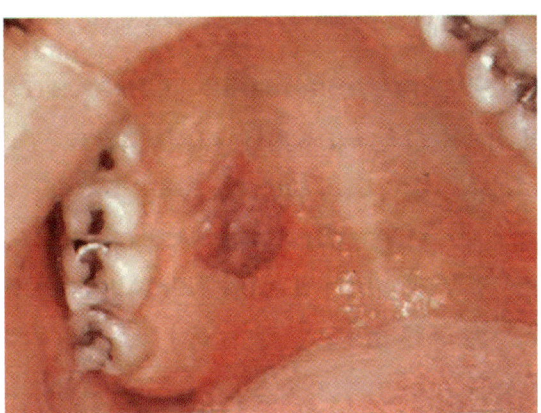

Fig. 10.77: Exophytic growth on palate shown to be Kaposi's sarcoma *(from Silverman S. jr; JADA, 1986)*

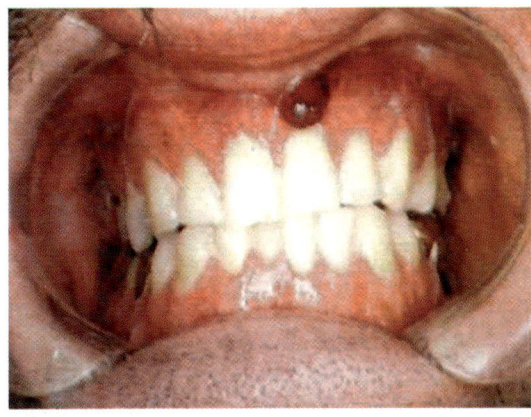

Fig. 10.79: Asymptomatic gingival lesion the first manifestation of Kaposi's sarcoma and AIDS

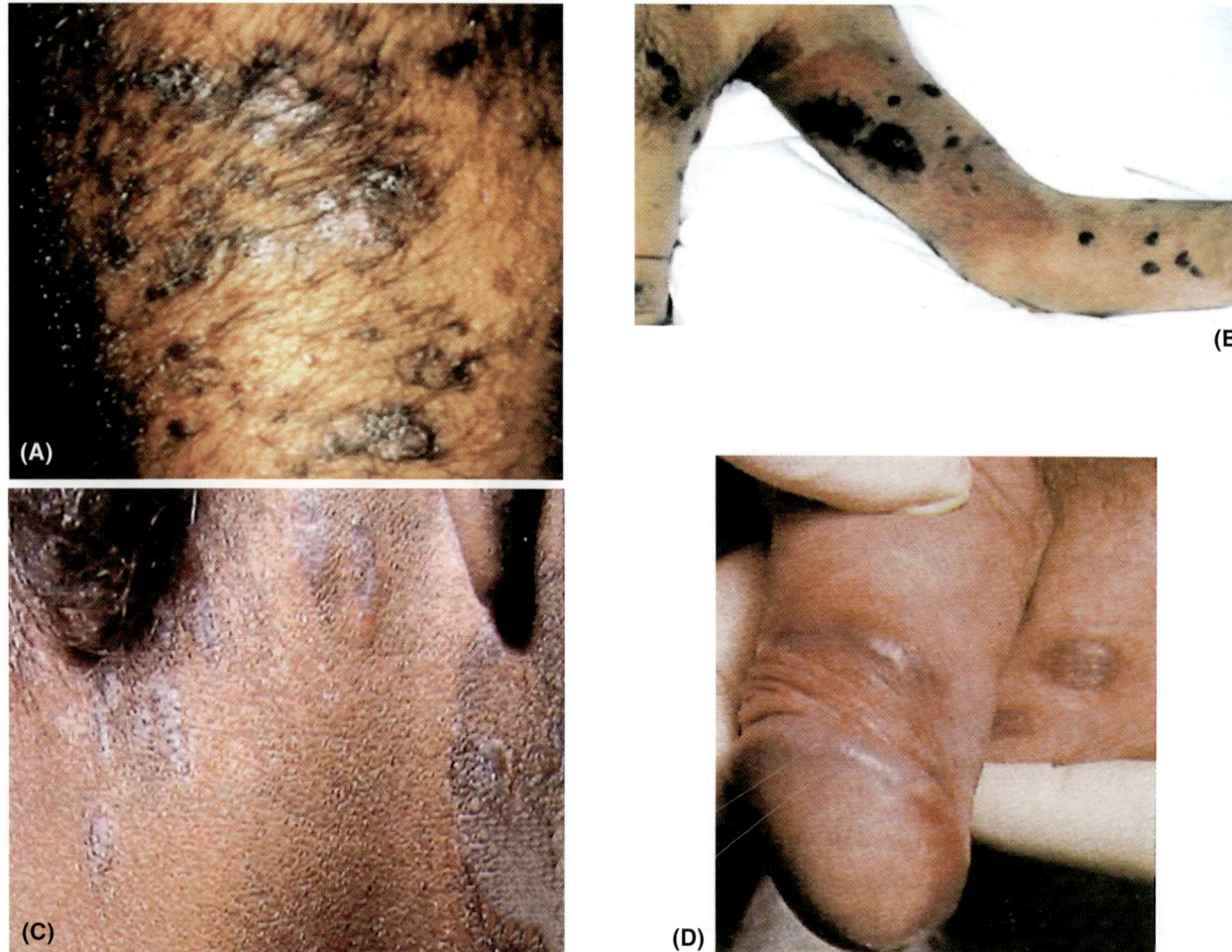

Fig. 10.80: Kaposi's sarcoma is a common complication of HIV infection. Kaposi's sarcoma usually appears as black lesions on the arm, chest and leg of darker-skinned individuals **(A, B, C)**. Kaposi's sarcoma developed in patients with AIDS may occur anywhere on the body surface including the penis and scrotum **(D)** *(Forbes and Jackson, 2003)*

to radiotherapy. Superficial skin KS can be treated with local laser resection or cryosurgery. Small intraoral KS interfering with function may be resected or debulked. Alternatively, chemotherapy (systemic and interalesional) or intralesional injection of vinblastine and 3% sodium tetradecyl sulfate is another option; one double-blind randomized control study demonstrated some efficacy with this approach (Baccaglini et al, 2007).

Linear Gingival Erythema

Characterized by an intense linear band of erythema along the gingival margin, which may also extend on to the attached gingivae. Severity of inflammation is out of proportion to the state of oral hygiene. Spontaneous gingival bleeding may also be a feature (Fig. 10.81).

Non-Hodgkin's Lymphoma

Uncommon but well-recognized complication of HIV infection. Typically presents as rapidly enlarging, firm, rubbery swelling. Common intraoral sites include fauces, palate and gingivae. Lesions can ulcerate and may be associated with destruction of tooth support. Treatment is generally with radiotherapy and/or chemotherapy.

Acute Necrotizing Ulcerative Gingivitis

Characterized by gingival pain, bleeding on probing or spontaneous bleeding and interdental ulceration with crater-like defects (Fig. 10.82).

Acute Necrotizing Periodontitis

Rapid localized or generalized periodontal destruction with severe pain, bone loss, tooth mobility and periodontal pocketing (Fig. 10.83).

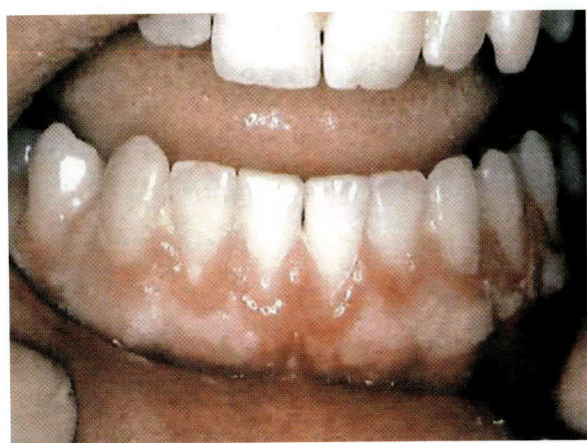

Fig. 10.81: Linear gingival erythema. Distinct linear band of erythema involving the free gingival margin *(AbouTable, 2006)*

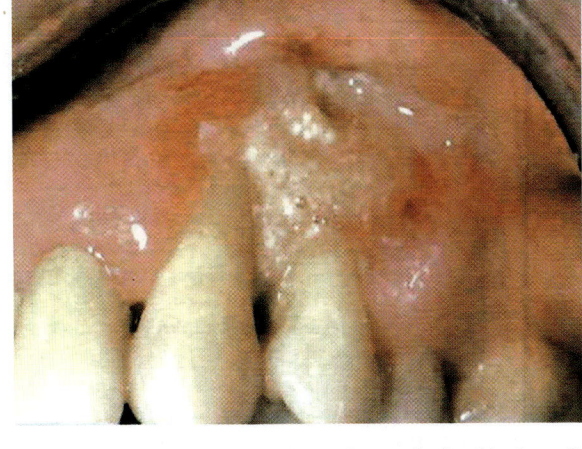

Fig. 10.83: Acute necrotizing ulcerative periodontitis. Localized loss of periodontal attachment with overlying necrosis of the gingival soft tissues *(AbouTable 2006)*

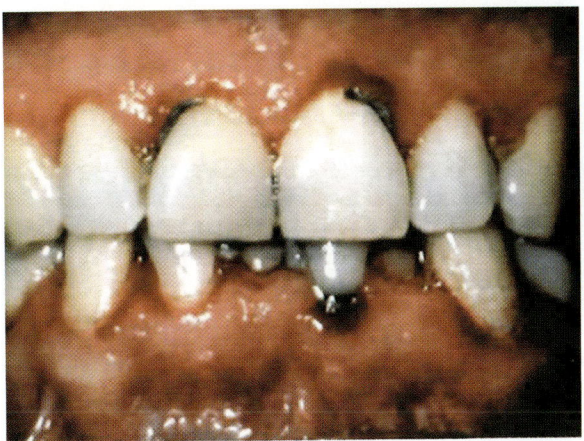

Fig. 10.82: Acute necrotizing ulcerative gingivitis (ANUG) (Vincent angina or trench mouth) caused by spirochetal and fusiform bacteria in an HIV patient. Note the punched-out ulceration of the interdental papillae, which are pathognomonic. (Courtesy of the Department of Dermatology. National Naval Medical Center, Bethesda, MD), *McGraw-Hill Co*

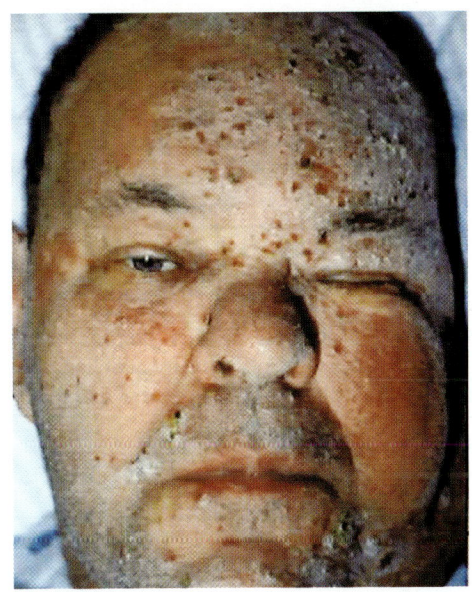

Fig. 10.84: Disseminated herpes zoster infection. Vesicles are seen over the entire face, representing disseminated HZV infection (multiple dermatomal distributions). *(Courtesy of Department of Dermatology, National Naval Medical Center, Bethesda, MD)*

Other Lesions

Other lesions are:
1. Herpes zoster (Fig. 10.84)
2. Herpes simplex (Figs 10.85A and 10.86)
3. Sessile nodules (condylomata) may develop intraorally (Figs 10.85 B and C and 10.87)
4. Molluscum contagiosum (Figs 10.88 and 10.89).

Molluscum Contagiosum

This is a contagious skin papular lesion caused by a large double-stranded DNA poxvirus, 300 nm in diameter. This virus is tropic for skin and rarely for mucosa. Molluscum contagiosum (MC) is transmitted by direct contact and by fomites. It has a worldwide distribution and is seen in conditions of crowding and poor hygiene; it may also be sexually transmitted.

Clinical course: MCs are small, discrete, flesh-colored, pearly papules, 2 to 6 mm, with characteristic small central umbilicated depressions or crusting (Figs 10.88 and 10.89). Cheesy keratinous infectious material can be expressed from the central depression. Sexually transmitted lesions are often located in the genitalia,

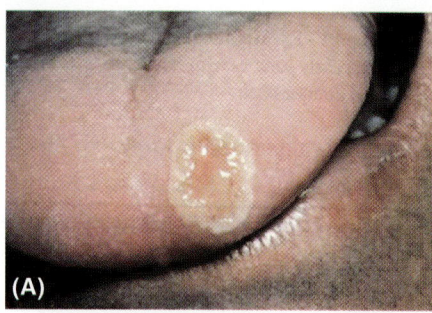 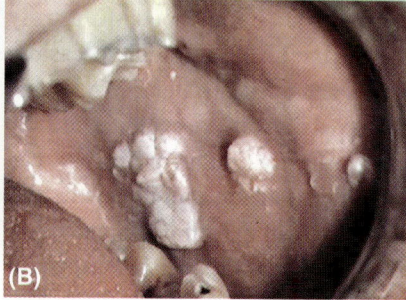 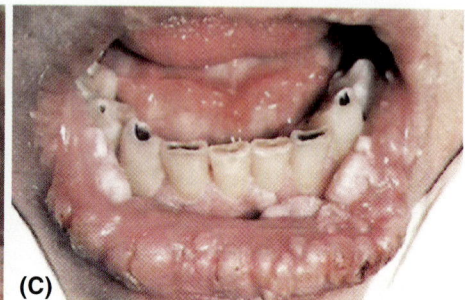

Fig. 10. 85: (A) Chronic herpes simplex infection. Mucosal erosion exhibiting cincinate dorsal surface of the tongue on the left side. Human papillomavirus infection. **(B)** Multiple sessile nodules of the left posterior buccal mucosa. **(C)** Multiple nodules of the labial mucosa and vermillion border of the lower lip *(Neville et al, 2009)*

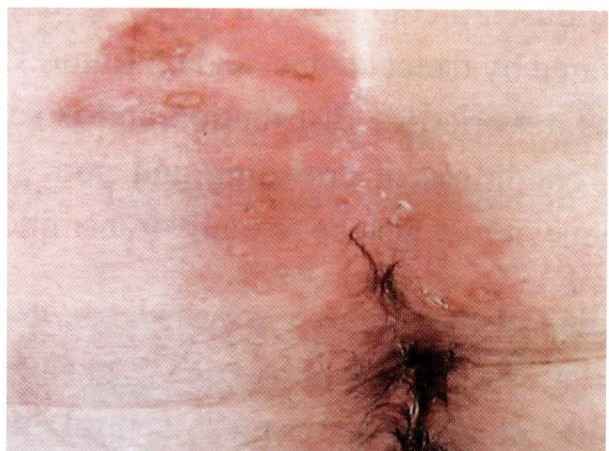

Fig. 10.86: Severe perianal herpes simplex is a common problem in homosexual patients with HIV infection. It may cause great discomfort but often responds to antiviral treatment

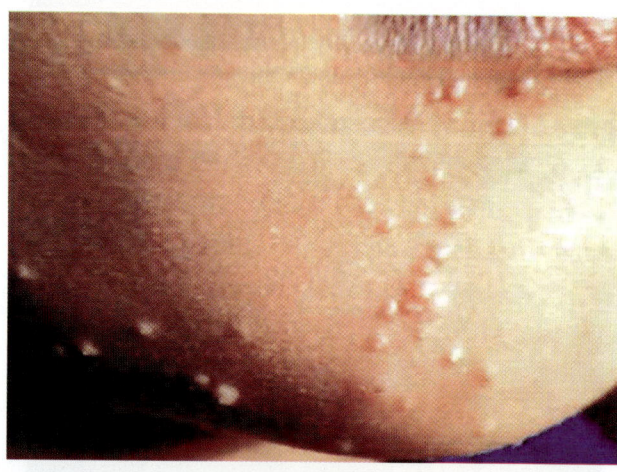

Fig. 10.88: Molluscum contagiosum. Cluster of small, pearly papules with characteristic umbilicated central compression

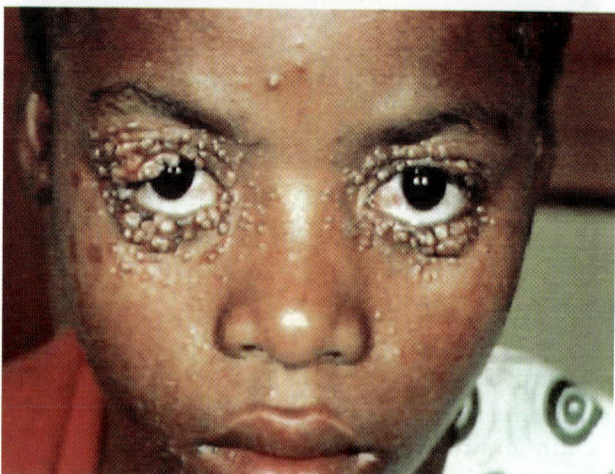

Fig. 10.89: Molluscum contagiosum. Patients with HIV/AIDS can have extensive multiple lesions

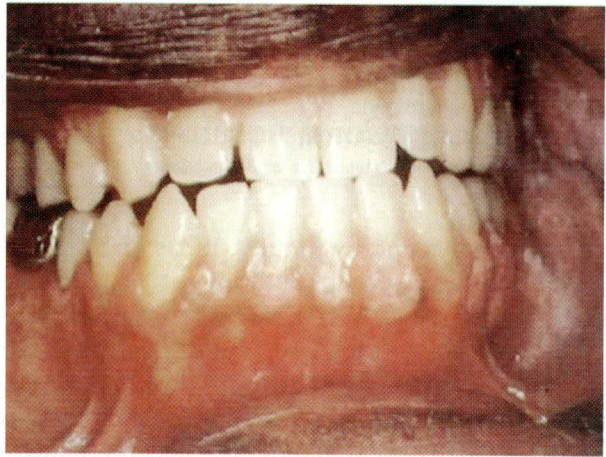

Fig. 10.87: Condylomata develops on gingiva of sexually active homosexual male who also had genital and skin warts

lower abdomen, and inner thighs. In children, MC is usually transmitted by direct contact or fomites (clothing, toys) (Nelson and Thompson Molluscum contagiosum, 2003). Childhood MC usually occurs on the limbs, neck, and occasionally face and eyelids (Dohil MA, Lin P, Lee J et al, 2006). Lesions are usually asymptomatic and nonpruritic but can become symptomatic after rupture or secondary bacterial infection. Immunosuppressed hosts (AIDS patients, renal transplant recipients, patients on steroids, etc.) may develop multiple lesions, which can become large and confluent (Mansur et al, 2004). MC in AIDS patients tends to occur on the facial skin and eyelids. Low CD4 cell counts have been associated with widespread facial MC, which serves as a marker for severe AIDS. Rarely, MC in immunosuppressed hosts can affect mucosal surfaces (Fornatora et al, 2001).

HIV Salivary Gland Disease

More common in HIV-infected children than adults. Characterized by xerostomia and/or swelling of major salivary glands. Clinical parallels with Sjögren's syndrome although characteristic autoantibody profile is lacking. Histological features—similar to Sjögren's syndrome.

MEDICAL TREATMENT

Highly active antiviral therapy signifies the use of combinations of antiviral drugs. The advent of HAART has dramatically shifted the infectious manifestations for HIV-seropositive patients.

Highly Active Antiretroviral Therapy (HAART)

HAART has been able to suppress the virus such that HIV is now considered a chronic disease. Once started, HAART has to continue for life, so the question is when to start the treatment. The benefits of HAART are that the levels of circulating vibrions may be lowered to undetectable levels and the variable levels of immune recovery may be evident. The result can be a striking fall in the incidence of opportunistic infections and regression of Kaposi's sarcoma, and retinitis.

The physician and the patient have to weight the short- and long-term risks or toxicity associated with HAART. The biggest benefit has been a 50% reduction in mortality. The drawbacks have been lipodystrophy and metabolic abnormalities increasing the risks for cardiovascular diseases.

Not all HIV-associated conditions are reduced with HAART. Suppression of HIV does not mean that there will be associated decline in the replication of hepatitis C virus. In fact, it may worsen hepatitis C coinfection.

HAART-Associated Lipodystrophy Syndrome and Metabolic Abnormalities

The resultant lipodystrophy syndrome is associated with abnormal fat accumulation causing central, intra-abdominal obesity and fat buildup around the back of the neck known as a "buffalo hump". Subcutaneous fat atrophy between the skin and the muscles mostly affect the face, arms and legs also occurs.

Organ Assessment Tests with Medication Intake

The following tests are required when the patient is on HIV/AIDS medications to detect adverse side effects with the medications:

1. *The CBC:* The CBC must be repeated every 3–6 months or sooner, if indicated.
2. *Liver function tests (LFTs):* LFTs are done to monitor the liver enzymes that may be affected.
3. *Renal function tests:* Urine analysis and serum creatinine are monitored while the patient is on the HIV/AIDS medications.
4. *Fasting blood sugar (FBS):* The FBS is monitored for patients on highly active antiretroviral therapy (HAART), because HAART can rise the blood sugar levels. The FBS must be repeated at 3–4 months.
5. *Lipid profile:* Lipid profile is monitored for patients on HAART because the lipid levels can be affected. The lipid profile must be repeated at 3–4 months.

An increased common disease caused by the HIV (HIV-1, HIV-2). T lymphocyte defect ensues with failure of (mostly) cell-mediated immunity. Although HIV exposure produces antibody response, the virus remains infective in the presence of antibody; it must be regarded as a marker of infectivity. Absence of HIV antibody does not, however, guarantee that person is not infected with HIV. HIV antibody positive patients are at risk of developing AIDS, usually after a prolonged latent period during which the T lymphocyte cells decrease in number.

HIV survives poorly outside the human body. It is destroyed by laundering, dish-washing, exposure to heat (50°C [135°F] for at least 10 minutes), chlorination of swimming pools and hot tubs, and disinfectants such as bleach, Lysol, hydrogen peroxide, rubbing alcohol, and germicidal skin cleansers (betadine and hibiclens, for example). A properly used, undamaged latex condom is an effective barrier to HIV, especially if augmented with the spermicide. Animal membrane condoms are not effective at blocking HIV transmission because the viruses are smaller than the gaps in the membrane.

About 1% of HIV's genes mutate every year. This rapid rate of mutation is a barrier to both natural immunity and development of a vaccine. Even when immune cells do become sensitized to HIV, the virus soon mutates and produces new surface antigens that escape recognition. The high mutation rate also would quickly make today's vaccine ineffective against tomorrow's strain of the virus. Another obstacle to treatment and prevention is the lack of animal models for vaccine and drug research and development. Most animals are not susceptible to HIV. The chimpanzee is an exception, but chimpanzees are difficult to maintain, and there are economic barriers and ethical controversies surrounding their use.

Until recently, the only anti-HIV drug approved by the Food and Drug Administration (FDA) was azidothymidine (AZT, or retrovir), which inhibits reverse transcriptase and prolongs the lives of some HIV-positive individuals. AZT is now recommended for any patient with a CD4 count below 500 cells/μL, but it has undesirable side effects including bone marrow toxicity and anemia. The FDA has approved other drugs, including dideoxyinosine (ddI) and dideoxycytidine (ddC) for patients who do not respond to AZT, but these drugs can also have severe side effects. Another class of drugs—protease inhibitors—inhibit enzymes (proteases) that HIV needs in order to replicate.

Dental Treatment for Patients with AIDS

Always obtain the following laboratory tests from the patient's physician using a signed consent from:

1. The CBC with platelet count: Megaloblastic anemia, neutropenia, and peripheral neuropathy (due to folic acid deficiency) are frequent side effects of anti-HIV medications. The use of opioids and block anesthesia is contraindicated when the hemoglobin is < 10 g/dL.
2. The CD4 count.
3. The viral load.
4. The PT/INR because the liver is frequently affected.
5. The liver function tests (LFTs).
6. Serum creatinine.
7. The fasting blood sugar (FBS), PPBS and HbA_1C.

The following are dental guidelines:

1. The patient is instructed to use mouth rinse prior to every appointment. Mouth rinse protocol should be prescribed daily as a home care.
2. Aggressive treatment of infections and antimicrobial prophylaxis are needed (Table 10.10)
3. Prior to treatment assess the current CD4 count and the WBC count. If the CD4 count is < 200 cells/μL and the WNC count is normal (3.5–11 K/mm^3), proceed with the dental management as in a normal patient.
4. In patients with a decreased WBC count (<3,500 cells/mm^3), calculate the absolute neutrophil count (ANC). ANC = total WBC × (neutronhils% + bands %). The average ANC is 1,500–7,200 μL.
5. As these patients are immunocompromised, any approach with a known risk of infective complications, e.g. extractions, should be covered with antiseptic, and any surgery should be as atraumatic as possible.
6. There may also be a slight tendency to bleeding in these patients, and local hemostatic measures may be needed.

Medications Contraindicated with HIV/AIDS

The following drugs are contraindicated:

1. Demerol, clarithromycin, tetracycliazole, ketoconazolene, doxycycline, metronidazole, diazepam, azole antifungals (clotrimazole, fluconazole, ketoconazole) should not be combined with protease inhibitors.
2. Antihistamines: Avoid asternizole, and terfenadine.

Table 10.10: Suggested anesthetic, analgesic, and antibiotic guidelines for patients on HIV/AIDS

Drug category	Drug	Comments
Anesthetics	2% Lidocaine (xylocaine)	Use maximum 2 carpules
	4% Prilocaine HCl (citanest)	Avoid with anemia
	0.5 Bupivacaine (marcaine)	Use maximum 2 carpules
	4% Septocaine (articaine)	Avoid with anemia
	2–3% Mepivacaine HCl (carbocaine)	Use maximum 2 carpules
Analgesics	Codeine + acetaminophen; tylenol	Use standard dose
	Meperidine (demerol)	Avoid
	Oxycodone + acetaminophen (percocet)	Use standard dose
Antibiotics	Penicillin	Use standard dose
	Amoxicillin (amoxil)	Use standard dose
	Amoxycillin + clavulanic acid	Use standard dose
	(augmentin)	Use standard dose
	Cephaloxin (keflex)	Use standard dose
	Cefadroxil (duricef)	Use standard dose
	Clarithromycin (biaxin)	Avoid
	Clindamycin	Use standard dose
	Tetracycline HCl	Avoid
	Doxycycline (vibramycin)	Avoid with protease inhibitors;
	Metronidazole (flagyl)	safe with other HIV drugs
Antivirals	Acyclovir (zovirax)	
	Valacyclovir (valtrex)	Use standard dose
Antifungals	Acyclovir (zovirax)	
	Valacyclovir (valtrex)	Use standard dose
	Mycostatin (nystatin)	
Benzodiazepines	Diazepam (valium)	Use lowest dose, if required
	Lorazepam (ativan)	after consultation

3. Psychotropics: Avoid midazolam, triazolam, alprazolam.
4. Antifungals: Avoid itraconazole, ketoconazole, voriconazole.
5. Anticonvulsants: Avoid phenobarbital.

INFECTION CONTROL

There have been no reports of immunodeficiency virus or HIV transmission from a patient to a health care worker or from a health care worker to a patient during dental invasive procedures. The recommendations for workers caring for AIDS patients are essentially the same as those for the prevention of spread of hepatitis B (Box 10.7).

In short, great care must be taken to prevent puncture wounds by objects potentially contaminated with infectious material. Gloves should be used when handling body fluids, and gowns should be employed when clothing could be soiled with contaminated material. Masks and protective eyewear should be worn when gross contamination may lead to aerosolization of blood.

Steam under pressure (autoclaving), dry heat (160°C for 2 hours), and boiling in water (100° C for 10 minutes) are effective measures for killing these viruses. AIDS (HIV) virus is easily inactivated by several common chemical germicides used in laboratory and health care facilities. Solutions of 25% ethanol, 1% alkaline glutaraldehyde, or 0.2% sodium hypochlorite (standard household bleach) for a minimum of 10 minutes may all be used for disinfection of medical instruments.

Sharp items must be considered potentially infective and should be handled and disposed of with extraordinary care to prevent accidental injuries. Blood and body fluids may be carefully poured down a drain that is connected to a sanitary sewer.

Box 10.7: Guidelines for prevention of transmission of AIDS in health care worker

Blood and body secretions are potentially infectious

1. Accidental wounds from instruments contaminated with blood, saliva, or exudates must be carefully avoided, as well as contact of open skin lesions with material from AIDS patient.
2. Gloves should be worn when handling blood or saliva, contaminated instruments, or specimens.
3. Gowns should be worn when the possibility of contaminating clothing with blood or secretions exists.
4. All blood specimens and biopsy specimens should be labeled "Blood precautions".
5. All blood spills should be promptly cleaned up with a disinfectant (1:10 dilution of 5.25% sodium hypochlorite with water).
6. Masks and protective eyewears should be worn, if aerosolization of blood and saliva is anticipated.
7. Needles should not be bent or resheathed after use, since this is a common cause of needlestick injuries. Instead, they should be placed in a puncture-resistant container.
8. Proper handwashing before and after treatment and cleaning of instruments are mandatory.
9. All health care workers who perform or assist in dental invasive procedures must be educated regarding epidemiology, modes of transmission, and prevention of AIDS infection and the need for routine use of appropriate barrier precautions during procedures and when handling instruments contaminated with blood after procedures.
10. Instruments contaminated with blood or body fluids should be decontaminated with a high-level chemical disinfectant.

C. HYPERSENSITIVITY (ALLERGY)

Introduction

The desirable effect of the immune system which eliminates the foreign antigen, is called immunity. The undesirable effect, which is the associated tissue damage, is called hypersensitivity.

Allergies may be treated with:
- Antihistamine drugs, to reduce the effect of histamine on the skin and blood vessels.
- Immunosuppressive drugs, such as cortisone or cyclosporine, to suppress the formation of antibodies, or
- Desensitization, a procedure in which first small doses and then progressively larger dose of allergens are injected into the body until the allergic response is minimized.

Hypersensitivity reactions or allergic diseases are immunologic reactions to a non-infectious foreign substance (antigen). They are unusual and perhaps damaging immune response to normally harmless substance.

Under some circumstances, repeated contact with or exposure to an antigen may cause an inappropriate response (hypersensitivity) that can be harmful or destructive to host tissues (Fig. 10.90). Foreign substances that trigger hypersensitivity reactions are called allergens or antigens. Hypersensitivity reactions can involve cellular or humoral components of the immune system. Two types of lymphocytes play central roles in the two branches of the specific immune system: B lymphocytes in the humoral branch, and T lymphocytes in the cellular branch. Reactions that involve the humoral system most often occur soon after contact has been made with the antigen. Allergic reactions that involve the cellular immune system often have delayed onset.

PATHOPHYSIOLOGY AND COMPLICATIONS

B lymphocytes recognize specific foreign chemical configurations via receptors on their cell membranes. For the antigen to be recognized by specific B lymphocytes, it must first be processed by T lymphocytes and macrophages. Each clone (family) of B lymphocyte recognizes its own specific chemical structure. Once recognition has taken place, the *B lymphocytes* differentiate and multiply, forming *plasma cells* and *memory B lymphocytes*. Memory B lymphocytes remain inactive until contact is made with the same type of antigen. This contact transforms the memory cell into a plasma cell that produces immunoglobulins (antibodies) specific for the antigen involved. Table 10.5 lists the functions of the five classes of immunoglobulins. Note that immunoglobulin E (IgE) is the key antibody involved in the pathogenesis of type I hypersensitivity reactions.

TYPES OF HYPERSENSITIVITY

As shown in Table 10.11, immunologic hypersensitivity includes four different types of reactions. The first three types of hypersensitivity reaction (types I, II, III) involve elements of the humoral system. Type IV hypersensitivity reactions involve the cellular immune system.

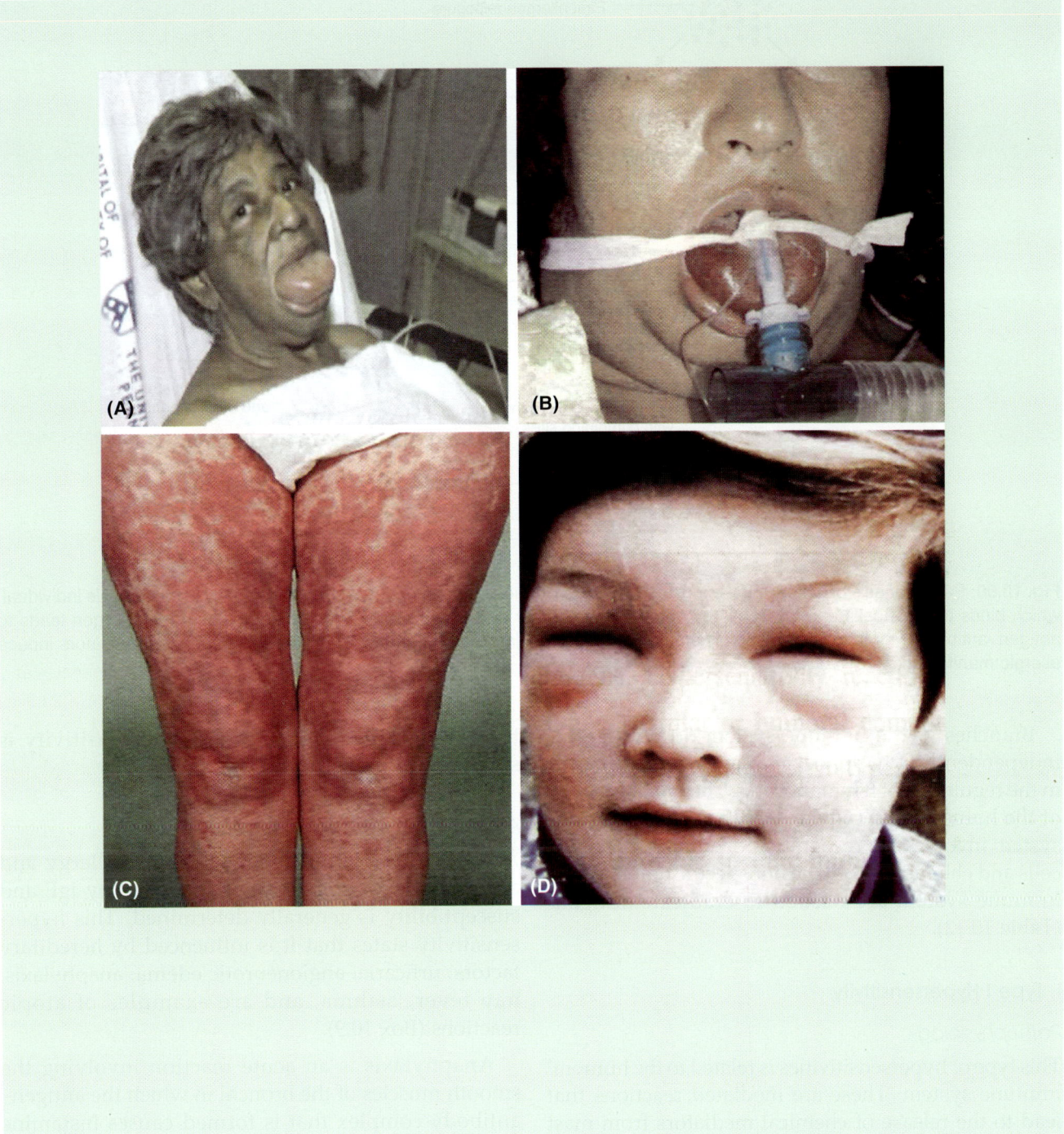

Plate XV: (A) Angioneurotic edema involving the tongue. The swelling of the tongue can compromise or obstruct the airway (Martini et al, 2008). **(B)** Severe angioedema in a 43-year-old woman with anaphylaxis. She required endotracheal intubation to overcome laryngeal obstruction. Note the edema of her mouth and face. **(C)** Ampicillin rash often presents as a symmetrical erythematous maculopapular eruption. This patient has a history of previous penicillin rashes, which had not been taken into account when the ampicillin was prescribed (Forbes and Jackson, 2003). **(D)** Severe angioedema in a 9-year-old boy after a bee sting

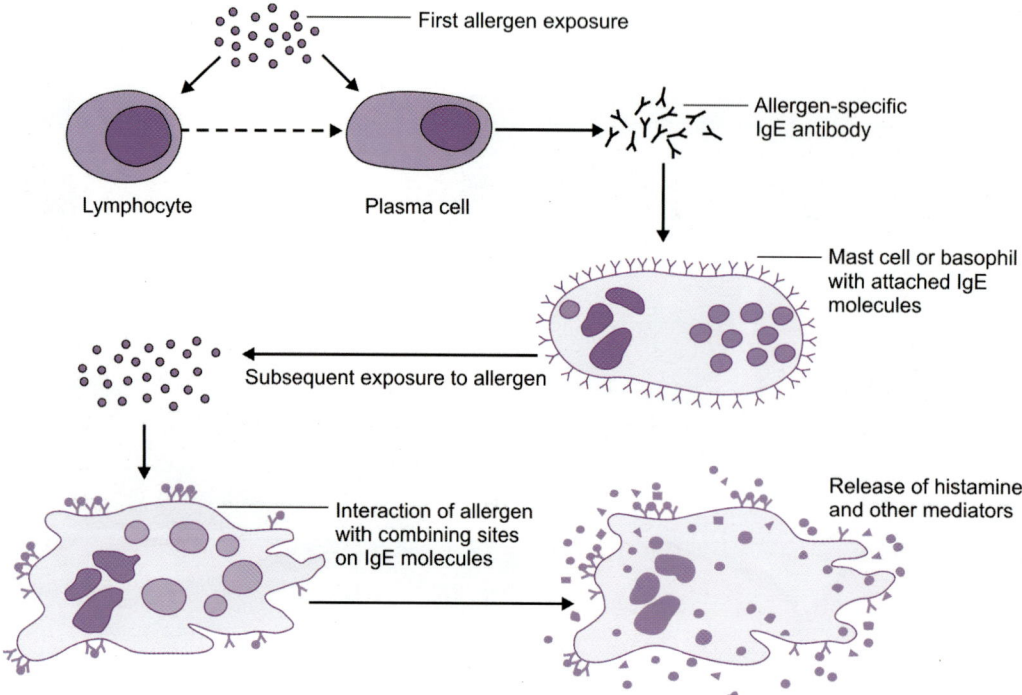

Fig. 10.90: Pathogenesis of allergy. First exposure to allergen induces formation of specific IgE antibody in susceptible individual, which binds to mast cells and basophils by nonantigen receptor end of molecule. Subsequent exposure to allergen leads to antigen–antibody interaction, liberating histamine and other mediators from mast cells and basophils. These mediators induce allergic manifestations *(Leonard and Crowley, 2004)*

Branches of the immune system do not operate independently. T lymphocytes play an important role in the regulation of B lymphocytes. The initial function of the humoral and cellular branches of the immune system involves the recognition of antigen; however, cells and chemicals from the nonspecific branch of the immune system are needed to eradicate antigens (Table 10.12).

i. Type I Hypersensitivity

Pathophysiology

This type of hypersensitivities is related to the humoral immune system. These are mediated reactions that lead to the release of chemical mediators from mast cells and basophils in various target tissues. It usually occurs soon after second contact with an antigen. In true allergic reactions, these lesions result from the effects of antigens and their antibodies (IgE) on mast cells in various locations in the body. Humoral antibodies involved in anaphylaxis and atopy are IgE antibodies that are fixed to and sensitize mast cells, so that when they encounter the antigen, they release

histamine (Fig. 10.91). Type I hypersensitivity is summarized in Box 10.8.

Atopy

Atopic disease is the common type of allergy and affects 1% of population. It is mediated by IgE and susceptibility is generally determined. This hypersensitivity states that it is influenced by hereditary factors, urticaria, angioneurotic edema, anaphylaxis, hay fever, asthma, and are examples of atopic reactions (Box 10.9).

Anaphylaxis is an acute reaction involving the smooth muscles of the bronchi in which the antigen–antibody complex that is formed causes histamine release from mast cells. The smooth muscle contracts, and this may lead to acute respiratory distress or failure. Urticaria, is a superficial lesion of the skin, while angioneurotic edema, is a lesion that occurs in the deeper layer of the skin or in other tissues such as the larynx or tongue. Agents that commonly cause acute urticaria include shell-fish, nuts, eggs, milk, antibiotic drugs, and insect bites (bee stings).

Table 10.11: Types of hypersensitivities*

Type	Example	Mechanism	Effects
I. Immediate hypersensitivity	Hay fever, anaphylaxis, angioneurotic edema, urticaria, insect venom, antisera.	IgE bound to mast cells; release of histamine and chemical mediators. Later contact with sensitizing antigen triggers mediator release and clinical manifestations.	Immediate (seconds to minutes): Localized response: hay fever, food allergy, urticaria. Systemic response: bee sting, penicillin anaphylaxis, angioneurotic edema.
II. Cyotoxic hypersensitivity reaction	Transfusion reaction, autoimmune hemolysis, hemolytic anemia, Rh hemolytic disease, certain drug reactions.	Antibody binds to cell or tissue antigen, and complement is activated, which damages cell, causes inflammation, and promotes destruction of antibody-coated cell by phagocytosis.	Cell lysis and phagocytosis
III. Immune complex disease	Autoimmune disorders: (systemic lupus erythematosus, glomerulonephritis, acute viral hepatitis. Rheumatoid arthritis.	Antigen–antibody complex deposits in tissue-complement activated	Six to eight hours later. Inflammation, vasculitis.
IV. Delayed (cell-mediated hypersensitivity)	Contact dermatitis; transplant rejection, infectious granulomas (tubercles, mycosis)	Antigen binds to T lymphocyte; sensitized lymphocyte, release lymphokines	Forty-eight hours later Delayed inflammation

* Modified from Krupp MA, Chatton MJ: Current Medical Diagnosis and Treatment, Los Alt CA, Lange Medical, 1984.

Table 10.12: Comparison of B cells and T cells

Property	B cell	T cell
Site of production of undifferentiated cell	Bone marrow	Bone marrow
Site of differentiation	Bone marrow	Thymus gland
Response after biniding to antigen	Become enlarged, multiply repeatedly to produce plasma cells; release specific antibodies	Become enlarged, multiply repeatedly, release cytokines
Antibody production	Synthesize and release specific antibodies	Stimulate B cells to produce specific antibodies
Type of immunity produced	Antibody-mediated (humoral) response	Cell-mediated response
Cytotoxic activity	None	Activated T cells kill specific antigen-bearing cells on contact
Factor influencing response to antigens	Macrophages	Macrophages
Effect on macrophages	None	Stimulate phagocytic activity
Basic functions	Release specific antibodies	Secrete specific toxins, stimulate production of specific antibodies by B cells, stimulate phagocytic activity of macrophages, produce cell-mediated immunity.

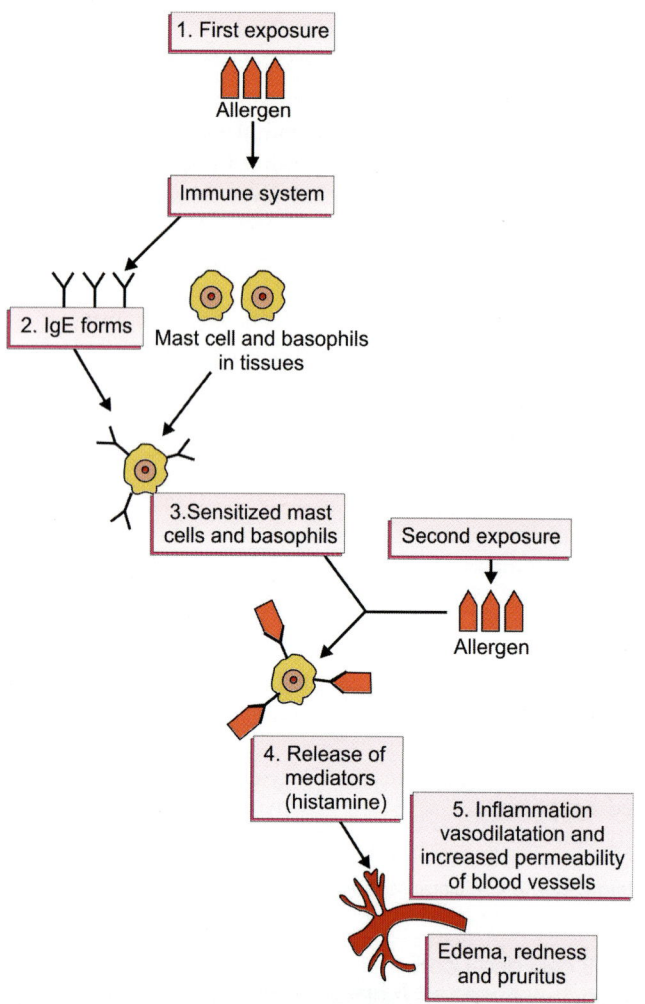

Fig. 10.91: Type I hypersensitivity-allergic reaction *(Gould, 2006)*

The antigen–antibody complex causes the release of mediators (histamine) from mast cells; these mediators then produce an increase in the

1. Immunoglobulin (Ig)E antibody mediated.
2. Immediate response.
3. Usual allergens (antigens)
   a. Dust
   b. Mites
   c. Pollens
   d. Animal danders
   e. Food
   f. Drugs (haptens)
4. Symptoms
   a. Anaphylaxis
   b. Hay fever
   c. Asthma
   d. Urticaria, angioedema
   e. Symptoms on occasion
5. Frequency: Affects about 10% of the population
6. Inherited tendency

* Modified from Thomson NC, Kirkwood EM, Levers RS. In Thomson NC, et al(eds). Handbook of Clinical Allergy. Oxford, Blackwell Scientific, 1990, pp 1–36.

permeability of adjacent vascular structures resulting in loss of intravascular fluid into surrounding tissue spaces. This reaction accounts for the edematous lesions of urticaria, angioneurotic edema, and secretions associated with hay fever.

The inflammation resulting from the release of chemicals from the activated mast cells may be mild or severe. Inflammation associated with the contraction of bronchial smooth muscles may be serious enough to interfere with breathing, as occurs in asthma. In most hypersensitivity reactions, the inflammation is localized. In allergies to pollen (popularly called hay fever), the inflammation is localized in the mucous membrane of the nose, where the allergens first make contact with the responsive tissue.

Box 10.9: Clinical examples of type I hypersensitivity reactions

Anaphylactic shock	Hay fever	Asthma
1st injection of antigen, e.g. penicillin or a bee sting general sensitization	1st contact with grass pollen → local sensitization of conjunctiva and nasal passages	1st contact with house dust or animal dander → local sensitization of bronchi
2nd injection of above → Acute collapse: bronchial constriction; vomiting; di-arrhea; a skin rash. May be fatal. Note that the antigens are injected: Enter bloodstream → Basophils affected → Widespread reaction	2nd contact with above → irritation or sweating of conjunctiva with excessive watery secretion	2nd contact with above → Bronchial constriction and secretion of thick mucus cause dyspnea (difficult breathing) Chronic asthma may involve cell-mediated immunity with destruction.

Widespread reaction: If an allergen enters the circulation, the effects may be distributed throughout the body, affecting several organ systems. Such a systemic reaction may result from insect stings, some therapeutic drugs (such as penicillin) (Fig. 10.92), and components of certain foods.

ANAPHYLAXIS

Anaphylaxis is a severe, life-threatening, systemic hypersensitivity reaction resulting in decreased blood pressure, airway obstruction, and severe hypoxia. The eliciting causes for the development of anaphylaxis are mentioned in Box 10.10. The reaction usually occurs within minutes of the exposure.

Pathophysiology

Large amounts of chemical mediators are released from mast cells into the general circulation very quickly, resulting in general vasodilation with sudden, severe decrease in blood pressure, edema of the mucosa and constriction of the bronchi and bronchioles with obstruction of the airflow (Fig. 10.93). The resulting marked lack of oxygen causes loss of consciousness within minutes.

Signs and symptoms: The initial manifestations of anaphylaxis include as generalized itching or tingling sensation over the body, coughing and difficulty in breathing. This is quickly followed by feeling of weakness, dizziness or fainting and a sense of fear and panic (Table 10.13). Edema may be observed around the eyes, lips, tongue, hands, and feet. Urticaria may appear on the skin. General collapse soon follows with loss of consciousness, usually within minutes.

Skin tests: Skin tests can be performed to determine the specific cause of an allergy. This procedure involves injecting a minute amount of antigen intradermally and observing the development of raised red itch wheal usually within 20 minutes, which indicates a positive skin reaction. In general, the larger the reaction, the more sensitive is the patient. A negative skin test means that the patient is not allergic to that particular antigen. Desensitization treatments involving repeated injections of very small amounts of antigen to create a blocking antibody may reduce the allergic response. Medications such as antihistamines or antidepressants, which interfere with allergy tests must be stopped from 2 days to 6 weeks or more before. A complication of skin testing is that it can induce sensitivity to the test compound;

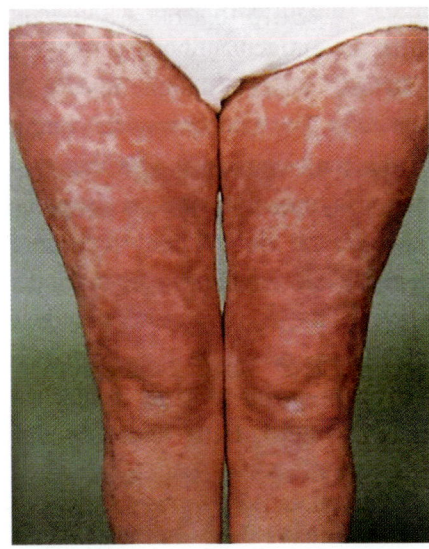

Fig. 10.92: Ampicillin rash often presents as a symmetrical erythematous maculopapular eruption. This patient had a history of previous penicillin rashes, which had not been taken into account when the ampicillin was prescribed *(Forbes and Jackson, 2003)*

anaphylaxis reactions can occasionally follow intradermal skin test doses, particularly of penicillin.

HAY FEVER (ALLERGIC RHINITIS)

People with hay fever react to one or more specific allergens such as pollen, mould, dust mites, and pet dander. These inhaled allergens inflame the nose, sinuses, eyelids and eyes. Hay fever can develop anytime during life but symptoms often fade with age. Signs are itchy eyes, nose, roof of the mouth and cough. Treatment includes the prescription of antihistaminics. Eyedrops containing antihistaminic and corticosteroid in nasal drops are the conventional medications used.

ANGIONEUROTIC EDEMA

Angioneurotic edema is an expression of type I hypersensitivity reactions. It is triggered when mast cells release histamine and other chemicals into the bloodstream. It may result in edema of tongue, pharyngeal tissues, or larynx and blocking the airway (Figs 10.94 and 10.95). Angioneurotic edema is precipitated by an allergic reaction to many allergens, such as latex, foods, shellfish, peanut, eggs and milk. Drugs such as penicillin, aspirin, ibuprofen, angiotensin converting enzyme inhibitors, and opioids may be responsible. Animal and plant antigens mainly pollens, animal dander, insect stings.

Box 10.10: Causes of human anaphyiactic reactions of importance to the dentist

Antibiotics
- Penicillins
- Sulfonamides
- Vancomycin
- Amphotericin B

- Cephalosporins
- Tetracyclines
- Streptomycin
- Chloramphenicol

Miscellaneous drugs/therapeutic agents
- Acetylsalicylic acid
- Succinylcholine
- Antitoxins
- Progestrone
- Thiopental

- Vaccine
- Nonsteroidal anti-inflammatory drugs (NSAIDs)
- Opiates

Diagnostic agents
- Radiographic contrast media

Hormones
- Insulin
- Parathormone

- Corticotropin
- Synthetic-adrenocorticotropic hormone (ACTH)

Enzymes
- Streptokinase
- Penicillinase

- Chymotrypsin
- Trypsin

Blood products
- Whole blood
- Plasma
- Gamma globulin

- Cryoprecipitate
- Immunoglobulin A(IgA)

Local anesthetics

Esters
- Procaine
- Propoxycaine
- Benzocaine
- Tetracaine

Antioxidant
  Sodium (meta) bisulfate

Parabens
  Methyl paraben

Angioedema is characterized by rapid development of oedematous swelling, particularly of the head and neck regions. It is the only type of allergy that can involve the oral tissues by causing swelling, particularly the lips, or the floor of the mouth (Fig. 10.94). Facial edema even though temporary can cause embarrassment, but when edema involves the neck and extends to the larynx, it can rapidly cause fatal respiratory obstruction. Acute allergic edema can develop alone or may be associated with anaphylactic reactions.

Treatment

Medication

- Systemic steroids are indicated to treat patients with asthma, immune complex injury, or cytotoxic immune reactions. Glucocorticoids or cortisone derivatives reduce the immune response and stabilize the vascular system. Give 100–500 mg of hydrocortisone sodium succinate or 50 mg methyl prednisolone IV every 6 hours up to 4 times.
- Antihistamines are indicated to treat patients with hay fever or urticaria.
- Immunosuppressive drugs and corticosteroids are given to patients who have received organ transplant.
- Topical steroids are used to treat patients with contact dermatitis.
    1. Place the patient in a supine position, i.e. lay the patient flat with the legs raised.
    2. Oxygen should be administered immediately.
    3. As in shock, keeping the patient warm.

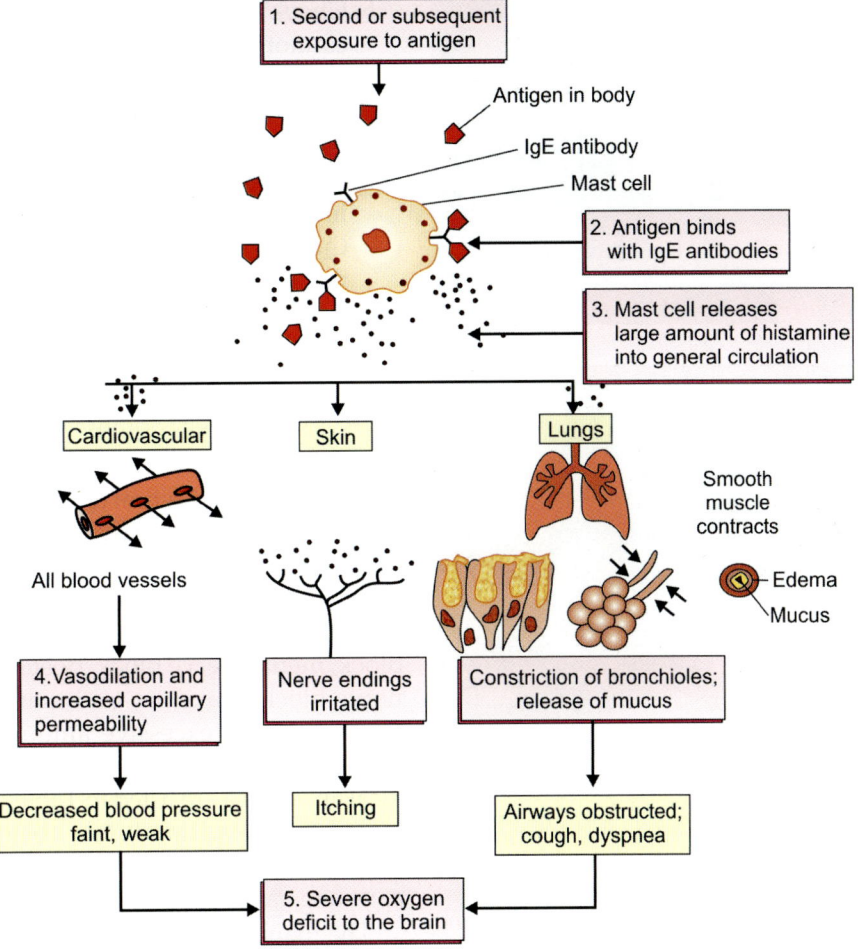

Fig. 10.93: The effects of anaphylaxis (type I hypersensitivity reaction) *(Gould BE, 2006)*

4. Inject epinephrine immediately. 0.3 of 1:1000 epinephrine through an IM (into tongue) or subcutaneously. The duration of action for epinephrine is relatively brief (10–30 min.). Repeat injection of 0.5 mL 1:1000 if no response. This drug acts to increase blood pressure by stimulating the sympathetic nervous system; it causes vasoconstriction and increases the rate and strength of the heart beats. This drug also relaxes the bronchiolar smooth muscle, opening the airway. The dosages may need to be repeated, if symptoms recur. Repeat every 10 min until recovery starts.

Table 10.13: Signs and symptoms of anaphylaxis

Manifestation	Rationale
Skin: Pruritis, tingling, warmth, hives	Histamine and chemical mediators irritate sensory nerves.
Respiration: Difficult in breathing, cough, wheezing, retrosternal tight feeling.	Chemical mediators cause contraction of smooth muscle in bronchioles, edema, and increased secretions leading to narrow airways and lack of oxygen
Cardiovascuilar: Decreased blood pressure with rapid, weak pulse; perhaps irregular, light headedness, generalized weakness, syncope, ischemic chest pain	Chemical mediators cause general vasodilation, leading to low blood pressure; sympathetic nervous responds by increasing heart rate
Central nervous system: Anxiety and fear (early); weakness; dizziness; and loss of consciousness	Early, sympathetic response; latter, lack of oxygen to the grain due to low blood pressure and respiratory obstruction

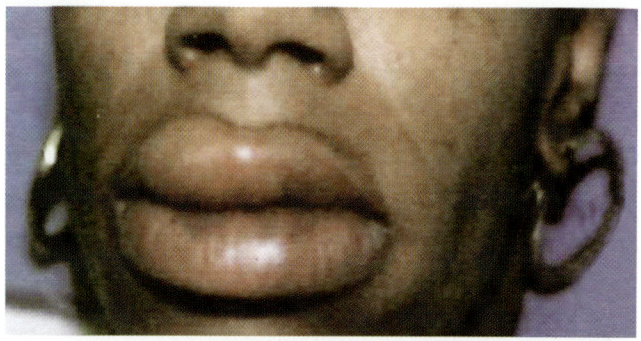

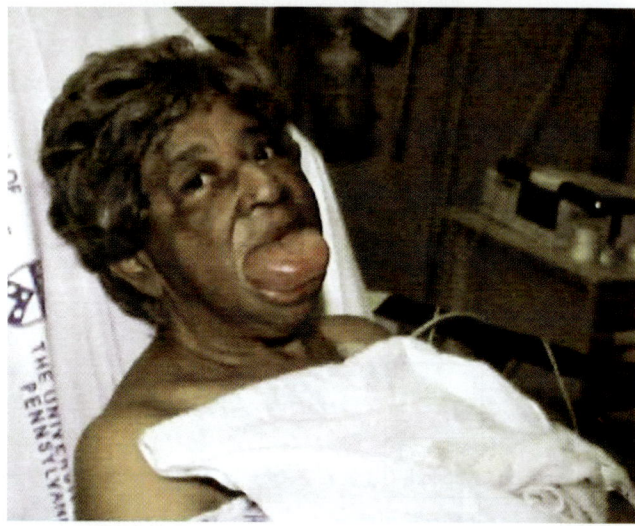

Fig. 10.94: (A) Angioneurotic edema involving the face and lips, **(B)** marked swelling of the tongue can compromise or obstruct the airway *(Martini et al, 2008)*

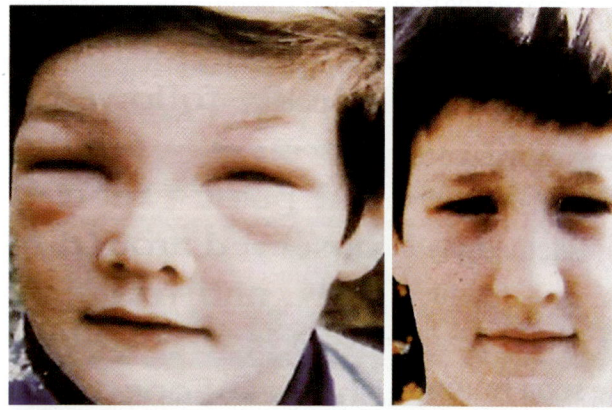

Fig. 10.95: (A) Severe angioedema in a 9-year-old boy after a bee sting. The patient required immediate treatment with adrenalin (epinephrine) to overcome a generalized anaphylactic response, and showed gross facial swelling. **(B)** shows the same patient without angioedema

5. Check the carotid or femoral pulse, if a pulse cannot be detected, closed chest cardiac massage should be initiated. Cardiopulmonary resuscitation may be necessary.

6. Antihistamine drug as diphenhydramine (Benadryl) or clorpheniramine slowly IV is useful in the early stages of an allergic reaction because they block the response of the tissues to the released histamine.

7. Summon help and transport to hospital.

ALLERGIC REACTIONS OF LOCAL ANESTHESIA

Syncopy developed following administration of local anesthesia is not an allergic reaction.

The reaction most often associated with local anesthetics is a toxic reaction. Development of toxicity following administration of local anesthetic is due to: (1) Intravenous injection of the local anesthetic agent, e.g. inferior alveolar nerve block, infraorbital nerve block, mental nerve block, posterior superior alveolar nerve block, maxillary and mandibular nerve block. (2) Injection of excessive amount of local anesthetic agent. The signs and symptoms of toxic reactions to local anesthesia are listed in Table 10.14. Toxic reactions may also developed due to the vasoconstrictor ingredient in the anesthetic carpules, these include sweating, tachycardia, apprehension and hyperactivity.

The management of intravascular injection of local anesthetic includes:

1. Stop the administration of the drug.
2. Lay the patient flat.
3. Reassure the patient.
4. Maintain the airway.

Most patients recover spontaneously within 30 minutes. Where possible, defer further treatment until another day.

If the history supports a true allergic reaction to a local anesthetic agent, the dentist should try to identify

Table 10.14: Signs and symptoms suggestive of an allergic reaction and toxic reaction to a given local anesthetic agent

Allergic reactions	Toxic reactions
1. Urticaria	Talkativeness
2. Swelling	Slurred speech
3. Skin rash	Dizziness
4. Chest tightnesss	Nausea
5. Dyspnea, shortness of breath	Depression
6. Rhinorrhea	Euphoria
7. Conjunctivitis	Excitement convulsions

the type of the anesthetic agent that was used. When the causative anesthetic is identified, resort to a new anesthetic with a different basic chemical structure can be used.

The two main groups of local anesthetics in dentistry consist of the following:

1. Ester group: Para-aminobenzoic acid (PABA) esters, e.g. procaine (novocaine), propoxycaine, tetracaine, benzocaine.
2. Amide group, e.g. lidocaine (xylocaine), mepivacaine (carbocaine), and prilocaine (citanest).

Allergy to local anesthetics occurs commonly in response to the ester group and not to the amide group of local anesthetics. However, true allergy to amide group may develop, although rarely, due to other components of the local anesthetic cartridge (Table 10.15). These components include the methylparaben and sodium metasulfite.

The parabens—methyl, ethyl, and propyle, are bacteriostatic agents and are added to many drugs, foods and cosmetics that are merant for multiple use. Parabens are structurally related to the ester local anesthetics, thus their increased allergenicity. Parabens are used increasingly in nondrug items, such as skin creams, hair lotions, suntan preparations, face powder, soaps, lip sticks, toothpastes, syrups, soft drinks, and candies. In response to the increasing incidence of allergic reactions to these products, certain products have been marked as "hypoaller-genic" and do not contain any parabens. Allergy to parabens is localized appearing as a localized skin eruption or as localized edema.

Allergy to sodium bisulfate or metabisulfite is being reported with increasing frequency. Bisulfites are antioxidants and are commonly used in restaurants where they are sprayed on fruits and vegetables as an antioxidants to prevent discoloration. For example, sliced apples sprayed with bisulfate do not turn brown (i.e. become oxidized). Bisulfites are also used to prevent bacterial contamination of wines, beers and distilled beverages. Patients with bisulfate allergy, frequently respond to contact with bisulfate with severe respiratory allergy, commonly bronchospasm. Within the asthmatic population, reports demonstrate that up to 10% are allergic to bisulfites. It is not known whether bisulfites are triggers of anaphylaxis. A history of bisulfate allergy should alert the doctor to the possibility of this same type of response, if sodium bisulfite or metabisulfite is included in the local anesthetic cartridge. Bisulfites are present in all local anesthetic cartridges that contain a vasoconstrictor. Local anesthetic solutions not containing vaso-constrictor additives do not contain bisulfites.

Management of Patients Allergic to Local Anesthesia

1. If allergy is limited to the ester group (e.g. procaine, propoxycaine, benzocaine or tetracaine), the amides (e.g. articaine, lidocaine, mepivacaine, or priolocaine) may be used because cross allergenicity, although possible, is quite rare.
2. If the local anesthetic allergy was actually an allergy to the paraben preservative, an amide local anesthetic may be injected, if it does not contain any preservative.
3. Where there is a questionable history of allergy to all the "caine" drugs, and where there is a dental emergency requiring immediate dental intervention, general anesthesia is resorted to.
4. Where general anesthesia is not a reasonable alternative, injectable histamine-blockers are used instead of local anesthetic agents. Most injectable

Table 10.15: Contents of local anesthetic cartridge

Ingredient	Function	"Plain" cartridge	Vasoconstrictor containing cartridge
Local anesthetic	Condition blockade	√	√
Vasconstrictor	Decrease absorption of local anesthetic into blood, thus increasing duration of anesthesia and decreasing local anesthetic toxicity	×	√
Sodium (metal) bisulfate	Antioxidant for vasoconstrictor	×	√
Sodium chloride	Isotonicity of solution	√	√
Sterile water	Diluent	√	√
Methylparaben	Bacteriostatic agent (to increase shelf life by maintaining sterility	×	×

histamine-blockers possess local anesthetic properties. Several are more potent local anesthetics than procaine has been the most commonly used histamine-blocker in this regard. 1% Diphenhydramine solution with 1:100,000 epinephrine is administered. Diphenhydramine produces pulpal anesthesia of up to 30 minutes duration, however, post-injection burning or stinging sensation is usually experienced. When the signs and symptoms of allergy to the injectable local anesthetic agents develop immediate treatment should be performed as mentioned in the management of anaphylaxis.

ii. Type II Hypersensitivity

Pathophysiology

The key elements involved in type II hypersensitivity are shown in Box 10.11. These reactions are IgG or IgM mediated (Fig. 10.96).

- This cytotoxic reaction causes some forms of hemolytic anemia (e.g. autoimmune HA), rhesus incompatibility and some blood transfusion reactions.
- In some autoimmune disorders, antibodies of this type are directed against specialized cell and surface receptors, e.g. Graves' disease or myasthenia gravis.

Cytotoxic T cells (Tc) have specific receptors for antigenic determinants. Cytotoxic T cells migrate from lymphoid tissue to the site of foreign invasion. There they make cell to cell contact with the foreign cells or virus. A cytotoxic T cell destroys a foreign cell by secreting a poreforming protein called perforin into the plasma membrane of the foreign cell. The perforin molecules create transmembrane pores in the foreign cells, causing them to rupture and die within 2 hours. This reaction is accomplished without the use of complement. T cells are the main cause of rejection of tissue or organ transplants from one person to another and are responsible for activity against tumors and

Box 10.11: Type II hypersensitivity

1. Antibody mediated
2. Cytotoxic hypersensitivity
   a. Antibodies combine with host cells recognized as foreign
   b. Foreign antigens bind to host cell membranes during induced hemolytic anemia or thrombocytopenia
3. Common examples
   a. Transfusion reactions from mismatched bloods.
   b. Rhesus incompatibility
   c. Goodpasture's syndrome

cancer cells. ABO blood incompatibility is a clinical example of type II sensitivity.

BLOOD TRANSFUSION

A. ABO Blood Group

If large quantities of blood are lost during surgery or in an accident, the blood volume must be increased, or a person can go into a shock and die. A transfusion is the transfer of blood, parts of blood, or solutions into a person's blood. In many cases, the return of blood volume to normal levels is all that is necessary. This can be accomplished by the transfusion of plasma or prepared solutions that have the proper amounts of solutes. When large quantities of blood are lost, however, erythrocytes must also be replaced so that the oxygen-carrying capacity of the blood is restored.

Early attempts to transfuse blood were often unsuccessful because they resulted in transfusion reactions, which included clumping of blood cells, rupture of blood cells and clotting within blood vessels. It is now known that transfusion reactions are caused by interactions between antigens and antibodies. In brief, the surfaces of erythrocytes have molecules called antigens, and in the plasma there are proteins called antibodies. Antibodies are very specific, meaning that each antibody can combine only with a certain antigen. When the antibodies in the plasma bind to the antigen on the surface of erythrocytes, they form molecular bridges that connect the erythrocytes together. As a result, agglutination or clumping of the cells occurs. The combination of the antibodies with the antigens also can initiate reactions that cause hemolysis or rupture of the erythrocytes. The debris formed from the ruptured erythrocytes can trigger clotting within small blood vessels. As a result of these changes, tissue damage and death may occur.

In humans, blood is categorized by the ABO blood group system. The ABO antigen appears on the surface of erythrocytes. Type A blood has type A antigens, type B blood has type B antigens, type AB blood has both types of antigens, and type O blood has neither A nor B antigens (Fig. 10.97, Table 10.16). In addition plasma from type A blood contains type B antibodies, which act against type B antigens, whereas plasma from type B blood contains type A antibodies, which act against type AA antigens. Type AB blood has neither type of antibody, and type O blood has both A and B antibodies. Each group

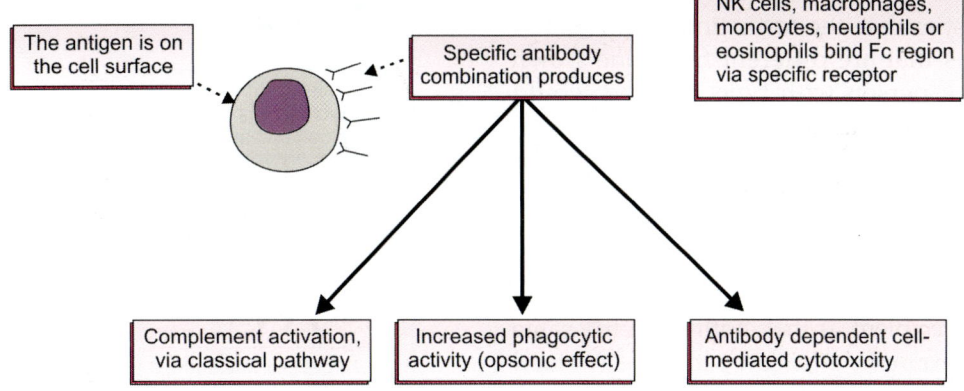

Fig. 10.96: Type II-cytotoxic type

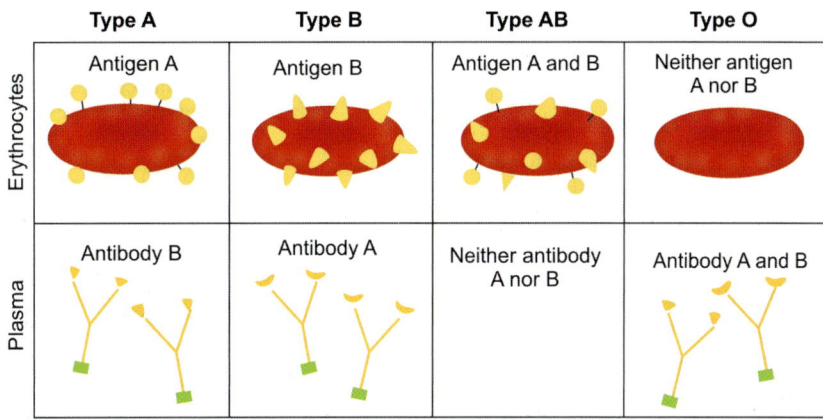

Fig. 10.97: ABO blood groups. The antigens found on the surface of the erythrocytes of each blood type and the antibodies found in the plasma of each blood type are shown *(Seeley et al, 1996)*

contains antibodies against foreign antigen, for example, group A blood possesses anti-B antibody. AB possesses no antibodies and is therefore the universal recipient. Group O individuals possess antibodies to both A and B.

It is essential that each patient is cross-matched correctly before transfusion (Fig. 10.96). Patients are grouped according to antigens expressed on their red blood cells as A, B, C, and O (Table 10.16).

The reason for the presence of A and B antibodies in blood is not clearly understood. Antibodies normally do not develop against an antigen unless the body is exposed to the antigen. This means that a person with type A blood should not have type B antibodies unless he or she has received a transfusion of type B blood, which contains type B antibodies, however, even though they never have received a transfusion of type B blood. One possible explanation

Table 10.16: ABO blood groups and transfusion compatibilities

Blood group	RBC antigen	Antibodies in plasma	For transfusion, can receive donor blood group
O	None	Anti-A and Anti-B	O
A	A	Anti-B	O or A
B	B	Anti-A	O or B
AB	A and B	None	O, A, B or AB

is that type A or B antigens on bacteria or food in the digestive tract stimulate the formation of antibodies against antigens that are different from one's own antigens. Thus a person with type A blood would produce type B antibodies against the B antigens on the bacteria or food. In support of this hypothesis is the observation that A and B antibodies are not found in the blood until about 2 months after birth.

A donor is a person who gives blood and a recipient is a person who receives blood. Usually, a donor can give blood to a recipient, if they both have the same blood type. For example, a person with type A blood could donate to another person with type A blood. There would be no ABO transfusion reaction because the recipient has no antibodies against the type A antigen. On the other hand, if type A blood were donated to a person with type B blood, an agglutination would occur because the person with type B blood has antibodies against the type A antigen, and "transfusion reaction" would result (Figs 10.98 to 10.101, Table 10.16). Signs of a transfusion reaction include a feeling of warmth in the involved vein, flushed face, headache, fever and chills, pain in the chest and abdomen, decreased blood pressure, and rapid pulse.

Historically, people with type O blood have been called universal donors because they usually can give blood to the other ABO blood types without causing an ABO transfusion reaction. Their erythrocytes have no ABO surface antigens and, therefore, do not react with the recepient's A or B antibodies. For example, if type O blood is given to a person with type A blood, the type O erythrocytes do not react with the type B antibodies in the recepient's blood. In a similar fashion, if type O blood is given to a person with type B blood, there would be no reaction with the recepient's type A antibodies.

However, it should be noted that the term universal donor is misleading. There are two circumstances in which transfusion of type O blood can produce a transfusion reaction. First, mismatching blood groups other than the ABO blood group can cause a transfusion reaction. To reduce the likelihood of transfusion reaction, all the blood groups must be correctly matched. Second, antibodies in the blood of the donor can react with antigens in the blood of the recipient. For example, type O blood has type A and B antibodies. If type O blood is transfused into a person with type A blood, the A antibodies, (in the type O blood) react against the A antigens (in the type A blood). Usually, such reactions are not serious

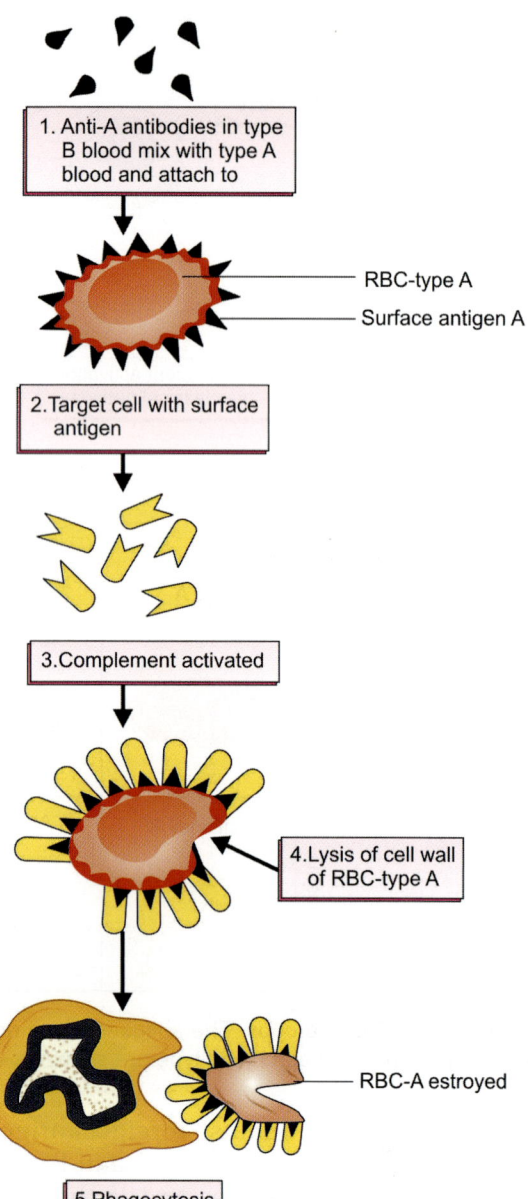

1. Anti-A antibodies in type B blood mix with type A blood and attach to

— RBC-type A
— Surface antigen A

2. Target cell with surface antigen

3. Complement activated

4. Lysis of cell wall of RBC-type A

— RBC-A estroyed

5. Phagocytosis

Fig. 10.98: The classic example of type II hypersensitivity (cytotoxic reaction) is transfusion reaction caused by mismatched blood *(Gould, 2006)*

because the antibodies in the donor's blood are diluted in the blood of the recipient and few reactions take place. However, because type O blood sometimes causes transfusion reactions in these situations, it is given to a person with another blood type only in life or death conditions.

B. Rh Blood Group

Another important blood group is the Rh blood group, so named because it was first studied in the rhesus

Donor blood type   +   Recipient blood type   =   Agglutination reaction

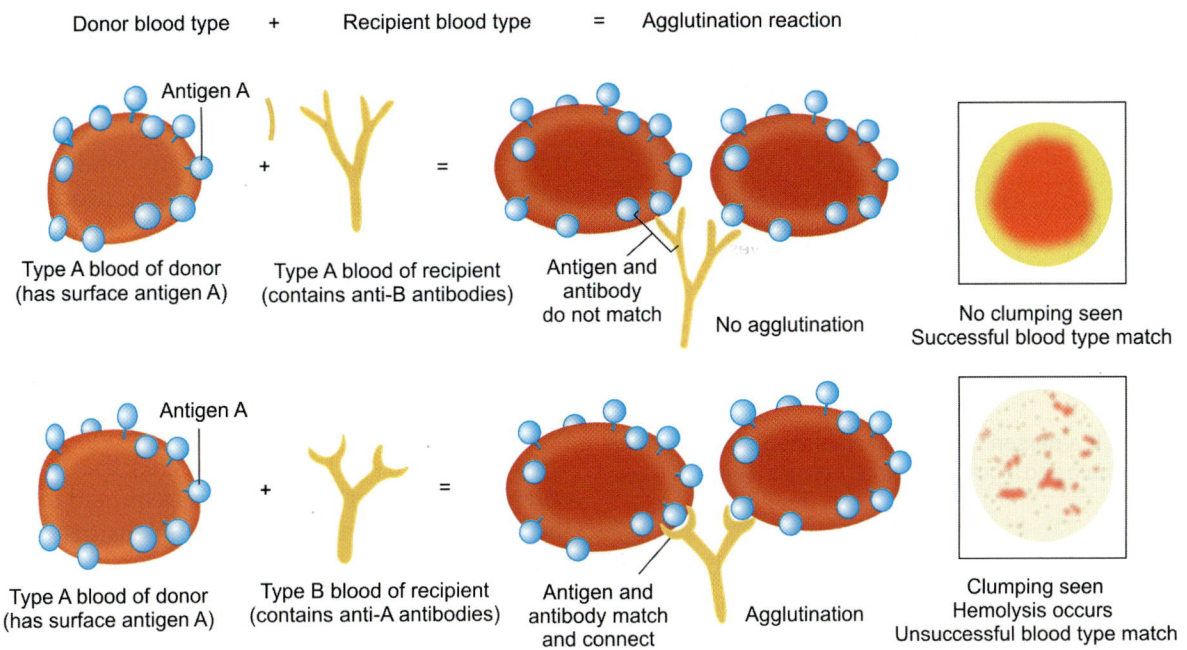

Type A blood of donor   Type A blood of recipient   Antigen and   No clumping seen
(has surface antigen A)   (contains anti-B antibodies)   antibody   Successful blood type match
  do not match   No agglutination

Type A blood of donor   Type B blood of recipient   Antigen and   Clumping seen
(has surface antigen A)   (contains anti-A antibodies)   antibody match   Agglutination   Hemolysis occurs
  and connect   Unsuccessful blood type match

Fig. 10.99: Agglutination reaction. Antibodies in the blood plasma bind to their corresponding surface antigens on the erythrocyte plasma membranes, causing agglutination *(McKliney& Louglin, 2006)*

monkey. People are Rh-positive, if they have certain Rh antigens on the surface of their erythrocytes, and they are Rh-negative, if they do not have these Rh antigens. The ABO blood type and the Rh blood type usually are designated together. For example, a person designated as A positive is type A in the ABO blood group and Rh positive.

Antibodies against the Rh antigen do not develop unless an Rh-negative person is exposed to Rh positive blood. This can occur through a transfusion or by the transfer of blood across the placenta to a mother from her fetus. When an Rh-negative person receives a transfusion of Rh-positive blood, the recipient becomes sensitized to the Rh antigen and produces Rh antibodies. If the Rh-negative person is unfortunate enough to receive a second transfusion of Rh-positive blood after becoming sensitized, a transfusion reaction results. Rh incompatibility can pose a major problem in some pregnancies, when the mother is Rh-negative and the fetus is Rh-positive (Fig. 10.102).

If fetal blood leaks through the placenta and mixes with the mother's blood, the mother becomes sensitized to the Rh antigen. The mother produces Rh antibodies that cross the placenta and cause agglutination and hemolysis of fetal erythrocytes. This disorder is called hemolytic disease of the newborn

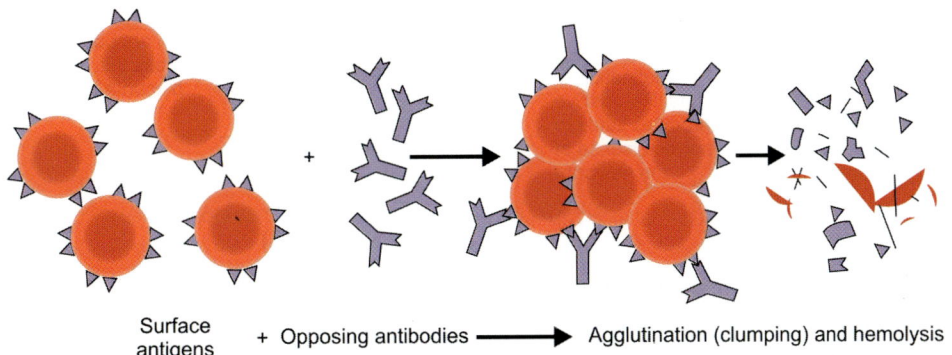

Surface   + Opposing antibodies ⟶ Agglutination (clumping) and hemolysis
antigens

Fig. 10.100: A cross-reaction occurs when antibodies in plasma encounter their target antigens on RBCs. The result is extensive clumping (agglutination) and hemolysis of the affected RBCs *(Martini et al, 2008)*

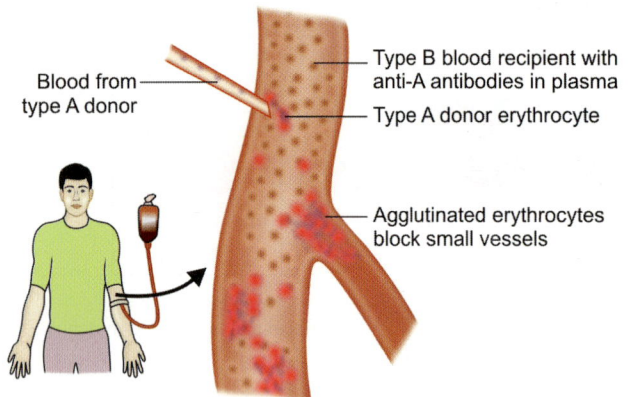

Fig. 10.101: If a person receives mismatched blood, erythrocytes agglutinate and block small blood vessels *(McKliney& Louglin, 2006)*

(HDN) or erythroblastosis fetalis and it can be fatal to the fetus. In the first pregnancy, there is often no problem. The leakage of fetal blood is usually the result of a tear in the placenta that takes place either late in the pregnancy or during delivery. Thus there

is not enough time for the mother to produce enough Rh antibodies to harm the fetus. In later pregnancies, however, there can be a problem because the mother has been sensitized to the Rh antigen. Consequently, if the fetus is Rh-positive and if any fetal blood leaks into the mother's blood, she rapidly produces large amounts of Rh antibodies and HDN develops.

Prevention of HDN is often possible, if the Rh negative woman is given an injection of a specific type of antibody preparation called anti-Rho(D) immune globulin (RhoGAM) immediately after each delivery or abortion. The injection contains antibodies against Rh antigens. The injected antibodies bind to the Rh antigens of any fetal erythrocytes that may have entered the mother's blood. This treatment inactivates the fetal Rh antigens and prevents sensitization of the mother.

If HDN develops, treatment consists of slowly removing the blood of the fetus or newborn and replacing it with Rh-negative blood. Exposure of the newborn's skin to fluorescent light is also used because

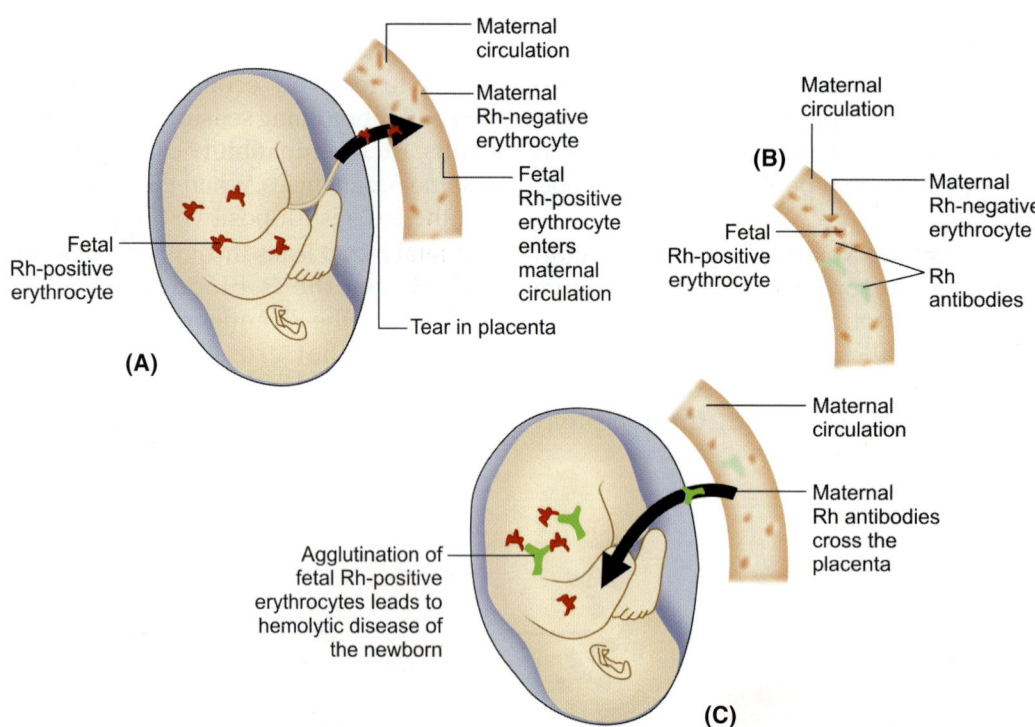

Fig. 10.102: Hemolytic disease of the newborn. **(A)** Before or during delivery, Rh-positive erythrocytes from the fetus enter the blood of an Rh-negative woman through a tear in the placenta. **(B)** The mother is sensitized to the Rh antigen and produces Rh antibodies. Because this usually happens after delivery, there is no effect on the fetus in the first pregnancy. **(C)** During a subsequent pregnancy with an Rh-positive fetus, Rh-positive erythrocytes cross the placenta and stimulate the mother to produce antibodies against the antigen. The Rh antibodies from the mother cross the placenta, causing agglutination and hemolysis of fetal erythrocytes, and hemolytic disease of the newborn develops *(Seeley et al, 1996)*

it helps to breakdown bilirubin in the blood as the blood flows through the skin. High levels of bilirubin are toxic to the nervous system and can cause destruction of brain tissue.

Type III Hypersensitivity

Type III hypersensitivity is summarized in Box 10.12. These reactions take place in blood vessels and involve soluble immune complexes (Fig. 10.103, Box 10.12). They constitute what is referred to as immune complex-mediated hypersensitivity. Their key feature is vasculitis.

- In most cases where there is Ag/Ab reaction, the immune complexes are removed from the circulation and hypersensitivity does not develop.
- Type III hypersensitivity may be a localized reaction, e.g. at the site of an insect bite or the development of a farmer's lung following inhalation of fungal antigens. When large amounts of circulating antigen enter the bloodstream and bind to antibody, circulating immune complexes are formed. Historically, serum sickness occurred in some individuals following administration of antitoxin in foreign serum.

Damage occurs particularly in the kidney when immune complexes aggregate in small vessels. Circulating immune complexes are important in the pathogenesis of systemic lupus erythematosus (SLE) and rheumatoid arthritis.

In this type of reaction, the antigen combines with the antibody, forming a complex, which is then deposited in tissue, often in blood vessel walls, and also activates complement (Fig. 10.104). This process causes inflammation and tissue destruction. Clinical examples include systemic lupus erythematosus and streptococcal glomerulonephritis. A number of diseases are now thought to be caused by immune complexes including glomerulonerphritis and

> **Box 10.12:** Type III hypersensitivity
>
> 1. Antibody mediated via immune complex formation.
> 2. Also known as immune complex-mediated hypersensitivity.
> 3. Immune complex formation
>   a. Hypersensitivity state: Complexes persist and lodge in blood vessel walls, initiating inflammatory reaction
>   b. Large complexes
>   c. Removed by neutrophils and macrophages
>   d. Soluble complexes (more antigen than antibody)
>   e. Complement is activated
>   - Vascular permeability increased
>   - Neutrophils attracted
>   - Neutrophils release enzymes
>   - Vasculitis results
> 4. Sensitive sites
>   a. Renal glomeruli
>   b. Synovial membranes
>   c. Examples
>   i. Systemic lupus erythematosus
>   ii. Poststreptococcal glomerulonephritis.

rheumatoid arthritis. Serum sickness refers to the systemic reaction that occurs when immune complex deposits occur in many tissues. With reduced use of animal serum for passive immunization, serum sickness is less common today. An Arthus reaction is a localized inflammatory and tissue necrosis that results when an immune complex lodges in the blood vessel wall, causing a vasculitis. One example is "farmer's lung", a reaction to molds inhaled when an individual handles hay.

Type IV Hypersensitivity

Type IV hypersensitivity which involve the cellular immune system, include infectious contact dermatitis, transplant rejection and graft-versus-host disease (Box 10.13).

The reaction is due to the consequences of specific direct antigen/antibody combination particularly complement activation and platelet aggregation. The antibodies involved are IgG or IgM.

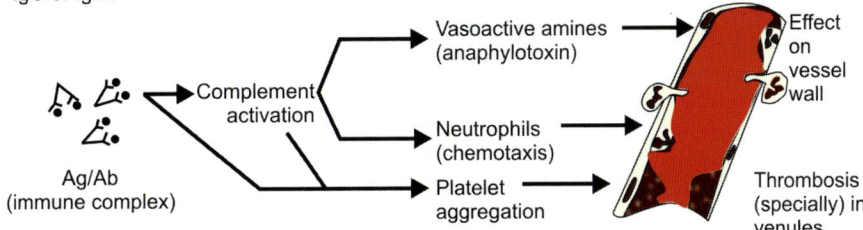

Fig. 10.103: Type III immune complex (Arthus) type

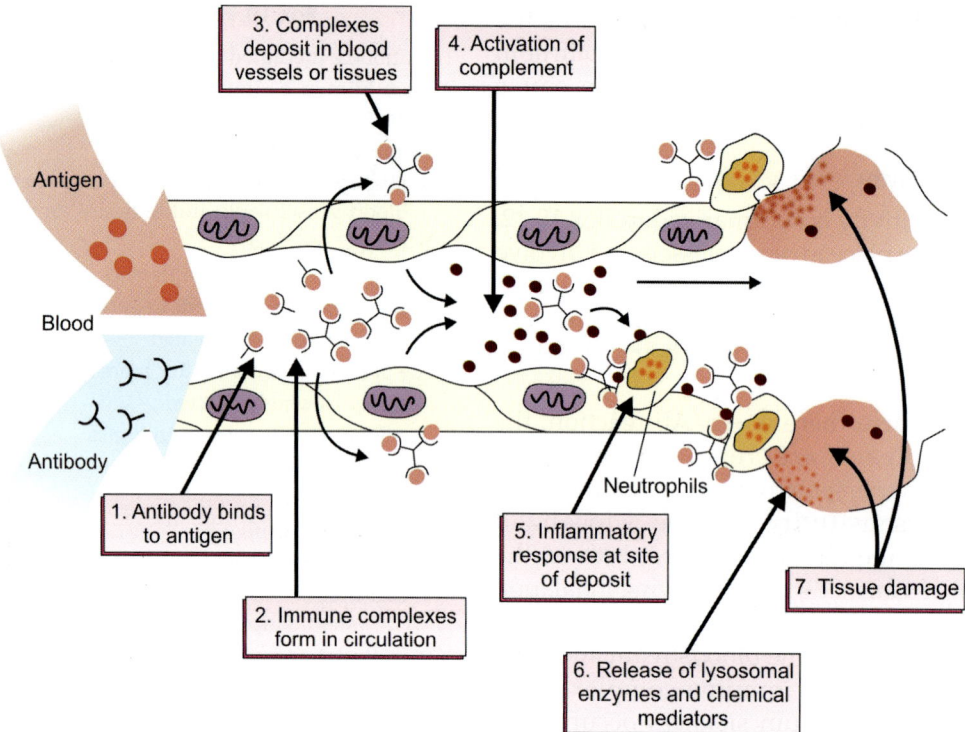

Fig. 10.104: Type III hypersensitivity—immune complex reaction *(Gould, 2006)*

Events in type IV hypersensitivity (contact dermatitis), which may involve dendritic cells and Langerhans cells, present the antigen to undifferentiated T lymphocytes. Some of the more common antigens that cause contact dermatitis include metal jewelry, perfuse, rubber products, chemicals such as formaldehyde and medicines such as topical anesthetics. Type IV hypersensitivity reactions usually are delayed and appear about 48 to 72 hours after contact has been with the antigen (Fig. 10.105).

Box 10.13: Type IV hypersensitivity*

Signs and symptoms of an allergic reaction
1. Mediated by T lymphocytes.
2. Does not involve antibodies.
3. Also called delayed-type hypersensitivity (response not seen until about 2 days after antigenic exposure).
4. Examples include the following:
   a. Contact dermatitis
   b. Graft rejection
   c. Some types of drug sensitivity.
   d. Some types of autoimmune diseases

*Modified from Thomson NC, Kirkwood EM, Lever RS: In Thomson NC, et al (eds.): Handbook of Clinical Allergy. Oxford, Blackwell Scientific, 1999, pp 1–36.

Infectious type allergic reactions are exemplified by the tuberculin skin test, in which a person who has previously been exposed to *Mycobacterium tuberculosis* develops, along with a second exposure in the form of an intradermal injection of altered bacteria a delayed response usually within 48–72 hours. This response is characterized by induration, erythema, swelling, and some time ulceration at the site of injection.

Contact allergy occurs when a substance of low molecular weight that is not antigenic by itself comes in contact with a tissue component (primarily a protein) and forms an antigenic complex. This small molecule is called a hapten (or one-half of an antigen), and the resulting complex causes sensitization of T lymphocytes (Fig. 10.106). Poisonivy is an example of a contact allergy where in the reaction is delayed (withy response occurring 48 to 72 hours after contact is made with the allergen).

Graft rejection occurs when organs or tissues from one body are transplanted into another body. Cellular rejection of transplanted tissue occurs, unless the donor and recipient are genetically identical or the host's immune response has been suppressed.

This reaction is an antigen-elicited cell-mediated immune response which produces tissue injury independently of the presence of antibody. The reaction is usally delayed taking 24–72 hours to develop. Classic examples include the tubercle follicle, graft rejection and contact dermatitis.

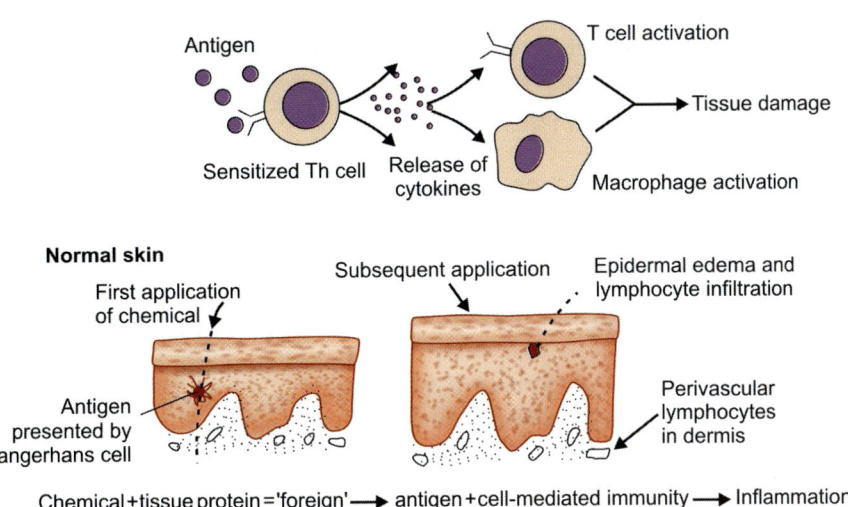

Chemical+tissue protein='foreign' → antigen+cell-mediated immunity → Inflammation

Fig. 10.105: Type IV hypersensitivity delayed type

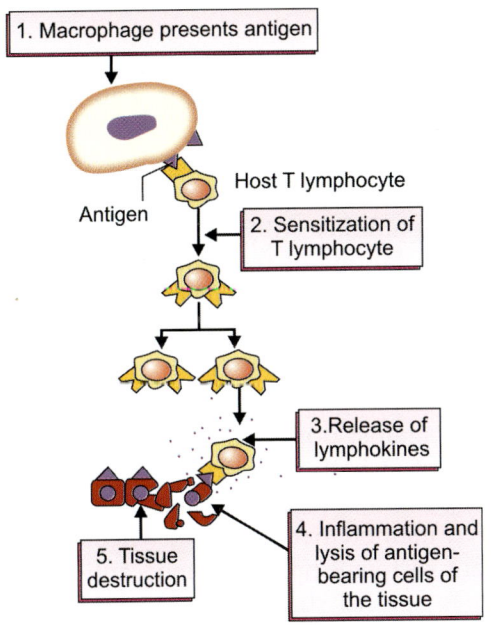

Fig. 10.106: Type IV hypersensitivity—cell-mediated delayed hypersensitivity *(Gould, 2006)*

Graft-versus-host reaction is an unusual phenomenon that occurs in bone marrow transplant recepients whose cellular immune system has been rendered deficient by whole body irradiation. Lymphocytes transferred to the host attempt to destroy host tissues.

TISSUE AND ORGAN TRANSPLANT REJECTION

Replacement of damaged organs or tissues by healthy tissues from donors is occurring more frequently as the success of such transplants improves. Skin, corners, kidneys, lungs, hearts, and bone marrow are among the more common transplants. Transplants differ according to donor characteristics as indicated in Table 10.17. The surface of nucleated cells in the human body contains antigens called human lymphocyte antigens (HLAs). The immune system can distinguish between self and foreign cells because self-cells have self-HLAs, whereas foreign cells have foreign HLAs. Rejection of a graft is caused by a normal immune system response to foreign HLAs.

Table 10.17: Types of tissue or organ transplants

Allograft (homograft)	Tissue transferred between members of the same species bit may differ genetically, e.g. one human to another human.
Isograft	Tissue transferred between two genetically identical bodies, e.g. identical twins.
Autograft	Tissue transferred from one part of the body to another part on the same individual, e.g. skin or bone.
Xenograft	Tissue transferred from a member of one species to a different species, e.g. pig to man.

In most cases, transplants, or grafts, involve the introduction of foreign tissue from one human, the donor, into the body of the human recipient (allograft). Because the genetic makeup of cells is the same only in identical twins, the obstacle to complete success of transplantation has been that the immune system of the recipient responds to the HLAs in foreign tissue rejecting and destroying the graft tissue.

The body recognizes the foreign antigens in the transplant, which becomes infiltrated by lymphocytes and macrophages and is eventually destroyed. This process is called rejection of the transplanted organ, and it is a manifestation of a cell-mediated immune reaction. Rejection is a complex process, primarily involving a type IV cell-mediated hypersensitivity reaction, but also involving a humoral response, both of which cause inflammation and tissue necrosis. The rejection process eventually destroys the organ, so that transplanted organs usually must be replaced after a few years. Rejection episodes may be mild or severe but, with time, will lead to failure or patient death. As surgical methods to transplant grafts improve, rejection becomes the major cause of graft failure. The other main cause of graft rejection is patient's failure to continue to take their immunosuppressive drugs. Of those awaiting organ transplantation, more than one-fourth of patients have already had at least one graft failure.

Graft-vs-host rejection: In graft-versus-host rejection, the transplanted donor, for example, bone marrow recognizes the recepient's tissue as foreign and the transplant rejects the recipient, causing destruction of the recepient's tissue and possibly death.

Host-vs-graft rejection: The recepient's immune system recognizes the donor's tissue as foreign and rejects the transplant.

Survival time of a transplant is increased when the HLA match is excellent, when the donor is living (less risk of damage to donor tissue) and when immunosuppressive drugs are taken on a regular basis. Corneas and cartilage lack a blood supply, and, therefore, rejection is not a problem with this transplanted tissues. With improved surgical techniques and better drug therapy, transplants are now lasting a long time. The success rates for organ transplants have increased tremendously with the discovery of immunosuppressants cyclosporine and tacrolimus (Prograf). These drugs have improved the survival rates in transplanted patients.

It now appears that neonates and young infants can receive heart transplants from donors without a good tissue match. Rejection does not occur because the infant's immune system is not yet mature and does not respond to the foreign tissue. The long-term effects are not known but the results to date are encouraging. Since heart transplants in infants are limited by organ size as well as by organ availability, the removal of the HLA restrictions would make more heart transplants available when needed and more donor hearts could be used rather than wasted.

IMMUNOLOGICAL EVALUATION

Immunological evaluation that primarily serves to avoid transplants that are at risk for antibody-mediated hyperacute rejection. The immunological evaluation includes: ABO blood group determination is used to determine, if the patient is a potential target of recipient circulating preformed cytotoxic anti-ABO antibody. Transplantation across incompatible blood groups may result in a humorally mediated hyperacute rejection. All transplant recepients and donors are tissue typed to determine the HLA class I and class II loci.

The degree of incompatibility between the donor and recipient is defined by the number of antigens that are mismatched at each of the HLA loci. All transplant candidates are screened to determine the degree of humoral sensitization to HLA antigens. Sensitization to histocompatibility antigens is of great concern in certain populations of transplant candidates. This happens when the recipient is sensitized because of receiving multiple blood transfusion, a previous organ transplant, or from pregnancy.

Transplantation of an organ into a recipient that is sensitized against donor class I HLA antigens puts the recipient at high risk of developing hyperacute antibody-mediated rejection. Crossmatching is an in-vitro assay method that determine whether a potential transplant recipient has performed anti-HLA class I antibodies against those of the organ donor. This immunologic test is conducted before transplantation. A negative crossmatch must be obtained before accepting an organ for transplantation.

KIDNEY TRANSPLANT

Dialysis is a very expensive option in the long run for renal failure patients. In dialysis, the functions of damaged kidneys are performed by a machine that facilitates diffusion between the patient's blood and a dialysis fluid whose composition is carefully regulated. The process, which takes several hours, must be repeated two or three times each week. A kidney transplant, the kidney of a healthy compatible donor is surgically inserted into the patient's body and connected to the circulatory system. If the surgical procedure is successful, the transplanted kidney(s) can take over all of the normal kidney functions. A kidney transplant is also expensive at first, but all in all it has a lower yearly maintenance cost, compared to dialysis. With kidney transplant, the quality of life improves for the patient and there is also an improvement of uremia, anemia, peripheral neuropathy, and autonomic neuropathy. A kidney transplant can double the lifespan of kidney failure patients. The transplanted kidney can be obtained from a cadaver-50% of transplants utilize this source— a live related donor, or a live distant/unrelated donor. Kidneys obtained from a live donor are much better than those obtained from a nonliving or cadaveric donor.

LIVER TRANSPLANT

Liver transplantation is the replacement of a native, diseased liver with a liver from a brain-dead donor (allograft). This operation allows a patient who otherwise would have died from liver failure to live a relatively full and normal life. The donor liver contains several tissue antigens that can induce an immune response in the recipient. Because of this, the donor and recipient must be checked for tissue antigen compatibility. A good match will decrease the likelihood of organ rejection. Patients who receive a liver transplant will be placed on immunosuppressive drugs and will remain on them for the rest of their lives.

Patients with fulminate liver failure, regardless of the cause, will die within hours or days, if a suitable organ donor cannot be located. In an extreme situation, a liver from a lower animal (xenograft), most commonly a pig, can be used temporarily until a human donor becomes available.

On rare occasions, liver tissue may be harvested from a suitable living donor. A lobe of the liver is taken from the donor and placed in the recipient. The liver is unique in that it will regenerate. Thus , in a living donor operation, the livers will grow to normal size in both the donor and the recipient within six to eight weeks.

A liver transplant is much more complicated than a kidney transplant because of the complexity of the surgical procedure. To prioritize a patient on the liver transplant list, the severity of a liver failure patient's status is assessed using the model of end-stage liver disease (MELD) criteria. The MELD criteria evaluate the following tests: bilirubin, PT/INR, and serum creatinine. The serum creatinine is the most sensitive mortality risk indicator of liver failure.

One type of rejection occurs when the host, or recipient's, immune system rejects the graft [host-versus-graft disease (HVGD)], a possibility with kidney transplants. Sometimes the graft tissue contains T cells that attack the host cells [graft-versus-host disease (GVHD)], as may occur in bone marrow transplants. Rejection may occur at anytime:

- Hyperacute rejection occurs immediately after transplantation, sometimes in the operating room, when circulation to the site is re-established, usually in patients, who for some reason, have pre-existing antibodies, perhaps from blood transfusions. The blood vessels are affected, resulting in lack of blood flow to the transplanted tissue.

- Acute rejection develops after several weeks when unmatched antigens cause a reaction.

- Chronic or late rejection occurs after months or years, with gradual degeneration of the blood vessels.

Immunosuppression techniques are used to reduce the immune response and prevent rejection. The common treatment involves drugs such as cyclosporine, azathioprine (Imuran) and prednisone, a glucocorticoid. The drugs must be taken on a continuous basis and the patient monitored for signs of rejection. The use of cyclosporine has been very successful in reducing the risk of rejection, but dosage must be carefully checked to prevent kidney damage. Also, many new drugs are under investigation in clinical trial. The major concern with any immuno-suppressive drug is the high risk of infection, because the normal body defenses are now limited.

Infections often are caused by opportunistic microorganisms, microbes which usually are harmless in healthy individual. Persons with diabetes frequently require transplants of kidneys and other tissues, and this group of patients is already at risk for infection because of vascular problems. Also of note is the increased incidence of certain cancers, including lymphomas, skin and lip cancers, and Kaposi's sarcomas in people taking immuno-suppressive drugs.

Dental professionals should be aware of the high incidence of gingival hyperplasia in patients taking cyclosporine.

Liver transplant recepients may be susceptible to recurrence of their original disease and may develop recurrence of hepatitis B or C, alcoholic liver disease, or, one of the autoimmune hepatitides. The severity of recurrence varies from mild to development of progressive allograft failure. HCV recurrence after transplantation is almost universal, but the extent of the graft damage is variable. The survival in the short term is not significantly affected, but concerns exist regarding long-term recurrence because the rate of developing cirrhosis at 5 years can be as high as 8–25.

Cells Responsible for Prevention of Organ Rejection

The following cells constitute the cell-mediated defenses for the prevention of organ rejection:

1. T cells: The most important cells.
2. Antigen-presenting cells.
3. Natural killer cells.
4. Monocytes.

DENTAL PROTOCOL FOR ORGAN TRANSPLANT PATIENTS*

1. Prior to the start of routine dental treatment always obtain laboratory tests to confirm that the transplanted organ is optimally functioning. Never presume that the transplanted organ works well.
2. Obtain a good dental history and perform a thorough dental examination, including full-mouth radiographs.
3. Prioritize the patient's dental problems. Those that are most likely to cause pain, infection, and/or bacteremia in the next 12 months should be taken care of immediately.
4. When treating a preliver transplant patient, follow the liver failure anesthetic, analgesic, antibiotic suggested guidelines during dentistry.
5. When treating a pre-renal transplant patient, follow the premedication protocol for shunts and renal failure anesthetic, analgesic, antibiotic (AAAs) suggested guidelines during dentistry.
6. Obtain the CBC and calculate the ANC count in any pre-transplant patient. Provide AHA recommended antibiotic premedication, if the patient has low ANC counts.

7. Premedication should also be provided in the presence of ascites in the pre-liver transplant patient.
8. In the patient awaiting a liver transplant, evaluate the PT/INR: fresh frozen plasma (FFP) transfusion will be needed, if the PT/INR is prolonged. Also evaluate the platelet count in the patient awaiting a liver transplant. Platelet replacement will be required, if the platelet count is < 50 K/mm^3.
9. Pre-transplant preparation of the oral cavity is the same as for patients who are to undergo chemotherapy or radiotherapy.
10. After transplantation, elective dental care is best deferred for at least 3 months, to avoid unnecessary complications. Infection is most likely at that time—the period of intense immunosuppression.
11. The anesthetics, analgesics, antibiotics (AAAs) used during dentistry will be determined by the current status of the transplanted organ. Obtain appropriate tests to evaluate the status of the transplanted organ and then proceed with dentistry.
12. General anesthesia should be avoided but if necessary, should only be given in hospital with appropriate expertise and facilities.
13. Avoid cimetidine (Tagamet), clarithromycin, corticosteroids, erythromycin and similar drugs in the presence of cyclosporine.
14. NSAIDs should be avoided since they potentiate the nephrotoxicity of cyclosporin and tacrolimus, may cause a bleeding tendency, and exacerbate ulcer, if the patient is on corticosteroids.
15. Avoid the following drugs in the dental setting in the presence of tacrolimus/prograf, antiacids, cimetidine (tagamet), clarithromycin, erythromycin, and methylprednisolone.
16. If macrolides are the only antibiotics that can be used in the first six months of the transplant because of allergy to penicillin, communicate with the patient's consultant. The consultant can assist with temporary lowering the cyclosporine doses so the macrolide can be safely used.
17. Patients may need steroid supplementation and cover during dental treatment. This applies probably for at least 2 years post-transplantation.
18. Bone marrow suppression is a genuine concern post-transplant, and these patients have an

---

* Modified from Ganada K: Dentist's Guide to Medical Conditions and Complications. 1st edn. Wiley-BlackWell, 2008

increased incidence of infection plus increased susceptibility to infections. Determine the ANC and provide appropriate antibiotics when needed. Treat infections aggressively.

19. Viral hepatitis B and C infections may be present, especially in older patients who have received blood transfusions before blood was routinely screened.

20. Herpangina occurs commonly post-transplant and is very aggressive when it occurs. Treat immediately with valacyclovir (Va Itrex) or acyclovir.

21. Gingival hyperplasia: cyclosporine is the leading cause for gingival hyperplasia, post-transplant.

22. Potential hypertension can occur with cyclosporine use, so always monitor the BP during dentistry.

23. Consider premedication for renal transplant patients that were on hemodialysis and still continue to have the shunt, even if the ANC is normal.

24. Consider premedication for any organ transplant patient with decreased immunity as indicated by assessment of the total WBC and the ANC counts. Follow the ANC guidelines, if the WBC count is below normal.

25. Look for oral sores and treat accordingly. Oral candidiasis may be persistent, or mixed bacterial plaques may develop on the oral mucosa. Oral candidiasis can usually be managed with topical nystatin, amphotericin, or miconazole.

26. Routine cancer surveillance is mandatory to assure rapid diagnosis and treatment of any malignancy, since patients on immunosuppressive treatment after organ transplantation have a greatly raised incidence of malignant disease, particularly lymphomas and, to less extent, skin, cervical and lip cancer. In other patients, hairy leukoplakia or Kaposi's sarcoma may be seen.

11

Neurosensory Deficit

"Facial Neuralgias"

I. Trigeminal Neuralgia
A. Idiopathic "Typical" Trigeminal Neuralgia
   Etiology
      Signs and Symptoms
      Trigger Zones
      Diagnosis
      Differential Diagnosis
   Treatment
      Medical
      Surgical
   Alcohol Injection
   Supraorbital and Supratrochlear
      Nerves
   Infraorbital Nerve
   Inferior Alveolar Nerve
   Mental Nerve
   Maxillary Nerve
   Mandibular Nerve
   Peripheral Neurectomy
      Supraorbital Nerve
      Infraorbital Nerve
      Inferior Alveolar Nerve
      Mental Nerve

      Avulsion of the Nerve by Cryoprobe
   Major Operative Procedures
      Rhizotomy
      Decompression of the Trigeminal Ganglion
B. Symptomatic "Atypical" Trigeminal
   Neuralgia
      Introduction
         Etiology
         Clinical Feature
         Investigations
         Anesthesia Dolorosa

II. Other Cranial Neuralgias
   i. Idiopathic Glossopharyngeal Neuralgia
   ii. Facial Nerve "Geniculate" Neuralgia
   iii. Great Auricular Neuralgia
   iv. Occipital Neuralgia

III. Other Neuropathic Facial Pain
   A. Post-herpetic Neuralgia
   B. Neuroma
   C. Burning Mouth Syndrome
   Taste Disorders

" FACIAL NEURALGIAS"

*If light stimulation produces a pain response out of proportion to the stimulus, a neuropathic process should be **considered**.*

Facial pain: The importance of the face to the individuals self-image and the vital functions of feeding and communication lend special psychosexual and social impact when pain is felt in that region. The clinical features of facial pain are unique in many ways and partly explainable on the basis of special anatomic characteristics. For example: (1) Many peripheral nerves and receptors are confined to non-distensible chambers or canals, such as the dental pulp chamber and the inferior alveolar and infraorbital canals, which may account for unusually intense responses to local pathology. (2) Explosive, paroxysmal pains like tic douloureux are not found outside of the cranial nerve distributions; although the precise etiology is still unknown, the relatively high proportion of large myelinated fibers that make up these nerves may be an, important factor. (3) Vascular pains, are not unique to the head and neck region, but their broad distribution and debilitating nature may be related to the high vascularity of mucous and respiratory membranes as well as the rich plexus of intra- and extracranial vessels.

The circumoral skin is richly innervated with thermoreceptors, nociceptors and mechanoreceptors, the latter including hair cells, touch receptors and pressure receptors. The lips in particular have great tactile sensitivity and a delicate touch or tickle at the edge of the vermilion border can be quite unpleasant even in normal circumstances. Pain in the face is referred to as typical trigeminal neuralgia, or atypical facial neuralgia.

RATIONALIZATION OF FACIAL PAIN

In an attempt to rationalize the language of facial pain, a new classification scheme that divides facial pain into distinct catigories was introduced by Broggi et al (2000).

- *Trigeminal neuralgia type I (TNI):* This is the classic form of trigeminal neuralgia in which episodic lancinating pain predominates.
- *Trigeminal neuralgia type II (TN2):* This is the atypical form of trigeminal neuralgia in which more constant pains (aching, throbbing, burning) predominate.
- *Trigeminal neuralgia pain (TNP):* This is pain that results from incidental or accidental injury to the trigeminal nerve or the brain pathways of the trigeminal system.
- *Trigeminal deafferentiation pain (TDP):* The pain that results from intentional injury to the system in an attempt to treat trigeminal neuralgia. Numbness of the face is a constant part of this syndrome, which has also been referred to as anesthesia dolorosa or one of its variants.
- *Post-herpetic neuralgia(PHN):* This is chronic facial pain that results from an outbreak of herpes zoster (shingles), usually in the ophthalmic division of the trigeminal nerve on the face and usually in elderly patients.
- *Geniculate neuralgia (GeN):* This is typified by episodic lancinating pain felt deep in the ear.
- *Glossopharyngeal neuralgia (GN):* This is typified by pain in the tonsillar area or throat, usually triggered by talking or swallowing.
- Other conditions that may mimic TN include odontogenic pain, temporomandibular disorders, cluster headache, and SUNCT (short-lasting, unilateral neuralgia from headache attacks with conjunctival injection and tearing) syndrome.

I. TRIGEMINAL NEURALGIA

Trigeminal neuralgia was first described at the end of the first century and was later given the name "tic douloureux" because of the distinctive facial spasms that often accompany the attacks.

Trigeminal neuralgia is one of the rare forms of Facial pain which is initially diagnosed in primary care both by doctors and dentists. Patients are often referred to secondary care where care will vary, depending on the specialty to which the patient is referred. Referrals can vary from neurologists, neurosurgeons and pain specialists through to oral and maxillofacial surgeons.

A zone of demyelination in the trigeminal root or pathway seems likely to be responsible for the generation of pain by allowing ephaptic transmissions (cross-talk) to take place between axons.

Basically trigeminal neuralgia is categorized as:

a. *Idiopathic trigeminal neuralgia:* Typical trigeminal neuralgia includes paroxysmal pain alone. No cause of the symptoms can be identified other than vascular compression.

b. *Symptomatic trigeminal neuralgia:* Atypical trigeminal neuralgia includes paroxysmal pain and

constant pain (Toda 2008). Another underlying cause is responsible for the symptoms as brainstem pathology including neoplasms, benign or malignant cysts, aneurysms or arteriovenous malformations, multiple sclerosis, and dental causes.

It is important to determine the type of pain in the face because the treatment of typical facial neuralgia is, in most cases, entirely different from that of atypical neuralgia.

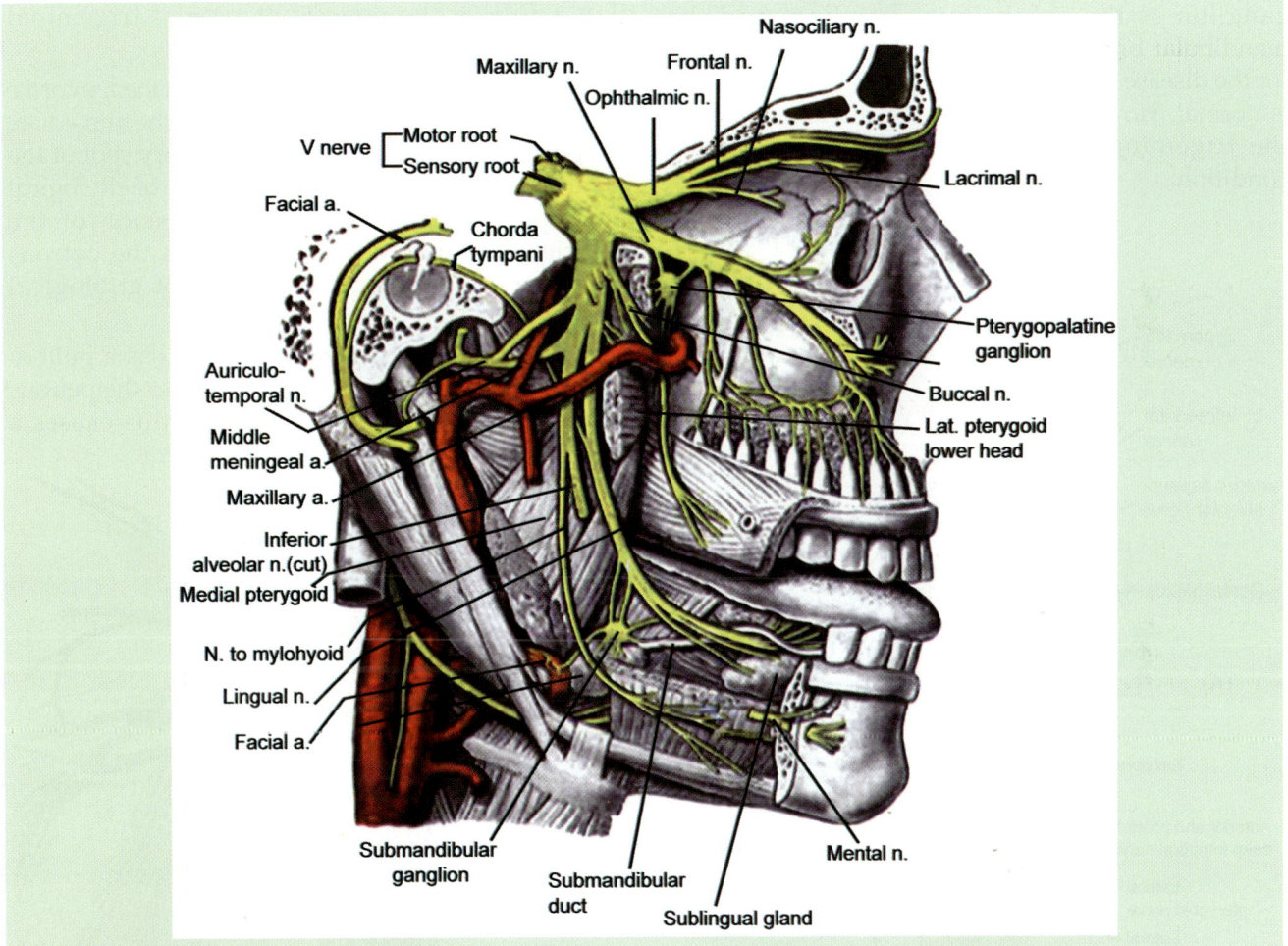

Plate (XVI). The trigeminal nerve and its ramifications into ophthalmic, maxillary, and mandibular branches

A. IDIOPATHIC TRIGEMINAL NEURALGIA

(TYPICAL–TIC–DOULOUREUX)

Trigeminal neuralgia literally signifies nerve pain arising from the trigeminal nerve. The International Association for the Study of Pain defines trigeminal neuralgia as "a sudden and usually unilateral severe, brief, stabbing, recurrent pain in the distribution of

one or more branches of the fifth cranial nerve" (Merskey and Bogduk, 1994).

Typical trigeminal neuralgia occurs more frequently in patients over 50 years age. However, it can occur in much younger patients. Males and females are about equally affected. The second and third divisions of the fifth cranial nerve are predominantly involved, and the right and left sides of the face are equally involved. The pain does not cross to the opposite side of the face, although the condition may affect the face bilaterally in as many as 3 to 5% of patients. The recurring bouts of pain seem to have a seasonal element. They occur particularly in the spring and fall of the year.

There is nothing wrong with the skin in idiopathic trigeminal neuralgia but sensory input is essential and this is conducted with along nerves with large myelinated axons; without it there is no pain. The trigeminal nerve branches (i.e. peripheral to the ganglion as the ophthalmic, maxillary and the mandibular branches) are not held to be responsible for the disease (Fig. 11.1). The neurologic examination is normal. However, a defect or a disease central to the trigeminal ganglion is the etiology of this condition.

ETIOLOGY

The cause of TN is not entirely clear but the consensus of opinion is that pressure on the root entry zone of the trigeminal nerve, in the middle cranial fossa, by a vascular loop leads to focal demyelination. This in turn precipitates ectopic or hyperactive discharge of the nerve. The site of demyelination determines the trigeminal division involved and hence the clinical presentation. Other diseases such as multiple sclerosis and tumors can produce pain similar to that produced by TN.

It is generally agreed that the following factors may play a role in the genesis of typical trigeminal neuralgia:

1. *Compression of the trigeminal nerve at the apex of the petrous ridge of the temporal bone.* The immediate postganglionic portion of the sensory root of the trigeminal nerve is considered to be of etiological importance (Fig.11.2). Compression of the trigeminal nerve where it crosses the petrous ridge of the temporal bone is of etiological importance.

This part of the trigeminal system has a built-in point of compression where it crosses the petrous ridge of the temporal bone and this causes a

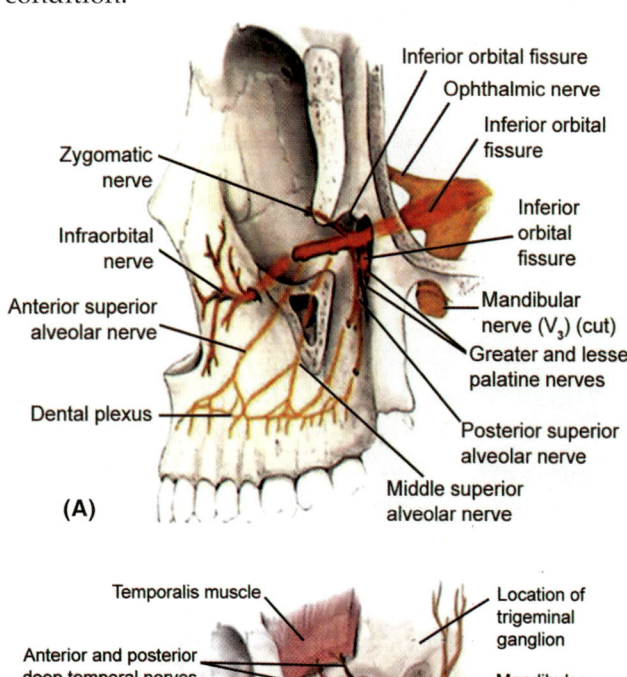

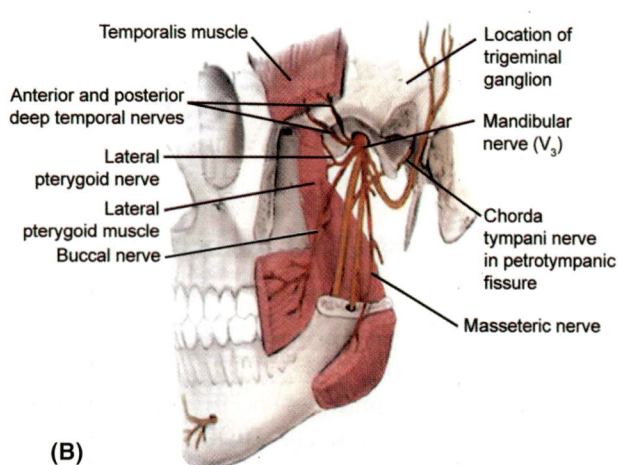

(A)

(B)

Fig. 11.1: The terminal ramifications of the maxillary. **(A)**, and mandibular divisions **(B)** of the trigeminal nerve

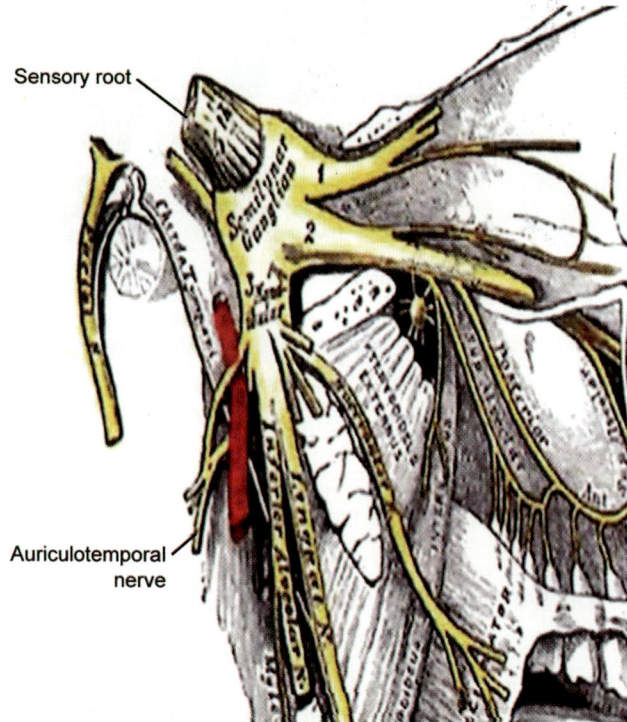

Fig. 11.2: Sensory and motor roots of the trigeminal ganglion are located in the trigeminal crypt (cavum trigeminale) in the middle cranial fossa

considerable bend in the mandibular and maxillary division, and much less change of direction for the fibers of the ophthalmic division (possibly a factor in why this division is less affected) (Fig. 11.3). The extra-compression at the petrous ridge might produce a lesion in the nerve fibers.

2. *Aging.* With aging, the brain tends to sink further into the posterior fossa. There can be a tension of

superficial petrosal sinus runs along the petrous ridge above the nerve roots, or between them and the bone (when it might act as padding). The internal carotid artery lies inferior to the ganglion, close to it, sometimes intimately so and pulsation might be a factor sensitizing the ganglion cells. However, the main vascular factor is thought by

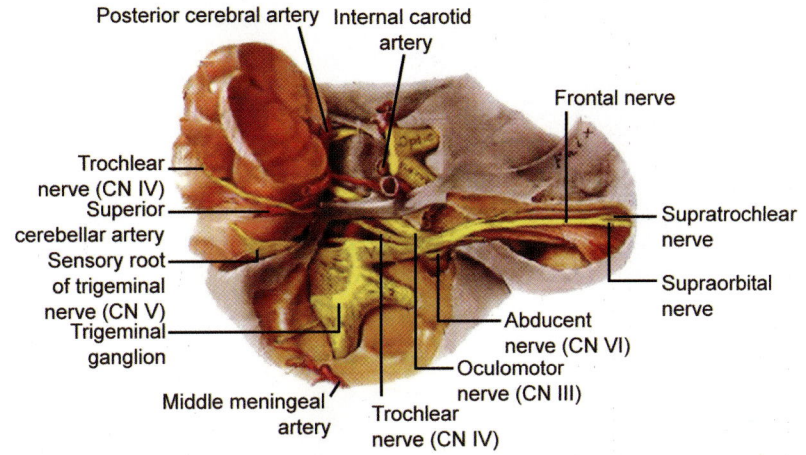

Fig. 11.3: Trigeminal nerve ganglion reveals the bend of the post-ganglionic fibers of the inferior aspect of the sensory root (where the maxillary and mandibular branches lie) while crossing the apex of the petrous ridge of the temporal bone *(Netter's: Atlas of Human Physiology, 1991)*

the axons with loss of myelin. Since the axons thus come to lie closer together, there is opportunity for ionic movements between adjacent fibers so that an impulse in one fiber could be communicated to another "cross-talk". The effect of this could be that neural impulses starting from mechanoreceptors in the skin and travelling in "A" fibers could set up impulses in the smaller "pain fibers" thereby increasing the total number of impulses to the level of a barrage which might be the basis of the shooting pain. Results from experimental studies suggest that demyelinated axons are prone to ectopic impulses, which may transfer from light touch to pain fibers in close proximity (ephaptic conduction) (Love and Coakham 2001).

3. *Neurovascular compression.* In this region, the vascular system may have an important influence. The major cause of trigeminal neuralgia is neurovascular compression, which can frequently be demonstrated by magnetic resonance imaging (MRI). Compression of the vessels on the trigeminal ganglion results in localized, but non-inflammatory sensory root demyelination. The

others to be pressure from a branch of the superior cerebellar artery (Figs 11.4 and 11.5).

The superior cerebellar artery is responsible in cases affecting the maxillary and mandibular divisions whereas the opthalmic division is affected by the inferior cerebellar artery. In one study, 64% of the compressing vessels were identified as an artery, most commonly the superior cerebellar (81%). Venous compression was identified in 36% of cases (Anderson et al, 2006). The relation of the vascular channels to the gasserian ganglion is usually detected in magnetic resonance imaging (Fig. 11.6).

Signs and Symptoms

Patients with typical trigeminal neuralgia describe the pains in various ways, depending on the descriptive adjectives at their command. Usually the pain is depicted as sharp, lancinating, shooting, searing, burning, lacerating, and stabbing. This discomfort resembles an electric shock. There may be only one jab of pain or several in quick succession, each lasting about a second or less. The classical features which help to distinguish trigeminal neuralgia from other

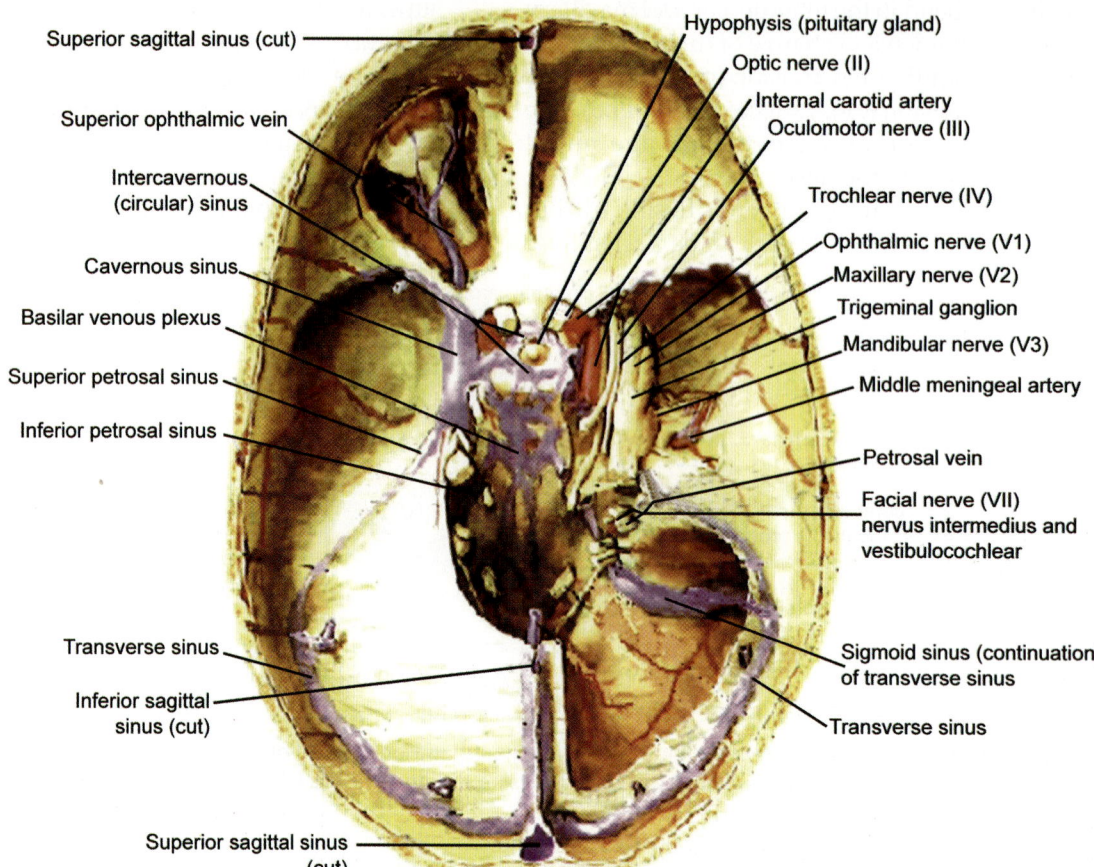

Fig. 11.4: The trigeminal ganglion lies in the trigeminal cave lateral to the apex of the petrous part of the temporal bone. The internal carotid artery lies medial to the ganglion, the petrosal sinus and the cerebral vein

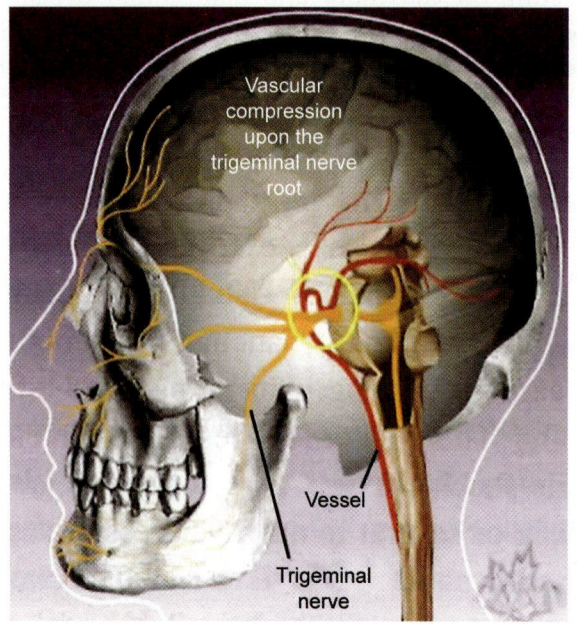

Fig. 11.5: Vascular loop located mesial to gasserian ganglion

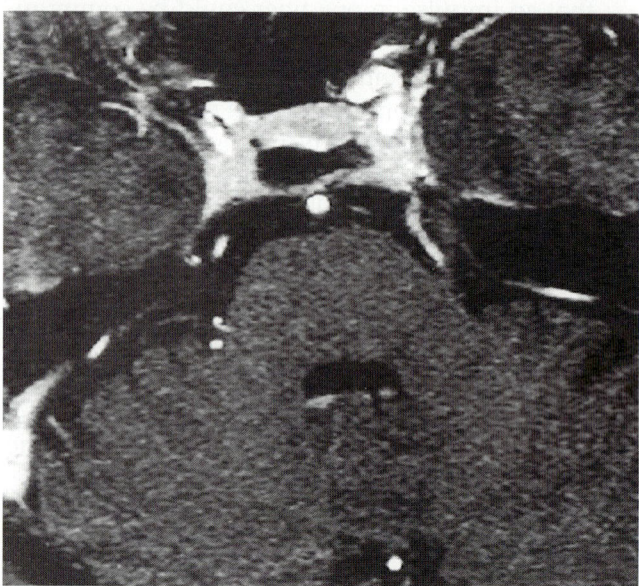

Fig. 11.6: T2-weighted MRI showing a prominent vascular loop passing superomedially to the root entry zone of the left trigeminal nerve suggesting decompression

facial pains of trigeminal neuralgia are summarized as follows (Zakrzewska, 2002; 2006):

1. Each single burst of pain lasts on average under 2 minutes.
2. There is no pain between bursts of pain.
3. Most patients will have complete remission of pain for weeks or months at least initially.
4. The pain is described as sharp, shooting, electric shock-like.
5. The pain is provoked by light touch activities but attacks of pain can also be spontaneous.
6. The pain is always located in the distribution of the trigeminal nerve and first division trigeminal pain is rare.
7. The severity of the pain can vary, especially if medication is used. However, when the disorder is at its peak the pain is suicidal, grossly impairs quality of life and leads to weight loss.
8. Sleep disturbance tends to occur, if the pain is severe.
9. Depression is often noted and there are reports of patients committing suicide or feeling suicidal.
10. Extremely rare to have any autonomic symptoms or signs.

In severe cases, pain can occur spontaneously but in most cases there is a recognizable stimulus. In these cases, the pain is initiated by some peripheral stimulation (external stimulus), such as washing or shaving the face, brushing the teeth, swallowing, yawning, chewing, talking, laughing, cold winds or draughts. It is because of this, the face of a patient suffering from tic douloureux is usually held immobile. The person appears transfixed, hardly daring to move until the attack ceases, this occurring either abruptly or more gradually. However, touch, even if wondrously light, is an effective stimulus rather than the stronger stimuli and a tickling sensation is even more effective. The intensity of an attack and its duration can vary from day to day or even hour to hour, so the case may seem different at different examinations.

Trigger Zones

The above mentioned tremendously light peripheral activities stimulate an area of skin or oral mucosa called a trigger zone causing a severe, unilateral, paroxysmal, shooting pain which seems to be superficial in most cases. Irrespective of the light stimulus, it seems essential that the trigger zone and the underlying tissues appear normal.

Trigger zones are an important feature of trigeminal neuralgia and can be located almost anywhere in the trigeminal receptive area but they are most common in the nasolabial fold, on the upper lip, the angle of the mouth and the lateral part of the lower lip (Figs 11.7 and 11.8). Sometimes the patient may delineate two trigger zones and sometimes a zone shift from one place to another during the course of the disease. Sometimes the trigger zone is large and diffuse but in most cases it is small and well defined, as little as 1 or 2 square millimeters. This is in accordance with the small area of receptor fields in the region. It has been suggested that the preponderance of mechanoreceptor fields in the perioral region could account for the high incidence of trigger points in this area.

The duration of an attack may be only seconds, but although the jabs of severe pain are thought to last only seconds, the effective duration of the attack is also described as one or two minutes or a quarter to half a minute still sounds good. After recognizing the jab as being only about a second, the patient may say that she has to wait 5–10 minutes while the pain dies.

There may be transient contractions at the angle of the mouth or of the eyelids, coincident with the attack, and these give the disease one of its namestic douloureux. There may also be increased lacrimation and associated rhinorrhea, but this is not peculiar to idiopathic trigeminal neuralgia for it occurs with other pain in the anterior part of the mouth and face.

True trigeminal neuralgia tends to become more severe with the passage of time. Only in rare cases, the pain is self-limited and seemingly permanently relieved. At times, a history can be obtained only while the patient is in acute pain. In such cases the examiner instructs the patient to nod his head for an affirmative answer and shake it for a negative response. This is necessary since movement of the jaw or tongue sets off the severe spasm. Considerable questioning is needed in some cases to elicit the information and it should not be forgotten that the patient may be very anxious, fatigued and upset, so care is needed. In one case, a patient had told me of the shooting pain and I asked, 'Where does it shoot to?' She fixed me with a withering look and replied, "I am suffering".

Patients react differently to the spasms of pain, so severe is the pain in some cases that the patient lives in fear of it and avoids activity that might provoke it, for example, the skin may not be washed or shaved, the teeth and gums not cleaned or the hair not

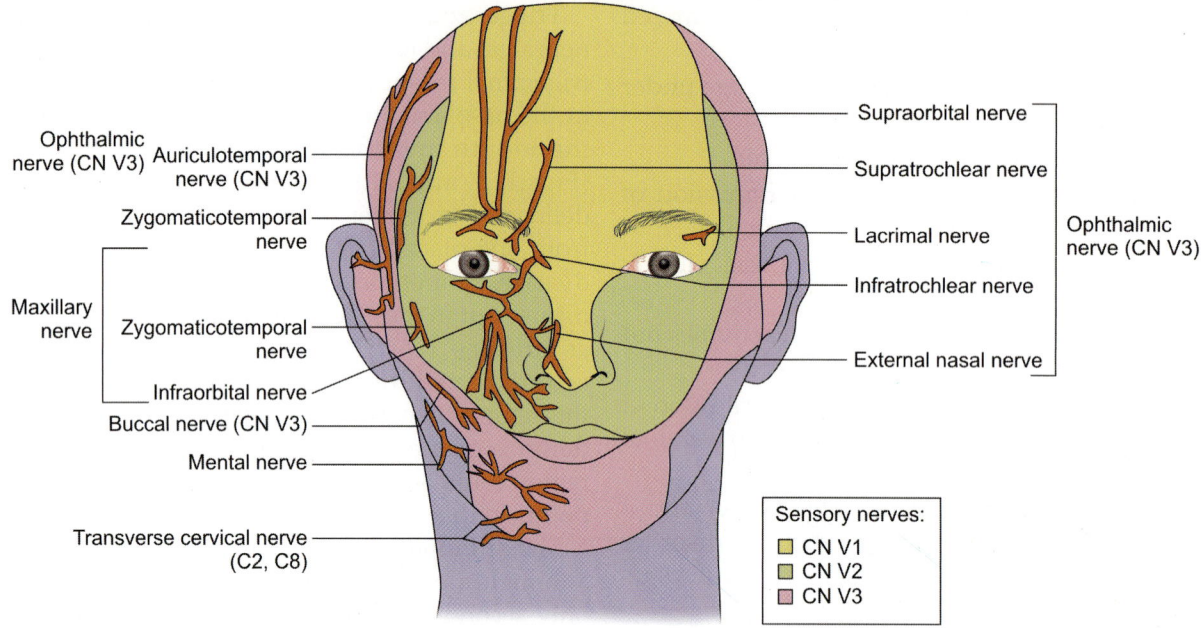

Fig. 11.7: Trigger zones may develop in any facial region supplied by the terminal ramifications of the maxillary or mandibular divisions of the trigeminal nerve

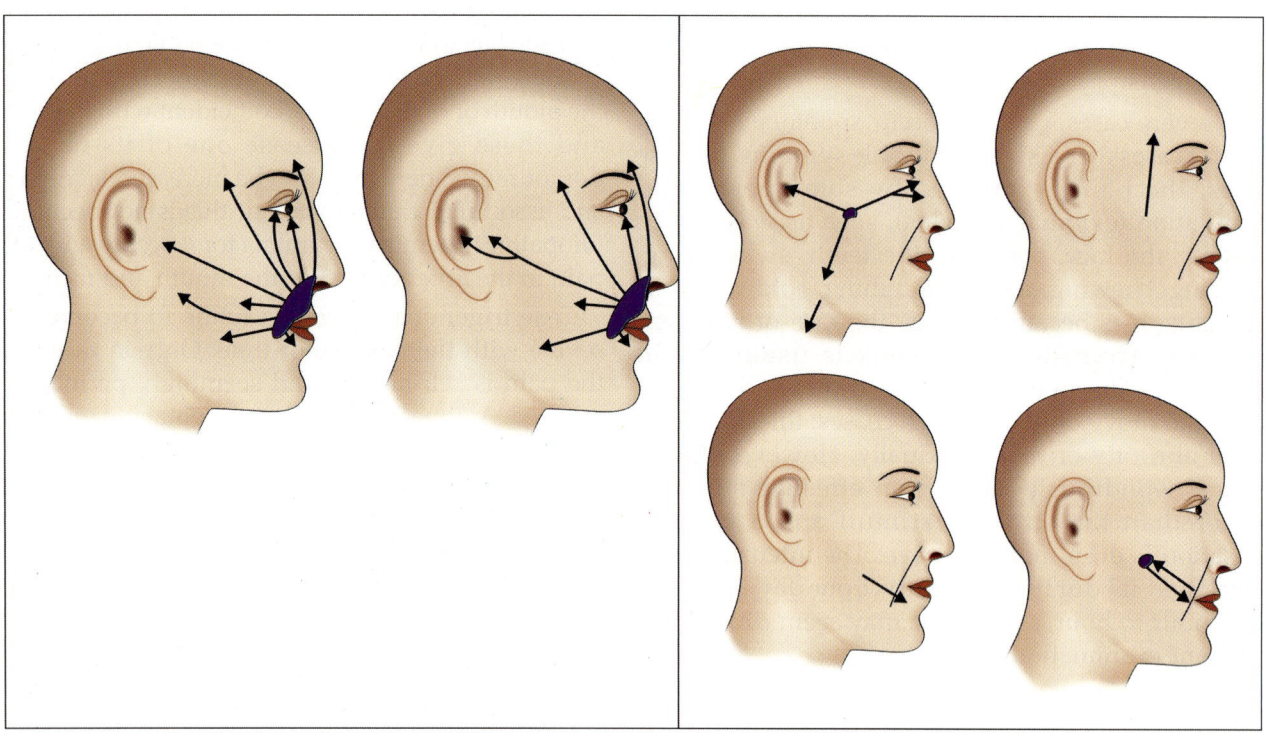

Fig. 11.8: Although the trigger zone of trigeminal neuralgia can be located almost anywhere in the trigeminal receptive area, however, but they are most common in the nasolabial fold, on the upper lip, the angle of the mouth and the lateral part of the lower lip

brushed. The patient may wear a scarf to protect the face against cold air or he may walk backwards into the wind. A few may throw themselves on the floor and scream during a violent spasm. Some remain absolutely immobile with no change in facial expression, even attempting to stop the spontaneous blinking of the eyes. Some patients use curious methods to relieve an attack. In one case, a lumberjack, who had spent most of his life in the deep woods, was able to obtain some measure of relief from the ticlike pains in his upper lip and ala of the nose by applying his tongue to these features. During each spasm, his tongue would appear in jerking movements, slapping the side of his nose. His tongue had attained such length of reach that it could easily touch the mid-portion of his nose.

In many cases, the attack is followed by a "refractory period", a period when triggering does not occur, so touching the trigger zone does not provoke an attack, and this is very variable, possibly lasting for weeks, days, hours, or may be only minutes. The remission periods of months or years sometimes supervene, during which attacks do not occur. Occasionally the patient will finger around the area 'searching' for the trigger, if the clinician asks. Patients report that they can eat alright or talk in this phase. These are the fortunate ones but others are scared to eat and some sufferers lose a great deal of weight.

Ancillary Testing

Laboratory studies generally are not helpful in patients with typical symptoms of trigeminal neuralgia. Occasionally, TMJ or dental radiographs may be useful when TMJ syndrome or dental pain is in the differential diagnosis.

Magnetic resonance imaging (MRI) of the brain is useful to look for multiple sclerosis, tumors, or other causes of symptomatic trigeminal neuralgia, and it should be performed in the initial evaluation of all patients presenting with trigeminal neuralgia symptoms. One recent study demonstrated that trigeminal reflex testing could distinguish classical from symptomatic trigeminal neuralgia with a sensitivity of 96% and a specificity of 93%. Trigeminal reflex testing involves electrical stimulation of the divisions of the trigeminal nerve and measurement of the response with standard electromyography apparatus. This testing is not readily available to most physicians (Cruccu et al, 2006).

Diagnosis

The diagnosis of trigeminal neuralgia should be considered in all patients with unilateral facial pain (Box 11.1). Accurate and prompt diagnosis is important because the pain of trigeminal neuralgia can be severe. Other diagnoses must also be considered, particularly in patients with atypical features of the disease or "red flags" in the history or physical examination. In addition, it is important to distinguish classical from symptomatic trigeminal neuralgia for the purpose of treatment. Symptomatic trigeminal neuralgia is always secondary to another disorder, and treatment should focus on the underlying condition.

Differential Diagnosis

Patients with trigeminal neuralgia have stereotyped attacks; a change in the location, severity, or quality of the pain should alert the physician to the possibility of an alternative diagnosis.

Some disorders that might be included in the differential diagnosis of trigeminal neuralgia are listed in Box 11.2. A careful examination may disclose local findings indicative of otitis, sinusitis, dental disorders, or TMJ dysfunction. A history of persistent pain or pain that occurs episodically in attacks lasting longer than two minutes eliminates classical trigeminal neuralgia and should lead to a search for other diagnoses. The pain of glossopharyngeal neuralgia, which may be triggered by talking or swallowing, is located in the tongue and pharynx. Symptomatic trigeminal neuralgia is usually caused by multiple sclerosis or by tumors arising near the trigeminal nerve root. A history of previous neurologic symptoms and typical findings on MRI assist with the diagnosis of multiple sclerosis. Tumors involving the trigeminal nerve usually cause additional symptoms or examination findings that suggest the diagnosis, and these tumors are generally visible on MRI.

TREATMENT

The treatment of idiopathic trigeminal neuralgia is either medical or surgical and both are associated with unfortunate side effects. Before embarking on long-term drug therapy or neurosurgical procedures, it is essential to be quite certain that there is no a more peripheral cause of the pain. For this reason, it is desirable that a meticulous examination should be made by a dentist. The dentist should preferably be a person who is interested in this subject because the large majority of cases will truly be medical or surgical problems and the tediousness of the dental examination will usually be fruitless and disheartening. Even when the dentist's efforts have no such dramatic result, it is still important to attend to the patient's oral hygiene. Unfortunately, this is often overlooked; yet the patient may be frightened. The

Box 11.1: Algorithm for the diagnosis and treatment of trigeminal neuralgia. (MRI = magnetic resonance imaging), *(Rudolph and Kraft 2008)*

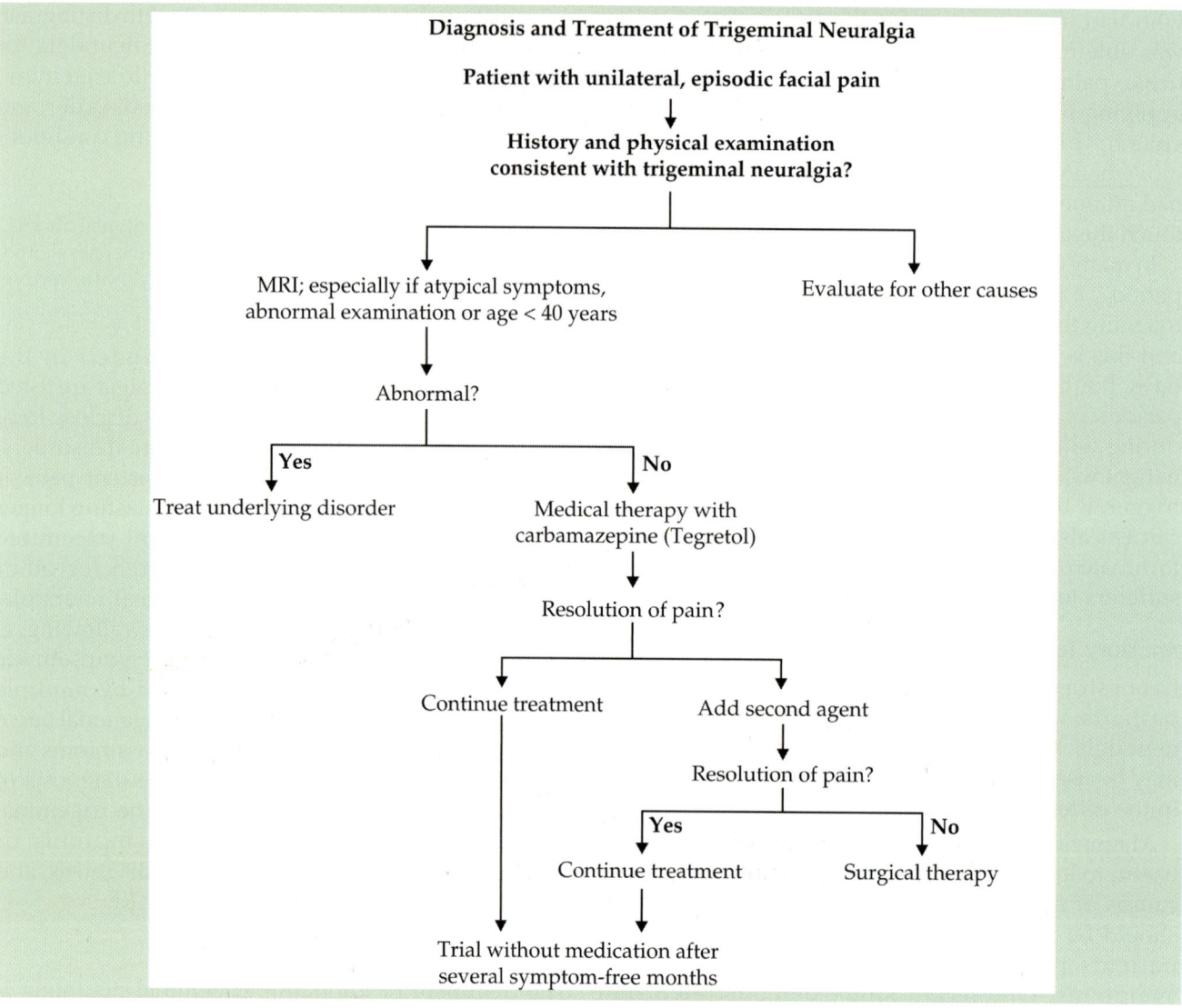

treatment of trigeminal neuralgia can be divided into two modalities—medical and surgical.

Medical Management

The initial choice of treatment for trigeminal neuralgia is medical therapy.

Medical therapy alone is adequate treatment for 75% of patients, however, pharmacological treatment does not cure trigeminal neuralgia, but only relieves pain while the medications are present. According to Dalessio (1982), medications work by interrupting the temporal summation of afferent impulses that precipitate the attack. Once a patient experience some relief of pain on a single agent, a second and even a third additional medication may be required to restore relief (Table 11.1). Medical therapy often is sufficient and effective, allowing surgical consideration only if pharmacologic treatment fails. Because this disorder may remit spontaneously after 6–12 months, patients may elect to discontinue their medication in the first year following the diagnosis and some restart medication in the future.

Medical treatment is generally undertaken with anticonvulsants. The classical medication for the condition is carbamazepine, but newer **anticonvulsants** (e.g. gabapentin, oxcarbazepine) and the **antispastic** baclofen are commonly used as well. These drugs are used to block nerve firing. Many of these

Box 11.2: Differential diagnosis of trigeminal neuralgia

Diagnosis	Features that differentiate from trigeminal neuralgia
Cluster headache	Longer-lasting pain; orbital or supraorbital; may cause patient to wake from sleep; autonomic symptoms
Dental pain (e.g. caries cracked tooth pulpitis)	Localized; related to biting or hot or cold foods; visible abnormalities on oral examination
Giant cell arteritis	Persistent pain; temporal; often bilateral; jaw claudication
Glossopharyngeal neuralgia	Pain in tongue, mouth, or throat; brought on by swallowing, talking, or chewing
Intracranial tumors	May have other neurologic symptoms or signs
Migraine	Longer-lasting pain; associated with photophobia and phonophobia; family history
Multiple sclerosis	Eye symptoms; other neurologic symptoms
Otitis media	Pain localized to ear, abnormalities on examination and tympanogram
Paroxysmal hemicrania	Pain in forehead or eye; autonomic symptoms; responds to treatment with indomethacin {indocin}
Post-herpetic neuralgia	Continuous pain; tingling; history of zoster; often first division
Sinusitis	Persistent pain; associated nasal symptoms
SUNCT	Ocular or periocular; autonomic symptoms
Temporo-mandibular joint syndrome	Persistent pain; localized tenderness; jaw abnormalities
Trigeminal neuropathy	Persistent pain; associated sensory loss

SUNCT= Shorter-lasting, unilateral neuralgiform, conjunctival injection and tearing (Zakrzewska, 2002).

medications have significant and even life-threatening side effects; therefore, only dentists focusing on orofacial pain diagnosis and management use them in dental practice. **Tricyclic antidepressants** such as amitriptyline or nortriptyline are used to treat pain described as constant, burning, or aching. Typical analgesics and opioids are not usually helpful in treating the sharp, recurring pain caused by trigeminal neuralgia.

1. *Carbamazepine* (Tegretol)

Some authors have suggested that carbamazepine is useful as a diagnostic trial for classical trigeminal neuralgia. Lack of response would suggest symptomatic trigeminal neuralgia or another diagnosis, both of which are less likely to respond to the drug.

Carbamazepine, being the most effective, should be the initial treatment for patients with classical trigeminal neuralgia. Other medications may be tried, if carbamazepine is unsuccessful or provides only partial relief.

The starting dosage is usually 100 mg or 200 mg twice daily; this is gradually increased by 200 mg every 2 to 3 days until the pain ceases or side effects ensue. The usual maintenance dosage is 600 to 1,200 mg/day in a divided-dose regimen. Most patients responding to 200 to 800 mg per day in two or three divided doses. A beneficial effect is often apparent within hours to a day or two of starting this medication.

The most common side effects of carbamazepine include drowsiness, dizziness, unsteadiness, nausea and anorexia. These are often transient, lasting weeks, and can be reduced by starting with a low does and increasing the, does slowly. Aplastic anemia is the most feared side effect of carbamazepine therapy but occurs rarely. Reversible leucopenia, neutropenia and/or thrombocytopenia occur in approximately 2% of patients and require periodic complete blood cell counts as well as hepatic and renal function tests. It has been recommended that complete blood cell counts be done every 2 weeks for the first 2 months and then quarterly thereafter, but these recommendations are undergoing re-evaluation given the relatively rare occurrence of serious side effects and the experience involved with frequent testing. From the practical standpoint, once a few months have passed, the frequency of routine testing can probably be reduced to yearly, if even that frequently. If there is a good response to the medication, it can be tapered slowly over 4 to 6 weeks after a patient has been symptom-free for a few months. Tolerance also develops so that this treatment may only be a means of delaying neurosurgery. Nevertheless, it may help the patient to reach a better frame of mind and helps the surgeon to plan the timing and type of surgery.

2. *Baclofen* (Lioresal)

It is another effective drug and some favor it over carbamazepine because it has fewer side effects and

Table 11.1: Common medications and suggested daily dose schedule for trigeminal neuralgia and neuropathic facial pains

Drug	Pretreatment precautions	Starting	Maintenance
Anticonvulsants Carbamazepine (Tegretol)	Electrocardiogram, hematological assessment, hepatic and renal biochemistry.	200 mg	1200 mg
	Side effects: Drowsiness, ataxia, headache, nausea, vomiting, constipation, blurred vision, rash, introduce slowly, drug interactions		
Oxcabamazepine (Trileptal)	Electrocardiogram, hematological assessment, hepatic and renal biochemistry	600 mg	1500 mg
	Side effects: Vertigo, fatigue, dizziness, nausea, hypotnatremia in high doses, no major drug interactions.		
Phenytoin (Dilantin)	**Side effects:** Ataxia, lethargy, nausea, headache, behavioral changes, nausea, headache, folate deficiency in prolonged use, gingival hypertrophy	100 mg	300–400 mg
Tricycline Antidepressants Amitriptyline		10	300
Doxypine			10–150
Nortriptyline Imipramine			10–300
Antispasitic Baclofen (Lioresal)	None *Side effects:* Atoxin, lethargy, fatigue, nausea, vomiting beware rapid withdrawal	10 mg	60 mg
Valproic acid (Depakene)	*Side effects:* Irritability, restlessness, tremor, confusion, nausea, rash, weight gain		

over phenytoin because it is more effective. The usual starting dosage is 5 to 10 mg three times a day, increasing the dose in 10 mg increments every other day until the patient is pain-free or side effects appear. The usual maintenance dosage is approximately 60 mg per day. The most common side effects include drowsiness, dizziness, and gastrointestinal distress. The medication can be slowly tapered after the patient is pain free for approximately 2 months. It should not be discontinued abruptly since hallucinations and seizures can occur. Baclofen has an additive effect with phenytion and carbamazepine.

3. Phenytoin (Dilantin)

It is a second-line drug for treatment of trigeminal neuralgia since it is not as effective as carbamazepine. If carbamazapine is not completely successful in relieving pain, it may be supplemented with analgesics, or phenytoin (Epanutin) in an equivalent dose. The usual maintenance dosage is 300 to 400 mg per day in two divided doses with an aim to achieve a therapeutic blood level and a positive clinical response. Rapid therapeutic serum levels can be achieved with an oral loading does of 20 mg/kg over a day. The most common side effects of phenytoin are drowsiness, dizziness, diplopia, ataxia, and cognitive dysfunction.

A variety of other medications and modalities have been tried for treatment of trigeminal neuralgia.

1. There are small studies reporting success with botulinum toxin type A (Botox) in some patients (Piovesan et al, 2005).
2. One case report of relief being experienced after an accidentally high discharge from a transcutaneous electrical nerve stimulation unit (Thorsen and Lumsden, 1997).
3. Topical capsaicin (Zostrix) was helpful for trigeminal neuralgia pain in one open-label trial (Epstein and Marcoe, 1994).
4. One recent study found that intranasal lidocaine (xylocaine) significantly decreased second-division trigeminal neuralgia pain for more than four hours (Kanai et al, 2006).
5. TN trigeminal nerve block with high concentrations of local anesthetics is considered as a percutaneous procedure in the management of

trigeminal neuralgia. The basic concept of applying high concentrations of lidocaine for the treatment of TN pain is its neurotoxic nature. Evidence indicates that lidocaine is perhaps more neurotoxic as a local anesthetic (LA) than other commonly used LAs, such as bupivacaine, tetracaine, mepivacaine and prilocaine (Rigler et al 1991, Drasner et al 1994). Nevertheless, it would be ideal to treat chronic pain with lidocaine, if such neurotoxicity leads to the blocking of pain-producing processes through nerve axons for a relatively long period without other functional abnormalities. Han et al (2008) studied the effects of trigeminal nerve block using high concentration (10%) lidocaine. They reported that trigeminal nerve blocks with 10% lidocaine were able to achieve considerably long duration of pain relief in certain TN patients who have relatively lower pain intensity and shorter duration of current pain attacks.

Surgical Management

Trigeminal neuralgia itself does not cause death, but the patient may be unable to eat or may die by self-inflicted means. A good policy is to describe the condition thoroughly to the patient, preferably in the presence of a close relative or friend, and then review in detail the various methods of treatment that may be instituted. The importance of a thorough discussion of the problem with the patient cannot be over-emphasized. The patient should be asked to express his opinions and to choose the type of treatment he wishes carried out. The consensus of opinions is to stress on the value of conservative procedures initially in most instances. Patients with trigeminal neuralgia are usually treated pharmacologically.

Indications for Surgical Management

Surgery is not right for everyone, and patients should be informed about their full range of choices. Usually Patients gain benefit from having surgery earlier than later in the disease process to improve quality of life, freedom from medication and need for regular follow-up (Zakrzewska and Patsalos, 2002). Surgical approaches are performed in the following conditions:

• When medication cannot control pain, i.e. when the patient does not attain pain relief after adequate trials of 2 or 3 medications.

• Patients cannot tolerate the adverse effects of the medication.

• In medically complex patients with polypharmacy for other conditions.

• When pain relief is attained but the patient requires medication dosing at levels that result in significant drug toxicity.

Non-pharmacological treatment includes:

I. *Alcohol injection "neurolytic block":* Neurolytic injections may be tried, using either absolute alcohol, phenol, or glycerol applied either to branches (supraorbital, infraorbital, inferior alveolar, or mental) or divisions (maxillary, mandibular) or even into the trigeminal ganglion "ganglionlysis", and these are effective for variable periods usually from months to about two years.

II. *Peripheral neurectomy:* Surgical transaction of the involved terminal branch of the trigeminal nerve, e.g. supraorbital, infraorbital, inferior alveolar, or mental.

III. *Major operative procedures*
  a. Rhizotomy.
  b. Balloon microcompression of the trigeminal ganglion.
  c. Microvascular decompression.

Zakrzewska and Lindsay (2009) categorized the surgical management of trigeminal neuralgia cases they performed, as shown in Table 11.2.

I. ALCOHOL INJECTION

For the dentist alcohol injection, freezing, or neurectomy of the involved trigeminal branch arrest the painful episode temporary, however, proper diagnosis of TN is essential so that unneeded dental treatment or extraction is avoided.

Of all the minor operative procedures instituted for the relief of pain in trigeminal neuralgia, alcohol injections into the various branches of the trigeminal nerve are the most helpful, and can usually be given quickly by trained individuals. The use of streptomycin as an alternative to alcohol has been reported. Here again, the pros and cons regarding the usefulness of alcohol injections must be thoroughly explained to the patient. The value of these injections is limited almost exclusively to neuralgia involving the second and third divisions of the fifth cranial nerve. Satisfactory injection of the first division, or supraorbital nerve, is difficult because, as the nerve emerges from

Table 11.2: Surgical management of trigeminal neuralgia, data on 5 years not available for some procedures

Procedure	%probability of being pain free	Mortality	Morbidity
Peripheral: neurectomy, cryotherapy, alcohol, injections, acupuncture	Two years—22	Nil	Low sensory loss, fronsient haematoma, oedema
Radiofrequency theramorhizotomy (RFT)	Two years—68 Five years—48	Low	Complications mainly relating to trigeminal nerve, dysethesia, anesthesia dolorosa, eye problems, masticatory problems, sensory loss over 50%.
Percutaneous glycerol rhizotomy	Two years—63 Five years—45	Low	Complications as for RFT but fewer cases of sensory loss
Balloon microcompression	Two years—79	Low	Complications as for RFT, with sensory loss but temporary mosticatory problems common.
Microvascular decompression	Two years—81 Five years—76 Ten years—70	0.4%	Overall 75% no complications, 16% transient cranial nerve 4th, 6th, 4% 8th dysfunction with 2% permanent deafness
Gamma knife surgery	Two years—58	Nil	Late onset of relief, may only be partial, 7% sensory loss up to 2 years post-treatment.

Adapted from Zakrewska and Linskey (2009)

the supraorbital notch, it divides almost immediately into fine branches.

Indications

The indications for alcohol injections are as follows:

1. When the diagnosis of tic douloureux is not certain, prolonged anesthesia of a branch of the trigeminal nerve may be helpful in making the correct diagnosis.

2. To give quick relief to the patient who has acute tic pain; this is of value particularly to the patient who must attend to pressing business efforts, or has important engagements that cannot be postponed.

3. To relieve elderly or debilitated patients suffering from other incurable disease, with a short life expectancy.

4. Patients who express reservations over the anesthesia which would result from root or ganglion destruction.

Alcohol injections have fallen into disrepute for a number of reasons.

- In the first place, formerly when performed without the aid of anesthesia, the injection was excessively painful. With the use of sodium thiopental (pentothal) intravenously, which induces light anesthesia, alcohol can be injected painlessly into the infraorbital nerve, branches of the second and

third trigeminal division, or the trunk of the second and third divisions of the trigeminal nerve as it emerges from the skull and the patient has complete amnesia regarding the injection.

- Secondly, it has been said that relief obtained by injections lasts only for a few months and, therefore is not worthwhile. In our experience, the period of relief is about a year, and many patients are relieved for much longer intervals. If the injection is not made properly— that is, if the needle does not enter the substance of the nerve— the injection may be completely ineffective, or relief may last only a few weeks.

Many patients ask to have the alcohol injection repeated. This has been accomplished in patients for many years even though a certain amount of scar tissue has formed in or around the nerve, thus making it more difficult to penetrate the nerve at the site of the previous injection due to fibrosis (Zakrzewska 1995).

After anesthesia in the correct region has been obtained and pain relief monitored with local anesthesia, 0.5 to 1.0 ml 100% absolute alcohol is injected. The average pain free time varies between one month to 22 months. The complications following alcohol injections include: sensory loss, skin necrosis, diplopia, burning sensation on the tongue and palate, avascular necrosis, infected hematoma, trismus, paresthesia, hypothesia, eye complaints (comprised of tearing, pain, reduced corneal sensitivity, and impaired vision).

The supraorbital, infraorbital, inferior dental, mental, maxillary, mandibular nerves and others are reported to be blocked with alcohol. The techniques used for alcohol injections of the various nerves are discussed below.

A. Injection of the Supraorbital and Supratrochlear Nerves

Clinically Relevant Anatomy

The supraorbital nerve arises from fibers of the frontal nerve, which is the largest branch of the ophthalmic nerve. The frontal nerve enters the orbit via the superior orbital fissure and passes anteriorly beneath the periosteum of the roof of the orbit (Fig. 11.9). The frontal nerve gives off a larger lateral branch, the supraorbital nerve and a smaller medial branch, the supratrochlear nerve (Fig. 11.10). Both exit the orbit anteriorly. The supraorbital nerve sends fibers all the way to the vertex of the scalp and provides sensory innervation to the forehead, upper eyelid and anterior scalp (Fig. 11.11).

Technique

The supraorbital notch on the affected side is identified by palpation. The skin overlying the notch is prepared with antiseptic solution, with care being taken to avoid

spillage into the eye. A 25-gauge, 1½-inch needle is inserted at the level of the supraorbital notch and is advanced medially approximately 15 degrees off the perpendicular to avoid entering the foramen (Fig. 11.12).

The needle is advanced until it approaches the periosteum of the underlying bone. A paresthesia may be elicited and the patient should be warned of such. The needle should not enter the supraorbital foramen, and should this occur, the needle should be withdrawn and redirected slightly more medially.

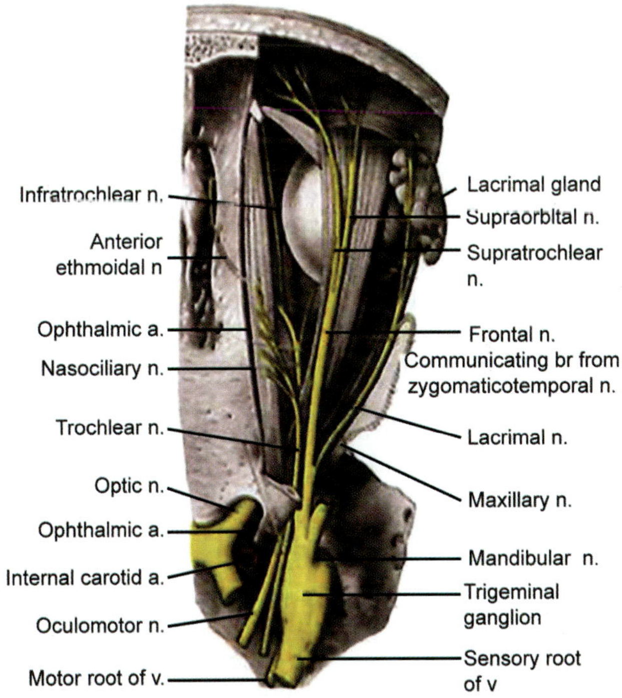

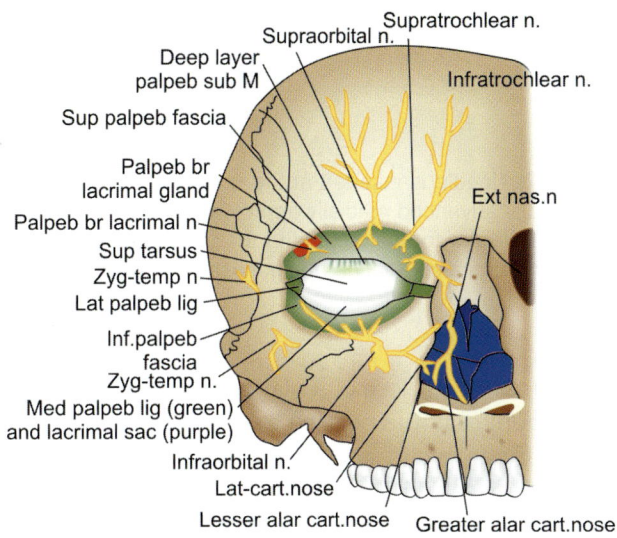

Fig. 11.10: Terminal branches of the frontal nerve

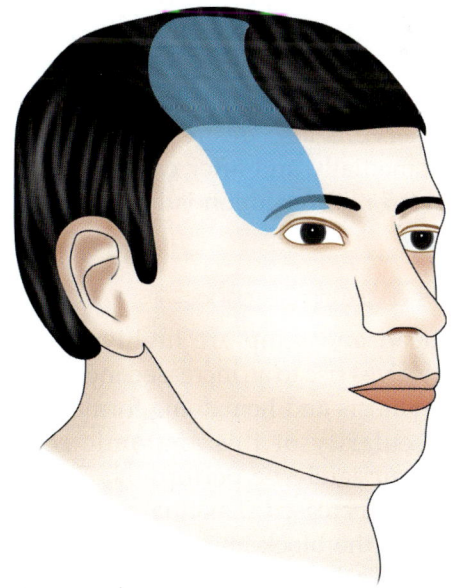

Fig. 11.9: The supratrochlear and supraorbital nerves are ramifications of the frontal division of the ophthalmic nerve

Fig. 11.11: Sensory distribution of supraorbital and supratrochlear nerves

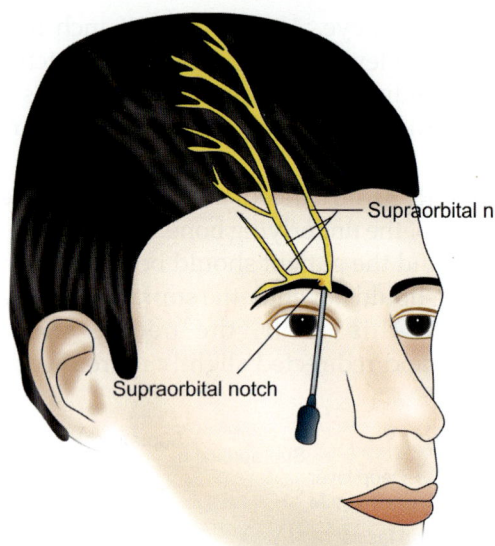

Fig. 11.12: Needle is inserted at the level of the supraorbital notch and is advanced medially approximately 15 degrees off the perpendicular to avoid entering the foramen. The needle is advanced until it approaches the periosteum of the underlying bone

Because of the loose alveolar tissue of the eyelid, a gauze sponge should be used to apply gentle pressure on the upper eyelid and supraorbital tissues before injection of solution to prevent the injection from dissecting inferiorly into these tissues.

This pressure should be maintained after the procedure to avoid periorbital hematoma and ecchymosis. After gentle aspiration, a 0.5 to 1 of absolute or 80% alcohol and 1% procaine are injected in a fan-like distribution. If blockade of the supra-trochlear nerve is also desired, the needle is then redirected medially and after careful aspiration, an additional 0.5 ml of solution is injected in a fan-like manner.

Side Effects and Complications

The forehead and scalp are highly vascular, this vascularity gives rise to an increased incidence of post-block ecchymosis and hematoma formation. In spite of the vascularity of this anatomic region, this technique can safely be performed. These complications can be decreased, if manual pressure is applied to the area of the block immediately after injection. Application of cold packs for 20-minute periods after the block also decreases the amount of post-procedure pain and bleeding the patient may experience.

B. Alcohol Injection of the Infraorbital Nerve

Clinically Relevant Anatomy

The infraorbital nerve is the terminal ramification of the maxillary nerver (Fig. 11.13). It emerges from the front of the maxilla through the infraorbital foramen. At this point, an infraorbital nerve block is readily administered as the fluid will difuse back through the canal to reach the anterior superior dental nerve.

The infraorbital nerve divides into its terminal branches which are shown in Fig. 11.14.

i. Palpebral branches passing to the skin of the lower eyelid and associated conjunctiva.

ii. Nasal branches to the skin of the side of the nose.

iii. Labial branches to the skin and mucous membrane of the upper lip, the labial gingiva and the vestibule of the nose.

The infraorbital foramen is located at the junction of the middle and inner thirds of the infraorbital ridge. A shallow depression can be felt which indicates the location of the infraorbital foramen (Fig. 11.15). This point is also on a line with the pupil of the eye when the patient looks straightforward (Fig. 11.16).

On palpation of the infraorbital ridge, a depression is felt below it. Move the palpating thumb or index finger 0.5 cm below the infraorbital ridge at the junction of its middle and inner thirds, now you are over the infraorbital foramen.

Intraoral Injection

The syringe and the needle are lined up parallel to the 2nd bicuspid and the needle is passed through the tensed tissue directly to the infraorbital foramen. The infraorbital foramen is configured such that its long axis is directed medially and caudally. Therefore, cannulation of the foramen requires that the needle be directed laterally and cephalad. The needle is inserted parallel to the long axis of the second premolar tooth (Fig. 11.17). The block can be accomplished by injecting 1 to 2 ml of anesthetic using a small-gauge needle at a point where the nerve exits the foramen. By gentle probing with the point of the needle, the infraorbital canal is entered and 0.5 to 1.0 cc. of alcohol injected.

Extraoral Injection

The needle is inserted in the nasolabial crease approximately one cm. below the medial third of the lower eyelid (Fig. 11.18). By gentle probing with the point of the needle, the infraorbital canal is entered and 0.5 to 1.0 cc. of alcohol injected. There should be immediate

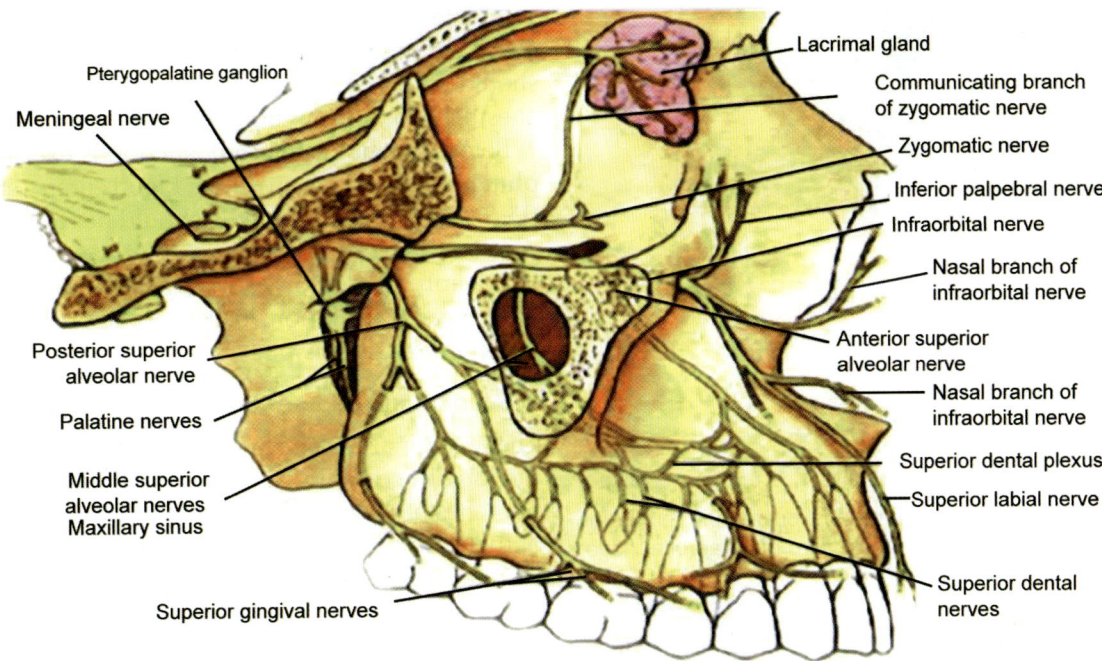

Fig. 11.13: The dental and paradental tissues supplied by the maxillary nerve

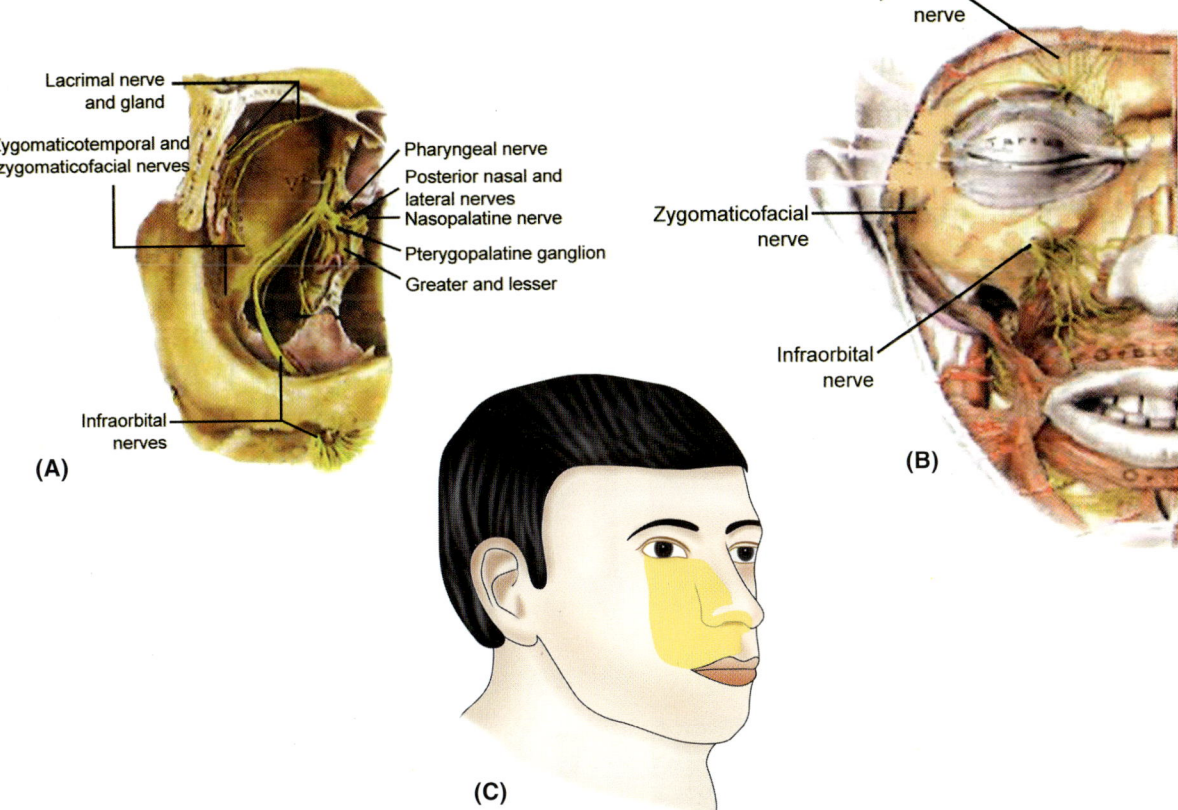

Fig. 11.14: (A) Pathway of the infraorbital nerve in the infraorbital groove. **(B)** Emergence of the infraorbital nerve on the face through the infraorbital foramen. **(C)** Approximate areas of the facial region (lower eyelid, anterior cheek, and upper lip) supplied by the infraorbital nerve

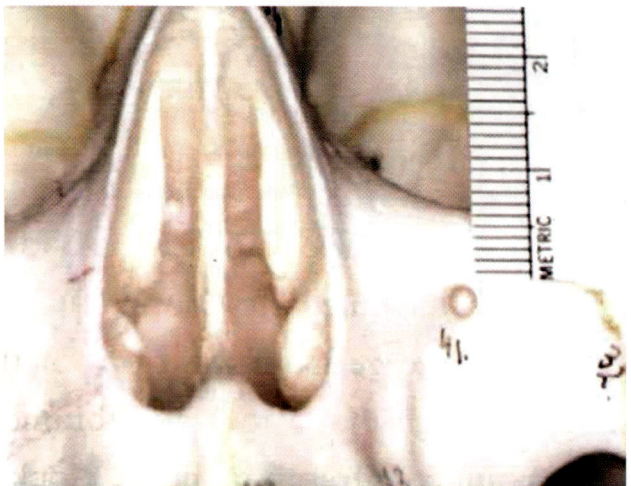

Fig. 11.15: The infraorbital foramen is located 0.5 mm below the junction of the inner and middle third of infraorbital ridge

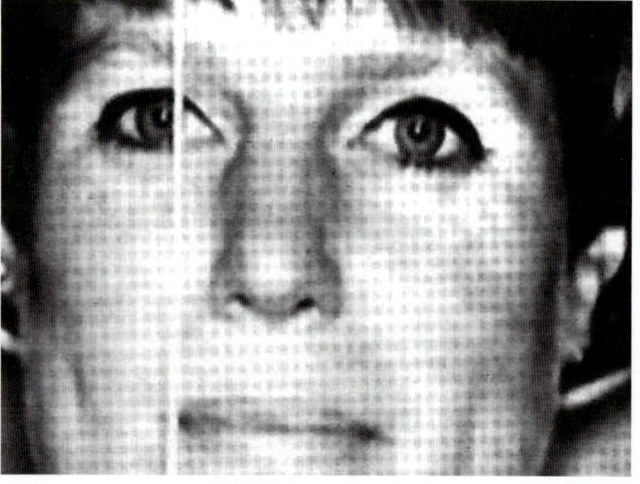

Fig. 11.16: Vertical alignment of the medial edge of the pupil with the infraorbital foramen (frontal view)

complete anesthesia of the infraorbital distribution. The ala of the nose and the medial portion of the upper lip should be tested for anesthesia. If they are completely anesthetized, the injection will be successful.

Before alcohol is injected, suction is exerted on the plunger to determine whether blood enters the syringe (Fig. 11.19). If so, the needle should be replaced in the proper position. The needle should not be inserted too deeply into the infraorbital canal, since the point may enter the inferior portion of the orbit because of a thin membranous plate.

C. Alcohol Injection of the Inferior Alveolar Nerve

The inferior alveolar (dental) nerve, the lingual nerve, the long buccal nerve as well as the mental nerve are branches of the mandibular nerve (Fig. 11.20). Because of their proximity, the inferior alveolar nerve injection results in anesthetization of the inferior alveolar nerve, the lingual nerve and occasionally the long buccal nerve. The inferior dental nerve block is by far the commonest used in dentistry, the reason being that it is the only satisfactory way of achieving analgesia in the area it supplies (Fig. 11.21).

A long needle (32 mm) must be used (Figs 11.22 and 11.23) because penetration to 25 mm may be needed. The needle should be inserted, from the contralateral side. When the needle is inserted as shown in Fig. 11.23, it contacts bone. This indicates that the needle points towards mandibular foramen. Prior to injection, aspiration is necessary to rule out intravascular injection. 0.5 to 1 ml of alcohol is injected.

Profound anesthesia develops within 2 to 5 minutes. The patient experiences the following subjective symptoms:

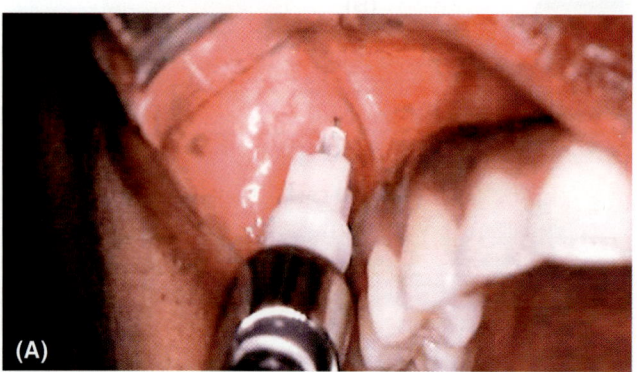

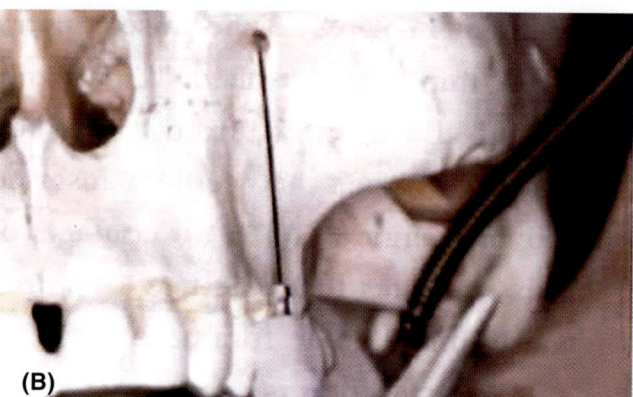

Fig. 11.17: (A) The needle is inserted 5 mm labial to the depth of the buccal sulcus parallel to the second bicuspid. **(B)** Clinical view showing the needle penetrating the tissues 5 mm buccal to the mucobuccal fold parallel to the long axis of the second premolar tooth

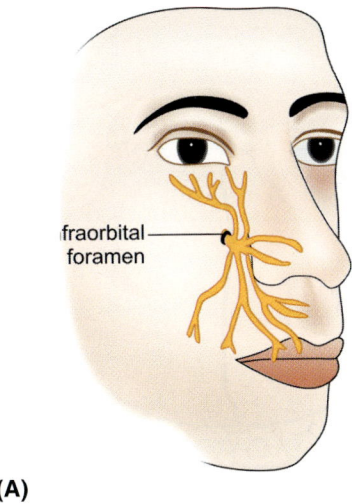

(A)

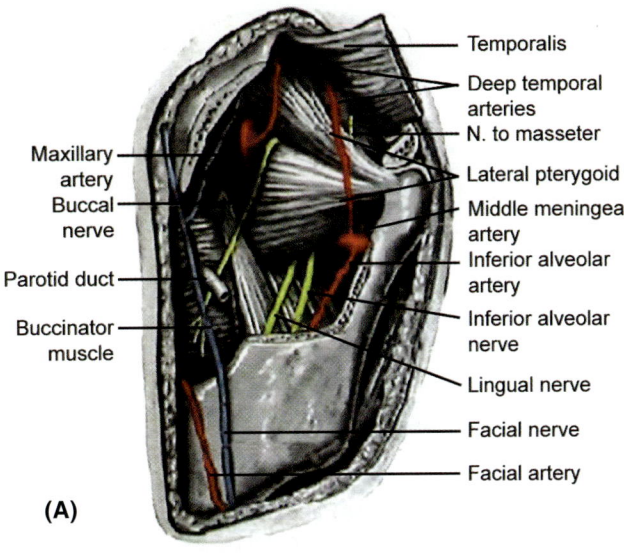

(A)

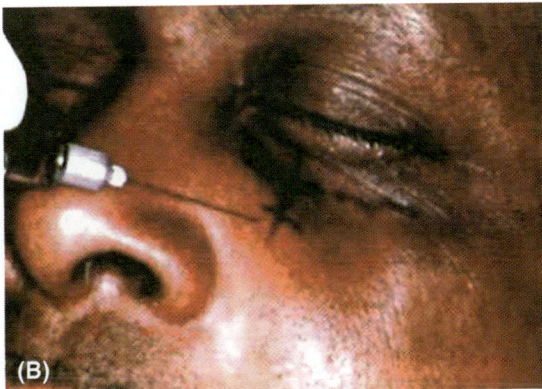

(B)

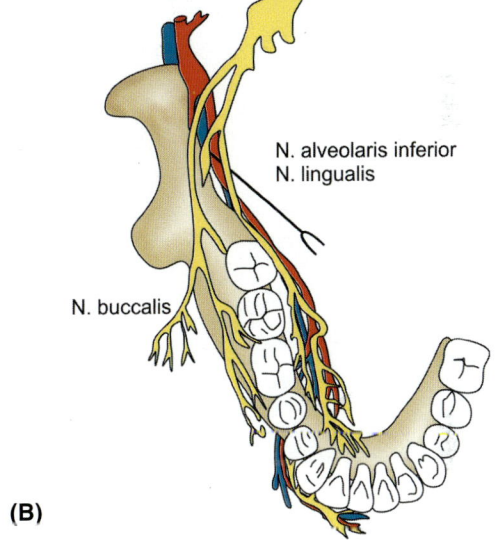

(B)

Fig. 11.18: **(A)** The infraorbital foramen lies approximately 0.5 cm below the infraorbital margin. The location of the infraorbital foramen is marked and the needle is inserted obliquely to the bone surface. **(B)** After feeling the infraorbital foramen with the needle, pass the needle gently 1–2 mm and inject slowly one ml of alcohol

Fig. 11.20(A and B): **(A)** Anatomic relation of the buccal, lingual, and inferior alveolar branches of the mandibular nerve. **(B)** The inferior alveolar, the lingual and the long buccal nerves are very proximate to each other

a. A feeling of warmth or a tingling sensation in the lip which starts at the corner of the mouth and spread until it reaches the midline of the lip. The tingling changes into a gradually increasing feeling of profound numbness; the lip may also feel very swollen.

b. The tip and side of the tongue tingle and then become numb.

D. Alcohol Block of the Mental Nerve

The mental nerve is a large branch of the inferior alveolar that leaves the interior of the mandible to

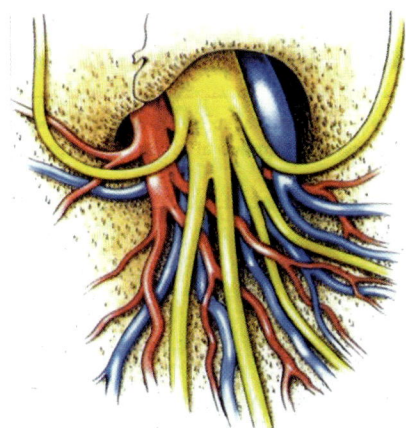

Fig. 11.19: Neurovascular bundle exits from the infraorbital foramen with the infraorbital nerve

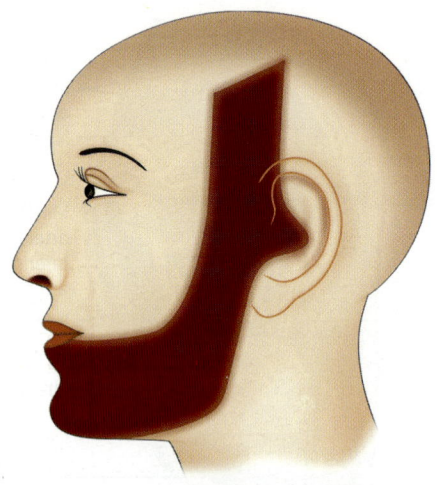
(A)

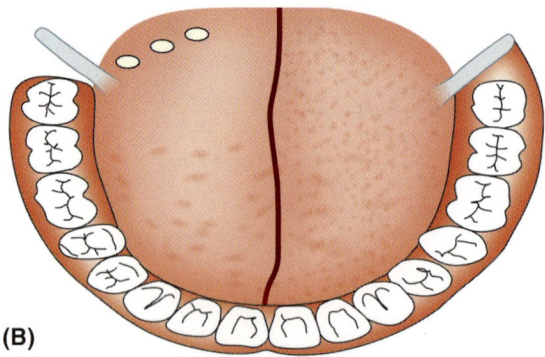
(B)

Fig. 11.21: The extraoral **(A)** and intraoral **(B)** anatomic regions supplied by the mandibular nerve which are anesthetized by alcohol injection of the inferior dental nerve

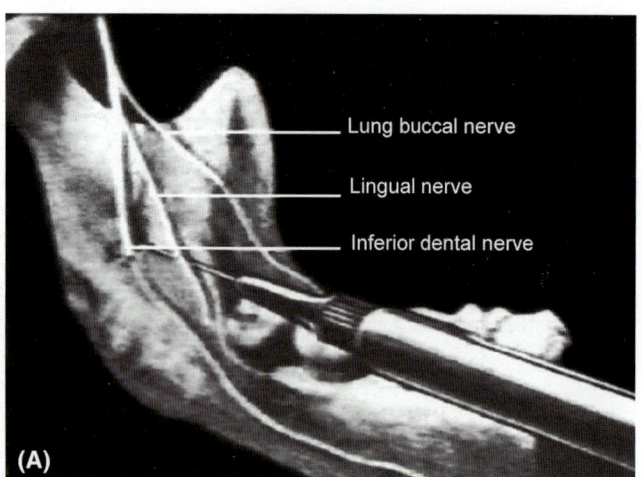
(A)

Lung buccal nerve

Lingual nerve

Inferior dental nerve

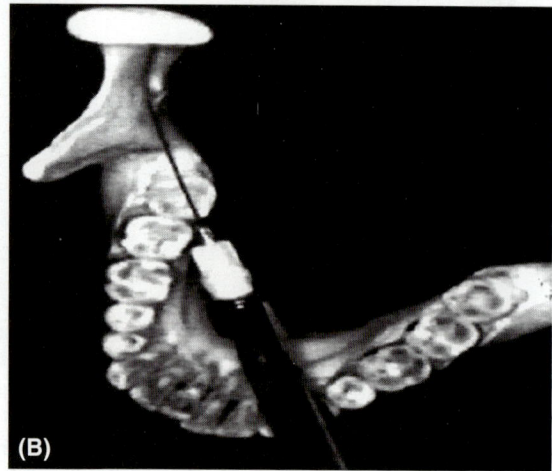
(B)

Fig. 11.22: (A) The needle points to the entrance of the inferior alveolar nerve into the mandibular canal. **(B)** The region where the local anesthetic agent should be deposited

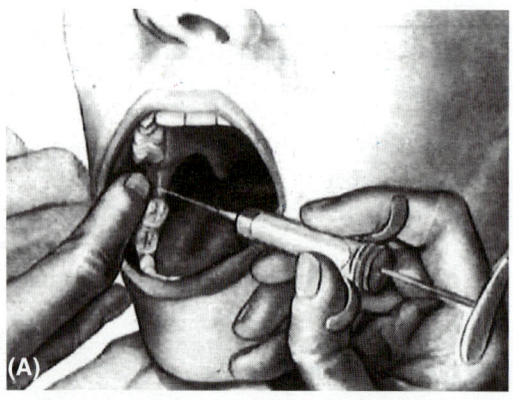
(A)

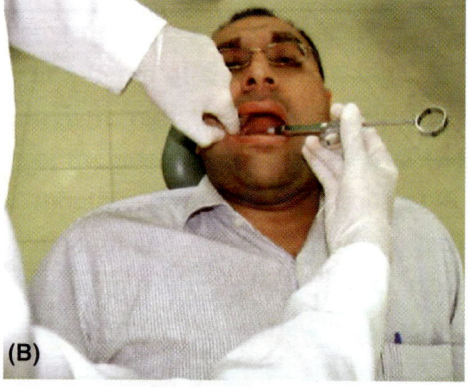
(B)

Fig. 11.23: (A) Right inferior alveolar nerve injection. With the left index finger delineating the site of the injection, keeping the barrel over the opposite bicuspid area and parallel to the occlusal plane of the mandibular teeth or ridge. **(B)** The needle is inserted in the deepest point of the retromolar triangle until it contacts bone at the point of entry of the inferior alveolar nerve into the mandibular foramen

supply the skin of the chin and lower lip, the mucosa of the lip and the adjacent gum to the midline (Fig. 11.24).

It is indicated when the trigger zone is present near the angle of the mouth, lower lip or chin region, i.e. anterior to the anatomic location of the mental foramen. The mental foramen may usually be found on the vertical line drawn downward from the supraorbital notch. It lies between the apices of the first and second premolar teeth. The needle is inserted into the opening of the mental foramen from the posterior superior direction (Fig. 11.25).

Intraoral Injection

The needle is inserted in the mucobuccal fold below the apex of the second premolar tooth (Fig. 11.25). Aspirate, if negative, slowly deposit 0.5 to 1 ml over 20 seconds. Tingling or numbness of the lower lip usually develops immediately.

Extraoral Injection

A 25-gauge, 1½-inch needle is inserted at the level of the mental notch and is advanced medially approximately 15 degrees off the perpendicular and the needle is advanced until it approaches the periosteum of the underlying bone (Fig. 11.26). Paresthesia is usually elicited and the patient should be warned of such. After gentle aspiration, 0.5 to 1 ml of alcohol is injected in a fan-like distribution.

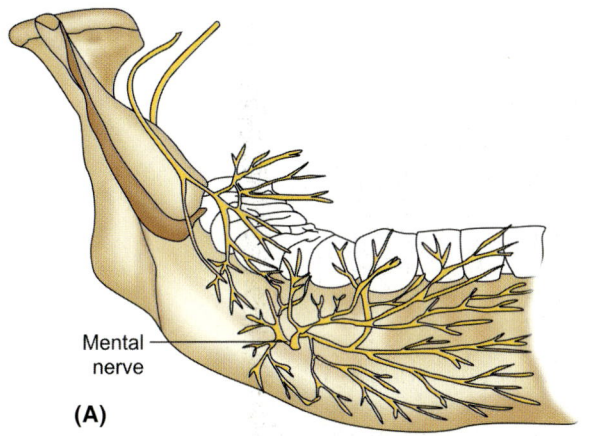

Mental nerve

(A)

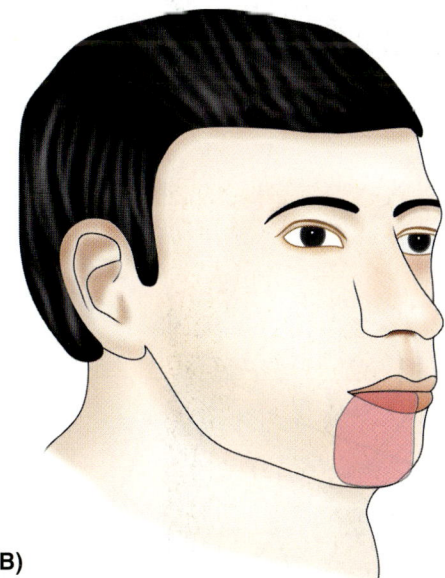

(B)

Fig. 11.24: (A) Emergence of the mental nerve through the mental foramen. **(B)** The mental nerve is responsible for sensory innervations of the lower lip and chin

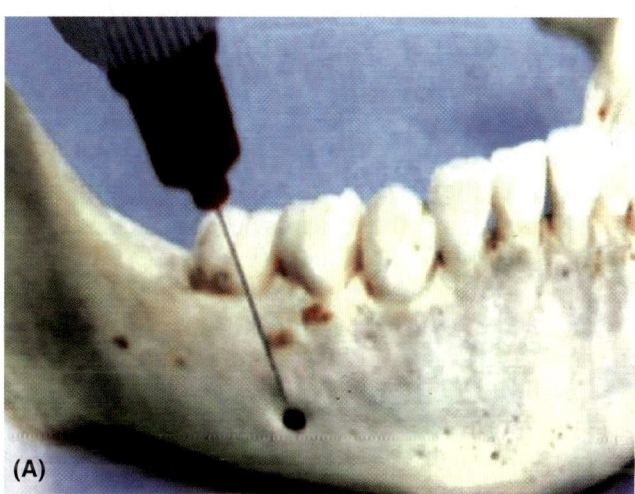

(A)

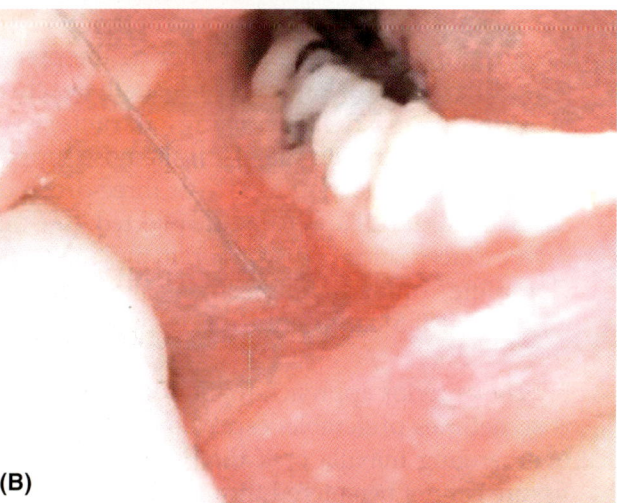

(B)

Fig. 11.25 (A and B): The needle is advanced toward the mental foramen from behind as the foramen faces posteriorly. The depth of penetration will be 5 to 6 mm

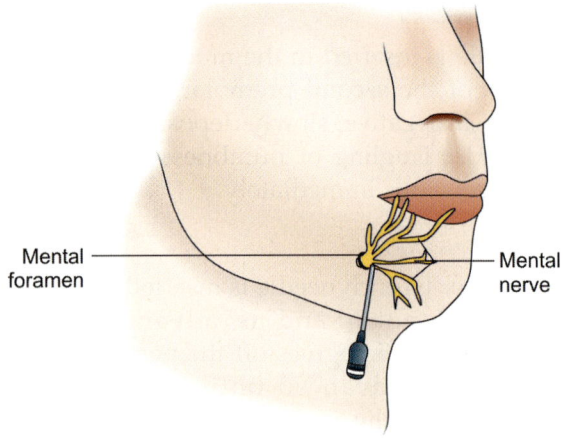

Fig. 11.26.

E. Alcohol Injection of the Maxillary Nerve at the Foramen Rotundum

Alcohol injection of the second division of the trigeminal nerve is used only if the pain involves the roof of the mouth. Otherwise, infraorbital nerve injection is adequate and is a simple procedure compared to the injection at the foramen rotundum.

A. The position of the patient's head and the position of the surgeon are identical with those used in the third division alcohol injection. The needle is marked at 6.0 cm, with a tiny piece of adhesive, and is directed slightly more anteriorly than in the third division in order to strike the external pterygoid plate.

B. a-1. Needle in contact with the external pterygoid plate.

a-2. Needle directed slightly more anteriorly and toward the base of the skull, entering the pterygomaxillary fissure. The nerve is usually reached at a depth of 5.5 cm, causing characteristic radiation of pain into the ala of the nose, upper lip and roof of the mouth. Two or three drops of 80% alcohol and 1% procaine are injected, causing severe exacerbation of discomfort in these regions. Complete, immediate anesthesia follows. An additional 0.5 cc. of solution is then injected (Fig. 11.27).

b. The anterior approach to the second division is sometimes preferable, especially if there is an overhanging maxilla or if the pterygomaxillary fissure cannot be entered through the zygomatic notch. The needle passes medially at a 40° angle, anterior to the coronoid process and immediately posterior to the maxillary process (Fig. 11.27).

As the needle enters the pterygomaxillary fissure (a narrow opening about 0.5 cm wide, as demonstrated), it usually strikes either the external pterygoid plate behind or the posterior border of the maxilla in front. As a rule, the nerve is reached at a depth of 5.5 cm, depending on the width of the skull. It is important not to go deeper than G.O cm. at any time, because of possible injury to important structures, especially the optic nerve.

If the external pterygoid plate is struck initially, it can be used as a valuable landmark. The foramen rotundum lies anteriorly and approximately 0.5 cm deeper.

If the posterior portion of the maxilla is reached before the pterygomaxillary fissure is entered, it will also servo as a guide: the fissure in which the nerve lies is bounded by the maxilla anteriorly and the external pterygoid plate posteriorly.

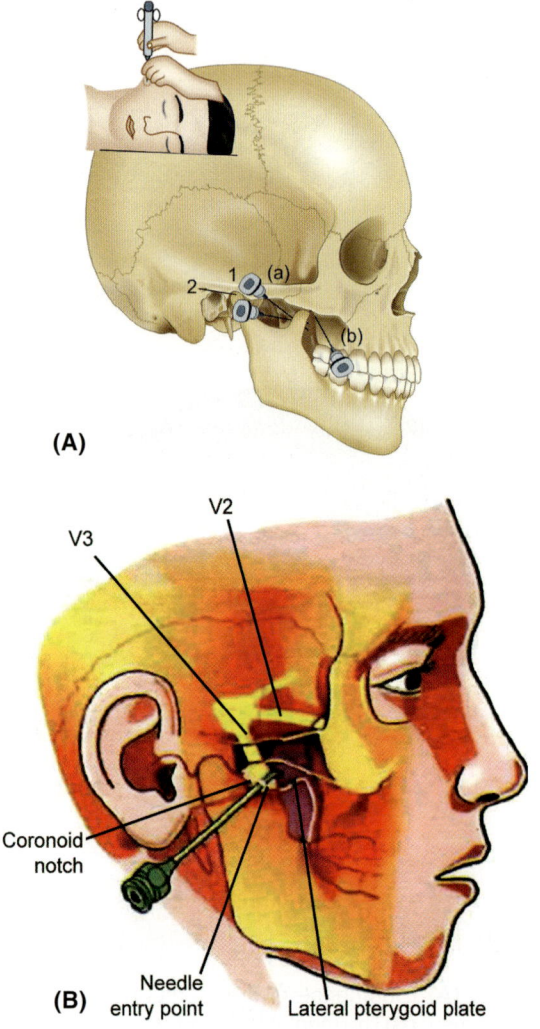

Fig. 11.27: Needle entry for injection of the maxillary nerve

The nerve will be reached by gentle manipulation of the needle, unless unusually bony prominences make it impossible. As soon as the needle enters the nerve tissue, a spray of pain will be felt along the course of the nerve. Here again only a few drops of alcohol are injected at a time. If complete immediate anesthesia of the upper lip, ala of the nose and roof of the mouth takes place with two or three drops of alcohol, another 0.5 cc. is injected slowly.

F. Alcohol Injection of the Mandibular Nerve at its Exit from Foramen Ovale

The procedure is illustrated in Figs 11.28 and 11.29.

1. a. Position of patient's head and surgeon: The patient's head is turned toward the left and the operator stands at the head of the table. A small area of skin immediately beneath the zygoma is sterilized. The inferior portion of the zygomatic notch is palpated firmly so that a small impression of the finger remains on the skin. The needle is first marked at 5.5 cm with a tiny piece of wax or adhesive, then inserted. The needle is directed slightly upward and backward to a depth of 4.5 cm (the usual depth, which varies with the width of the skull). Immediate reaction is noted with the patient under light anesthesia, depending on the depth of anesthesia. The corner of the mouth is usually drawn up as the nerve is reached. If the nerve is not reached at the usual depth, the needle is slightly withdrawn.

   b. The needle is redirected slightly forward to contact the external pterygoid plate. This is an

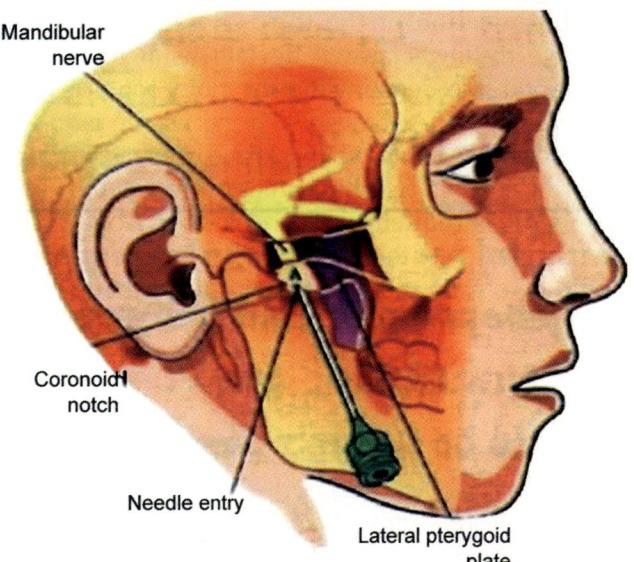

Fig. 11.29: Following contact with the lateral pterygoid plate, the needle is redirected posteriorly and inferiorly to bypass the inferior margin of the lateral pterygoid plate

essential landmark because the foramen ovale lies just posterior and slightly medial to it.

2. When the pterygoid plate is located, the needle is again slightly withdrawn and directed backward at a minimal degree until the nerve is entered, as evidenced by pain radiation.

   It may be necessary to repeat this process several times and the variation in depth of the foramen must also be considered. In some patients, the foramen may be reached at a depth just under 4.5 cm—and rarely, even at a depth as great as 5.0 cm—from the skin.

3. When the nerve trunk has been entered and a few drops of alcohol injected, the plunger of the syringe is withdrawn to ensure that the point of the needle is not in an artery. The patient's lower lip near the median line is tested for anesthesia. If the nerve has been struck properly, the sensory loss is immediate in this portion of the lip, the lower gum and half of the anterior two-thirds of the tongue.

4. When the level of anesthesia has been determined, another 0.5 to 1.0 cc of alcohol is slowly injected. The needle is then withdrawn and pressure is applied with sterile gauze over the point of entrance, to prevent oozing from the skin. The patient is now asked to open his mouth.

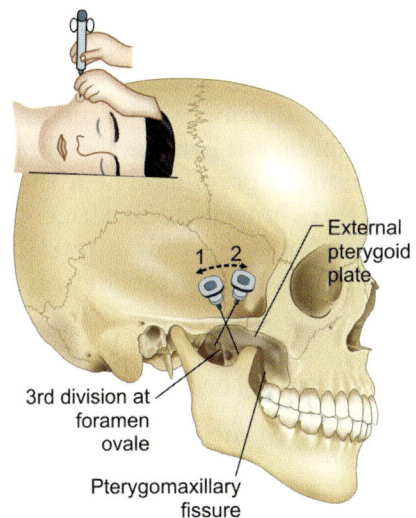

Fig. 11.28: Blockage of the mandibular nerve.

If the injection of the third division has been complete, the lower jaw will deviate distinctly toward the affected side, denoting that the motor root has been affected as well. At times when the needle is in the proper position and depth there is no extension of pain down the jaw, but a severe pain is present at the tip of the needle. Frequently, there is radiation to the external portion of the ear anteriorly, but the operator should be certain that the patient does not complain of pain deep in his ear canal.

II. PERIPHERAL NEURECTOMY

Pain relief from peripheral neurectomy may be complete, but it is generally not permanent, and recurrences almost invariably occur. Peripheral neurectomy is still appropriate and should be strongly considered in a selected subgroup of patients.

Peripheral neurectomy is effective because it eliminates the nociceptive afferent input to the spinal trigeminal nucleus and tract. In addition, there is evidence that trauma to peripheral branches of the trigeminal nerve also produce temporary degenerative changes in trigeminal ganglion cells, which also may contribute to the pain relief that occurs following neurectomy.

Indications

1. A neurectomy is sometimes utilized when repeated alcohol injections of a peripheral nerve have become difficult because of the formation of scar tissue. Most patients prefer the localized and transient numbness of such an operation to the widespread permanent anesthesia that follows partial or total root section, even though they realize that an operation on the sensory root will have to be performed at some future time when the pain recurs.
2. Peripheral neurectomy is indicated for an aged or severely debilitated patient in whom MVD or percutaneous ablative procedures are contra-indicated.

Advantages

1. Technically simple as long as one has an understanding of the pertinent anatomy of the trigeminal nerve.
2. Low morbidity procedure that can be especially beneficial in an elderly and in firm patient who might not otherwise tolerate a more involved procedure.
3. It is particularly useful in patients who suffer from trigeminal neuralgia involving the first division because there is no risk of producing corneal anesthesia as there is with retrogasserian procedures, especially radiofrequency lesions.
4. Peripheral neurectomy also may prove beneficial in the treatment of selected patients with trigeminal neuropathic pain syndromes caused by dental surgery, surgery on the paranasal sinuses, and injury to peripheral branches from facial trauma.
5. Lack of need for any special intraoperative imaging such as biplane fluoroscopy, which is essential in performing retrogasserian procedures.
6. A neurectomy is sometimes utilized when repeated alcohol injections of a periphery nerve have become difficult because of the formation of scar tissue. Most patients prefer the localized and transient numbness of such an operation to the widespread permanent anesthesia that follows partial or total root section, even though they realize that an operation on the sensory root will have to be performed at some future time when the pain recurs.

The outcome varies widely in literature, Freemont and Millac (1981) reported that a single neurectomy yielded on average 26.5 months free of pain and serial neurectomies gave on average a 59-month pain-free period. Quinn and Weil (1975) found that there was a pain-free mean period of 37.5 months after mental neurectomy, 38 months after inferior alveolar neurectomy, 44 months after lingual neurectomy, and 38.5 months after infraorbital neurectomy. To generalize, temporary relief may be obtained for 1 or 2 years or more by peripheral neuroctomy of one or more of the three branches of the trigeminal nerve. The techniques for supraorbital, infraorbital and inferior dental and mental neurectomy are illustrated.

NEURECTOMY OF THE SUPRAORBITAL NERVE

The procedure is illustrated in Fig. 11.30.

NEURECTOMY OF THE INFRAORBITAL NERVE

The procedure is illustrated in Fig. 11.31.

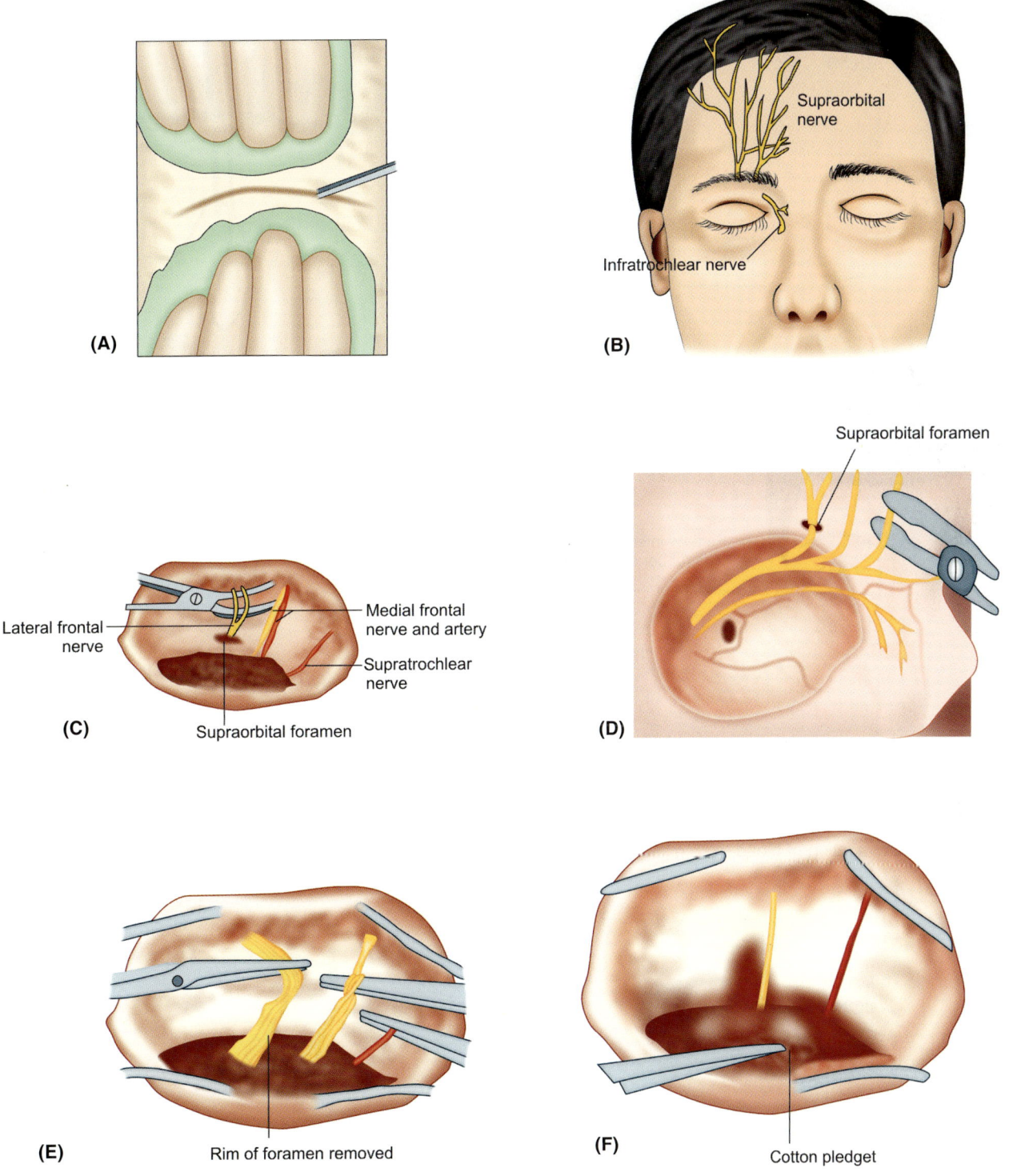

Fig. 11.30: Supraorbital neurectomy. **(A)** Semicurved incision through shaved eyebrow. **(B)** Relation of the supraorbital branches and the infratrochlear branch to the line of incision. **(C)** The main trunk of the supraorbital nerve extends through the bony foramen. **(D)** The thin, bony ledge of the orbital rim is removed with small rongeurs. **(E)** Avulsion of distal branches. **(F)** Orbital fat is separated from the orbital roof by thin cotton pledgets

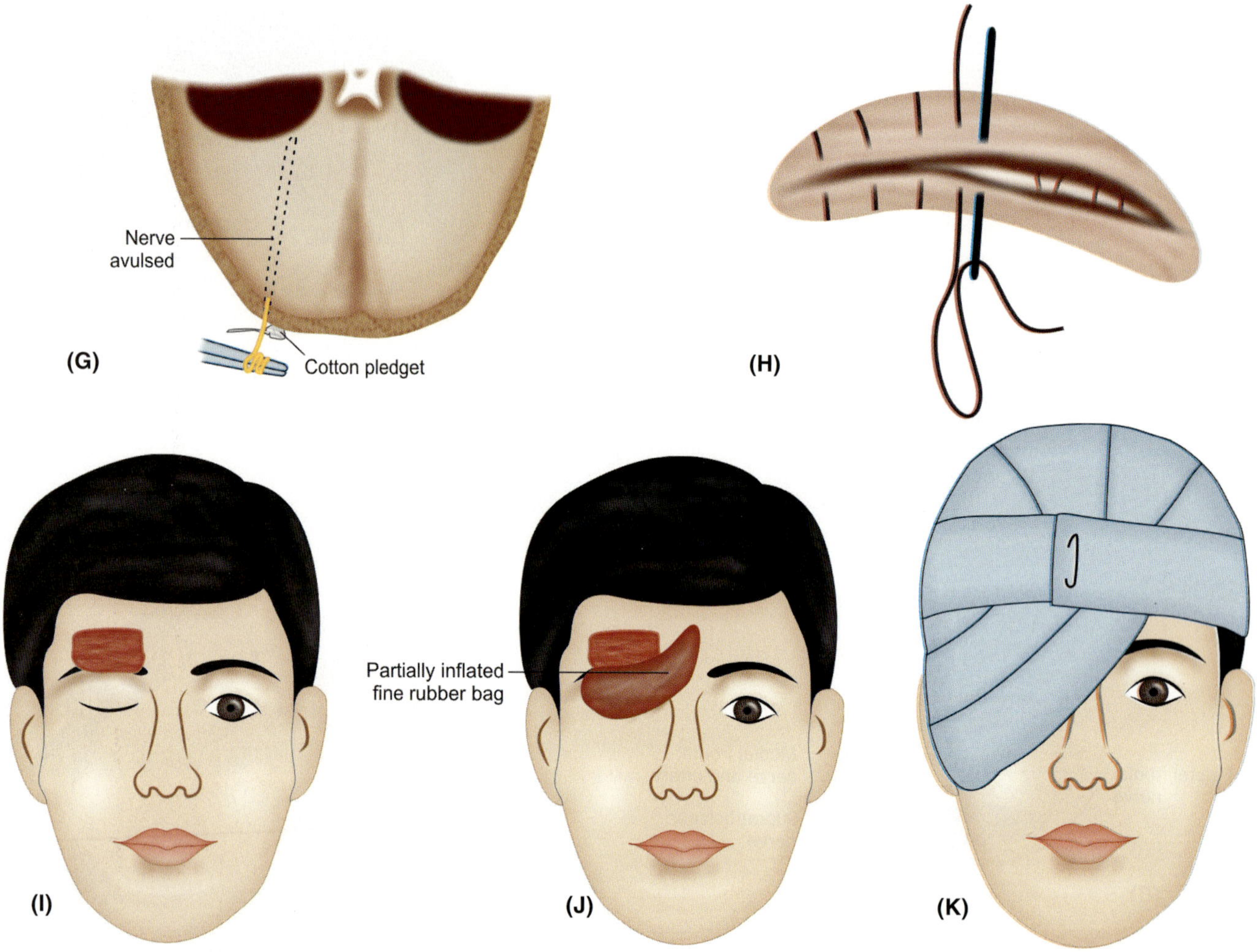

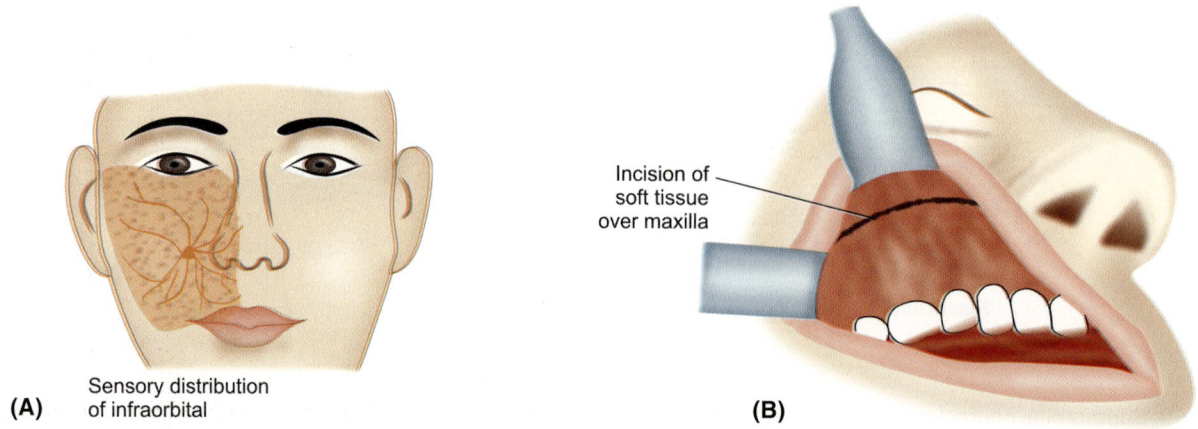

(G)

Nerve avulsed

Cotton pledget

(H)

(I)

Partially inflated fine rubber bag

(J)

(K)

Fig. 11.30: (continued) Supraorbital neurectomy. **(G)** The nerve is dissected and avulsed intraorbitally. **(H)** Closure. **(I)** Bandage. **(J)** Rubber bag partially inflated with air placed over orbit. **(K)** Light pressure bandage applied over rubber bag to prevent swelling and extravasation of blood

Sensory distribution
of infraorbital

(A)

Incision of
soft tissue
over maxilla

(B)

Fig. 11.31: Infraorbital neurectomy. **(A)** Infraorbital nerve distribution. **(B)** Incision is made just above the gingival mucous membrane

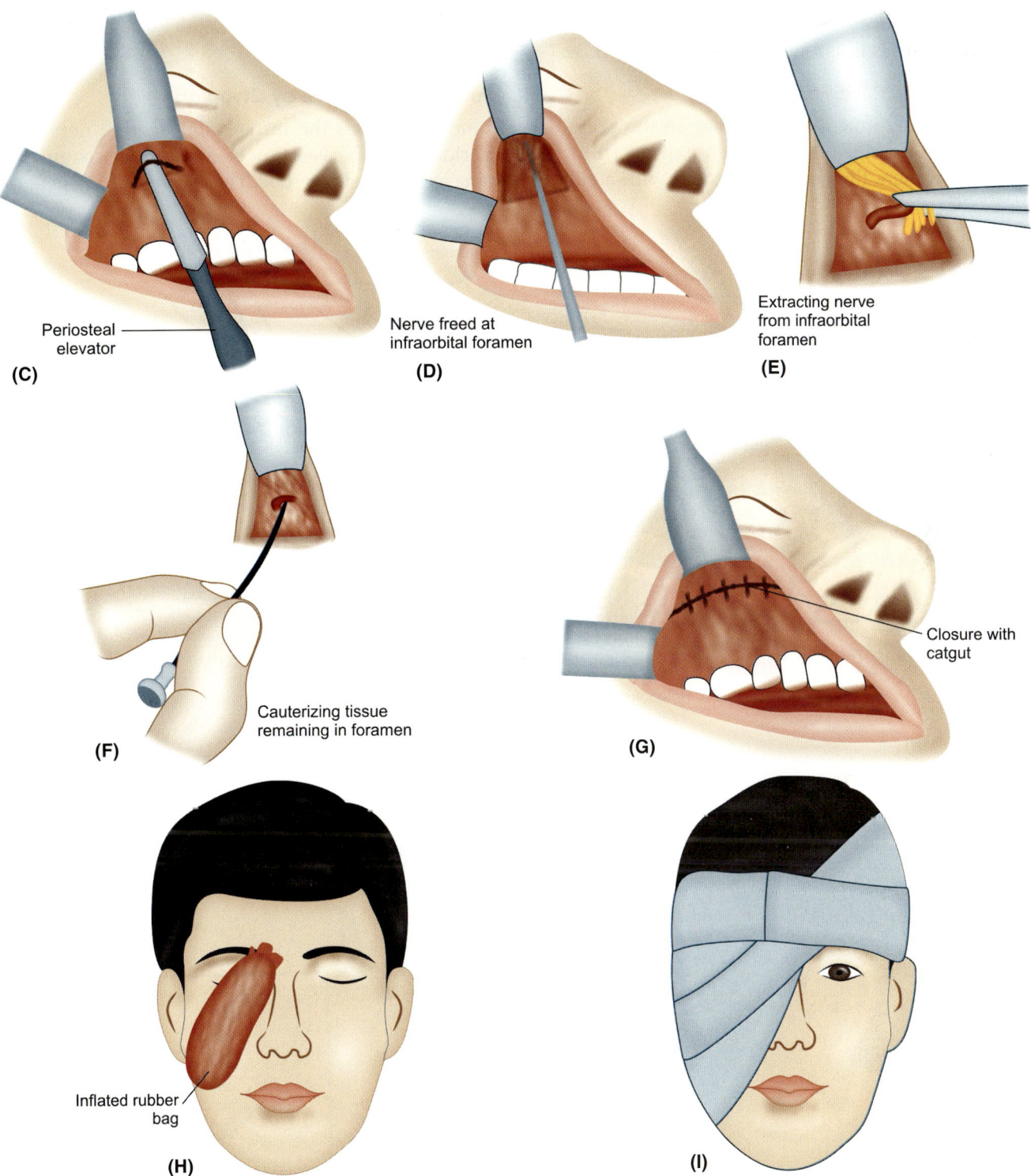

Periosteal
elevator
(C)

Nerve freed at
infraorbital foramen
(D)

Extracting nerve
from infraorbital
foramen
(E)

Cauterizing tissue
remaining in foramen
(F)

Closure with
catgut
(G)

Inflated rubber
bag
(H)

(I)

Fig. 11.31: (continued) Infraorbital neurectomy. **(C)** The mucous membrane and periosteum are elevated from the maxillary bone to the infraorbital foramen. **(D)** The nerve is separated and traction maintained with nerve hook. **(E)** Nerve branches can be separated from the soft tissues for a considerable distance with a periosteal elevator/the nerve is avulsed from the infraorbital foramen. **(F)** A small metal probe is inserted into the infraorbital foramen and coagulation applied; the distal portion of the smaller branches is avulsed. **(G)** Closure is made with fine catgut which can be let in situ. **(H)** A loosely inflated bag is inserted over the maxilla. **(I)** A light pressure bandage is applied for a period of 12 to 24 hours

NEURECTOMY OF THE INFERIOR ALVEOLAR NERVE

The procedure is illustrated in Figs 11.32 to 11.39.

NEURECTOMY OF THE MENTAL NERVE

After reflecting mucoperiosteal flap in the premolar region, the mental nerve is seen exiting from the mental foramen, the nerve is grasped with a curved

hemostat. By rotating the hemostat, the nerve will turn around its tip and avulsed (Fig. 11.40).

Avulsion of the Nerve by Cryoprobe

Branches such as the infraorbital, mental nerves or inferior dental nerves may be avulsed, or coagulated using a cryosurgical probe. These methods are usually

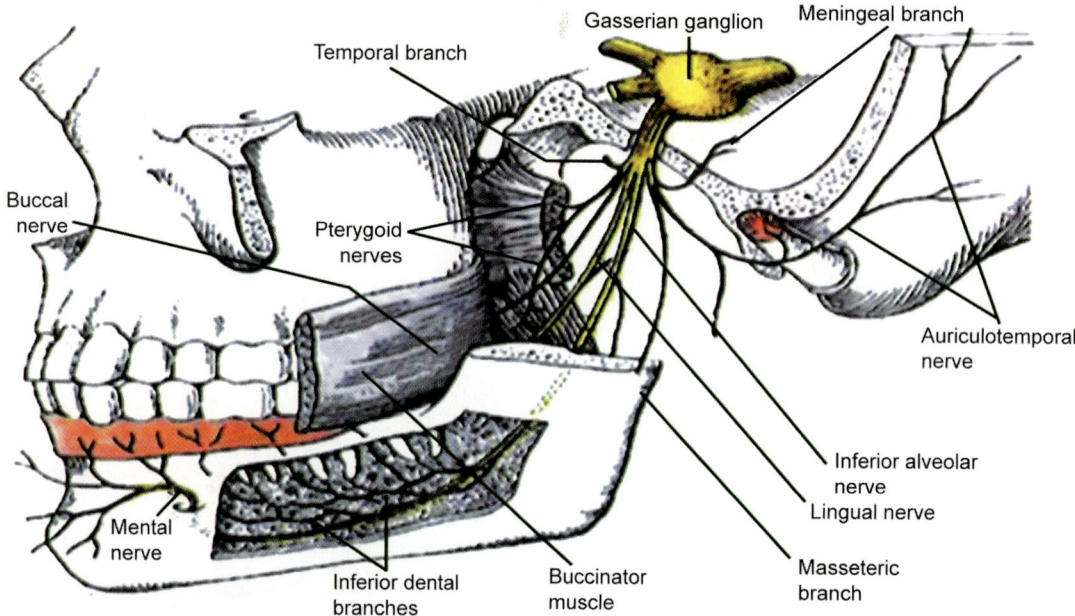

Fig. 11.32: Anatomy of the inferior alveolar nerve

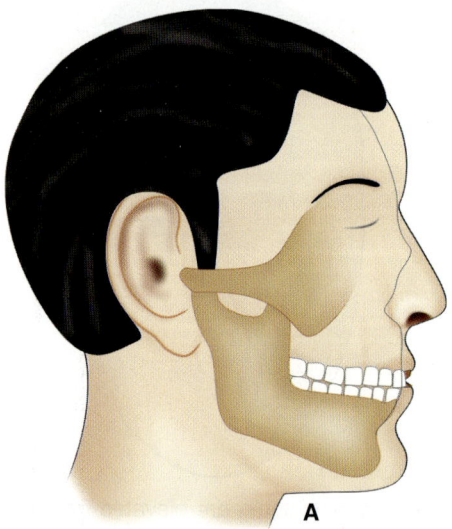

Fig. 11.33: The skin crease (A) is the most appropriate location for an incision to be carried out. Incising the skin and subcutaneous fascia along this crease avoids injury to the mandibular branch of the facial nerve, and hides the resulting scar

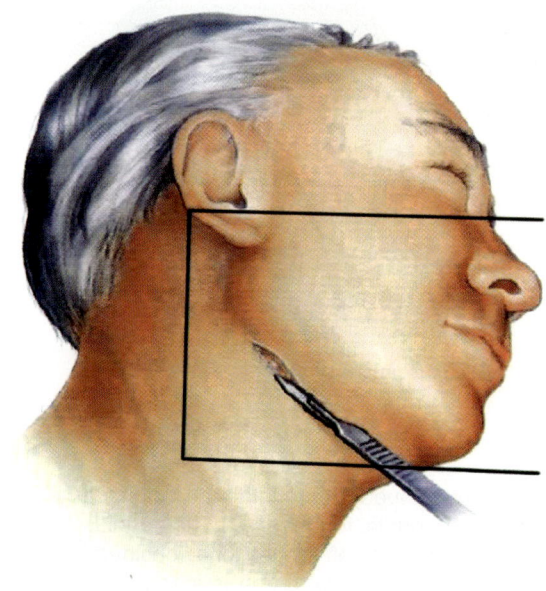

Fig. 11.34: Bard Parker scalpel number 10 is used to carry out an incision through the skin and subcutaneous fascia, crease

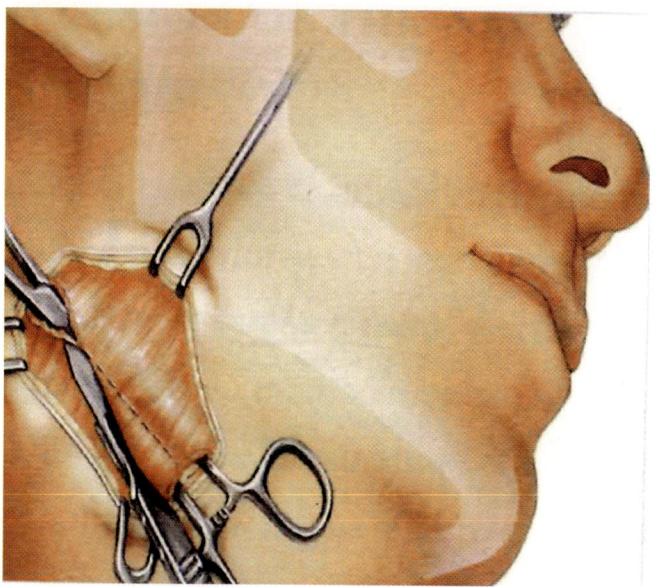

Fig. 11.35: During retraction, the position of the tissues may be distorted so that an incision through the platysma may lie directly over the mandibular branch of the facial nerve

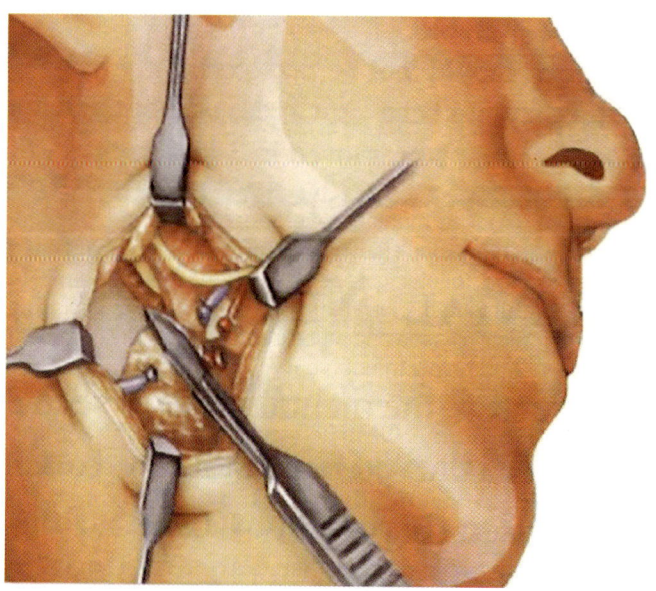

Fig. 11.36: The facial artery (external maxillary artery and the vein may be seen crossing the surgical field. In such instance, they should be ligated and transected. A stimulator is helpful in locating the mandibular branch of the facial nerve so that it will not be injured. If identified, this nerve should be retracted upward with a smooth retractor. The masseter muscle and the periosteum are incised along the inferior border of the mandible

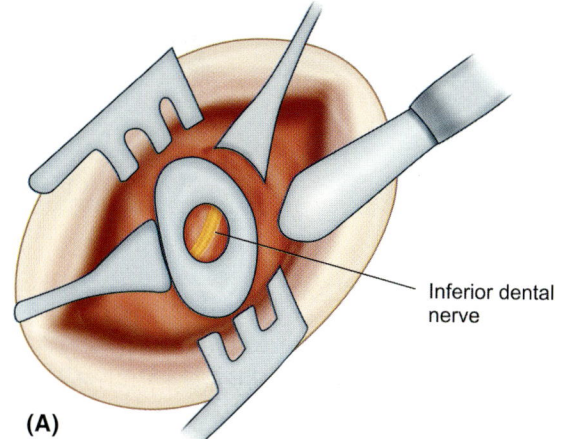

(A)

Inferior dental nerve

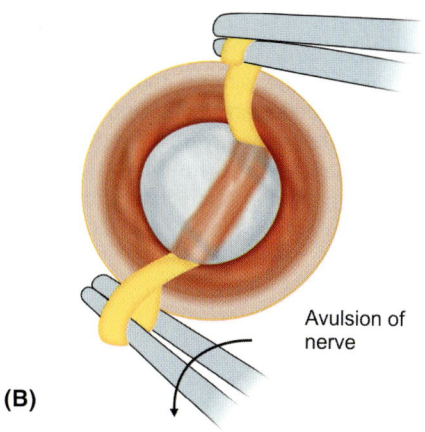

(B)

Avulsion of nerve

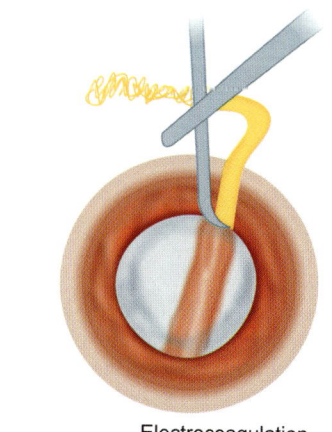

(C)

Electrocoagulation

Fig. 11.37: (A) A bur opening made through the central portion of the mandible, exposing the inferior dental nerve. **(B)** The nerve is divided and avulsed as far as possible. The ends of the nerves usually break off at the edge of the bone that is exposed. **(C)** A nerve hook is inserted into the foramen cephalad and distally; coagulation is applied

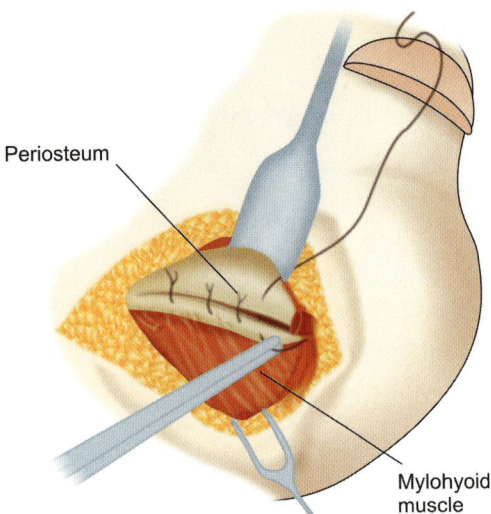

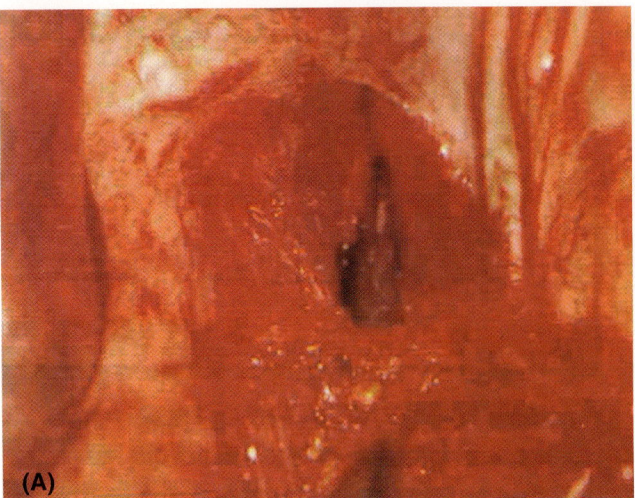

(A)

Fig. 11.38: The periosteum is closed with 0000 absorbable sutures cut out at the knot. To minimize the possibility of adhesions of the skin to bone with an immovable depressed scar, accuracy in replacement and suture of the periosteum, musculature, and subcutaneous layers is important. If gross contamination is suspected, or if haemorrhage cannot be controlled adequately, a small rubber drain should be placed in the wound, it may be removed in 24 to 48 hours

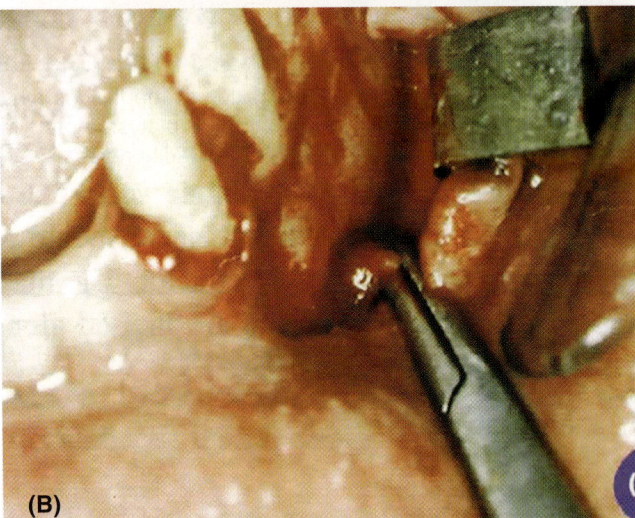

(B)

Fig. 11.40: (A) The mental nerve is exposed intraorally and grasped with hemostat. **(B)** The mental nerve trunk is attached to scar formed following repeated alcohol injections. The tissues surrounding the nerve are undermined by the scissors so that connective tissue and muscle can be carefully dissected from above and below the nerve

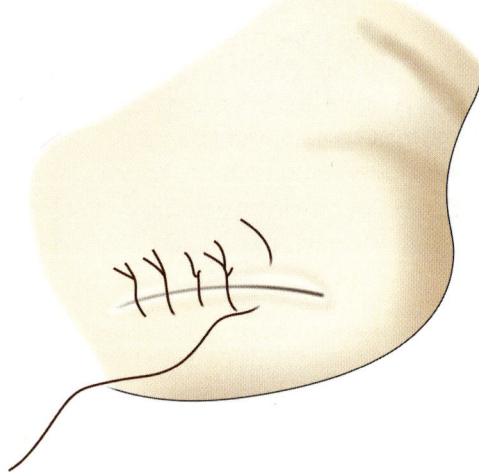

Fig. 11.39: The tension is moved from the wound margins by use of subcutaneous sutures. Approximation of the skin edges is accomplished by interrupted single strand nylon sutures or by subcuticular sutures. To avoid scarring due to suture marks along the line of approximation of the wound edges

1. Interrupted single strand synthetic (nylon) sutures are preferable.
2. Sutures should not be tied too tightly.
3. Knots should be kept at the side of the wound.
4. Knots should be removed in 3 to 4 days.
5. Subcuticular closure is preferable.

successful for a time. Destruction of the axon by cooling below minus 40°C, without interruption of axons, is carried out. After months the axons regenerate with recovery of sensibility. Cryotherapy is usually performed in patients who wish to avoid MVD or when MVD is contraindicated. It affords a patient an interim period of pain relief after which the patient is able to make a rationale choice about the surgical management of his or her condition. Cryotherapy is a simple and repeatable procedure. Pain abolition demonstrated by localized injections of a local anesthetic solution determines which nerves require cryotherapy.

- The procedure can be performed transmucosally or after surgical exposure of the affected nerve. In the "open" technique, the involved nerve is frozen by direct application of a fine cryoprobe under general or local anesthesia, with or without sedation in outpatients. Poon (2000) exposed the nerve surgically under general anesthesia or local anesthesia and a cryoprobe (–120°C) was applied directly on to the exposed nerve for a standard 3 cycles of 2-minute freeze and 5-minute thaw. Rahnama and Gaweda 184 used peripheral cryotherapy with liquid nitrogen (–180°C) in local anesthesia. The freezing-defreezing cycle was repeated 2 to 3 times (Rahnama M, Gaweda A, 2003). Pradel et al 187 reported transmucosal cryosurgery under nerve block at the infraorbital foramen (infraorbital nerve) and/or mental foramen (inferior alveolar nerve) by an intraoral approach. The diameter of frozen gelatin in front of the cryoprobe was only up to 4 to 5 mm and the maximum freezing temperature ranged from –40 to –120°C in tissue. Nally 188 performed some procedures and reported that the best results were probably achieved with a temperature of –100°C or lower for three 2-minute freezes, with a 5-minute defrost between freezes.

Pradel et al (2002) designed a newly developed cryoprobe for peripheral nerves allows surgeons to freeze branches of the trigeminal nerve at the infraorbital or the mandibular foramen without exposing the nerve or damaging the surrounding tissue, i.e. transmucosally. The probe has an outer diameter of 2.7 mm and a vacuum-insulated shaft to protect the adjacent tissue (Figs 11.41 and 11.42).

The cooling system works with liquid nitrogen through a hand spraying device (IKG 3) at a pressure of 0.4 mPa. Although ice balls with a diameter of up to 10 mm were achieved in water (Fig. 11.41 D), the freezing efficacy of the probe in tissue is more likely to be characterized by the data in gelatin. The diameter of frozen gelatin in front of the cryoprobe was only up to 4–5 mm and the maximum freezing temperatures ranged between –40 and –120°C.14. This has to be taken into account when inserting the cryoprobe, which has to be placed with extreme accuracy. Freezing of the branches of the trigeminal nerve at the infraorbital or the mandibular foramen is illustrated in Figs 11.42 and 11.43, as reported by Pradel et al (2002).

They reported, "This cryosurgical method reliably eliminated attacks of pain. However, recurrences were observed as early as 6–8 months after treatment, which is early compared with other surgical methods. An important advantage, in contrast to other surgical methods is the restoration of sensation, which is the experience of some authors. Sensation was lost in the affected region for only 3–4 months. The duration of loss of sensation and elimination of pain depend on the temperature achieved at the nerve. Therapeutic efficacy might be improved by placing the cryoprobe more accurately by using intraoperative radiography. Lower temperatures at the tip of the cryoprobe and greater freezing capacity may also lengthen the pain-free interval".

III. MAJOR OPERATIVE PROCEDURES

When neurovascular compression is caused by an artery, the vessel is mobilized, displaced and fixed to dura with shredded Teflon wool aligns reinforced with fibrin glue. When veins are discovered, they should be coagulated and divided. When the trigeminal sensory root appears normal, with no signs of extrinsic compression, a partial sensory rhizotomy is performed with sectioning of the inferior half to two-thirds of the trigeminal nerve close to the pons.

Approximately 30% of patients with trigeminal neuralgia will ultimately fail medical treatment. A variety of surgical approaches have been advocated for treatment. Before any surgical procedure, it may be desirable to give an ordinary local anesthetic nerve block so that the patient gets a reasonable idea of the area and sense of 'decadness'. Some might prefer the pain.

The method of choice for many years has been open operation to cut the sensory root, approaching the root via either the middle cranial fossa or the posterior cranial fossa, the choice depending partly on technical factors and partly on any suspected abnormality in either fossa. The sensory root can be completely divided, taking care to preserve the motor root, or partly divided so as to retain the fibres of the ophthalmic division, this being of great importance to maintain the corneal reflex functioning properly. Introduction of the operating microscope has greatly improved the safety of the posterior fossa approach. This can also be used when the intention is to mobilize the posterior superior cerebellar artery.

The surgical interference can be categorized as: (a) Rhizotomy, (b) balloon microcompression of the trigeminal nerve and (c) decompression of the trigeminal ganglion. Apart from microvascular decompression, all the other surgical procedures rely

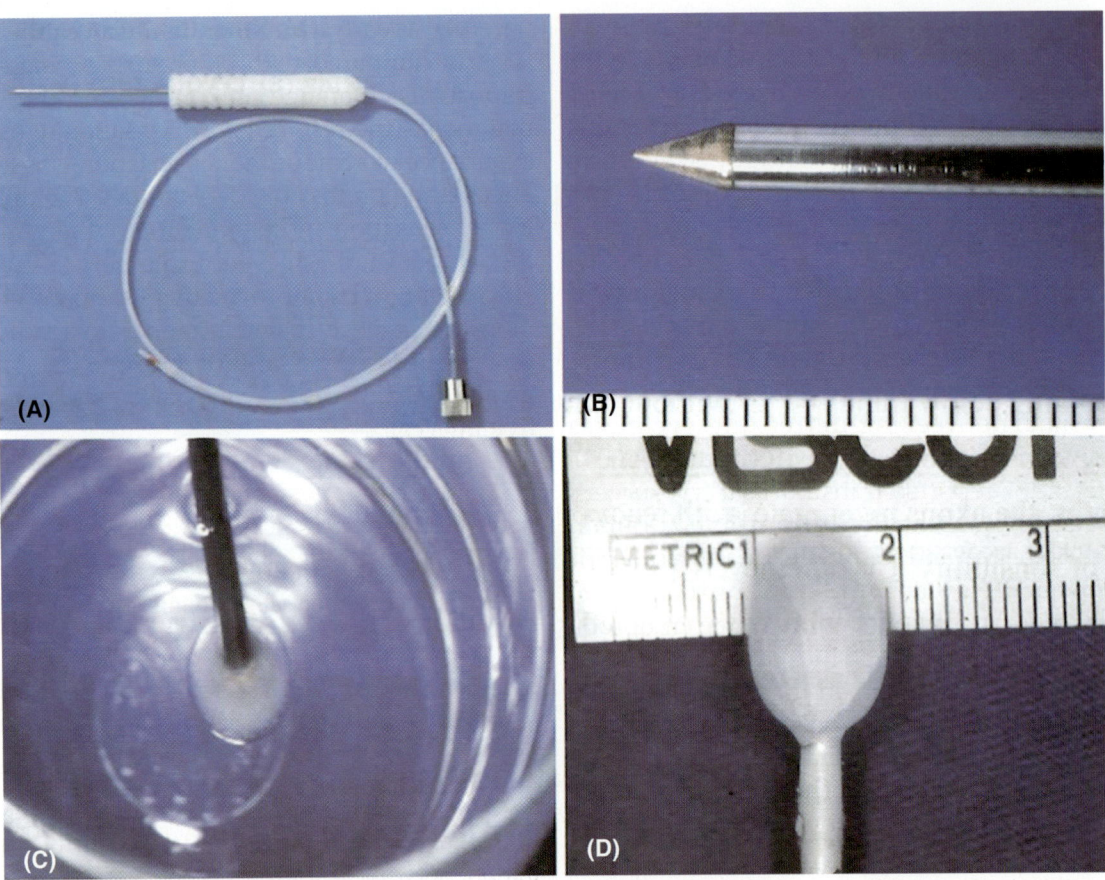

Fig. 11.41: (A) Transmucosal vacuum-insulated cryoprobe. **(B)** Cryoprobe: Construction of tip of cryoprobe containing outer vacuum insulation (chromium, nickel, strontium), inner vacuum insulation; tube for returning nitrogen liquid-gas mixture; feeding tube for liquid nitrogen; and copper tip. **(C)** Cryoprobe in water. **(D)** Formation of ice ball at tip of probe in water *(Pradel et al., 2002)*.

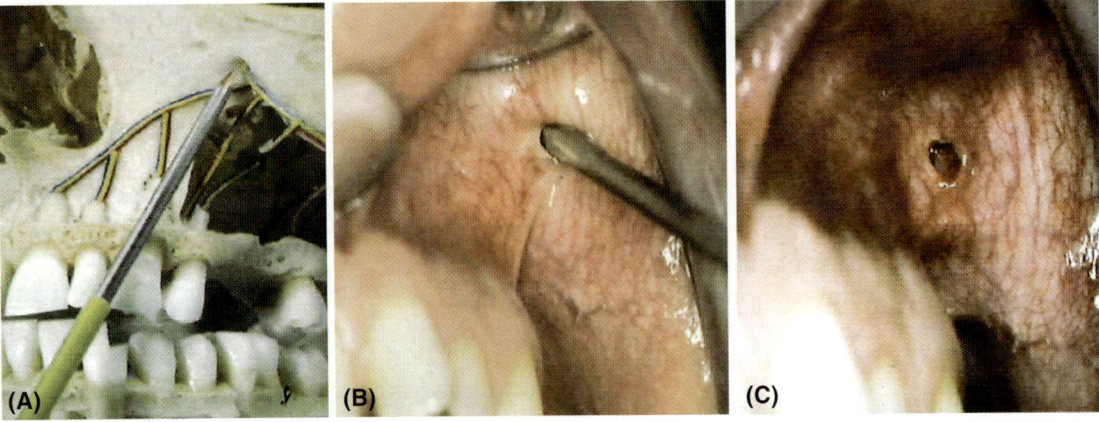

Fig. 11.42: (A) Distribution of the infraorbital nerve. **(B)** Cryoprobe inserted transmucosally advanced to the infraorbital foramen during cryosurgery. **(C)** Site of insertion of the cryoprobe for freezing of the infraorbital nerve *(Pradel et al., 2002)*.

on destruction of the sensory fibers of the trigeminal nerve and hence result in varying degrees of sensory change postoperatively.

A. Rhizotomy

It is a neurosurgical procedure by which selected nerve fibers near or within the gasserian ganglion are either

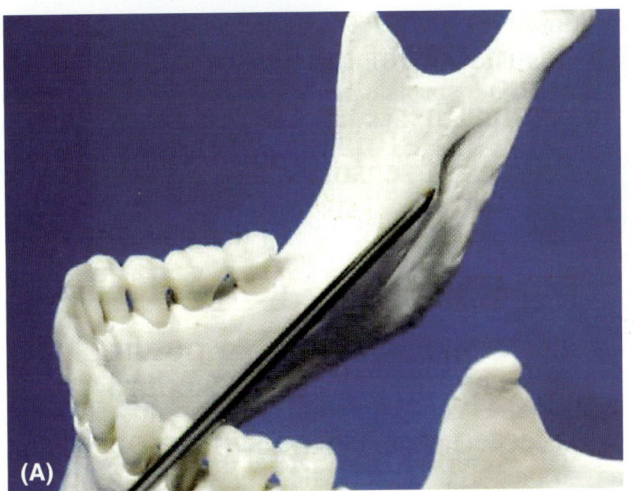 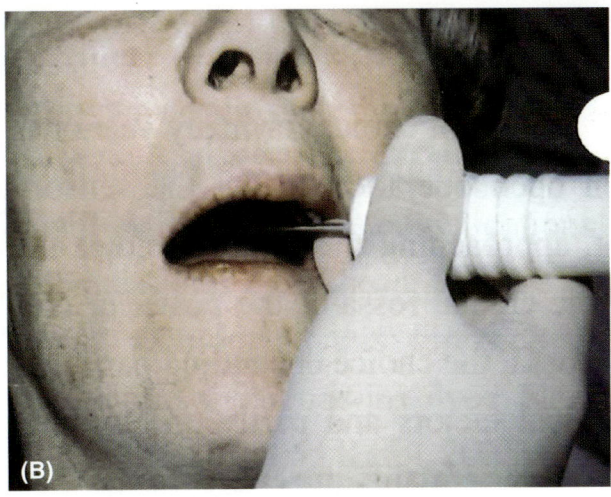

Fig. 11.43: (A and B): Site of insertion of the cryoprobe for freezing of the inferior alveolar-lingual and possibly buccal nerves

traumatized or destroyed. Rhizotomy is a procedure in which select nerve fibers are destroyed to block pain. Gudmundsson et al (1971) reported that the fibers from the third division remained ventrolateral throughout the interval from the ganglion to the pons, the first division dorsolateral, with the second division fibers being in an intermediate position. Intraoperative topographic mapping of the trigeminal nerve root using electrophysiological methods might be used as a guide for performing PSR (Stechison et al, 1996).

Rhizotomy is reported by neurosurgeons as "partial sensory rhizotomy" (PSR) is performed in the following instances:

1. Patients in whom posterior fossa exploration fails to reveal significant compression of the trigeminal sensory root, PSR is indicated or performed instead of microvascular decompression (MVD).
2. Patients in whom MVD is technically infeasible.
3. Patients in whom MVD results poor and no significant vascular contact was present at the time of reoperation (Delitala et al, 2001; Howng and Chang, 12998; Young and Wilkins,1993; Klun 1992).

Bederson and Wilson (1989) reported that patients with distortion of the trigeminal nerve root caused by vascular compression underwent MVD, those with no compression underwent PSR, and those with vascular contact but no distortion of the nerve root underwent MVD and PSR.

The percutaneous procedures can usually be performed on an outpatient basis under local or brief general anesthesia at acceptable or minimal risk of morbidity. For these reasons, they commonly are performed in debilitated persons or those older than 65 years. Rhizotomy causes some degree of permanent sensory loss and facial numbness.

This is accomplished by introducing a trocar or needle lateral to the corner of the mouth and guided by radiographic fluoroscopic guidance into the gasserian ganglion through the ipsilateral foramen oval of the sedated patient. After careful manipulation and feedback from the patient, the selected nerve fibers involved in the pain condition are located. At that time, the selected nerve fibers are destroyed by:

i. *Percutaneous radiofrequency rhizotomy* (thermocoagulation of the gasserian ganglion, radiofrequency thermocoagulation). In this procedure, a needle is inserted through the cheek and the foramen ovale and an electrical impulse is applied to the ganglion. An electric current is passed through a needle placed into the gasserian ganglion to produce thermal lesion in the ganglion. To avoid the complications of numbness and dysesthesia, some experts do not recommend this approach when ophthalmic division is involved. Karol et al (Karol et al, 2005; Karol, 2005) made a somatotopic map of the human gasserian ganglion and it may reduce unnecessary morbidity from percutaneous thermocoagulation.

ii. *Percutaneous glycerol rhizotomy* (depositing a toxic substance such as glycerol). A lumbar puncture needle is inserted via the foramen ovale into the trigeminal cistern under intermittent fluoroscopic control. Bennett and Lunsfors 92 proposed that glycerol more specifically affected the damaged myelinated axons than normal myelinated axons. Small doses of glycerol are reported to be worthwhile to relieve pain without significant sensory loss (Hakanson, 1983; Lunsford and Bennett, 1984).

B. Percutaneous Balloon Microcompression of the Trigeminal Ganglion

Under fluoroscopic control, a Fogarty balloon catheter is inserted and slowly inflated with a water-soluble contrast agent for 1 to 7 minutes to compress the trigeminal ganglion. Balloon compression is technically easier than radiofrequency thermo-coagulation, which shows similar outcomes. The rate of initial pain relief is approximately 95%, and recurrence rate is estimated, in large number of reports, to be 20 to 30% at 5 years. The longer compression time causes the greater rate of complete pain relief (Meglio et al, 1990; Lee and Chen, 2003) but shorter durations of compression have fewer side effects.

C. Microvascular Decompression of the Trigeminal Ganglion

Surgeons perform the operation under general anesthesia, incising the skin behind the ear and performing a 3 cm craniotomy. After retracting the dura to expose the trigeminal nerve, they identify an arterial loop compressing the nerve as it enters the pons. The superior cerebellar artery is the most common offending vessel. When this is the case, the vessel is carefully dissected from the trigeminal nerve and a sponge or Teflon is placed between these structures. Remarkable success has immediately followed this procedure.

Although this neurosurgical procedure appears to have great long-term success, a major surgical procedure is required with its accompanying morbidity and mortality. Mobidity associated with trigeminal nerve decompression stems from hemorrhage, infection, and possible damage to the brainstem around the area of decompression. Patient selection is, therefore, extremely important. Relatively young, healthy patients are obviously the best candidates.

Some authors thought that MVD alleviated pain by causing injury to the trigeminal nerve rather than by removing neurovascular compression (Adams, 1989; Tenser, 1998). Therapeutic success is greater when vascular contact is arterial in comparison to venous or mixed arterial and venous contact (Piatt and Wilkins, 1984; Sun, 1994; Barker et al, 1996; Li et al, 2004; Hamlyn and King, 1992).

When other surgical procedures have been tried and failed the neurosurgeon can resort to cutting the spinal tract of the trigeminal system (trigeminal tractotomy). It should rarely be the initial procedure.

B. ATYPICAL TRIGEMINAL NEURALGIA

Introduction

The information elicited from the case history may prove valuable since patients report shooting pains in many other conditions besides idiopathic trigeminal neuralgia. Even though the pain of atypical neuralgia may appear to be spasmodic, it never comes and goes in a few seconds. The pain of atypical facial neuralgia usually intensifies gradually and works up to a peak in a few minutes; it remains at a plateau for half an hour to several hours and then gradually subsides. In idiopathic trigeminal neuralgia, the pain is momentary and is of sudden severe intensity "electric shock". In idiopathic trigeminal neuralgia, there are no abnormal neurological findings such as loss of corneal reflexes, anesthesia, paresthesia, muscular atrophy or muscle weakness. If such features are present, it is not a case of idiopathic trigeminal neuralgia but a secondary neuralgia, symptomatic of some other conditions.

Atypical trigeminal neuralgia or type II occurs in patients who still have fairly classical features of trigeminal neuralgia but also report a background burning, dull type of pain which persists for some time after an attack of pain and is often not as responsive to the usual mainstream medications (Limonadi et al, 2006).

The International Headache Society has published criteria for the diagnosis of classical and symptomatic trigeminal neuralgia (Box 11.3). In classical trigeminal neuralgia, no cause of the symptoms can be identified other than vascular compression. Symptomatic trigeminal neuralgia has the same clinical criteria, but another underlying cause is responsible for the symptoms.

Trigeminal neuralgia can present with principally intraoral symptoms and so toothache needs to be considered as a differential. Temporomandibular disorders, especially if they are unilateral and the pain is centred in the preauricular area, can also be confused with trigeminal neuralgia (Drangsholt and Truelove, 2001). Other neuropathic pain to be considered includes, sinus disease, head and neck neoplasms, infections, post-herpetic neuralgia

Box 11.3: Diagnostic criteria for classical (idiopathic) and symptomatic trigeminal neuralgia*

Classical

A. Paroxysmal attacks of pain lasting from a fraction of a second to two minutes, affecting one or more divisions of the trigeminal nerve, and fulfilling criteria B and C

B. Pain has at least one of the following characteristics:
1. Intense, sharp, superficial, or stabbing.
2. Precipitated from trigger zones or by trigger factors

C. Attacks are stereotyped in the individual patient.

D. There is no clinically evident neurologic deficit

E. Not attributed to another disorder.

Symptomatic

A. Paroxysmal attacks of pain lasting from a fraction of a second to two minutes, with or without persistence of aching between paroxysms, affecting one or more divisions of the trigeminal nerve, and fulfilling criteria B and C

B. Pain has at least one of the follwoing characteristics:
1. Intense, sharp, superficial, or stabbing.
2. Precipitated from trigger zones or by trigger factors.

C. Attacks are stereotyped in the individual patient.

D. A causative lesion, other than vascular compression, has been demonstrated by special investigations and/or posterior fossa exploration.

* Reported by International Headache Society (HIS)

traumatic neuropathic trigeminal pain, cluster headache and migraine (especially lower half headache) (Box 11.4).

If symptoms are predominantly in the first division of the trigeminal nerve, then the rarer group of disorders known as the trigeminal autonomic cephalalgias such as cluster headache, paroxysmal hemicranias, SUNCT (short unilateral neuralgiform pain with conjunctival redness and tearing) and SUNA (short unilateral neuralgiform pain with autonomic

Box 11.4: Atypical features suggesting symptomatic trigeminal neuralgia or alternative diagnosis

Abnormal neurologic examination	Hearing loss or abonormality
Abnormal oral, dental, or ear examination	Numbness
Age younger than 40 years	Pain episodes persisting longer than two minutes
Bilateral symptoms	Pain outside of trigeminal nerve distribution
Dizziness or vertigo	Visula changes

symptoms) need to be considered (Cohen et al, 2006). Temporal arteritis or giant cell arteritis can cause unilateral or bilateral aching, throbbing pain most frequently around the temples and must be diagnosed rapidly to prevent blindness.

Etiology

Among the most common etiologic factors responsible for the genesis of atypical neuralgia are the following:

1. *Multiple sclerosis (MS)*

   Risk factors for trigeminal neuralgia include multiple sclerosis and hypertension (Zakrzewska and Hamlyn, 1999). MS may cause hyperexcitability of the trigeminal nucleus (Meaney et al, 1994).

   Multiple sclerosis is a chronic disease of unknown etiology characterized by the development of focal areas of degeneration of the myelin sheaths of the nerve fibers in the brain and spinal cord. The lesion develops in a random manner throughout the brain and spinal cord. The areas of demyelination eventually heals by forming masses of glial scar tissue. The name of the disease is derived from the characteristic multiple areas of involvement that heal by sclerosis (another form of scarring).

   The cause of pain in trigeminal neuralgia which develops in cases of multiple sclerosisis thought to be due to inflammatory demyelination in the trigeminal root entery zone, disturbing (the balance between abnormal and physiological inputs) or central pathways (modified excitability of neurons of the trigeminal nucleus). The trigeminal neuralgia that occurs in multiple sclerosis sufferers poses a number of therapeutic problems: it may occur in young patients, it can be bilateral, there may be significant neurological morbidity and there may be an increased intolerance of carbamazepine side effects.

2. *Tumor compression, e.g.* acoustic neuroma. Acoustic neuroma is an intracerebral tumor involving the vestibulocochlear nerve (cranial nerve VII), which is often called by its older name of acoustic nerve. The nerve exits the brain at the junction between the pons, medulla and cerebellum. Frequently, the tumor compresses the adjacent brain and the nearby cranial nerves as it grows, and it may also erode the adjacent temporal bone. Clinically, the tumor causes ringing in the ear (tinnitus) on the affected side.

Compression of the nerve causes partial hearing loss on the affected side, the symptoms related to pressure on the adjacent cranial nerves, e.g. trigeminal nerve and the brainstem.

3. *Deficiency of inhibitory transmitter:* An important factor could be the failure of inhibition. Since gammaaminobutyric acid (GAB A) is the commonest inhibitory transmitter in the central nervous system, it is conceivable that deficiency of this could be a factor. Also it has been suggested that there might be such extensive presynaptic inhibition of small fibers that the threshold of excitation was actually exceeded leading to both orthodromic and antidromic transmission. It has been suggested that carbamazapine might work by decreasing presynaptic inhibition.

4. *Damage to the afferent nerves (deafferentiation)*

> *Chronic irritation of the peripheral nerve leads to ectopic action potentials and also failure of segmental inhibition in the trigeminal nucleus (Fromm et al, 1981).*
>
> *An increased afferent input from primary nociceptive afferents, activating second-order neurones, may cause sensitization and hyperexcitability (Bartsch, 2003).*

Pain secondary to deafferentiation refers to pain that occurs when there has been damage to the afferent pain transmission system. Usually this condition is secondary to trauma or surgery, including extraction and endodontic treatment. By definition, extraction and endodontics are deafferentiating, because they both involve amputation of tissue that contains the nerve supply of a human structure, the tooth. Limb amputation is another example of a "deafferentiation" procedure. As with phantom limb pain, a similar picture of oral deafferentiation pain may occur, but only in a small subset of patients are the symptoms severe enough to warrant treatment. These pains may be maintained by various mechanisms, some readily appreciated and others quite complex and not yet completely understood.

Peripheral hyperactivity at the site of nerve damage is quite easily understandable. At the site of alveolar nerve damage, neuronal hyperactivity leading to persistent pain occurs. In this form, the pain is frequently arrested with local anesthetic block.

CNS hyperactivity can, however, also be responsible for persistent pain experienced in the tooth site. In this model, peripheral pain damage leads to changes in the second-order neuron in the trigeminal nucleus that synapsed with the primary peripheral

nociceptor. Changes occur centrally in which ongoing pain transmission to higher centers can occur despite minimal or even no peripheral input. Local anesthetic does not arrest pain in these circumstances.

Additionally, patients may exhibit both forms of compromise simultaneously (i.e. only portion of pain may be arrested by local anesthetic block). Sympathetic nervous system activity has also been shown to augment some of these complex neuropathic processes.

Clinical Feature

The clinical feature of deafferentiation pains is mentioned in Box 11.5:

Box 11.5: Clinical feature of deafferentiation pains

Burning or aching pain is continuous or almost continuous. Sharp paroxysms may occur.
Allodynia, hyperesthesia, or hypoesthesia may be present. No dentoalveolar cause is found.
History of surgery or other trauma exists.
History of symptoms greater than 4 to 6 months exists.
Local anesthetic block equivocal.

The key to recognize all of these conditions and avoiding unnecessary and potentially harmful dental treatment, frequently lies in obtaining an excellent description of the chief complaint, including quality of pain, duration, alleviating factors and aggravating factors. The history of the complaint and how the symptoms have changed over time can also be quite valuable.

Concerning dentistry, the sites and directions of dental neuralgic pain seem some-what different from comparable ones in idiopathic trigeminal neuralgia.

Dental neuralgic pain may be elicited due to:
a. Acute pulpitis of upper second molar and second premolar.
b. Deep caries of upper canine, and sinus near lateral incisor.
c. Dry socket after extraction of lower second molar.
d. Shooting from upper molar and back to it. Acute pulpitis.
e. Herpetic neuralgia.
f. Masticatory dysfunction syndrome.
g. Pressure on the mental foramen from a denture or residual cyst.
h. Abrasion cavity or a leaking filling.
i. Malignancy.

Moreover, dentists tend to be, quite rightly, conservative; for example, when working on deep dental cavities, the dentist probes gently to avoid exposing the pulp, but in cases with pain of unknown origin, the probe should be applied strongly so that it can penetrate a thin layer of dentin when the underlying pulp may be diseased. Fillings that might otherwise be left may be better removed. It is hoped that teeth will not be uselessly extracted causing unnecessary mutilation but pulps can be extirpated and the teeth restored after endodontic procedures. In a few cases, the dentist's contribution to the problem meets with success and these may involve dentinal faults, pulp disease, retained roots, cysts, impacted teeth, faulty dentures and masticatory dysfunction. Pathological lesions within the bone itself may also be found. This means, of course, that the condition was not idiopathic trigeminal neuralgia but some cases are presented which are more surprising. The following are examples of atypical trigeminal neuralgia:

A female patient, aged 36 years, had a generalized discomfort of the right side of her face, which never completely ceased, with severe attacks of shooting pain. When the pain shot to the ear it always left a sense of deafness and tenderness of the ear. For both the latter reasons, she took to holding the telephone against her other ear. Examination revealed that she was somewhat deaf and the neurosurgeon considered the possibility of an acoustic neuroma. Fortunately, a bitewing radiograph revealed deep dental caries in two teeth. Removal of the fillings and caries revealed that both dental pulps were exposed. Both teeth were extracted and histological examination showed acute inflammation of the pulp in each case. Pain ceased, and it transpired that deafness was coincidental.

An edentulous patient was diagnosed as having idiopathic trigeminal neuralgia affecting the third division but radiographic examination revealed a residual cyst close to the mental foramen. This was removed and pain ceased.

Another patient diagnosed as having idiopathic trigeminal neuralgia had a shooting pain just above his left eyebrow. Radiographic examination of this middle-aged man revealed an unexpected impacted lower left second premolar. This was removed with even more care than usual since levering it might have compressed the inferior dental nerve. Pain ceased.

Among the other possible dental reasons of atypical trigeminal neuralgia are the following:

a. *Tooth extraction.* Considering next the central connections of the trigeminal nerve, an interesting point may be made about the effect of tooth extraction. Idiopathic trigeminal neuralgia can occur whether the teeth are present or absent, and the teeth are not considered to be a factor in themselves. However, they have a rich nerve supply so extraction is associated with considerable deafferentation in terms of both pulpal and periodontal nerve fibers. It might be expected that degeneration of the nerve fibers would be confined to the parts peripheral to the trigeminal ganglion but degeneration proximal to the ganglion also occurs—transganglionic degeneration and involves restricted areas of the spinal nucleus of the trigeminal nerve. If deafferentation from loss of teeth were proved to be an important factor, it would partly explain the preponderance of the disease in the maxillary and mandibular divisions as opposed to the ophthalmic division.

b. *Roughness of the foramina of exit of the trigeminal divisions.* A common cause of pain in the middle and anterior portion of the mandible is an injury or abnormality of the inferior alveolar nerve or its largest terminal branch, the mental nerve. Procedures such as implant placement, simple and complex oral surgical procedures, or improper retraction of a tissue flap containing the mental nerve are all known causes for injury to the mental nerve. In addition, crushing injuries, producing permanent nerve injury, is another recognized cause of mental nerve pain. Trigeminal neuralgia-like pain is often seen in the mental nerve region of the mandible, but frequently, there is no radiographic evidence for the source of such *pain (Altay et al 1997, Shankland, 2009).* Irregularities in the lip of the mental foramen may cause severe irritation to produce a chronic, atypical type of trigeminal neuralgia of the mental nerve distribution, which is not amenable to treatment with medications. *A case was reported by Shankland (2009) whereby the patient's mental* nerve pain was caused by an irregular surface of the anterior portion of the mental foramen. Successful treatment was provided by surgically recontouring the edge or lip of the mental foramen without injury to the mental nerve.

Investigations

The preferred imaging investigation is magnetic resonance imaging, as this will also show up whether there is neurovascular contact between the cerebral vessels and the trigeminal nerve, especially in the root entry zone. Currently magnetic resonance imaging does not have sufficient positive or negative predictive value to assess vascular compression as an etiological factor for this syndrome. Neurophysiological testing such as quantitative sensory testing and evoked potentials (available only in larger centres) can predict symptomatic cases of trigeminal neuralgia (Cruccu et al, 2008; Gronseth et al, 2008). Hematological and biochemical investigations are useful as baselines when using medical therapies. A psychological assessment which includes quality of life and mood is a useful tool in predicting the need for future neurosurgical interventions.

Anesthesia Dolorosa

Following major operations dividing the trigeminal nerve, there are occasional fatalities or various other complications including keratitis following corneal insensitivity. Amongst these is anesthesia dolorosa which occurs in about 3% of cases and as its name implies, is a painful area in a part that is anesthetic. However, anesthesia dolorosa also occurs, some touch sensation being preserved. There may be nothing to see but, after many years, the sufferer may contemplate suicide.

A possible method of investigation is by thermography which shows that the temperature in the area is raised by about 1°C. This does not help treatment but it does help the patient who likes to think the doctor knows that there is objective evidence and the pain is not just imagined. It may also prove of value in attempting to understand the cause of the pain. One possibility, from animal experiments, is that the unpleasant sensation is due to activity in the cut and sprouting nerve fibers. Some cases which seem to be closely related are seen quite often in dental practice after the inferior dental nerve has been damaged in various operative procedures. These patients complain of a burning, tingling sensation in the lower lip which can be so unpleasant as to interfere with eating and cause loss of weight. This condition usually resolves in several months but may take 2 or 3 years. Anesthesia dolorosa is difficult to treat but combinations of analgesics and psychotropic drugs may be tried, clonazepam being most favored.

II. OTHER CRANIAL NEURALGIAS

As, with trigeminal neuralgia, any of the cranial nerves (CNs) with a sensory component appears capable of a neuralgic presentations, e.g. glossopharyngeal neuralgia, facial nerve (VII) (geniculate neuralgia) and greater occipital neuralgia. The most common is the glossopharyngeal nerve (IX) involvement.

   i. Idiopathic glossopharyngeal neuralgia
  ii. Facial nerve "geniculate" neuralgia
 iii. Great auricular neuralgia
 iv. Greater occipital neuralgia

I. IDIOPATHIC GLOSSOPHARYNGEAL NEURALGIA (MIXED NERVE)

Clinically Relevant Anatomy

The glossopharyngeal nerve contains both motor and sensory fibers. The motor fibers innervate the stylopharyngeus muscle. The sensory portion of the nerve innervates the posterior third of the tongue, palatine tonsil, and the mucous membranes of the mouth and pharynx. Special visceral afferent sensory fibers transmit information from the taste buds of the posterior third of the tongue. Information from the carotid sinus and body that helps control blood pressure, pulse, and respiration is carried via the carotid sinus nerve, which is a branch of the glossopharyngeal nerve.

Parasympathetic fibers pass via the glossopharyngeal nerve to the otic ganglion. Postganglionic fibers from the ganglion carry secretory information to the parotid gland. The glossopharyngeal nerve exits from the jugular foramen in proximity to the vagus and accessory nerves and the internal jugular vein (Fig. 11.44). All three nerves lie in the groove between the internal jugular vein and internal carotid artery. The nerve proceeds inferiorly and courses medially, where it lies submucosally behind the palatine tonsil, allowing easy access via the intraoral approach.

Signs and Symtoms

The pain of glossopharyngeal neuralgia is similar to that of trigeminal neuralgia and the paroxysm is

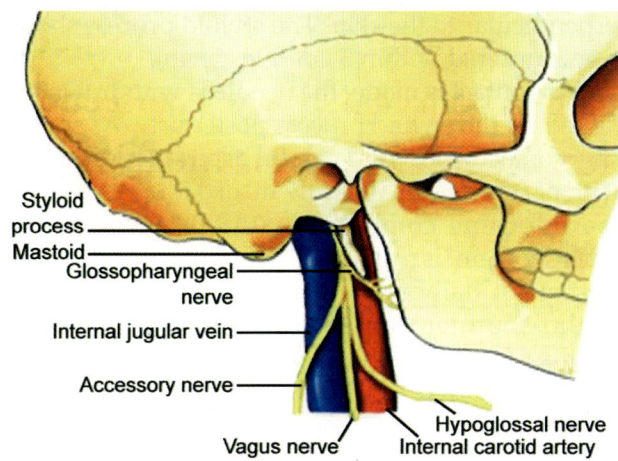

Styloid process
Mastoid
Glossopharyngeal nerve
Internal jugular vein
Accessory nerve
Vagus nerve
Hypoglossal nerve
Internal carotid artery

Fig. 11.44: The glossopharyngeal nerve exits from the jugular foramen in proximity to the vagus, accessory nerves, and the internal jugular vein

similarly triggered by swallowing, chewing, talking, yawning, coughing or sneezing. As might be expected, eating is an ordeal so there is likely to be loss of weight. Kerr (1967) stated that idiopathic trigeminal neuralgia was 100 times more common than idiopathic glossopharyngeal neuralgia and this proportion seems acceptable. The two conditions may be present simultaneously according to Petr (1970) who found 5 such combined cases in a series of 480 cases of trigeminal neuralgia (1%); the pain of both ceased after transection of the sensory root of the trigeminal nerve.

The trigger zones and the pain are in the tonsils, the pharyngeal wall, the base of the tongue and the ears. The pain of glossopharyngeal neuralgia usually starts in the tonsillar fossa and extends to the ipsilateral ear. The timing of the pain is similar to that of trigeminal neuralgia. Paroxysms of pain of increasing intensity last 20–30 seconds and are often followed by a burning sensation for 2–3 minutes. The clinician's finger on the tonsil provokes the pain and the only case who came directly to the author actually lost consciousness on one occasion—according to the patient and his wife. The explanation of this is said to be that neural impulses from the tonsillar trigger point proceed centrally and are interpreted as coming from the carotid sinus, also innervated by the glossopharyngeal nerve, and the heart slows reflexly.

The pain of glossopharyngeal neuralgia usually starts in the tonsillar fossa and extends to the ipsilateral ear. Paroxysms of pain of increasing intensity last 20–30 seconds and are often followed by a burning sensation for 2–3 minutes.

Reichert's syndrome is an " incomplete" neuralgia affecting the tympanic branch of the glossopharyngeal nerve. It may be relieved by intracranial section of the glossopharyngeal nerve.

The glossopharyngeal nerve is rarely involved alone (e.g. by neuralgia), but generally together with the vagus and accessory nerves by compression, inflammation, or trauma. Lesion which may involve the ninth nerve include bulbar diseases, syphilis, tuberculosis, basal tumors, jugular vein thrombosis, trauma in the retroparotid space, aneurysm of the circle of Willis, and diphtheritic neuritis.

The pharyngeal (gag) reflex depends on the ninth nerve for its sensory component; stroking of the affected side does not produce gagging, if the nerve is injured. Vernet's Rideau phenomenon (constriction of the posterior pharyngeal wall in saying, "Ah") is absent when the ninth nerve is involved. The carotid sinus reflex depends on the ninth nerve for its sensory component. Pressure over the sinus normally produces slowing of the heart and a fall in blood pressure.

The dentist will have to consider the problem/occasionally when a patient complains of a pain near the tonsil or the posterior part of the lower alveolar ridge and mylohyoid ridge. The likely cause of this is from an over-extended flange of a lower denture which could be stimulating the lingual nerve. Such a denture has the flange reduced and repolished and pain should cease. Also the denture can be left out for a while. Such a case is possible when a patient has worn the same denture for many years and the alveolar ridge has been resorbed, thus allowing the denture to settle lower in the mouth.

Treatment

Glossopharyngeal nerve block is a simple technique that can produce dramatic relief for patients suffering from the previously mentioned pain complaints. The management of glossopharyngeal neuralgia aims at achieving long-term relief and includes:

1. Carbamazepine is given as for trigeminal neuralgia.

2. Neurolytic block with small quantities of alcohol, phenol, and glycerol. Neurolytic block with small quantities of alcohol, phenol and glycerol has been shown to provide long-term relief for patients suffering from glossopharyngeal neuralgia and cancer-related pain who have not responded to more conservative treatments.

3. Destruction of the glossopharyngeal nerve can also be carried out by creating a radiofrequency lesion under biplanar fluoroscopic guidance.

4. Injection of lidocaine and methyl prednisolone. 7 ml of 0.5% preservative-free lidocaine combined with 80 mg of methyl prednisolone is injected in incremental doses. Subsequent daily nerve blocks are carried out in a similar manner, substituting 40 mg of methylprednisolone for the initial 80 mg dose.

5. If this fails the glossopharyngeal nerve is cut, approaching via the posterior cranial fossa or via the neck.

Injection of Neurolytic Agents (Alcohol)

A. *Extraoral Approach*

The key landmark for extraoral glossopharyngeal nerve block is the styloid process of the temporal bone. This osseous process represents the calcification of the cephalad end of the stylohyoid ligament. Although usually easy to identify, the styloid process may be difficult to locate with the exploring needle, if ossification is limited.

The patient is placed in the supine position. An imaginary line is visualized running from the mastoid process to the angle of the mandible (Fig. 11.45). The styloid process should lie just below the midpoint of this line. The skin is prepped with antiseptic solution. A 22-gauge, 1½-inch needle attached to a 10 ml syringe is advanced at this midpoint location in a plane

perpendicular to the skin. The styloid process should be encountered within 3 cm (Fig. 11.46).

After contact is made, the needle is withdrawn and walked off the styloid process posteriorly. As soon as bony contact is lost and careful aspiration reveals no blood or cerebrospinal fluid, 7 ml of 0.5% preservative-free lidocaine combined with 80 mg of methyl prednisolone is injected in incremental doses. Subsequent daily nerve blocks are carried out in a similar manner, substituting 40 mg of methyl prednisolone for the initial 80 mg dose. This approach may also be used for breakthrough pain in patients who previously experienced adequate pain control with oral medication.

B. *Intraoral Approach*

The patient is placed in the supine position. The tongue is anesthetized with 2% viscous lidocaine. The patient opens the mouth wide and the tongue is then retracted inferiorly with a tongue depressor or laryngoscope blade. A 22-gauge, 3½ inch spinal needle that has been bent approximately 25° is inserted through the mucosa at the lower lateral portion of the posterior tonsillar pillar (Fig. 11.47).

The needle is advanced approximately 0.5 cm. After careful aspiration for blood and cerebrospinal fluid, 7 ml of 0.5% preservative-free lidocaine combined with 80 mg of methylprednisolone is injected in

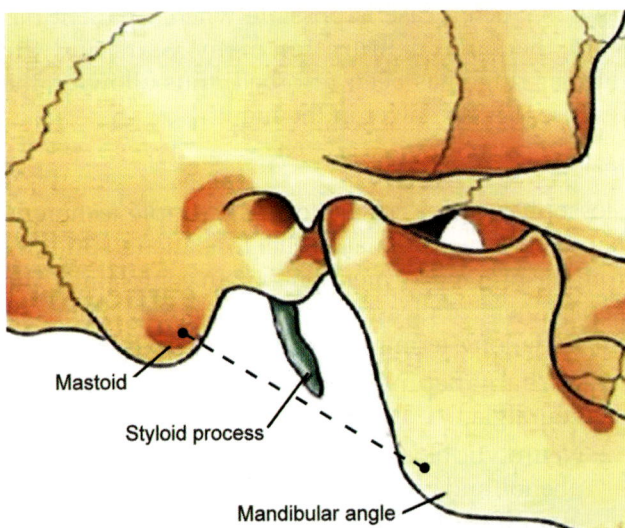

Fig. 11.45: Extraoral approach. The key landmark for extraoral glossopharyngeal nerve block is the styloid process. The styloid process lies below a midpoint of a line connecting the mastoid process and angle of the mandible

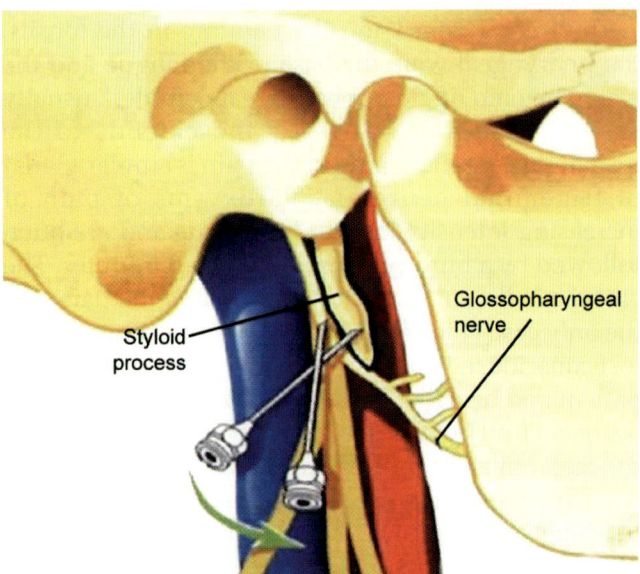

Fig. 11.46: The needle is inserted at the midpoint of the mastoid–mandibular angle plane perpendicular to the skin for 3 cm to contact the styloid process. The needle is then slightly withdrawn and injection is carried out

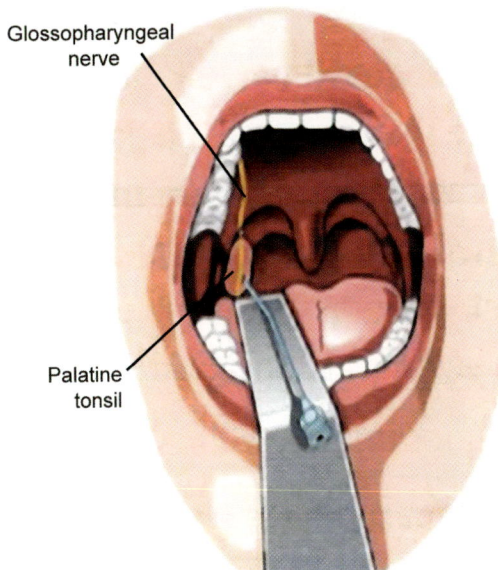

Glossopharyngeal nerve

Palatine tonsil

Fig. 11.47: Intraoral approach. A needle bent 25° is inserted through the mucosa at the lower lateral portion of the posterior tonsillar pillar. The needle is then advanced 0.5 cm to approximate the glossopharyngeal nerve

incremental doses. Subsequent daily nerve blocks are carried out in a similar manner, substituting 40 mg of methylprednisolone for the initial 80 mg dose.

Side effects and complications
1. As mentioned earlier, the proximity of the glossopharyngeal nerve to major vasculature (the internal jugular vein and carotid artery):
   a. Makes post-block hematoma and ecchymosis a distinct possibility. While these complications are usually transitory in nature, their dramatic appearance can be quite upsetting to the patient, and, therefore, the patient should be warned of such prior to the procedure.
   b. The vascularity of this region also increases the incidence of inadvertent intravascular injection. Even small amounts of local anesthetic injected into the carotid artery at this level will result in local anesthetic toxicity and seizures. Incremental dosing while carefully monitoring the patient for signs of local anesthetic toxicity helps avoid this complication.
2. Blockage of the motor portion of the glossopharyngeal nerve can result in dysphagia secondary to weakness of the stylopharyngeus muscle.
3. If the vagus nerve is inadvertently blocked, as is often the case during glossopharyngeal nerve block.

   a. Dysphonia secondary to paralysis of the ipsilateral vocal cord may occur.
   b. A reflex tachycardia secondary to vagal nerve block is also observed in some patients.
4. Inadvertent block of the hypoglossal and spinal accessory nerves during glossopharyngeal nerve block results in weakness of the tongue and trapezius muscle.
5. A small percentage of patients who undergo chemical neurolysis or neurodestructive procedures of the glossopharyngeal nerve experience post-procedure dysesthesias in the area of anesthesia. These symptoms range from a mildly uncomfortable burning or pulling sensation to severe pain. When this severe post-procedure pain occurs, it is called anesthesia dolorosa.

II. GENICULATE NEURALGIA

This is the analagous condition affecting the seventh cranial nerve and is also known as intermediate neuralgia, the intermediate nerve being the sensory root of the facial nerve. Pain is usually felt deep in the ear, the trigger zone being near the eardrum on the posterosuperior wall of the external auditory meatus (Cohen, 1959). The condition is rare.

III. GREAT AURICULAR NEURALGIA

There is pain behind the ear and it may be felt at the angle of the jaw (Cohen, 1959), though Kerr (1967) said that idiopathic neuralgia did not occur in the first, second and third cervical nerves.

IV. OCCIPITAL NEURALGIA

Clinically Relevant Anatomy

The greater auricular nerve arises from fibers of the primary ventral ramus of the second and third cervical nerves. The greater auricular nerve pierces the fascia inferior and lateral to the lesser occipital nerve. It passes superiorly and forward and then curves around the sternocleidomastoid muscle, moving more superficially to provide cutaneous sensory innervation to the ear, external auditory canal, angle of the jaw, and the skin overlying a portion of the parotid gland (Figs 11.48 and 11.49).

The term greater occipital neuralgias (GON) encompasses a collection of signs and symptoms that develop secondary to a variety of different diseases

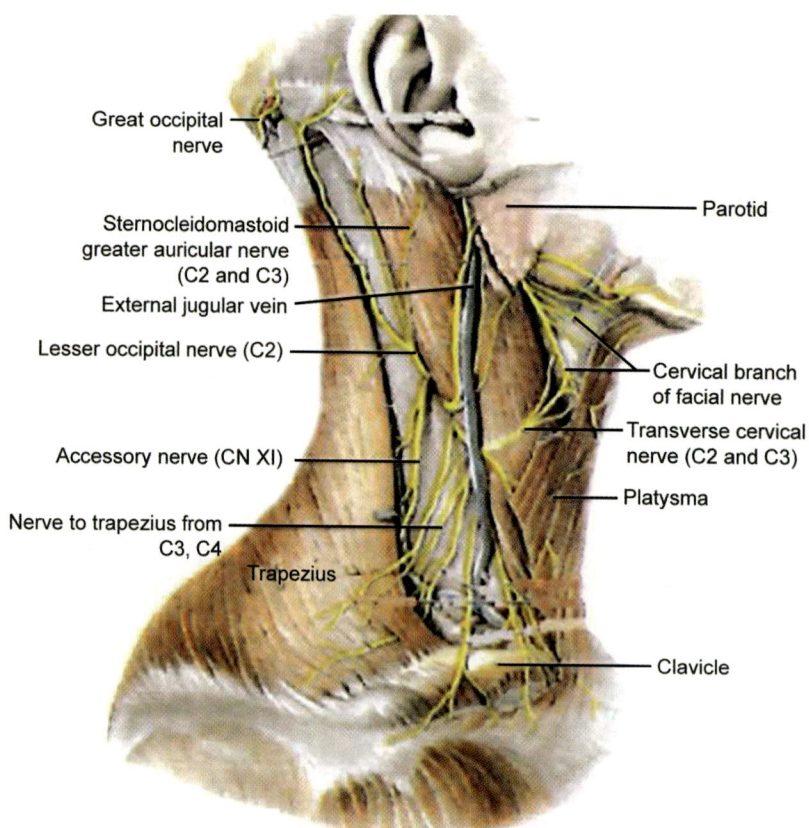

Great occipital nerve

Sternocleidomastoid greater auricular nerve (C2 and C3)

External jugular vein

Lesser occipital nerve (C2)

Accessory nerve (CN XI)

Nerve to trapezius from C3, C4

Trapezius

Parotid

Cervical branch of facial nerve

Transverse cervical nerve (C2 and C3)

Platysma

Clavicle

Fig. 11.48: The greater auricular nerve curves around the sternocleidomastoid muscle, passes upward and forward in the subcut, fascia to provide cutaneous sensation to the ear, external auditory canal, angle of the mandible, and skin covering the parotid gland

such as occipital osteolytic lesions, upper cervical cavernous angioma, cervical osteochondroma, giant cell arteritis, exuberant callus formation and C1-C2 arthrosis syndrome.

Greater occipital neuralgia (GON), apparently more frequent in women, manifests as a paroxysmal, sharp or electric-like pain, unilateral or bilateral in the distribution of the greater, lesser or third occipital nerves, that can be triggered by movement, specifically hyperextension, with or without pain between paroxysms. Occasionally, the pain radiates into the arms and shoulders. The physical examination is usually normal or may show cervical tenderness, limitation of motion and decreased sensation over the C2 dermatome.

Occipital neuralgia has often been implicated in headache syndromes associated with tenderness in the suboccipital area (Bogduk 1989; Anthony 1992; Elias and Burchiel). Trigeminal neuralgia (TN) may be associated with other primary headaches (clustertic and migrainetic syndromes). It is possible that in migraine patients, neuralgias may contribute to headache chronification (Bartsch and Goadsby 2002; Drummond and Granston, 2004).

Pathophysiology

An increased afferent input from primary nociceptive afferents, activating second-order neurons, may cause sensitization and hyperexcitability (Bartsch and Goadsby 2003). This process is thought to involve the release of neuropeptides, including calcitonin gene-related peptide (CGRP), glutamate and substance P. The sensitization may also be the result of decreased local segmental spinal inhibition in response to afferent stimulation (Bartsch and Goadsby 2003; Woolf 2000). In addition to these factors, dysfunctional brainstem pain—modulatory structures could trigger the development of central sensitization.

Clinically, this would explain the phenomenon of hypersensitivity, spread, and referred pain to and from trigeminal and cervical dermatomes, and worsening in the migraine pattern with the

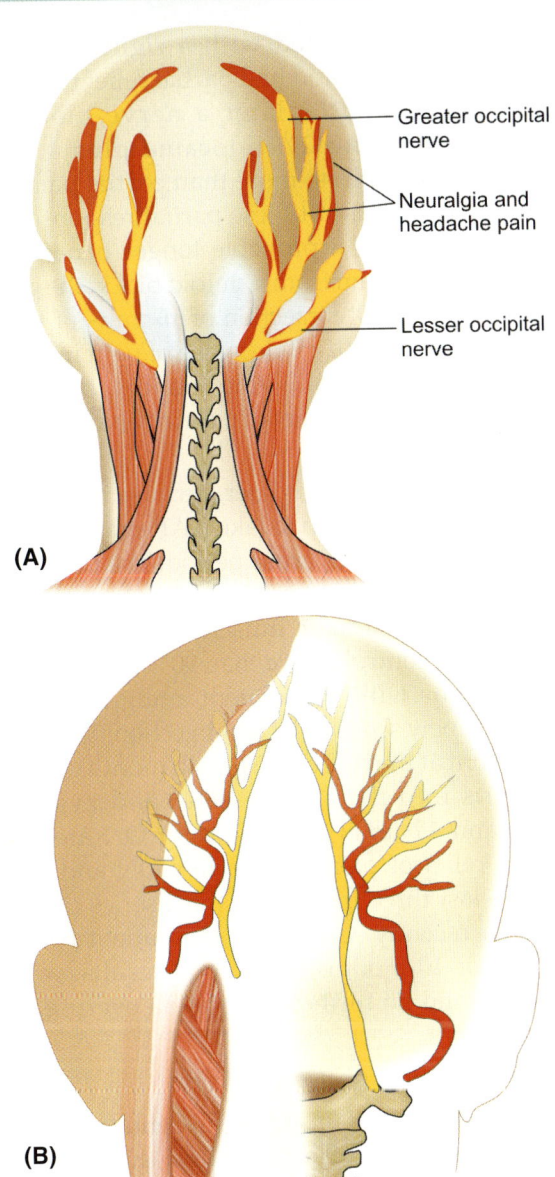

(A)

(B)

Fig. 11.49: Illustration of occipital nerve and artery, superior trapezius and cervical vertebrae

supratentorial dura mater, and ipsilateral, as well as contralateral occipital nerve (Piovesan et al, 2003; Bartsch and Goadsby, 2003). Neuronal convergence with subsequent central sensitization also could partially explain the relationship between TN and migraine refractoriness.

Treatment

1. Injections of local anesthetics and corticosteroids into the region of the occipital nerve (ON) are usually the treatment of choice for ON (Fig.11.50) (Gawel 1992; Rothbart; Terzi et al, 2002).

2. Neurosurgical procedures including nerve resection have been suggested as alternative therapies for the treatment of refractory GON.

3. BTX-A was effective in the local treatment of GON and TN. Several blocks with corticosteroids and other local analgesic substances were less effective than BTX-A (Volcy et al, 2005).

BTX-A proves effective in the local treatment of GON and TN. Several blocks with corticosteroids and other local analgesic substances were less effective than BTX-A.

BTX-A is used to treat various neurological disorders associated with pathologically increased muscle tone. It is of value for the following reasons:

BTX-A inhibits the release of the neurotransmitter acetylcholine at the neuromuscular junction thereby inhibiting striatal muscle contractions. Besides the reduction in muscle tone, BTX-A tends to reduce pain in pain syndromes associated with muscle spasm through the release inhibition of nociceptive

development of secondary medication overuse. The association between occipital neuralgia and migraine could be explained by several factors. On the one hand, the occipital nerve contains fibers from the C2 and C3 dorsal root ramus that emerges through the trapezius and sternocleidomastoid muscles (Vital et al, 1989; Bovim et al, 1991; Bogduk, 1980 and 1989). The trigeminocervical complex neurons are the major relay neurons for nociceptive afferent input from the meninges and cervical structures from the level of the caudal trigeminal nucleus to at least the C2 segment, which allows for a synaptic convergence input from

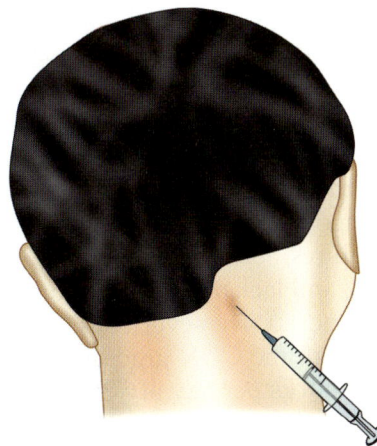

Fig. 11.50: A needle is injected at the base of the skull and the medication is injected around the origin of the occipital nerve

neuropeptides and/or postganglionic sympathetic neuropeptides (norepinephrine and ATP) (Mense, 2004). In addition, BTX-A has been proposed as an analgesic, suggesting alternative noncholinergic mechanisms of action (Dolly, 2003; Dodick et al, 2004; Blumenfeld, 2004; Mathew et al, 2002; Gobel 2004). Indeed, a recent study found evidence that BTX-A can directly decrease the amount of calcitonin gene-related peptide (CGRP) released from afferent nerve terminals of the trigeminal neurons (Durham et al 2004).

Case Report

Volcy et al (2005) under the title of " Botulinum toxin A(BTX-A) therapy for the treatment of trigeminal neuralgia" described a case of 44-year-old white male with a history of migraine with and without aura since the age of 12, characterized by unilateral throbbing pain, predominantly on the left side, of one-day duration. The initial headache frequency was less than three attacks per week of moderate intensity and one severe attack every 6 months.

Since the age of 22, temporally related to a dental procedure, the patient developed severe short-lasting (from 20 s to 2 min) episodes of stabbing pain over the left cheek, of variable frequency (from two per week to four per day). Shaving, talking and local touch triggered the pain. Four years ago, the patient also developed unilateral pain in the left temporo-mandibular joint (TMJ), and was diagnosed with TMJ dysfunction (TMD). At that time, the patient began to overuse aspirin/acetaminophen/caffeine (AAP) (more than 5 pills per/day) and developed daily, diffuse headaches. After the daily headaches were established, the patient had his initial evaluation at our headache centre.

Two years ago, the patient suddenly developed severe, intermittent, stabbing, side-locked right occipital pain, which recurred five to 20 times per day. Duration was one to five minutes. On physical examination, he had significant tenderness in the territory of the right occipital nerve, as well as decreased range of movement of the neck. Based on the clinical features, absence of neck clinical or imaging abnormalities, and lack of pain abolition with blocks, GON was diagnosed. The severity of the pain, as well as the duration of the GON gradually increased, up to 3–4 severe attacks per day of at least 1-h duration.

The GON was treated with a right superficial cervical plexus block and had partial relief for several weeks; seven months later a nerve block was performed injecting 2% lidocaine plus 4 mg of dexamethasone with no more than partial pain relief for 2 months. Because of these partial responses, and taking into account a probable longer benefit from BTX-A treatment than from a steroid block, the patient was given a right ON injection of 15 units of BTX-A. The patient had a gradual decrease of pain in the first 10 days. In the two following months, the patient experienced complete relief of pain in the right greater ON distribution.

However, a few months later, because of persistent left V2 TN pain, he began to take AAP again, resulting in a third medication overuse period. The patient was given an additional 7.5 units of BTX-A into the left masseter and zygomatic muscles, which gave him excellent pain control (more than 90% relief) over the next 2 months with consequent analgesic overuse cessation. A new series of BTX-A injections were given to the patient at the end of the fourth month of follow-up, 6 units into the left masseter and zygomatic muscles and 12 units over the right ON area, with complete relief of pain both from GON and left V2 TN in the last three months. A third series of BTX A was given recently. Currently, the patient has been followed for 10 months, with good results, without side effects and no further medication overuse.

Past medical history and investigation

He underwent several unsuccessful dental procedures for the TMD and the left V2 neuralgia, such as electric stimulation (was successful just for 1 week) and two series of nerves blocks with mepivacaine/ steroid with partial benefit(last time in August 2003). The patient had two normal brain MRIs with and without contrast (July 2000 and August 2001).

The case reported herein has several particularities. Of particular note: In a patient with episodic migraine, poor control of GON and TN were associated with increase in migraine frequency and development of medication overuse headache; effective treatment of both disorders was associated with reduction in headache frequency and analgesic use.

III. OTHER NEUROPATHIC FACIAL PAIN

A. Post herpetic neuralgia
B. Neuroma
C. Burning mouth syndrome.

A. POSTHERPETIC NEURALGIA

Postherpetic neuralgia (PHN) is a potential sequelae of herpes zoster infection. Shingels, or herpes zoster, may occur at any stage in a person's life. By far the greater number of cases of herpes zoster heal completely and remain pain free. Unfortunately, in about 20% of cases pain persists as postherpetic neuralgia, perhaps for months and may even last for years. Herpes zoster is the clinical manifestation of the reactivation of a lifelong latent infection with varicella-zoster virus, usually contracted after an episode of chickenpox in early life. Herpes zoster occurs more commonly in later life and in immuno-compromised patients.

Varicella-zoster virus tends to be reactivated only once in lifetime, with the incidence of the second attacks being less than 5%. PHN occurs after reactivation of the virus, which can lay dormant in the ganglia of a peripheral nerve. Most commonly this is a thoracic nerve, but approximately 10 to 15% of the time the trigeminal nerve is involved, with the VI dermatome affected in approximately 80% of cases. When reactivated, the virus travels along the nerve and is expressed in that nerves cutaneous dermatome. For a thoracic nerve, for example, the patient develops a unilateral patch of vesicular eruption closely outlining the classical dermatome for that nerve. In the ophthalmic division of the trigeminal nerve, the VI dermatome is outlined by rash. In the V2 and V3 distribution, both intraoral and cutaneous expression is commonly seen (Figs 11.51 and 11.52). The acute phase is quite painful but subsides within approximately 2 to 5 weeks.

However, a subset of patients develops a deafferentiation pain that, as discussed previously, can have peripheral, central or mixed features. The pain is typically burning, aching or shock-like consistent with a pain caused by a neuropathic condition. It occurs spontaneously but is made worse by contact, with the result that the patient may withdraw from the clinician's examining hand, i.e. there is hyperalgesia. There may be paresthesia and some weakness of the masseter and pterygoid muscles on

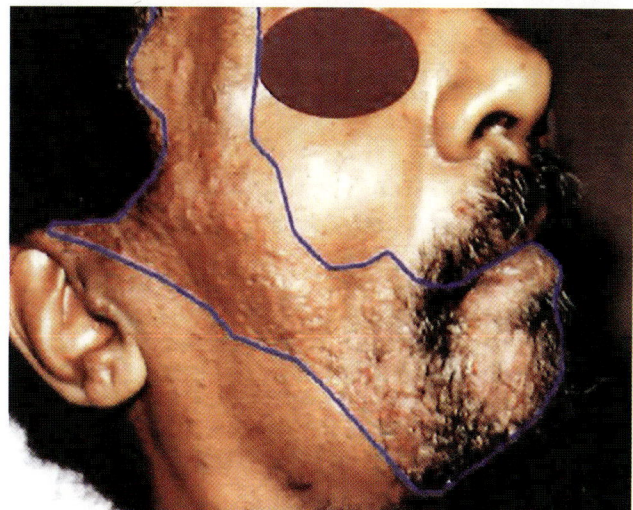

Fig. 11.51: Herpes zoster involving the distribution of the mandibular nerve

the affected side. In this disease, there is a loss of the larger diameter nerve fibers via which an inhibitory effect is usually exerted over the smaller diameter fibers which are important in the mediation of pain. Since the larger diameter fibers are lost and they can no longer exert this influence there is less presynaptic inhibition and the area becomes painful.

Treatment

The reason for early treatment is that once the postherpetic neuralgia starts it has a tendency to become intractable. Various treatments for this have been tried, including acupuncture, transcutaneous neural stimulation, and nerve blocks. Treatment is undertaken with anticonvulsant or the tricyclic or other antidepressants. Tramadol, a mild opioid with mild antidepressant effects can be useful adjunct. Local injection of painful sites, sympathetic block, or both is sometimes of value. Most importantly, preventive treatment of PHN with antivirals, analgesics, and frequently corticosteroids very early after rash presentation can significantly reduce the expression of PHN.

A related condition, **Ramsay-Hunt syndrome,** is a herpes zoster infection of the sensory and motor

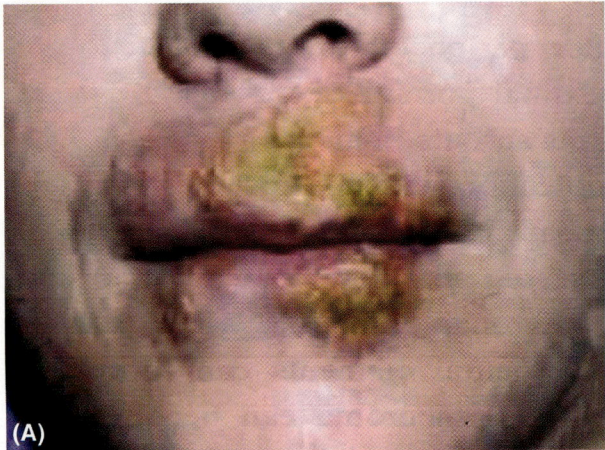

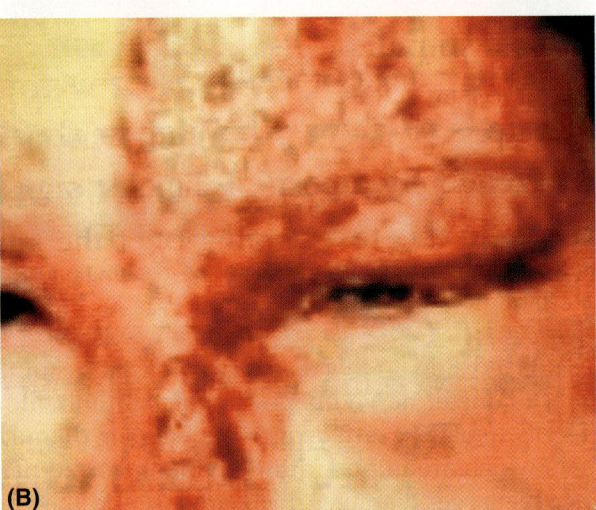

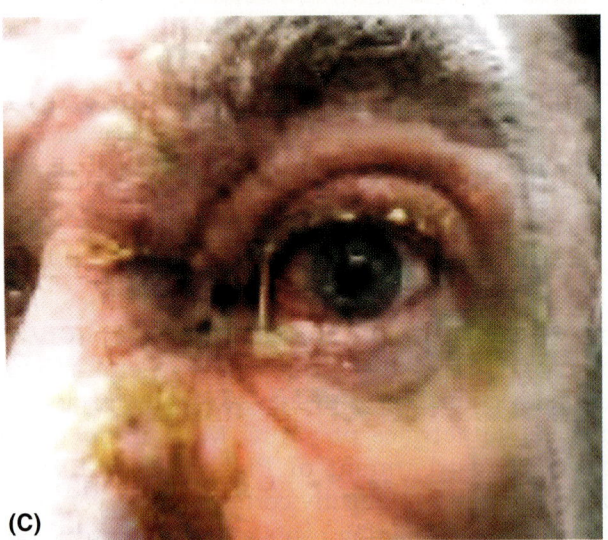

Fig. 11.52: **(A)** Vesicular eruption of heres zoster develops in the upper and lower lips, **(B)** the frontal region, and **(C)** the nose bridge

branches of the facial nerve (VII) and in some cases the auditory nerve (VIII). Symptoms include facial paralysis, vertigo, deafness and herpetic eruption in the external auditory meatus.

B. NEUROMA

After peripheral nerve transection, the proximal portion of the nerve generally forms sprouts in an effort to regain communication with the severed distal component. When sprouting occurs without distal segment communication, a stump of neuronal tissue, Schwann cells, and other neural elements can form. This stump, or neuroma can become exquisitely sensitive to both mechanical and chemical stimuli.

The pain is commonly burning or shock-like. Frequently a positive Tinel's sign is present. In this test, tapping over the suspected neuroma produces sharp shooting electric shock-like pain. Damage to the mandibular or lingual nerve after third molar surgery is another source for neuroma formation. Some oral and maxillofacial surgeons provide microneurosurgical treatment, which can be beneficial for some patients.

Although it is difficult to predict which patient will benefit from nerve repair, it is clear that neurosurgical intervention should be accomplished within 3 to 6 months to improve the likelihood of success.

C. BURNING MOUTH SYNDROME *(Glossodynia, oral dysesthesia, stomatodynia)*

Burning mouth syndrome is a common dysesthesia (distortion of sense) characterized by burning sensation, experienced in the absence of identifiable organic etiological factors. The International Association for the Study of Pain defined it as "A distinctive nosological entity characterized by unremitting oral burning or similar pain in the absence of detectable mucosal changes".

Etiology

Current literature favors the following etiologic factors:

1. *Hormonal imbalance:* The fact that most patients are post-menopausal women has led to the common belief that estrogen or progesterone deficit is responsible, but a strong correlation between such deficits and burning tongue syndrome has not been established.

2. *Autoimmune origin:* Some evidence exists for an autoimmune origin. Abnormal levels of

antinuclear antibody (ANA) and rheumatoid factor (RF), for example, are found in the serum of more than 50% of patients, although these may also be found in older persons without burning mouth syndrome.

3. *Psychogenic cause:* Such as anxiety, depression, or cancerphobia, can be identified in about 20% of cases.

4. *Neurological disturbance:* The cause is unknown but a defect in pain modulation may be the most promising theory. Changes in the dopaminergic system result in trigeminal excitability or loss of central inhibition from taste damage in the chorda tympani and/or glossopharyngeal nerve (Fig. 11.53), or asymptomatic activity-mediated neuropathic disorder induced by traumatic trigeminal nerve injury or varicella-zoster infection.

Dopamine is secreted by neurons that originate in the substantia nigra and extend into the basal ganglia. The normal effect of dopamine is inhibitory.

Although no precipitating cause for burning mouth syndrome can be identifies in a great percentage of cases, however, in some patients local or systemic factors may be identifiable.

The local precipitating causes: Allergies bruxism, tongue thrust, candidiasis dermatoses, e.g. lichen planus, dry mouth erythema migrains, geographic tongue and fissured tongue.

The systemic precipitating factors include hematinic deficiency of vitamin B_{12}, folate and iron drugs, hormonal diabetes, hypothyroidism and HIV.

The substances implicated in causing oral burning sensation include food and additives, e.g. benzoic acid chesnuts cinnamonaldehyde instant coffe nicotinic acid peanuts sodium metabisulpite scorbic acid, metals as cadmium cobalt chloride mercury nickel pallidium, platics as benzoyl perioxide epoxy resins methyl methacrylate.

In the postmenopausal sufferers, hormone replacement therapy does not consistently affect symptoms. Approximately 50% of patients improve without treatment over a 2 years period indicating the importance of placebo-controlled trials when scientifically testing any treatment modality. The predominant treatment approach is with antidepressants or anticonvulsants, although neither avenue, even in combination, shows consistent results.

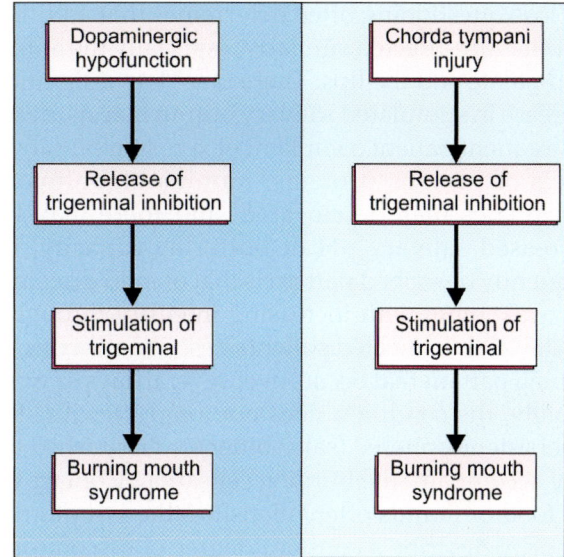

Fig. 11.53: Burning mouth syndrome may have a neurological basis

Clinical Features

The disorder has a typically spontaneous onset, although it may be quite gradual. In this condition, the patient perceives a burning or aching sensation in all or part of the oral cavity. The tongue is the most frequently involved site. Although the tongue is most commnoly affected (glossopyrosis), other mucosal surfaces may also be affected (stomatopyrosis). Women are 4 to 7 times more likely to have burning tongue syndrome than men. The onset in women usually occurs within 3 to 12 years after menopause. The syndrome is rare before the age of 30 years, is especially seen in middle-aged or elderly patients.

The dorsum of the tongue develops a burning, scalded, tingling sensation usually bilateral and sometimes is strongest in the anterior third. These abnormal sensations are not worsened by eating. Rather it is often relieved by eating and drinking, in contrast to pain caused by organic lesions, which is typically aggravated by eating. Alcohol may reduce the symptoms.

Mucosal changes are seldom visible, although some patients will show diminished numbers and size of filiform papillae and individuals who rub their tonguer against the teeth often have erythematous and edematous papillae on the tip of ther tongue. If the dorsum is significantly erythematous and smooth, an underlying systemic or local infectious process, such as anemia or erythematous candidiasis, should be suspected.

Close questioning often determines that additional oral sites are affected similarly, especially the anterior hard palate and the lips. There is seldom a significant decrease in stimulated salivary output in tests, despite the frequent patient complaint of xerostomia. Salivary levels of various proteins, immunoglobulins and phosphates may be elevated, and there may be a decreased salivary pH or buffering capacity. One frequently described pattern is that of mild discomfort on awakening, with increasing intensity throughout the day. Other affected patients describe a waxing and waning pattern that occurs over several days or weeks. Usually, the condition does not interfere with sleep. A persistently altered (salty, bitter) or diminished taste may accompany the burning sensation. Contact with hot food or liquids often intensifies the symptoms. A minority describe a constant degree of discomfort.

As with other chronic disorders, affected patients frequently demonstrate psychologic dysfunction, usually depression, anxiety, or irritability. The dysfunction often disappears, however, with resolution of the burning or painful tongue condition, and there is no correlation between duration and intensity of the burning sensation and the amount of psychologic dysfunction.

Management

It is important to clearly acknowledge the reality of the patient's symptoms and distress and never to trivialize or dismiss them. Active dental or oral surgical treatment or attempts at hormone replacement in the absence of any specific indication should be avoided. Try and explain the psychosomatic background to the problem, ascribing the symptoms to causes for which the patient cannot be blamed. Help the patient to cope with the symptoms, rather than attempt any impossible cure. Describe one of the mood altering drugs, e.g. clonazepam tablets 0.5 mg. Take one tablet, then adjust dose after 3 day intervals. This therapy is probably best managed by an appropriate specialist or the patient's physician at this time. Other antidepressant drugs include amitriptyline tablets 25 mg, one tablet at bedtime for one week, then 2 tablets hs. Increase to 3 tablets hs after 2 weeks and maintain at that dosage or titrate as appropriate. Explain that antidepressants, if prescribed, are being used to treat the symptoms not depression and that antidepressants have been shown in controlled trials to be effective for the problem, whether or not the patient is depressed. The pain reduction achieved with antidepressants exceeds that produced by the placebos, but antidepressants must be given for at least 3–4 weeks to achieve any antidepressive effect.

The long-term prognosis for idiopathic burning tongue or mouth syndrome is variable. Some patients experience a spontaneous or gradual remission months or years after the onset of symptoms. However, other patients may continue to experience symptoms throughout the rest of their lives. Even though the condition is chronic and may not always respond to therapy, patients should be reassured that it is benign and not a symptom of oral cancer.

DISORDERS OF TASTE

Taste (**gustation**) is a sensation that results from the action of chemicals on the **taste buds.** There are about 4,000 of taste buds, located not only on the tongue but also inside the cheeks and on the soft palate, pharynx, and epiglottis.

Anatomy

The tongue, where the sense of taste is best developed, is marked by four types of bumps called lingual papillae (Fig. 11.54):

1. *Filiform* * *papillae* are tiny spikes without taste buds. They are responsible for the rough feel of a cat's tongue and are important to many mammals for grooming the fur. They are the most abundant papillae on the human tongue, but they are small and play no gustatory role. They are, however, important to appreciation of the texture of food.

2. *Foliate* ** *papillae* are also weakly developed in humans. They form parallel ridges on the sides of the tongue about two-thirds of the way back from the tip. Most of their taste buds degenerate by the age of 2 or 3 years.

3. *Fungiform* *** *papillae* are shaped somewhat like mushrooms. Each has about three taste buds, located mainly on the apex. These papillae are widely distributed but especially concentrated at the tip and sides of the tongue.

---

* *fili = thread, form = shaped.*
** *foli = leaf, ate = like.*
*** *fungi = mushroom, form = shaped.*

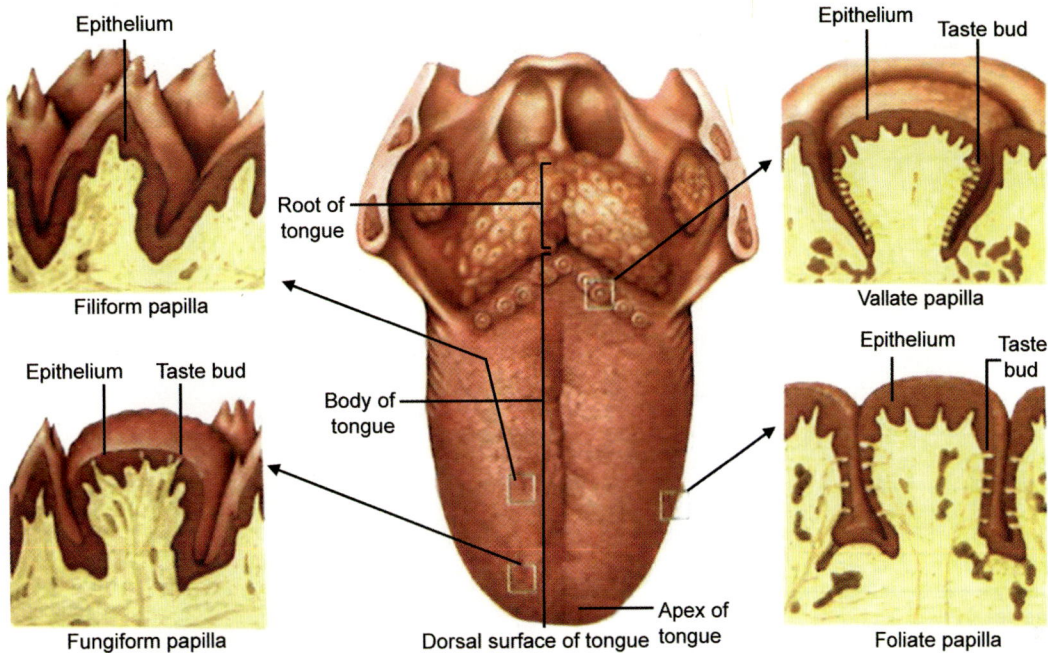

Fig. 11.54: Tongue papillae. Papillae are small elevations on the tongue surface that exist in four types: filiform, fungiform, vallate and foliate. In adults, only fungiform and vallate papillae contain taste buds for gestation; in infants and young children; the foliate papillae have a few taste buds *(McKinely and O'Loughlin 2006)*.

4. *Vallate**** (circumvallate) papillae* are large papillae arranged in a V at the rear of the tongue. Each is surrounded by a deep circular trench. There are only 7 to 12 of them, but they contain about half of all our taste buds— around 250 each, located on the wall of the papilla facing the trench. Regardless of location and sensory specialization, all taste buds look alike. They are lemon-shaped groups of 40 to 60 cells of three kinds— *taste cells, supporting cells* and *basal cells.*

Taste (gustatory) cells are more or less banana-shaped and have a tuft of apical microvilli called taste hairs that serve as receptor surfaces for taste molecules (Fig. 11.55). The hairs project into a pit called a taste pore on the epithelial surface of the tongue. Taste cells are epithelial cells, not neurons, but they synapse with sensory nerve fibers at their base. A taste cell lives 7 to 10 days and is then replaced by mitosis and differentiation of basal cells. Supporting cells have a similar shape but no taste hairs. They lie between the taste cells.

Physiology

Taste buds are present on the tongue mainly, but also on the soft palate, uvula, epiglottis, pharynx, larynx and esophagus. Taste perception can be tested with salt (NaCl), sweet (saccharin), acidic (citrus) and bitter (quinine), or by electrogustometry. The complex process of tasting begins when molecules stimulate special sensory cells in the nose, mouth, or throat. These gustatory or taste cells react to food and beverages. Another chemosensory mechanism, the common chemical sense, contributes to appreciation of food flavor, especially to sensation like the sting of ammonia, the coolness of menthol and the irritation of chili peppers. Human can commonly identify at least five different taste sensations: sweet, sour, bitter, salty and umami (the taste elicited by glutamate, found in chicken broth, meat extracts and some cheeses). Flavors are recognized mainly through the sense of smell.

To be tasted, molecules must dissolve in the saliva and flood the taste pore. On a dry tongue, sugar or salt has as little taste as a sprinkle of sand. Physiologists currently recognize five primary taste sensations (Fig. 11.56):

1. *Salty,* produced by metal ions such as sodium and potassium. Since these are vital electrolytes, there is obvious value in our ability to taste them and

---

**** *vall = wall, ate = like, possessing.*

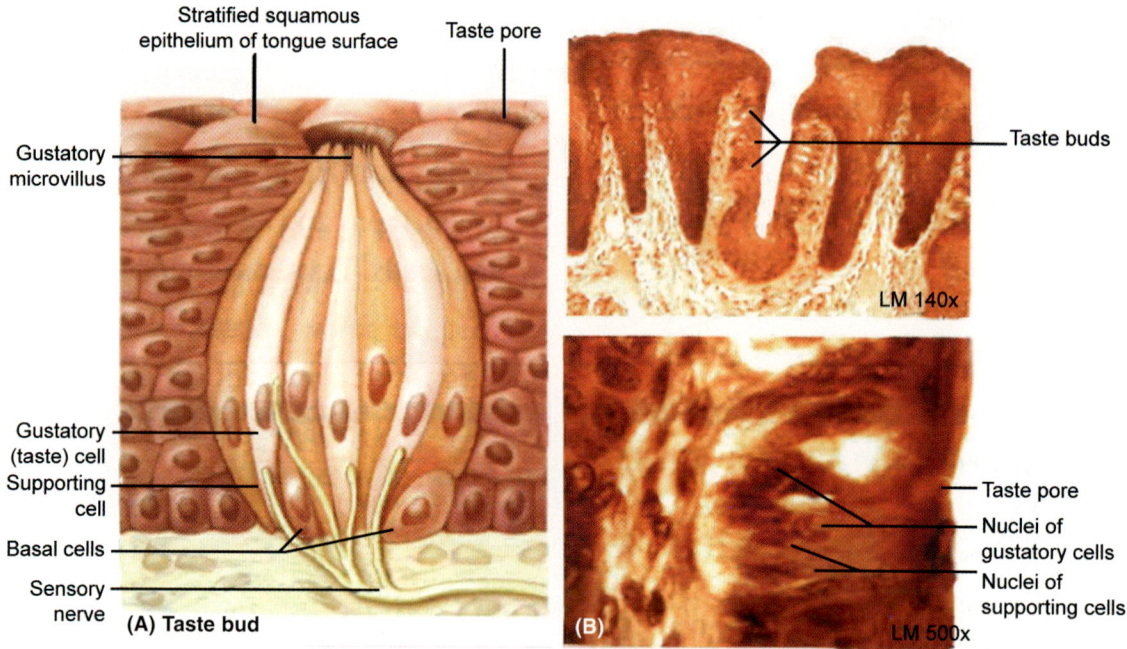

Fig. 11.55: Taste buds, **(A)** The detailed structure of a taste bud and its organization in the wall of a papilla, **(B)** Photomicrographs show the histologic structure of taste buds *(McKinely and O'Loughlin 2006)*

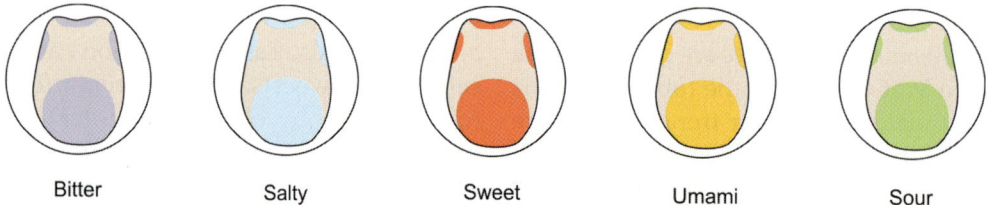

Fig. 11.56: Regions of the tongue sensitive to different categories of taste

in having an appetite for salt. Electrolyte deficiencies can cause a craving for salt; many animals such as deer, elephants, and parrots thus seek salt deposits when necessary. Pregnancy can lower a woman's electrolyte concentrations and create a craving for salty food.

2. *Sweet*, produced by many organic compounds, especially sugars. Sweetness is associated with carbohydrates and foods of high caloric value. Many flowering plants have evolved sweet nectar and fruits that entice animals to eat them and disperse their pollen and seeds. Thus, our fondness for fruit has coevolved with plant reproductive strategies.

3. *Sour*, usually associated with acids in such foods as citrus fruits.

4. *Bitter*, associated with spoiled foods and with alkaloids such as nicotine, caffeine, quinine and morphine. Bitter alkaloids are often poisonous, and this sensation usually induces a human or animal to reject a food. While flowering plants make their fruits temptingly sweet, they often load their leaves with bitter, toxic alkaloids to deter animals from eating them.

5. *Umami*, is a "meaty" taste produced by amino acids such as aspartic and glutamic acids. The taste is best known from the salt of glutamic acid, monosodium glutamate (MSG). Pronounced "oohmommy," the word is Japanese slang for "delicious" or "yummy."

All of the primary tastes can be detected throughout the tongue, but certain regions are more sensitive to one category than to others. The tip of the tongue is most sensitive to sweet tastes, which trigger such responses as licking, salivation, and swallowing. The lateral margins of the tongue are the most sensitive areas for salty and sour tastes. Taste buds in the vallate papillae at the rear of the tongue are especially sensitive to bitter compounds, which tend to trigger rejection responses such as gagging to protect against the ingestion of toxins. The threshold for the bitter taste is the lowest of all—that is, we can taste lower concentrations of alkaloids than of acids, salts and sugars. The senses of sweet and salty are the least sensitive. It is not yet known whether umami stimulates any particular region of the tongue more than other regions. Sugars, alkaloids and glutamate stimulate taste cells by binding to receptors on the membrane surface, which then activate G proteins and second-messenger systems within the cell. Sodium and acids penetrate into the cell and depolarize it directly. By either mechanism, stimulated taste cells then release neurotransmitters that stimulate the sensory dendrites at their base.

The many flavors we perceive are not simply a mixture of these five primary tastes but are also influenced by food texture, aroma, temperature, appearance, and one's state of mind, among other things. Many flavors depend on smell; without its aroma, cinnamon merely has a faintly sweet taste, and coffee and peppermint are bitter. Some flavors such as pepper are due to stimulation of free endings of the trigeminal nerve. Food scientists refer to the texture of food as *mouthfeel.* Filiform and fungiform papillae of the tongue are innervated by the *lingual nerve* (a branch of the trigeminal) and are sensitive to texture.

Projection Pathways

Taste buds stimulate (Fig. 11.57):

- The facial nerve (VII) in the anterior two-thirds of the tongue. Taste fibers of the facial nerve run in the chorda tympani to the lingual nerve and supply the receptors of the fungiform papillae on the anterior two-thirds of the tongue.

- The glossopharyngeal nerve (IX) in the posterior one-third, taste fibers of the glossopharyngeal nerve run in the lingual branches of the glossopharyngeal nerve to the posterior third of the tongue and supply the receptors of the vallate papillae. In the tonsillar branches of the glossopharyngeal nerve, taste fibers run to the soft palate.

- The vagus nerve (X) in the palate, pharynx, and epiglottis. Taste fibers of the vagus nerve reach the epiglottis and the epipharynx through the pharyngeal branches of the vagus nerve.

The fibers originate from pseudounipolar neurons in the cranial nerve ganglia, namely:

- The *geniculate ganglion*
- The *petrosal ganglion* (inferior ganglion of the glossopharyngeal nerve) and
- The *nodose ganglion* (inferior ganglion of the vagus nerve).

All taste fibers project to the *solitary nucleus* in the medulla oblongata. Second-order neurons from this nucleus relay the signals to two destinations: (1) nuclei in the hypothalamus and amygdala that activate autonomic reflexes such as salivation, gagging and vomiting and (2) the thalamus, which relays signals to the insula and postcentral gyrus of the cerebrum, where we become conscious of the taste.

Causes of Hypogeusia

1. Upper respiratory infections
2. Head injury
3. Chemicals such as insecticides
4. Some drugs
5. Oral health problems
6. Surgery with nerve damage (third molar extraction and middle ear surgery)
7. Radiation therapy
8. Diabetes
9. Hypertension
10. Malnutrition

Disorders of taste are fairly common and can have a wide range of causes (Table 11.3). Similar conditions to those that cause halitosis can cause a bad taste in the mouth (dysguesia). The sense of taste can also be temporarily disturbed by the use of chemicals such as chlorhexidine. Gymnemic acid abolishes the perception of sweet tastes while amiloride abolishes salt perception. Loss of taste can be due to medical disorders, or anesthesia of the nerves involved, particularly damage to chorda tympani (from herpes zoster oticus, otitis media, mastoiditis, or cholesteatoma). The most common taste complaint is of phantom taste perceptions. Additionally, testing may demonstrate a weakened ability to taste sweet, sour, bitter, salty and umami (ageusia). Rarely there is complete lack of taste perception (ageusia). Perceived loss usually reflects a smell loss, which is often confused with a taste loss. In odor disorders of the chemical senses, the system may misread and/or distort an odor, a taste or a flavor. Alternatively, a person may detect a foul taste from a substance that is normally pleasant tasting (Table 11.3).

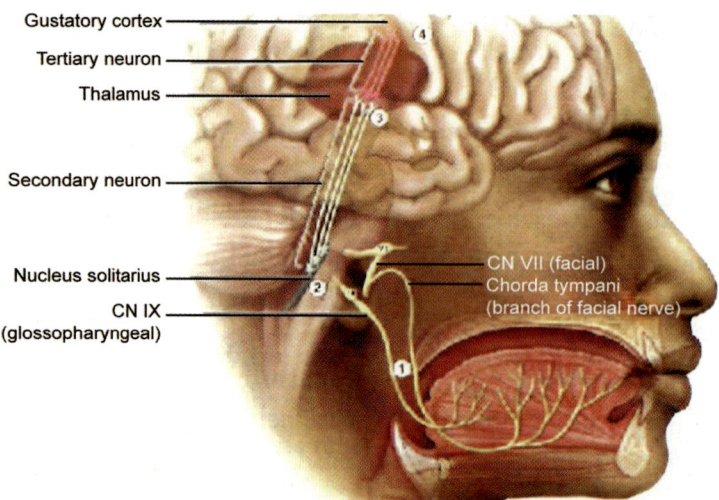

Fig. 11.57: Gustatory pathway. Taste sensations are carried by the paired facial nerves (CN VII) from the anterior two-thirds of the tongue and by the glossopharyngeal nerves (CN IX) from the posterior one-third of the tongue. These taste sensations enter the brainstem and travel to the nucleus solitarius before being conducted to the thalamus and finally entering the gustatory cortex of the cerebrum *(McKinely & O'Loughlin 2006)*

1. Primary (sensory) neuron axons from gustatory cells pass from the tongue through cranial nerves VII and IX.
2. Primary neurons synapse in the nucleus solitarius of the brainstem.
3. Secondary neurons travel from the nucleus solitarius and synapse in the thalamus.
4. Tertiary neurons travel from the thalamus and terminate in the gustatory cortex of the cerebrum

Table 11.3: Causes of taste loss or change

Ageing	
Local causes	Xerostomia
	Irradiation of the oral cavity
	Antihistamines
	Antihypertensives
Drugs	Antidepressants
	Cytotoxic agents
	Protease inhibitors
	Alzheimer's disease
	Chorda tympani damage
	Facial palsy
Neurological causes	Head trauma
	Multiple sclerosis
	Parkinson's disease
	Riley-Day syndrome
	Temporal lobe epilepsy
	Cancer
Nutritional defects	Zinc deficiency
	Vitamin B deficiency
	Addison's disease
	Diabetes
Endocrinopathies	Cushing's syndrome
	Hypopituitarism
	Hypothyroidism
Metabolic disorders	Chronic renal failure
	Hepatic disease
Viral infections	

Neuromotor Deficits

Motor Unit
Neuromuscular Junction
- Myasthenia Gravis
  Etiology
  Signs and Symptoms
  Diagnostic tests
  Treatment
  Dental Management
- Multiple Sclerosis
  Incidence
  Etiology
  Pathophysiology
  Signs and Symptoms
  Dental Management
- Facial Paralysis
  Pathophysiology

Upper and Lower Motor Neuron Lesion
Bell's Palsy
General Management
Dental Aspects
- Epilepsy
  Pathophysiology
  Types
  Signs and Symptoms
  Medical Management
  Dental Management
  Oral Complications
- Parkinson's Disease
  Etiology
  Signs and Symptoms
  Pathophysiology
  Medical Management
  Dental Management

NEUROMOTOR DEFICITS

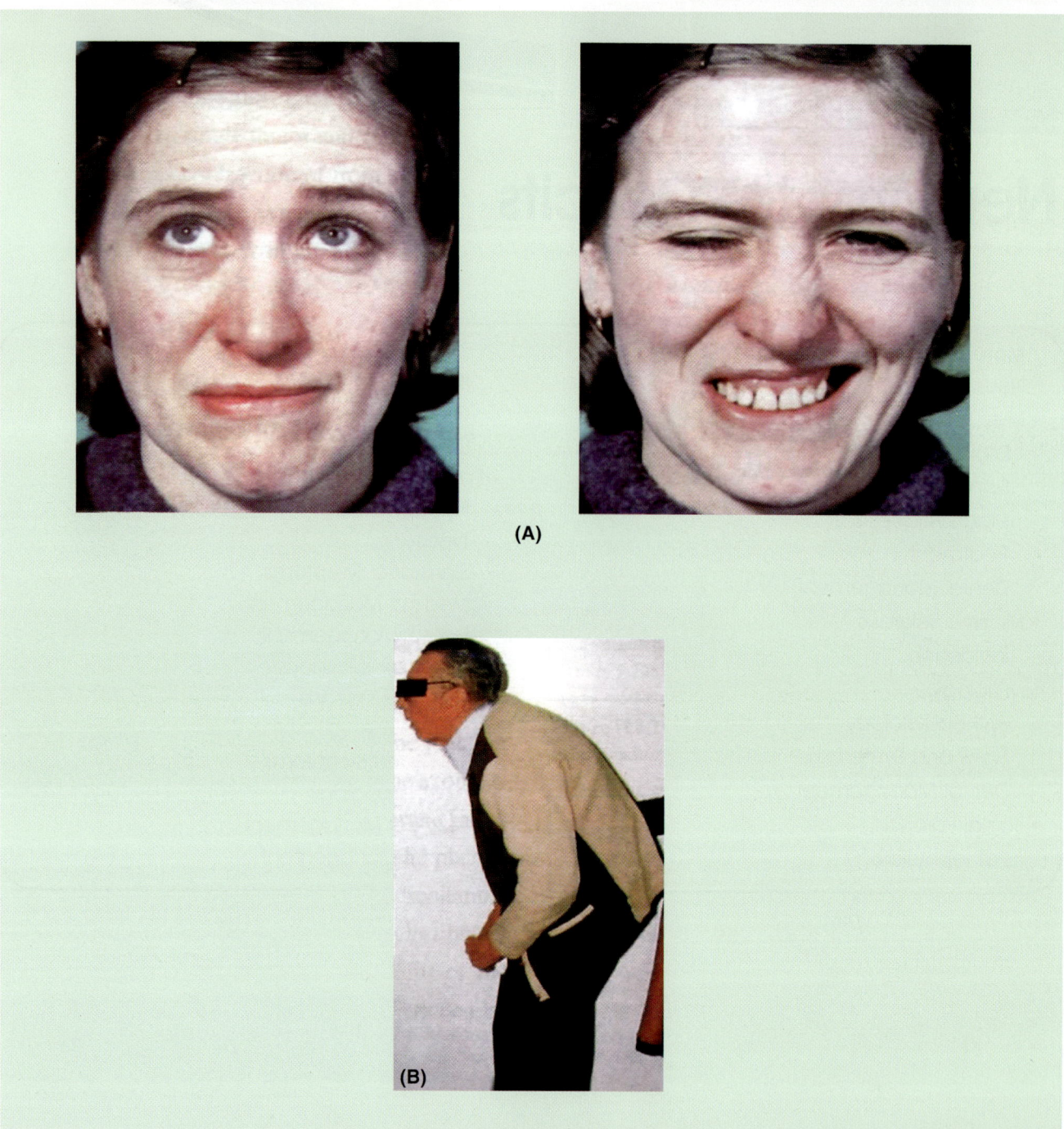

(A)

(B)

Plate (XVII). **(A)** Lower motor neuron palsy of the right fascial nerve (Bell's palsy). The face may look almost normal at rest, but this patient is unable to wrinkle her brow fully on the affected side, the right corner of her mouth droops and there is a prominent right nasolabial fold. When the patient is asked to close her eyes and slow her teeth, the difference between the unaffected left side becomes more obvious. In upper motor neuron lesions, the weakness is less evident and the brow muscles function normally. **(B)** Parkinson's disease–typical posture. Note the stooped posture and the typical position of his arms, which are held slightly flexed at the side *(Forbes & Jackson, 2003)*

MOTOR UNIT

Contraction of skeletal muscle is under nervous control that is, the muscle tissue alone cannot contract. Its contraction is initiated by a chemical released from a nerve cell, or neuron. A motor neuron, together with the muscle fibers it innervates, is called a motor unit (Figs 12.1 and 12.2). In humans, a single motor unit causes the simultaneous contraction of about 6 to 30 fibers (in some eye muscles) to over 1000 fibers (in powerful leg muscles).

Neuromuscular Junction

The junction between a motor neuron ending and a muscle fiber is called a neuromuscular (nerve + muscle) junction (Figs 12.3 and 12.4). The end branches of the motor neuron, known as axon terminals, gain access to the muscle fiber through the endomysium. At the junction between the muscle fiber and the axon terminals, the muscle fiber membrane forms a motor end plate. The motor end plate is the specialized portion of the sarcolemma (plasma membrane) of a muscle fiber. It surrounds the synaptic end bulbs of the axon. Each muscle fiber is innervated by only one axon terminal.

At the motor end plate, nerve endings are separated from the sarcolemma of the muscle fiber by a tiny gap called a synaptic cleft (Fig. 12.4). The chemical transmitter acetylcholine is synthesized in the cytoplasm of the neuron and then packaged in the synaptic vesicles.

The acetylcholine is released from the synaptic vesicles of the nerve endings, where it diffuses across

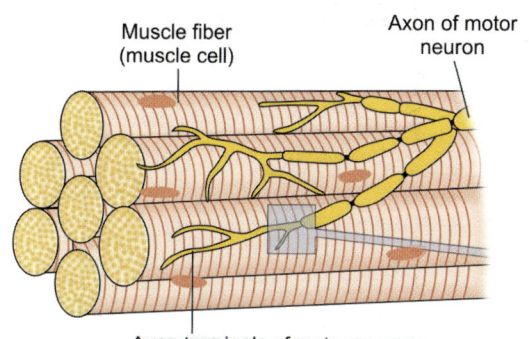

Fig. 12.2: Schematic drawing of a neuromuscular junction *(Wynsberghe et al, 1995)*

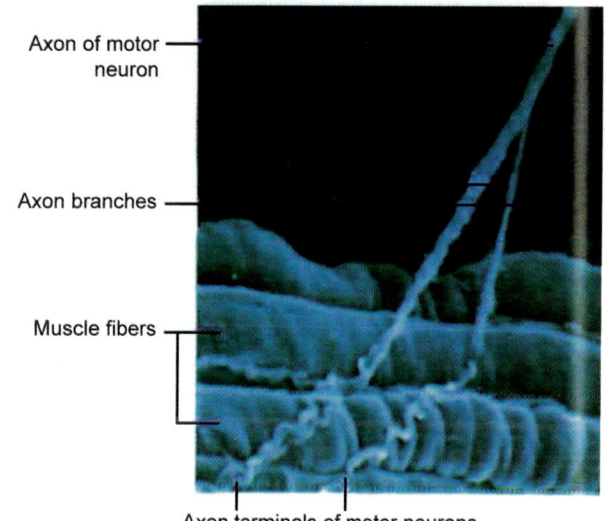

Fig. 12.3: Neuromuscular junction. Scanning electron micrograph of a motor neuron fiber terminating on several muscle fibers. The neuromuscular junction consists of a synaptic end bulb at the end of an axon terminal branch and a motor end plate on the surface of the muscle fibers *(Donna V, 1995)*

the synaptic cleft and flows into the folds of the sarcolemma. Some acetylcholine then becomes attached to the receptor sites in the sarcolemma, initiating an electrochemical impulse across the sarcolemma of the muscle cells, so that sodium ions move into the sarcoplasm and potassium ions move out. The result of this action of acetylcholine is a temporary disturbance in the permeability of the sarcolemma that leads to muscle contraction.

The sequence of events at the neuromuscular junction is shown in Fig. 12.5 and Box 12.1, which is numbered to correspond to the following account:

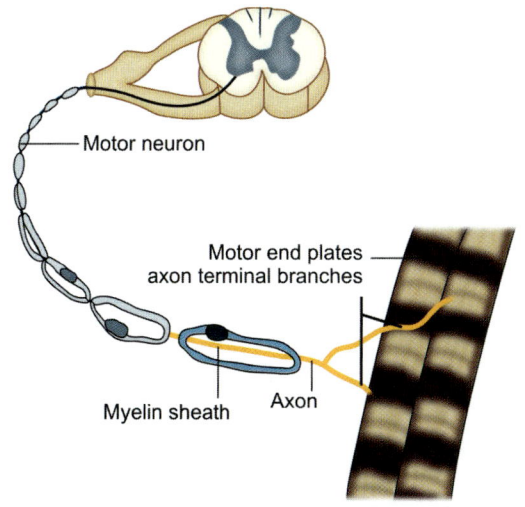

Fig. 12.1: Motor unit

Axon

Synaptic
end bulb

Sarcolemma

(A)

Muscle fiber
(muscle cell)

Muscle fiber
nucleus

Axolemma

Synaptic cleft

Mitochondria

Synaptic end bulb

Sarcolemma

Sarcoplasm

(B)

Synaptic vesicles

Junctional folds in
sarcolemma

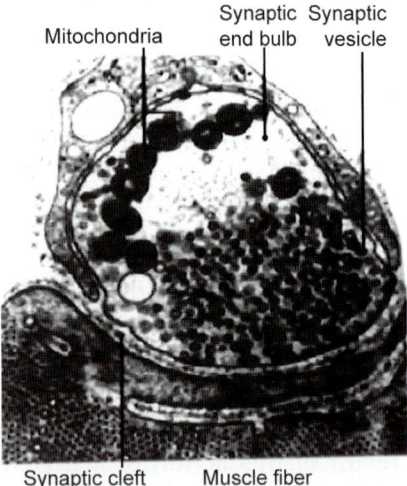

Mitochondria

Synaptic
end bulb

Synaptic
vesicle

(C)

Synaptic cleft

Muscle fiber

Fig. 12.4: (A) Enlarged drawing of the muscle fiber and the axon terminal. **(B)** Enlarged drawing showing the motor end plate in detail. **(C)** Electron micrograph of a neuromuscular junction 17,400× *(Wynsberghe et al, 1995)*

1. A nerve impulse (action potential) is propagated along the axon of a motor neuron, triggering the opening of voltage-gated calcium channels. Channel proteins in plasma membranes are usually involved with transporting ions across the membrane, and so they are called ion channels. These channels are selective, allowing some ions to pass but blocking others. The channels are not always open. Because the channels have gates that open and close with changes in voltage along the plasma membrane, they are called voltage-gated channels.

2. The opening of the calcium channels causes calcium ions (Ca^{2+}) to flow into the synaptic end bulb of the axon terminal.

3. The increase in Ca^{2+} concentration stimulates the exocytosis of the neurotransmitter acetylcholine from vesicles in the synaptic end bulb into the synaptic cleft.

4. Acetylcholine diffuses across the synaptic cleft at the neuromuscular junction and binds to specific receptor sites on the motor end plate of the muscle cell plasma membrane. (Each motor end plate may have 20 to 40 million acetylcholine receptor sites.)

5. When acetylcholine binds to the receptor sites, sodium and potassium channels in the plasma membrane of the motor end plate open. The flow of sodium ions (Na^+) into the muscle fiber is greater than the flow of potassium ions (K^+) out.

The resulting change in the concentration of Na^+ and K^+ causes a depolarization (the reversal of

Box 12.1: Sequence of events at the neuromuscular junction

Motor neurons carry nerve impulses
from brain and spinal cord to muscle
↓
Each motor neuron releases
acetylcholine into synaptic cleft
↓
Acetylcholine binds to
receptor sites on sarcolemma
↓
Acetylcholine increases sarcolemma
permeability to sodium and potassium ions
↓
Production of end plate potential
↓
End plate potential depolarizes
sarcolemma, producing action potential
↓
Myofibril contraction

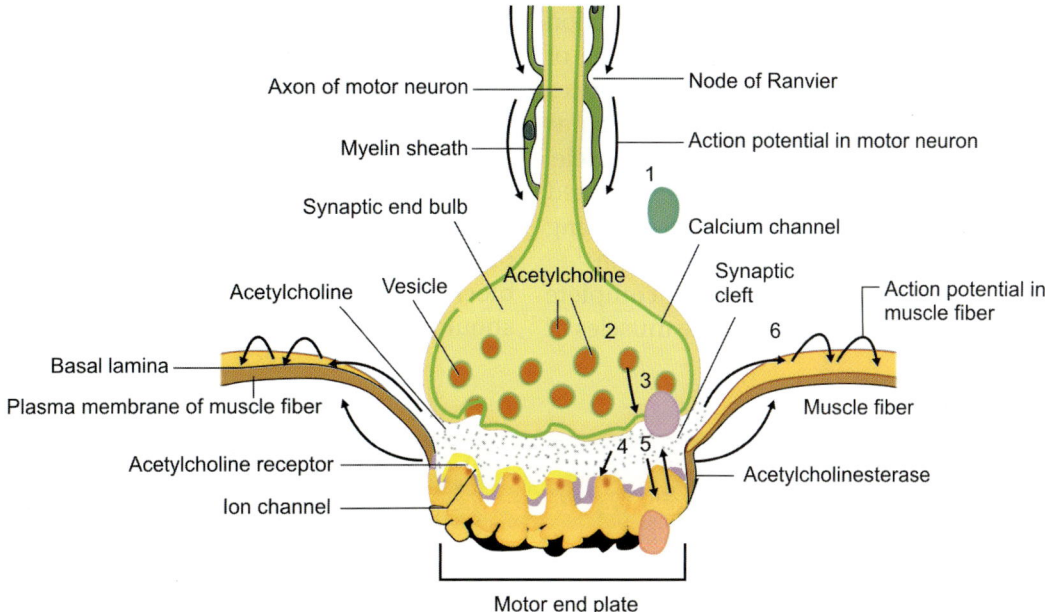

Axon of motor neuron — — Node of Ranvier

Myelin sheath — — Action potential in motor neuron

Synaptic end bulb

— Calcium channel

Acetylcholine   Vesicle   Acetylcholine

Acetylcholine

Synaptic cleft — Action potential in muscle fiber

Basal lamina

Plasma membrane of muscle fiber

Acetylcholine receptor

Ion channel

Muscle fiber

Acetylcholinesterase

Motor end plate

Fig. 12.5: An activated neuromuscular junction. The numbered sequence follows the discussion in the text *(Wynsberghe et al, 1995)*

the electrical charge across the plasma membrane) called an end-plate potential at the motor end plate.

6. The end-plate potential depolarizes the adjacent plasma membrane, which reaches its threshold potential, a degree of depolarization adequate to initiate an action potential. The action potential propagates over the surface of the entire muscle fiber and continues into the fiber along transverse tubules. In the transverse tubes, it causes the release of Ca^{2+} from the sarcoplasmic reticulum; these ions stimulate all the myofibrils in the muscle cell to contract at the same time.

7. Acetylcholinestrase, an enzyme found on muscle fiber membranes, then breaks down acetylcholine into acetate and choline. When the receptor sites no longer contain bound acetylcholine, the ion channels in the motor end plate close; the plasma membrane of the motor end plate returns to its resting potential and can respond to another stimulus.

Neuromuscular Blockage

Acetylcholine combines with receptor substances at the membranes of skeletal muscles and nerve cells. The drug-receptor interaction sets of biochemical changes that result in the contraction of muscle cells and impulse propagation in nerve cells. A drug such as atropine is capable of combining with the

acetylcholine-receptor substance to form a complex that prevents the access of acetylcholine to the same receptors. The antagonist (atropine) thus competes for the acetylcholine receptor substance—a process known as competitive antagonism.

Certain emergency situations require chemically paralyzing the patient so that an endotracheal tube can be placed to assist or manage breathing. This procedure, referred to as rapid sequence intubation (RSI), involves the use of medications that act on the neuromuscular junction. Nerve impulses travel down the nerve and release a chemical transmitter that stimulates (depolarizes) the associated skeletal muscle fibers, which result in contraction. Acetylcholine is the principal neurotransmitter in the neuromuscular junction. Blocking its action results in relaxation of skeletal (voluntary) muscles.

There are two ways to block the neuromuscular junction. One is by the administration of depolarizing agents act over a prolonged time, which results in continued muscle depolarization and muscle paralysis. Because they have a stimulating effect, they often produce fasiculations (generalized involuntary muscle twitching), especially in children, immediately after administration. The depolarizing neuromuscular blocker is succinylcholine. It is the most commonly used neuromuscular blocker for rapid sequence intubation.

The other way to block the neuromuscular junction is to administer a drug that blocks the reuptake of acetylcholine into the nerve terminal. This produces an excess of acetylcholine into the neuromuscular junction and inhibits the stimulation of the muscle. Because these drugs do not depolarize the affected muscle fibers, they are referred to as non-depolarizing blockers. They do not cause muscle fasciculation.

Chemically, palarizing a patient causes complete voluntary muscle relaxation, including the muscles of respiration. This allows caregivers to take control of the airway and provide unimpeded mechanical ventilation. Esophageal and stomach muscles, and therefore, sphincter tone, also relax, which increases the risk of vomiting and aspiration. Because neuromuscular blocking agents do not affect mental status or pain sensation, patients should be sedated or put to sleep before administration of neuromuscular blockers. If pain is present or expected, an analgesic should be administered.

MYASTHENIA GRAVIS
(GRAVE MUSCLE WEAKNESS)

The motor end-plate is the specialized neuromuscular junction situated at the middle of each muscle fiber. The nerve impulses cause release of acetylcholine at the specialized nerve endings—depolarisation at this site is the stimulus to contraction. The sarcolemma at this site contains abundant cholinesterase. In myasthenia gravis, the essential disorder is at the motor-end-plate where there is a defect in the action of acetylcholine.

Myasthenia gravis is a condition associated with weakness and muscle fatigue of voluntary muscle, due to poor response of the muscle receptor to the neurotransmitter acetylcholine. It is an autoimmune disease caused by antibodies (molecules that defend against a foreign substance) directed against acetylcholine receptors. The antibodies reduce the number of functional receptors or impede the interaction between acetylcholine and its receptors at the motor end plate. As a result, skeletal muscles become chronically weak and even the slightest muscular exertion causes extreme fatigue.

The weakness and fatigue of affected muscles is gradual or insidious in onset. The weakness may be localized or more generalized, when several muscles are affected. It is often unmasked and/or exacerbated by certain stress factors such as infection, pregnancy, or menstrual periods. Muscle weakness becomes more pronounced as the day progresses. Although myasthenia may become progressively worse, it is usually not fatal unless the respiratory muscles fail and breathing becomes impossible.

Myasthenia gravis can occur at all ages, but it is most commonly affects women between the ages of 20–40 and men over 40. It is between the three times as common in women as in men.

Etiology

This is essentially an autoimmune disease.

1. Antibodies (an IgG antibody) to acetylcholine receptors at the ACh binding site on the postsynaptic membrane, are present in 90% of cases.
2. There is strong association with thymic abnormalities.
3. Myasthenia gravis can occasionally be associated with other conditions such as rheumatoid arthritis and thyrotoxicosis (this has an autoimmune basis).

Signs and Symptoms

Myasthenia gravis typically has an insidious onset. Clinical manifestations may first appear during pregnancy, during the postpartum period, or in conjunction with the administration of certain anesthetic agents. The foremost complaint is muscular fatigue and progressive weakness. The individual often complains of fatigue after exercise and has a recent history of recurring upper respiratory tract infections. The muscles of the eyes, face, mouth, throat and neck usually are affected first. The extraocular muscles and the levator muscles are most affected.

Symptoms experienced are associated with the muscles involved:

- Involvement of the ocular muscles results in ptosis, diplopia, ocular palsies and vision problems.
- The muscles of facial expression, mastication, swallowing, and speech are the next most affected. The results are facial droop, and an expressionless face, difficulty chewing and swallowing associated with dietary changes and weight loss, drooling, episodes of chocking ; and a nasal low-volume but high-pitched monotonus speech pattern. Difficulty in swallowing with nasal regurgitation of food and drink may develop. The gag reflex can be absent or poor, and the ability to cough may be compromised in the myasthenia gravis patient, causing an increased risk of aspiration.
- A very lax jaw can be found on physical examination.
- The respiratory muscles of the diaphragm and chest wall become weak and ventilation is impaired.
- The muscles of the neck, shoulder girdle and hip flexors are affected less frequently. When these muscles become involved, however, the person experiences fatigue requiring period of rest, weakness of the arms and legs that improved with rest, and difficulty in maintaining head position.

Myasthenia Crisis

Myasthenia crisis occurs when severe muscle weakness causes extreme quadriparesis or quadriplegia, respiratory insufficiency with shortness of breath, and extreme difficulty of swallowing. The individual in myasthenia crisis is in danger of respiratory arrest. Myasthenia crisis usually occurs 3 to 4 hours after the person takes medication.

Diagnostic tests

The following are tests to diagnose myasthenia gravis:
1. *Endrophonium (tensilon) injection test:* The diagnosis of myasthenia gravis is confirmed by demonstration of improved patient response to IV endrophonium, a short-acting anticholinesterase.
2. *Acetylcholine receptor antibody test:* Blood tests showing elevated levels of circulating acetylcholine receptor antibodies confirms the diagnosis of myasthenia gravis.

Treatment

Myasthenia gravis treatment considerations are the following:
1. Oral anticholinesterase, neostigmine, and pyridostigmine (60 mg tablets) are the drugs most widely used. Their duration of action is 3–4 hours. The dose (usually 4–16 tablets daily) is determined by the patient's response. Anticholinesterases increase the amount of available acetylcholine (ACh) at the myoneuronal junction by inhibiting the degradation of ACh (inhibit cholinesterase). This allows acetylcholine to remain in the synaptic cleft and influence receptor sites on the postsynaptic membrane of a muscle fiber for a longer time than usual, thus relieving some of the muscle weakness.
2. *Neostigmine (prostigmin) and pyridostigmine (mestinon):* These drugs are used alone or in combination and provide symptomatic relief by enhancing neuromuscular transmission, but they do not affect the course of the disease.
3. *Immunosuppressant drugs (corticosteroids or cyclosporine or azathioprine):* Occasionally, the treatment is supplemented with corticosteroids or cyclosporine or azathioprine to suppress the abnormal antibody production and provide symptomatic relief.
4. *Surgery (thymectomy):* Thymectomy improves prognosis, particularly in women below 40 years with positive receptor antibodies and a history of myasthenia of less than 10 years. Some 60% of non-thymoma cases improve, the precise reason is unclear. If a thymoma is present, surgery is necessary to remove a potentially malignant tumor, it is less unusual for myasthenia to improve.

Dental Management

1. Always confirm the extent of the disease affecting the entire body and particularly the head and neck regions.
2. Check for the gag reflex plus the ability to cough and confirm that both are adequate before you begin treatment.
3. Anticholinesterases increase salivation, and you may often have to provide active suction during dental treatment.
4. Follow the rule of "two's", if the patient is currently on steroids or has been on steroids for two weeks or longer within the past two years.
5. Any form of infection, emotional stress, or certain medications can worsen the status of the disease. Explain the procedure for the day to help relax the patient and decrease any anxiety.
6. Avoid macrolides, tetracycline, aminoglycosides (but penicillin or erythromycin can safely be used) and fluoroguinotones, diazepam (valium),

lorazepam (ativan) and general anesthesia because these drugs can aggravate myasthenia gravis symptoms.

7. Avoid all types of muscle relaxants.
8. Dental treatment is best carried out during a remission.
9. Morning appointments are recommended because the weakness is least in the morning and worsens as the day progresses. Treatment is best carried out 1–2 hours of routine medication with anticholinesterases, with short appointment.
10. Local anesthesia is preferred. Lidocaine, priolocaine, or mepivacaine can be safely used. Use a minimal dose of local anesthesia, limit it to 2 carpules only, and avoid lidocaine.
11. Weakness of the masticatory muscles causing the mouth to hang open is characteristic and patients typically tend to support the jaw with their hand.

MULTIPLE SCLEROSIS

Incidence

Multiple sclerosis is a chronic debilitating disease affecting the central nervous system (brain and spinal cord). The disease usually affects young adults between ages 18 and 40 and is five times more prevalent in whites than in blacks. The name of the disease is derived from the characteristic multiple areas of involvement that heal by sclerosis (another name of scarring).

Etiology

The specific cause of MS is not known, but two theories are currently held:

1. A slow acting virus infects the CNS, and
2. It has been suggested that MS is related to consumption of large quantities of animal fats.

Survey in Norway has shown that MS is distinctly uncommon in coastal fishing communities compare with agricultural communities. The role of diet is particularly difficult to evaluate. The body's immune system attacks its own central nervous system (an autoimmune response). The autoimmune upset is directed against proteins in the myelin sheath, which causes inflammation and damage to the sheath with multiple areas of scarring (sclerosis), which slow or block muscle coordination, visual sensation and other nerve signals.

Pathophysiology

Multiple sclerosis (MS) is a progressive demyelination of neurons in the central nervous system accompanied by the destruction of oligodendrocytes that interferes with the conduction of nerve impulses and results in impaired sensory perceptions of nerve impulses and motor coordination. The glial scarring in this disease is produced by a type of neuroglial cell called an astrocyte and differs somewhat from the usual fibrous scar produced by connective tissue cells. The discrete areas of myelin loss with glial scarring are called multiple sclerosis plaques. They are readily demonstrated within the nervous systems of affected persons by means of magnetic resonance imaging (Figs 12.6 and 12.7).

Signs and Symptoms

The neurological signs reflect white matter damage, upper motor neurone weakness and paralysis; incoordination; visual disturbances; paresthesia. (Gray matter's signs, e.g. apahsia, fits and muscle atrophy are rare.)

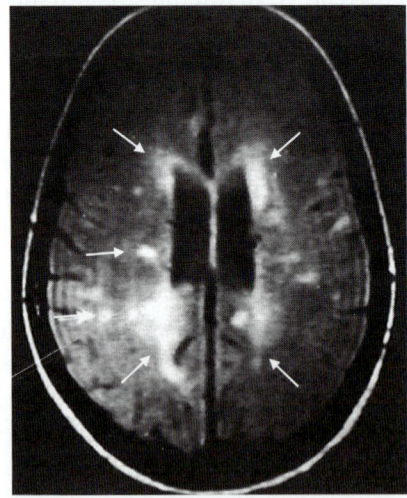

Fig. 12.6: Multiple sclerosis, demonstrated by magnetic resonance imaging (MRI). Ventricular system is well demonstrated in the center of the photograph. Dense white areas adjacent to posterior horns of the ventricles and scattered throughout the brain lateral to the ventricles (arrows) are multiple plaques

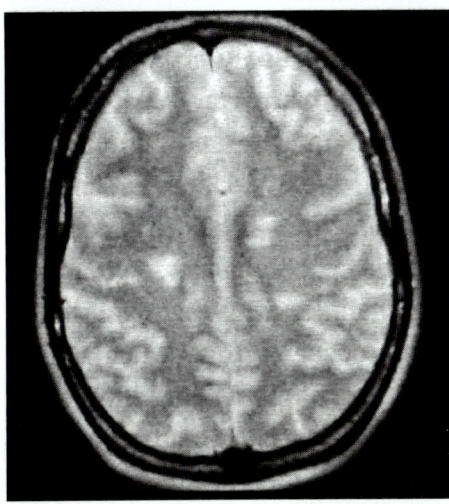

Fig. 12.7: Multiple sclerosis. This MRI picture shows multiple "high signal" lesions in the white matter of both hemispheres. These represent multiple areas of demyelination *(Chabner, 2001)*

Because almost any myelinated site in the brain or spinal cord may be involved and the nerve conduction is disrupted, the effects depend on what part of the CNS is involved. The symptoms of the disease are diverse—double vision—abnormal eye movements (nystagmus and blindness), jerky speech defects, neurosis, and numbness. Motor disturbances affect walking and the use of hands (incoordination, spasticity, difficulty in walking, tremor, weakness or paralysis of one or more limbs). Sensory disturbances include loss of touch, pain, temperature, and proprioception (numbness, pins and needle sensations), urinary infections, bladder incontinence, and drastic mood changes. Occasionally, mental changes such as forgetfulness or confusion occur. With repeated attacks of inflammation at myelinated sites, scarring (sclerosis) takes place and some permanent loss of function occurs.

Patients experience variable cycles of milder and worse symptoms until they eventually become bedridden. Most die from 7 to 32 years after the onset of the disease. The cause of MS remains uncertain; most theories suggest that it results from an immune disorder triggered by a virus in genetically susceptible individuals.

There are no specific oral manifestations of MS but this diagnosis should always be considered in:

1. A young patient presenting with trigeminal neuralgia, particularly if bilateral or if there have been other neurological disturbances, or if the pain lasts minutes or hours. It may respond to carbamazepine. Some patients may have difficulty localizing orofacial pain.
2. Facial palsy not associated with retroaural pain or with loss of taste sensation such as may be seen in Bell's palsy.
3. Abnormal perioral sensation, such as extreme hypersensitivity or facial anesthesia. Facial myokymia (worm-like movements) or hemispasm, abnormalities of speech.

There is no cure. The following procedures should be followed.

1. *Steroids:* Steroids when given, are used to reduce the severity and duration of attacks. Occasionally, a patient experiencing troublesome optic symptoms can benefit from a short course of IV methylprednisolone (Solu-Medrol) followed by oral steroids. Interferon administration reduces antigen presentation, proliferation of T cells, and the production of tumor necrosis factor and have been shown to slow the progression of the disease. Interferon reduces the relapse rate by one-third and prevents an increase in lesions seen on MRI over time.
2. *Muscle relaxants:* Belcofen and tizanidine muscle relaxants are dispensed for the treatment of muscle stiffness, muscle spasms and increased muscle tone. Be aware that these drugs can cause drowsiness and xerostomia.
3. *Anticonvulsants:* The patient may be on carbamazepine (tegretol) or phenytoin sodium (dilantin) for the treatment of trigeminal neuralgia or neuropathy.
4. *Antidepressants:* Serotonin reuptake inhibitors and tricyclic antidepressants: Tricyclic antidepressants are often prescribed to overcome the associated depression.
5. *Physical therapy and exercise:* Physical therapy and exercise is provided to help maintain muscle function and mobility.

Dental Management

Limited mobility and psychological disorders may interfere with routine dental treatment. Patients with severe MS are best treated fully supine, as respiration may be embarrassed. Treatment is best carried out under local anesthesia, if possible. Nitrous oxide is probably best avoided since it may theoretically cause demyelination. Some patients are on corticosteroids, with their attendant complications:

1. Patients with severe MS will need shorter appointments because they are unable to keep their mouth open for a longer duration.
2. It is best to treat these patients during morning appointments because fatigue experienced is more pronounced in the afternoon.
3. These patients may need assistance with transfer from the wheelchair to the dental chair.
4. Evaluate the CBC, serum creatinine, prior to the start of dental treatment.
5. The patient can experience abnormal facial pain or intraoral pain and discomfort that may be localized or generalized. The patient must be thoroughly evaluated to determine the cause and be referred to the medical side for further evaluation. Incomplete assessment could lead to unnecessary extractions or endodontic treatment.
6. MS can trigger the development of trigeminal neuralgia that is often bilateral. It causes paroxysmal pain that stimulates electrical shocks, and it can be brought on by chewing or stroking of the cheek. The pain when it occurs is severe and recurring.
7. The trigeminal sensory neuropathy-associated paresthesia is progressive and the maxillary and mandibular divisions of the trigeminal nerve are frequently affected.
8. Significant facial anesthesia can also occur in the severe cases of MS.
9. Numbness of the lower lip and chin with or without pain can occur, if the mental nerve is involved.
10. A significant number of patients may be affected with facial palsy, which occurs later in the disease.
11. Severe respiratory problems can occur when the respiratory muscles are affected. The gag reflex may be lacking or impaired. These patients can also suffer from vertigo, which can worsen in the lying-down position. For all these reasons, the patient should be treated in a semisitting position. The rubber dam should be used, only if the patient can adequately breathe through the nose.
12. There is high incidence of caries in patients with MS because there is significant xerostomia.
13. It is not uncommon to find stomatitis, ulcerations, gingivitis, herpes infection, candidiasis and parotid gland enlargement.
14. Dentistry for severe cases may have to be done under general anesthesia in a hospital setting.
15. Interferon and many of the immunosuppressive drugs can cause changes in the CBC affecting the WBCs (neutropenia and/or lymphopenia, hemoglobin, hematocrit, and platelets). Always evaluate the CBS prior to dentistry. All infections should be aggressively treated because infections can worsen the status of the disease. Also adequately compensate for thrombocytopenia, when present. Interferon beta-Ia (avonex/rebif) causes leucopenia, anemia, thrombocytopenia, and alternation of the LFTs. All hepatotoxic drugs must be avoided with this drug. Interferon beta-Ib (beta-aseron) causes significant lymphopenia and neutropenia.
16. Copolymer-1/glatiramer acetate (capoxone) can cause enlargement of the parotid glands and severe stomatitis.
17. Evaluate the oral cavity for Candida infection in patients on steroids.
18. Follow the "rule of two's" during major dentistry if the patient is currently on steroids or has been on steroids for 2 weeks or longer within the past 2 years. Always provide antibiotic coverage for 5 days, following major dentistry to prevent any possible infection.
19. Steroids mask the symptoms and signs of infection; be extravigilant. Carefully examine and treat any infection found in the oral cavity.

FACIAL PARALYSIS

Bell's palsy is a degenerative disorder of the facial nerve, probably due to a virus. It is characterized by paralysis of the facial muscles on one side with resulting distortion of the facial features, such as sagging of the mouth or lower eyelid. The paralysis may interfere with speech, prevent closure of the eye, and cause excessive tear secretion. There may also be a partial loss of the sense of taste. Bell's palsy may appear abruptly, sometimes overnight and often disappears spontaneously within 3 to 5 weeks.

Pathophysiology

The facial nerve is the motor supply to the muscles of the facial expression. It also carries taste sensation from the anterior two-thirds of the tongue (via the chorda tympani) secretomotor fibers to the sub-mandibular and sublingual salivary glands and to the lacrimal glands and branches to the stapedius muscle in the middle ear. The neurons supplying the lower face receive upper motor neurons from the contralateral motor cortex, whereas the neurons to the upper face receive bilateral upper motor neuron innervations.

The concept of upper and lower motor neuronal activity, based on anatomical and physiological evidence, has great clinical value in diagnosis. The upper motor neurons (UMN) synapse with the lower motor neurons (LMN). It will be appreciated that in its long course from the cerebral cortex to the anterior horn, the upper motor neuron is susceptible to damage from a variety of disease process acting at various sites. The lower motor neuron may be damaged in the cord or in the peripheral nerve (Table 12.1, Fig. 12.8).

Upper motor neuron lesion, such as stroke, weakness of the lower part of the face on the side opposite the lesion, causes unilateral facial palsy with some sparing of the frontalis and orbicularis oculi muscles because of the bilateral cortical representation. Thus the normal furrowing of the brow is preserved, and eye closure and blinking are not affected. Although voluntary facial movements are impaired, the face may still move with emotional responses, for example, on laughing and smiling. Paresis of the ipsilateral arm (monoparesis) or arm and leg (hemiparesis), or dysphagia, may be associated because of more extensive cerebrocortical damage.

Table 12.1: Differentiation of upper from lower neuron lesions of the facial nerve

	Upper motor lesion	Lower motor lesion
Emotional movements of face	Retained	Lost
Blink reflex	Retained	Lost
Ability to wrinkle forehead	Retained	Lost
Drooling from commissure	Uncommon	Common
Lacrimation, taste and hearing	Unaffected	May be affected
Tongue protrusion	Normal	Deviates to unaffected side

Lower motor neuron lesion causes weakness of all the muscles of facial expression on the same side. The face, especially the angle of the mouth, falls and dribbling occurs from the corner of the mouth (Fig. 12.9). There is weakness of frowing (frontalis) and of eye closure since the upper facial muscles are weak. Corneal exposure and ulceration, if the eye does not close during sleep. The platysma muscle is weak.

Bell's Palsy

Dr. Charles Bell of Edinburgh first described the condition which is termed Bell's palsy in 1882. Inflammation of the facial nerve in the stylomastoid canal with demyelination and edema further hazards the blood supply. Bell's palsy is more common in pregnancy, diabetes, influenza, a cold or another respiratory illness. There is acute onset of unilateral paralysis over a few hours, maximum within 48 hours. Pain in the region of the ear or in the jaw may proceed the paralysis by one or two days. Occasionally, hyperacusis (oversensitivity to sound, due to loss of function of nerve to stapedius). Lower motor neuron facial palsy, such as Bell's palsy is characterized by unilateral paralysis of all muscles of facial expression for both voluntary and emotional responses.

In facial palsy, the forehead is unfurrowed, the patient unable to close the eye on that side and attempted closure causes the eye to roll upwards (Bell's sign). Tears tend to overflow onto the cheek (epiphora), the corner of the mouth droops and nasolabial fold is obliterated (Plate XVII - A, Fig. 12.9). Saliva may dripple from the commissure and may cause angular stomatitis. Food collects in the vestibule and plaque accumulates on the teeth on the affected side. Depending on the site of the lesion, other defects such as loss of taste may be associated.

Facial weakness is demonstrated by asking patients to close their eyes against resistance, to *raise the eye brows, to whistle or to show their teeth. Lacrimation is diminished in a* VIIth nerve lesion. Schirmer's test, carried out by gently placing a strip of filter paper on the lower conjunctival sac and comparing the wetting of the paper with that on the other side, may be helpful. Taste is diminished in a VII nerve lesion and is tested by applying sugar, salt, lemon juice or vinegar on the tongue and asking the patient to identify each of them.

The most commonly injured branches of the facial nerve are the buccal and mandibular; they also have few interconnections with other branches. The facial

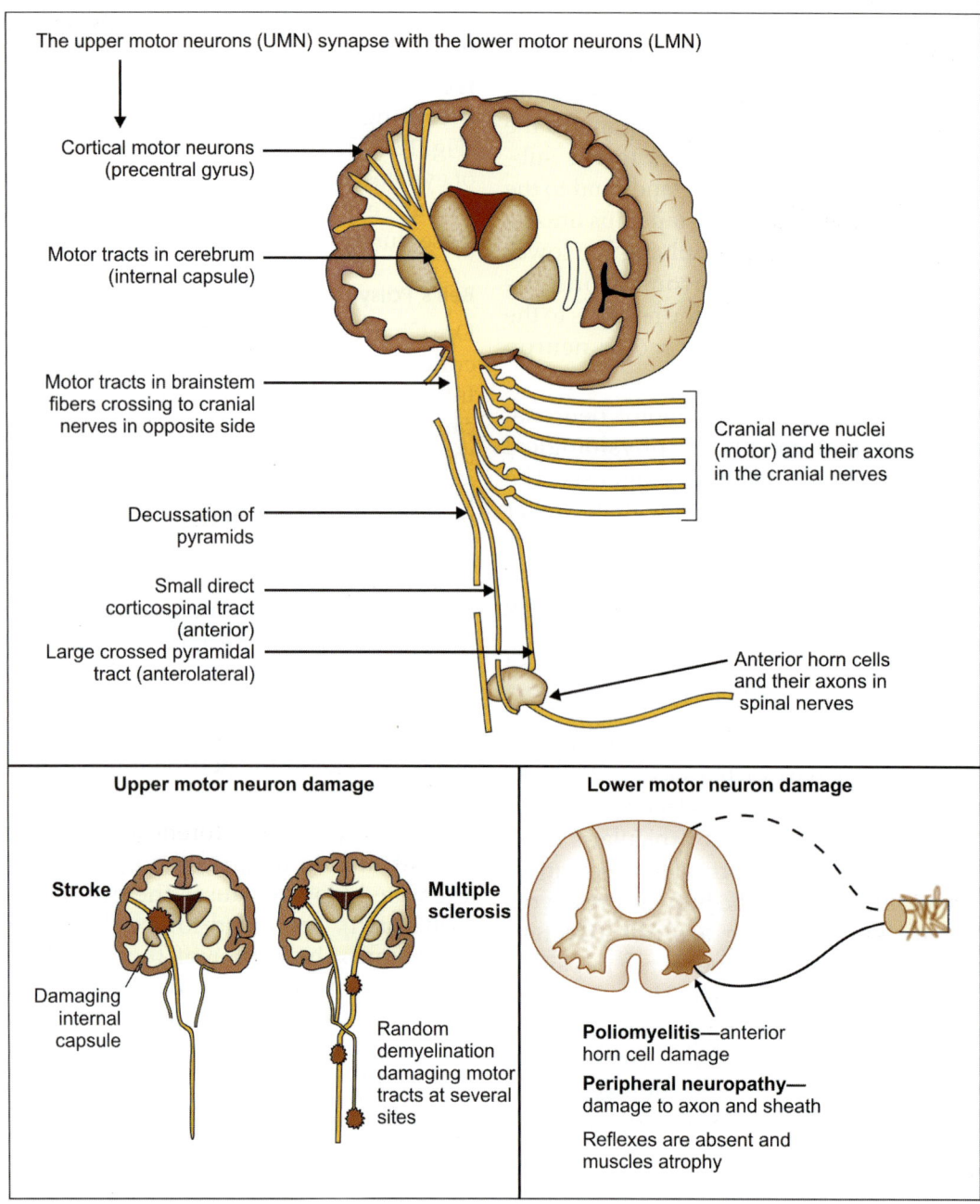

Fig. 12.8: Reid and Roberts, 2005

nerve and its branches are obviously in danger during parotidectomy. They can be preserved only by careful observation and awareness of the anatomy. A stimulating electrode can be employed in verifying facial motor branches, causing muscle spasms when a nerve is contracted. The facial trunk is large enough for anastomosis of the cut end, should this be necessary. The smaller branches are injured more often and are much less easily sutured. No repair will completely restore function. A traction injury may result in temporary paresis or permanent injury. Injury to the auriculotemporal nerve can produce Prey's syndrome, in which the skin anterior to the ear sweats during eating (gustatory sweating).

General Management

Eighty-five percent of patients make a total, spontaneous recovery within a few weeks but some

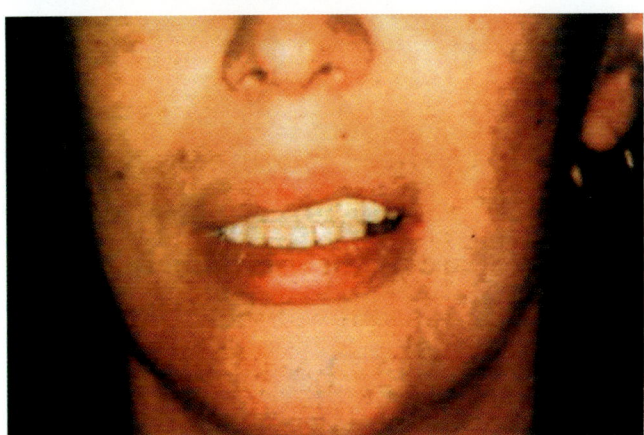

Fig. 12.9: Facial nerve palsy in a 30-year-old woman with AIDS

have residual permanent palsy. Where paralysis is complete, only 50% recover completely within one week, but few who have not recovered by 2 weeks will do so. Favorable prognostic signs are incomplete paralysis in the first week and persistence of the stapedial paralysis in the first week and persistence of the stapedial reflex, measured by electroneurography. Bad prognosis signs are hyperacusis, severe taste impairment and/or diminished lacrimation or salivation, especially in older, diabetic or hypertensive patients.

1. Anti-inflammatory medication. A short course of prednisolone may reduce inflammation and swelling in the narrow stylomastoid canal. Corticosteroids result in 80–90% complete recovery compared with about 50–60% in the absence of such treatment. Prednisolone 20 mg four times a day for 5 days, then off over the succeeding 4 days is often recommended.

2. Antiviral medication with acyclovir may limit damage to the nerve from herpetic infection. The combination of oral acyclovir 400 mg five times daily with oral prednisolone 1 mg/kg daily for 10 days is more frequently effective.

3. Facial massage may help prevent permanent contractures of the paralyzed muscles before recovery takes place.

4. In chronic cases, surgical decompression of the nerve in the stylomastoid canal may be attempted.

5. During the acute phase, suturing of the upper to lower lid (tarsorrhaphy) is essential to prevent prolonged corneal exposure, if the eye cannot be closed. Adhesive tape to hold the eye closed is an invaluable temporary protective measure.

6. If paralysis persists and function remains incomplete, the palpebral fissure may narrow, the nasolabial fold deepen and facial spasm may develop. If there is severe late residual paralysis, cosmetic surgery is sometimes helpful.

Dental Aspects

Facial palsy may lead to poor oral cleansing and accumulation of food debris in the vestibules and of plaque on the teeth on the affected side. Saliva may leak from the affected side and cause angular stomatitis.

Construction of a splint to support the angle of the mouth may improve the esthetics to some degree. In chronic palsy, a facial graft or other maneuvers such as facial-hypoglossal nerve anastomosis may ameliorate the cosmetic deformity, but the results are not always entirely satisfactory.

EPILEPSY

Epilepsy derived from the Greek term *epilepsia*, meaning "to take hold of". The World Health Organization defines epilepsy as "a chronic brain disorder of various etiologies characterized by recurrent seizures due to excessive discharge of cerebral neurons. In epilepsy, there is a disturbance of movement, sensation, behavior, perception, and/or consciousness. Epileptic seizures develop due to excessive focal neuronal discharge that spreads to the thalamic and brainstem nuclei. The excessive discharge may be due to altered neuronal membrane potentials, altered synaptic transmission, diminution of inhibitory neurons, increased neuronal excitability.

Epilepsy or seizure may be defined as uncontrolled motor activity, sensation, behavior, consciousness, or a combination of these, produced by abnormal electrical activity in the brain. Seizures may be either convulsive (i.e. uncontrolled motor activity accompanied by motor manifestations) or manifested by other changes in neurologic function (i.e. sensory, cognitive, emotional).

Pathophysiology

A seizure results from a sudden, spontaneous uncontrolled depolarization of neurons, which causes abnormal motor or sensory activity and possibly loss of consciousness. The neurons in the epileptogenic focus are hyperexcitable and have lowered threshold for stimulation. Any physiologic changes, such as alkalosis or other sensory stimulus—for example, flashing lights—can easily activate the irritable neurons. These focal cells stimulate the surrounding normal cells, spreading the activity. There are various theories about the specific mechanism for seizure activity, including altered permeability of the neuronal membrane, reduced inhibitory control of neurons, or a transmitter imbalance.

Spread of electrical activity between cortical neurons is normally restricted. Synchronous discharge of neurons in normal brain takes place in restricted groups whose limited discharge are responsible for the normal EEGT rhythm. During a seizure, large groups of neurons are activated repetitively and hypersynchronously. There is failure of inhibitory synaptic contact between neurons.

A partial epilepsy is epileptic activity confined to one area of cortex with a recognizable clinical pattern. This activity either remains focal or spreads to generate epileptic activity in both hemispheres and thus a generalized seizure. An area of brain is or becomes epileptogenic either because neurons have a predisposition to be hyperexcitable, for example following abnormal migration patterns in utero, or because they acquire this tendency. Trauma or brain neoplasms are examples of acquired conditions that alter the seizure threshold of neurons.

Types

Epilepsy is categorized as:

a. *Grand mal epilepsy:* This is the most dramatic type. It is major motor seizure. It is more properly known as generalized tonic-clonic seizure (GTCS). Grand mal epilepsy occurs equally in both sexes and in any age-group, although more than two-thirds of cases occur by the time the individual reaches puberty. Causes include drug withdrawal, photic stimulation, menstruation, fatigue, alcohol, or other intoxications, and falling asleep or awakening. The entire seizure lasts 5 to 15 minutes, but a complete return to normal may take up to a 2 hours. It is characterized by

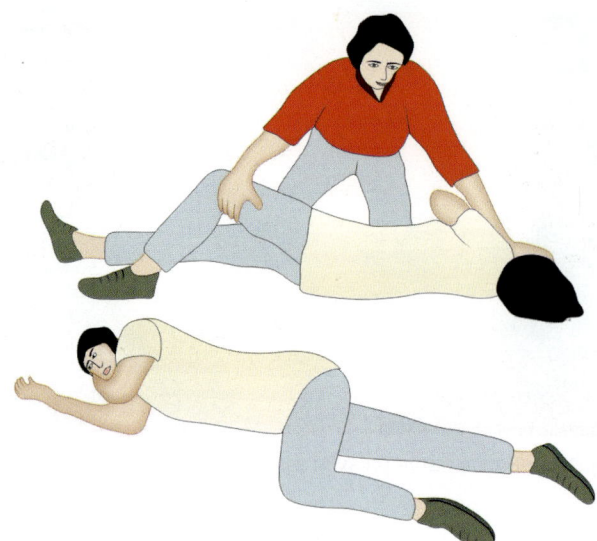

Fig. 12.10: Patient with epileptic seizure should be placed in a supine position with the head tilted to the side

generalized convulsions and loss of consciousness, and is sometimes herald by the so-called "aura", or peculiar sensation, which warns the patient of an impending attack. During the fit, the pulse and blood pressure remain normal but muscle contractions may affect respiration causing cyanosis and the tongue may be bitten, if not protected. Generally, a single episode in an otherwise healthy person is not a life-threatening event, especially if it is observed and supportive care can be rendered.

b. *Petit mal epilepsy:* Also known as absence seizures. Almost always occur in children and adolescents between 3 and 15 years. The incidence of petit mal seizures decreases with age and its persistence beyond 30 years is rare. Petit mal seizures tend to occur shortly after awakening or during periods of inactivity. Clinically, a petit mal seizure consists of a brief lapse of consciousness, normally lasting from 5 to 10 seconds and only rarely beyond 30 seconds. The individual exhibits no movement during the episode other than perhaps a cyclic blinking of the eyelids. The episode usually terminates just as abruptly as it began. If the individual is standing at the onset of the seizure, the posture usually remains erect throughout the episode.

c. *Status epilepticus:* Defined as repetitive seizures or a seizure that persists for more than 1 hour without intervening return of consciousness can be life-threatening, mainly because of hypoxic brain damage. It may occur secondary to: (i) Loss of control of the thoracic respiratory muscles, (ii) Upper airway obstruction by foreign bodies (e.g. denture or food). Seizures are most common during childhood. The most common factor precipitating status epilepticus is failure of the epileptic patient to take antiepileptic drugs. The etiology of epilepsy is known in many patients. Common causes include head trauma, intracranial neoplasm, hypoglycemia, drug withdrawal and febrile illness.

Many patients, however, have epilepsy for which there is no known cause. This is termed **idiopathic epilepsy.** Although the underlying cause of idiopathic generalized epilepsy is unknown, seizures can sometimes be evoked by a specific stimulus. Approximately 1 out of 15 patients reports that seizures follow exposure to a specific circumstance—such as flickering lights, monotonous sounds, music, or a loud noise.

Signs and Symptoms

There is a pattern for the grand mal (tonic-clonic) seizures, which usually ends spontaneously by: Prodromal signs occur in some individuals, such as nausea, irritability, depression, or muscle twitching some hours before the seizure. An aura, such as a peculiar visual or auditory sensation, immediately precedes the loss of consciousness in many persons. Loss of consciousness occurs, and the individual falls to the floor. Strong tonic muscle contraction, resulting briefly in flexion, is followed by extension of the limbs and rigidity in the trunk.

Aery escapes as the abdominal and thoracic muscles contract, forcing air out of the lungs. The jaws are clenched tightly and respiration ceases. The clonic stage follows. Clonic means intermittent muscular contraction and relaxation. This results in a series of forceful jerky movements that involves the entire body. Increased salivation (foaming at the mouth) and bowl and bladder incontinence may occur.

Contractions gradually subside spontaneously in several minutes; the body is limp and consciousness slowly returns and the person is confused and fatigued, with aching muscles and falls into a deep sleep.

Medical Management

The medical management of epilepsy is based on drug therapy. Phenytoin (dilantin) is the anticonvulsant drug that is still most commonly used as a first line of treatment; however, there are several other drugs in common use. Table 12.2 is a list of the more commonly used drugs for control of generalized tonic-clonic epilepsy. Attempts are made to use single-drug therapy to avoid adverse drug interactions and facilitate compliance.

Unfortunately, it is frequently necessary to use combination therapy.

Patients who are taking anticonvulsants may suffer from the toxic effects of these drugs. And the dentist must always be sensitive to their manifestations. Among the more common adverse effects are drowsiness, slow mentation, dizziness, ataxia and gastrointestinal upset. Occasionally, allergy may be seen as a rash or an erythema multiforme-like reaction. Phenytoin, carbamazepine, and valproic acid all can cause leukopenia and/or thrombocytopenia resulting in an increased incidence of microbial infection, delayed healing and gingival bleeding. In addition, valproic acid can cause decreased platelet

Table 12.2: Anticonvulsants used in the management of generalized tonic-clonic (grand mal) seizures

Generic name	Trade name	Usual daily adult dose (mg)	Drug interactions	Dental considerations
Phenytoin	Dilantin	300 to 400	———	Gingival hyperplasia, increased incidence of microbial infections, delayed healing, gingival bleeding (leukopenia)
Carbamazepine	Tegretol	600 to 1200	Propoxyphene, erythromycin	Xerostomia, increased incidence of microbial infection, delayed healing, gingival bleeding (leukopenia and thrombocytopenia)
Phenobarbital	Luminal	60 to 120	———	
Valproic acid	Depakene	750 to 1250	Aspirin NSAIDs	Excessive bleeding and petechiae, decreased platelet aggregation, increased incidence of microbial infection, delayed healing, gingival bleeding (leukopenia and thrombocytopenia).

aggregation, lending to spontaneous hemorrhage and petechiae.

Propoxyphene and erythromycin should not be administered to patients taking carbamazepine because of interference with metabolism of carbamazepine, which could lead to toxicity. Aspirin and non-steroidal anti-inflammatory drugs (NSAIDs) should not be administered to patients taking valproic acid; they can further decrease platelet aggregation, leading to hemorrhagic episodes.

Dental Management

The following explains how to deal with epileptic patient requiring dental treatment (Box 12.2):

1. Well-controlled epileptic patients withstand routine oral surgery as well as the average patient. Anxiety may be a precipitating factor in unstable or poorly controlled epileptics but is not a major factor in well-controlled patients. Sedation may be a useful adjunct to therapy for the same indications as would apply in normal patients.

2. In spite of appropriate preventive measures taken by the dentist and patient, there is always the possibility that an epileptic patient may have a generalized tonic-clonic convulsion in the dental office. The dentist and staff should always anticipate this occurrence and be prepared to deal with it. Boxes 12.2 and 12.3 outline the steps to follow in the management of petit mal and partial seizures.

The primary task of management is to protect the patient and try to prevent injury. If the patient has a seizure while in the dental chair, no attempt should be made to move him or her to the floor. Instead, the chair should be placed in a supported supine position (Fig. 12.11) and the patient should, if possible, be

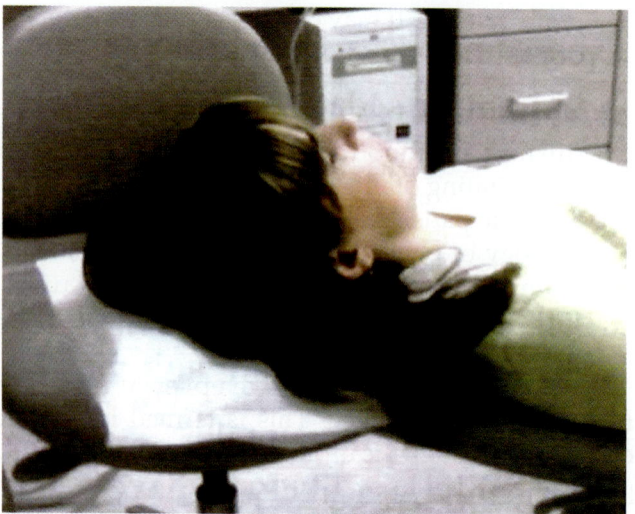

Fig. 12.11: Dental chair in the supine position with the back supported by the operator's or by the assistant

turned to the side to control the airway and minimize aspiration of secretions. No attempt should be made to restrain or hold the patient down. Passive restraint should be used only to prevent injury from hitting nearly objects or from falling out of the chair.

One often is counseled to place a padded tongue blade between the teeth to prevent tongue biting (Fig. 12.12). In reality, this is nearly an impossible task once the seizure has begun, and it may damage the teeth or oral soft tissue. Therefore, it is not advised. An exception to this would be if the patient senses a pending seizure and can cooperate. In this case, a padded tongue blade or folded towel may be placed between the teeth before they are clenched.

Seizure generally do not last more than a few minutes. Afterwards the patient will fall into a deep sleep from which he or she cannot be aroused. Then in a few minutes the patient will gradually regain consciousness but may be confused, disoriented and embarrassed. Headache is a prominent feature of this period.

No further treatment should be attempted although any injuries sustained (e.g. lacerations or fractures) should received immediate attention. In the event of avulsed or fractured teeth or a fractured alliance, an attempt should be made to locate the tooth or fragments to rule out aspiration. A chest radiograph may be required to locate a missing fragment or tooth.

1. In the event, a seizure becomes prolonged or is repeated (status epilepticus), intravenous diazepam 10 mg, is effective in controlling it.

Box 12.2: Management of petit mal and partial seizures

1. Terminate dental procedure
2. *Positioning the patient* "leave patient alone during seizure"

Seizure ceases	*Seizure continues (> 5 minutes)*
Reassure patient Allow patient to recover before discharge	Summon medical assistance

3. Basic life support as needed "A- B- C"

A, airway; B, breathing; C, circulation.

Box 12.3: Dental management of the epileptic patient

1. *Identification of patient by history*
   a. Type of seizure
   b. Age at time of onset
   c. Cause of seizures (if known)
   d. Medications
   e. Frequency of physician visits (name and phone number)
   f. Degree of seizure control
   g. Frequency of seizures
   h. Date of last seizure
   i. Known precipitating factors
   j. History of seizure-related injuries

2. *Provide normal care:* Well-controlled seizures pose no management problems.

3. *Consult with the physician:* If questionable history or poorly controlled seizures, consult with physician before dental treatment— may require modification of medications

4. *Be alert to adverse effects of anticonvulsants*
   a. Drowsiness
   b. Slow mentation
   c. Dizziness
   d. Ataxia
   e. Gastrointestinal upset
   f. Allergic signs (rash, erythema multiform)

5. *Bleeding tendency:* Patients taking valproic acid (depakene) may have bleeding tendencies because of platelet interference- order pretreatment bleeding time; if grossly abnormal, consult with physician

6. *Be prepared to manage grand mal seizure*
   a. Chair back in supported supine position
   b. Patient turned to side (to avoid aspiration)
   c. Do not attempt to use padded tongue blade

2. Measures for respiratory support should be available since respiratory function may be depressed. So the major priority is to establish an adequate airway. If this cannot be secured by positioning the patient properly or by use of an oral airway, then endotracheal intubation is required. Endotracheal intubation has the advantage of allowing mechanical ventilation and it prevents aspiration of gastric contents.

3. An IV line should be established, but before infusion of any medications is started, a blood sample should be drawn for determination of antiseizure medication and serum glucose levels (hypoglycemia being a precipitating factor that is easily correctable). A glucose infusion (50 Ml of 50% solution) can be given immediately after the blood sample is drawn. More detailed information as regard anticonvulsants is mentioned in Chapter 15, A: Anticonvulsants, page 434.

4. Avoid centrally acting pain medications, sedatives, hypnotics, narcotics and sedating antihistamines with anti-seizure medications because they enhance sedation. Use regular— strength acetaminophen (tylenol) only.

5. Drug therapy includes:
   a. *Diazepam (valium)* is a rapid acting and effective agent in all forms of epilepsy. It has less of a respiratory depressant effect than do the barbiturates, which are also used for acute management.
   b. *Phenytoin (dilantin)* is used but is less effective than diazepam. It has the advantage of minimal respiratory depressant and sedative effect. Given the short duration of diazepam's anti-seizure effect, phenytoin may be given adjunctively for long-term seizure control. Most of the seizure medications cause xerostomia. Phenobarbital and primidone (mysoline),

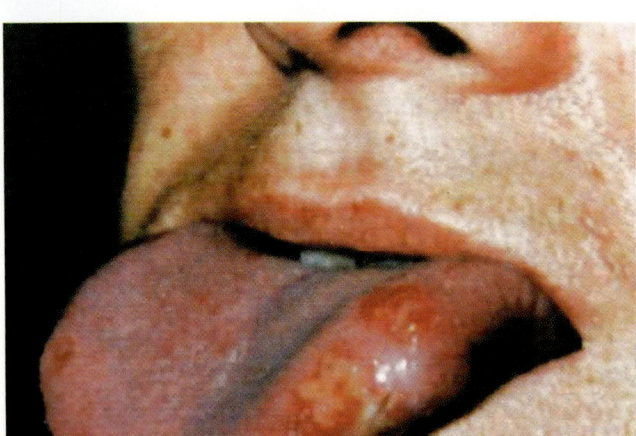

Fig. 12.12: The bitten tongue as a sign of epilepsy. Damage to the tongue is a common complication of generalized seizure and may be helpful evidence where there is doubt about the diagnosis. During epileptic attacks, the patient should be protected from harm, if possible; but forcible attempts to open the mouth or restrain the patient often do more harm than good

depress the CNS and the patient could be sleepy in the chair.

All antiseizure drugs can increase the effectiveness of pain medications and muscle relaxants, causing drowsiness.

c. On occasion, *general anesthesia* is called for in the attempt to break status epilepticus and it has the advantage of allowing use of muscle relaxants. This helps prevent physical exhaustion from persistent violent muscular activity. It also allows good control of respiration.

Some additional considerations in the management of the patient with seizures include:

1. A patient with poorly controlled disease may require additional anticonvulsant or sedative medication, as directed by the physician.

2. General anesthesia is not contraindicated. For unstable patients, a hospital setting or day care unit may be the preferable site. An epileptic patient is probably less likely to have a seizure during general anesthesia than at any other time. An IV dose of phenytoin may be given intraoperatively to ensure that post-anesthetic excitement does not initiate seizure activity.

3. IMF increases the risk of upper way obstruction and aspiration of gastric contents. Consideration should be given to the use of rigid fixation for fractures, osteotomies or bone grafts to avoid IMF in any patient with a history of a seizure disorder.

4. A missing tooth or teeth should be replaced if possible to prevent the tongue from being caught in the edentulous space during a seizure (as commonly happens). Generally, a fixed prosthesis is preferable to a removable one. The removable prosthesis is more easily dislodged. For fixed prostheses, all metal units should be considered when possible to minimize the chance of fracture. When placing anterior castings, the dentist may wish to consider using three-quarter crowns or retentive acrylic facings in lieu of porcelain to facilitate repair, if fracture occurs. Removable prostheses are nevertheless, sometimes constructed for epileptic patients. Metallic palates and bases are preferable to all-acrylic ones. If acrylic is used, it should be reinforced with a wire mesh.

5. Careful monitoring of the antiseizure medication blood levels is indicated. It may be worth discussing with the patient's physician a temporary increase in dosage during a period of unavoidable IMF.

6. Pulse oximetry should be considered mandatory for any patient with a seizure disorder and the potential for upper airway obstruction.

Syncopal episodes occur in many nonepileptic patients and may be accompanied at times by short bursts of seizures like tonic or clonic movement of the extremities. Seizure patients also experience syncope, and this may occur without provoking a seizure. However, transient hypotension and cerebral hypoxia, which account for loss of consciousness in syncope, may initiate seizure activity, especially in the poorly controlled epileptic patient.

Most syncopal episodes occur after an injection of a local anesthetic agent or venipuncture. Careful observation of the patient will normally reveal premonitory signs before syncope occurs—dizziness, slowing of the pulse, sudden thirst, blurring of vision.

Raising the feet, lowering the head, use of spirits of ammonia, and inhalation of oxygen, if rapidly available, may help abort a syncopal episode and are particularly useful in epileptics.

Oral Complications

The most significant oral complication seen in epileptic patients is gingival hyperplasia associated with phenytoin (Figs 12.13 to 12.15). The incidence of this in epileptics is difficult to ascertain because of the variable criteria used in studies reported incidences range from 0 to 100% with an average of approximately 42%. There seems to be a greater tendency for youngsters than for adults to develop hyperplasia. The anterior labial surfaces of the maxillary and mandibular gingivae are most commonly and severely affected.

Some disagreement exists in the literature as the relationship between drug dosage and severity of hyperplasia, but the majority of studies do not support a statistically valid connection. Another area of controversy is the effectiveness of oral hygiene in preventing gingival hyperplasis; however, the preponderance of evidence suggests that meticulous

oral hygiene will prevent or significantly decrease its severity. Good home care must always be combined with the removal of irritants such as overhanging restorations and calculus. Frequently, hyperplastic tissues will become large enough to interfere with function or appearance and surgical reduction will become necessary.

Because gingival hyperplasia is associated with phenytoin administration, every effort should be made to maintain a patient at an optimum level of oral hygiene. This may require frequent visits for monitoring progress. If significant hyperplasia exists, surgical reduction will be necessary; however, this must be accomplished by an increased awareness of oral hygiene needs and a positive commitment by the patient to maintain oral cleanliness.

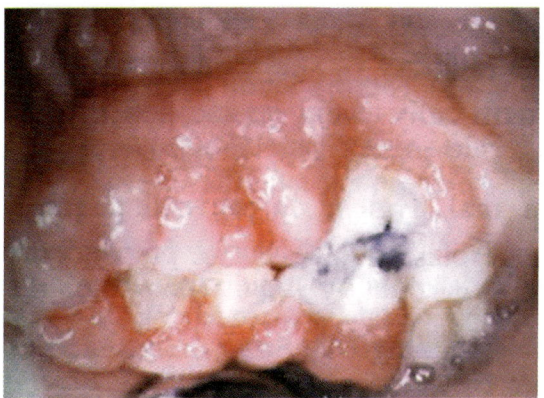

Fig. 12.13: Phenytoin-related gingival hyperplasia. Significant gingival hyperplasia almost totally covers the crowns of the posterior maxillary dentition.

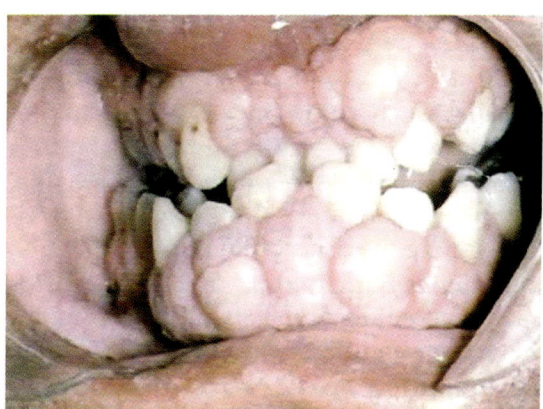

Fig. 12.14: An example of gingival hyperplasia associated with the medication phenytoin (dilantin) used to treat seizures.

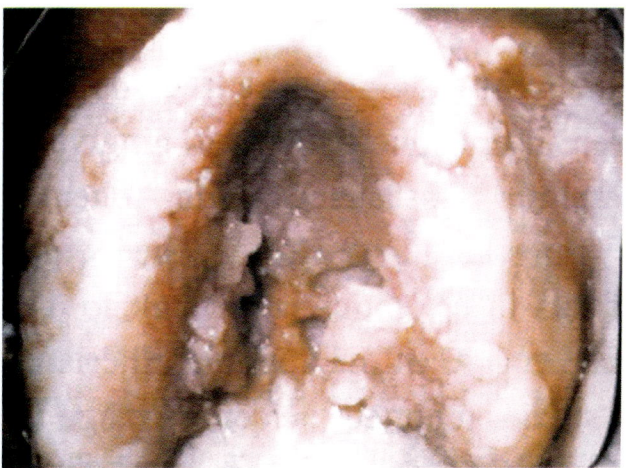

Fig. 12.15: Phenytoin-related palatal hyperplasia. Extensive hyperplasia of palatal mucosa in an edentulous patient with poor denture hygiene.

PARKINSON'S DISEASE

- Is a disease of the extrapyramidal system which links the higher motor centers and effector motor cells of the spinal cord. Important neurotransmitters are dopamine and γ-aminobutyric acid (GABA).
- Parkinson's disease is a progressive degenerative disorder of neurons of the basal ganglia that produce dopamine. Dopamine modulates the activity of adrenergic neurons. It is involved in arousal and motor activity.
- Unlike the cerebellum, the basal ganglia do not receive an input from the spinal cord, but they do receive direct input from the cerebral cortex. The main action of the basal ganglia is on the motor areas of the cortex by way of the thalamus. In addition to the role in motor control, the basal ganglia contribute to affective and congnitive functions. Lesions of the basal ganglia produce abnormal movements and posture.
- The deficits seen in the various basal ganglion diseases include abnormal movements (dyskinesias), increased muscle tone (cogwheel rigidity) and slowness in initiating movements (bradykinesia). Abnormal movements include tremor and dystonia among other movements. The tremor of the basal ganglia disease is a "pill-rolling" tremor that occurs, when the limb is at rest (Fig. 12.16). Dystonic movements are slow truncal movements that distort the body positions.
- In Parkinson's disease, there is a reduction in the neurotransmitter dopamine in the neurons with cell bodies in the substantia nigra and axons that terminate in the caudate nucleus and putamen. The resulting reduction in the inhibitory activity of dopamine elicits the symptoms of Parkinson's disease, which is characterized by rigidity, tremor and akinesia.

Etiology

1. *Genetic:* Most Parkinson's disease is idiopathic. People who have a first-degree relative with idiopathic Parkinson's disease, such as parent, sibling or child, are at three times greater risk of developing the disease themselves.
2. *Environmental:* Toxins such as pescticides, manganese, heavy metals or carbon monoxide have been implicated.
3. *Cerebrovascular disease.*
4. *Head injury,* particularly in boxers.
5. *Drugs* (particularly phenothiazine) and dopamine receptor blockers, valproate, and prochloro-perazines.

Signs and Symptoms

Parkinson's disease is an ailment that usually appears between ages 55 and 70 and it occurs more often in men than in women. Parkinson's disease is more common in people who are involved in farming, live in a rural area or drink well water. Parkinson's disease is a motor disability, commonly called *shaking palsy* because it is characterized by resting tremors, rigidity and aknesia. *Rigidity* is increased tonus in the skeletal muscles, tremor is rhythmic oscillatory trembling movements, especially of the forearm and hand and aknesia is the tendency to be immobile, the facial muscles may become rigid and produce a staring, expressionless face with a slightly open mouth. With rigidity, the arms are flexed and held stiffly at the sides. Tremors of the head and hands, slow movements, rigid joints, handwriting becomes cramped and eventually illegible.

Tasks such as buttoning clothes and preparing food become increasingly laborious. Speech becomes slurred. He or she takes smaller steps and develops a slow, shuffling gait with a forward bent posture and a tendency to fall forward. Gait disturbance with shuffling short steps and a tendency to turn en bloc is a prominent feature. Freezing of gait occurs commonly at the onset of locomotion (start hesitation), when attempting to change direction or run around and upon entering a narrow space such as a doorway.

Abnormalities of balance and posture tend to increase in prominence as the disease progresses. Flexion of the head, stooping and tilting of the upper trunk and a tendency to hold the arm in a flexed posture while walking are common, as are changes in the posture of the fingers and hands. Postural instability is one of the most disabling features of advanced Parkinson's disease, contributing to falls and injuries and leading to major morbidity and mortality.

The non-motor signs and symptoms include depression and anxiety, cognitive impairment, sleep disturbances, sensory abnormalities and pain, loss of smell (anosmia), and disturbances of autonomic function.

The tremor, which is rhythmic and fine and is best seen in the extremity at rest, produces a "pill-rolling rest tremor" and hand writing changes. Cogwheel-type rigidity (decreased arm swing with walking and foot dragging). The neck and shoulders are rigid causing a stooped posture, unsteadiness, imbalance (gait instability) and falls also are common features. Slowness (bradykinesia) in the initiation and execution of movements and poverty of spontaneous movements. The patient may be slow at starting to walk, but then runs forwards (festinant gait) or shuffles with slow, short steps (Figs 12.16 and 12.17).

This can make performing the simplest tasks difficult and time-consuming. In addition, pain, musculoskeletal, sensory (burning, numbness, tingling). Parkinson's disease may cause either urinary incontinence or urine retention and certain medications used to treat the disease, especially anticholinergic drugs, also make it hard to urinate. Orthostatic hypotension and bowel and bladder dysfunction occur in approximately 50% of patients. Cognitive impairment of memory and concentration occurs to varying degrees. Mood depression, anxiety, insomnia and dementia. The blackness of expression and the apparent unresponsiveness of Parkinson's patient should not be mistaken with lack of reaction or intelligence.

Pathophysiology

Deep within each cerebral hemisphere is a group of five subcortical nuclei called the basal ganglia. The basal ganglia are composed of several nuclei which include the caudate (tail-shaped) nucleus, putamen,

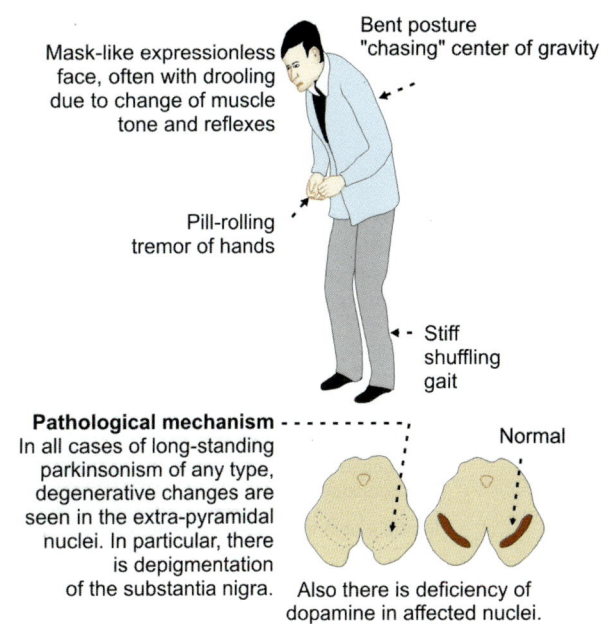

Bent posture "chasing" center of gravity

Mask-like expressionless face, often with drooling due to change of muscle tone and reflexes

Pill-rolling tremor of hands

Stiff shuffling gait

Pathological mechanism
In all cases of long-standing parkinsonism of any type, degenerative changes are seen in the extra-pyramidal nuclei. In particular, there is depigmentation of the substantia nigra.

Normal

Also there is deficiency of dopamine in affected nuclei.

Fig. 12.17: Characteristic features and the underlying pathological mechanism of Parkinson's disease. Gait with rapid, short, shuffling steps and reduced arm swinging, bend posture, pill-rolling tremor of hands *(Reid and Roberts, 2005)*

globus pallidus (pale ball), subthalamic nucleus and substantia nigra (Figs 12.18 and 12.19).

These nuclei are intimately involved in coordinating cerebral activities with other brainstem functions. Along with the cerebellum, the basal ganglia act at the interface between the sensory systems and many motor responses, affecting motor, emotional and cognitive behaviors. The basal ganglia are important in controlling background gross body movements, whereas cerebral cortex is necessary for performance of the more precise movements of the arms, hands, fingers and feet. When the hand is performing some precise activity that requires a background stance of the body the basal ganglia provides the body movements, while the cerebral cortex provides the precise movements. Clinically, the term movement disorders and malfunctioning of the basal ganglia are essentially synonymous. Parkinson's disease is a basal ganglia disturbance.

The basic circuitry associated with the basal nuclei may be summarized as follows: The basal ganglia receive information from many areas of the cerebral cortex, process and integrate these inputs and then relay them to the thalamus, which in turn projects its output to the motor, premotor and limbic cortical areas. These areas then exert their influences on the

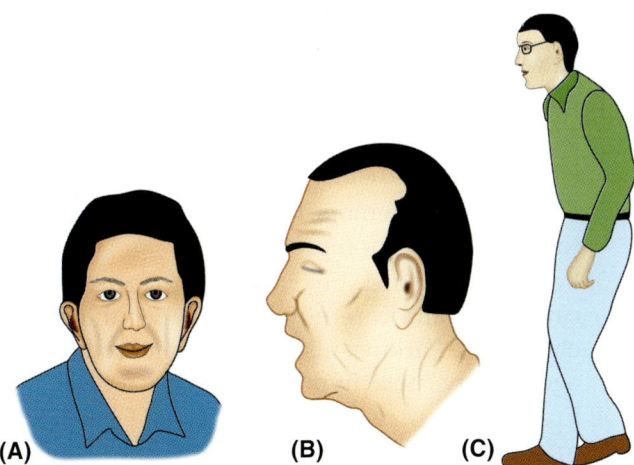

Fig. 12.16: Characteristic features of Parkinson's disease. **(A)** Mask-like appearance, stare and excessive sweating. **(B)** Drooling with excess saliva. **(C)** Gait with rapid, short, shuffling steps and reduced arm swinging *(From Seidel HM, Ball JW, Dains JE, et al. Mosby's Guide to Physical Examination, 6th ed. St. Louis, Mosby, 2006)*

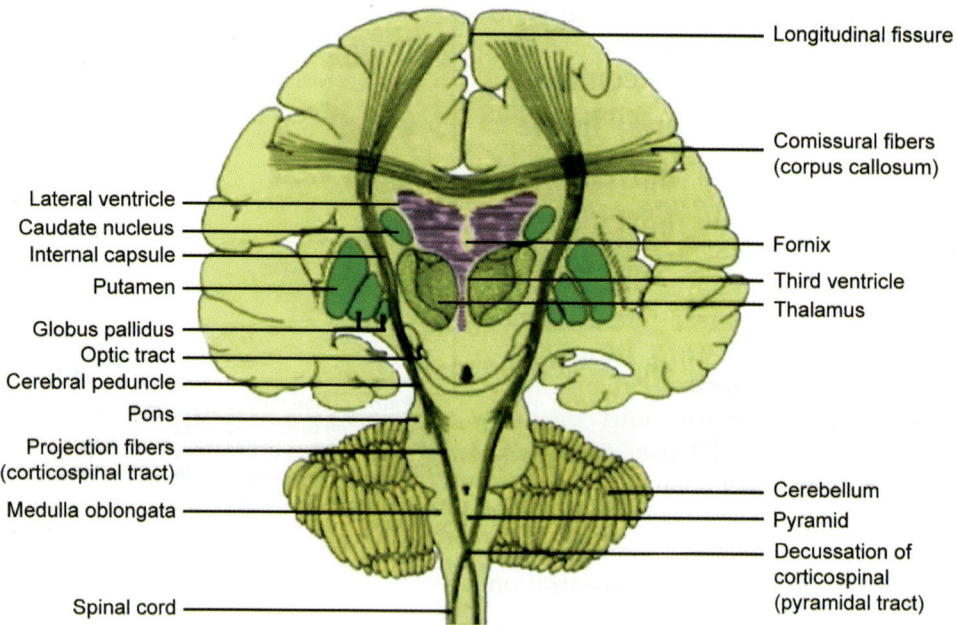

Fig. 12.18: Anterior view of fiber tracts in the white matter of the cerebrum *(Donna VW, 1995)*

upper motor neuron pathways and other systems that affect motor, emotional and cognitive behaviors.

Dopamine (DA) is an inhibitory neurotransmitter that normally prevents excessive activity in motor centers of the brain called the *basal nuclei*. Degeneration of the dopamine-releasing neurons leads to an excessive ratio of ACh to DA, leading to hyperactivity of the basal nuclei. As a result, a person with PD suffers involuntary muscle contractions.

Medical Management

Patients cannot be expected to recover from PD, but its effects can be alleviated with drugs and physical therapy. Treatment with dopamine is ineffective because it cannot cross the blood-brain barrier. Before the dopaminergic neurons are completely lost, administration of L-dopa is prescribed and it can cross the blood-brain barrier. This drug is metabolized into dopamine. Anticholinergic drugs are of value to block the effect of another brain neurotransmitter (acetylcholine) to rebalance its levels with dopamine. L-Dopa affords some relief from symptoms, but it does not slow progression of the disease and it has undesirable side effects on the liver and heart. L-dopa is converted within the brain into dopamine. The drug therapy alleviates symptoms because it raises the concentration of dopamine in the basal ganglia, thereby supplying the neurotransmitters that is deficient. It is effective for only 5 to 10 years of treatment. A newer

drug, Deprenyl, is a monoamine oxidase (MAO) inhibitor that retards neuronal degeneration and delays the development of symptoms. Modest improvement has been obtained by implanting other dopamine producing tissues into the brains of PD patients—namely, adrenal medulla and fetal brain tissue. Even though the latter tissue has not come from elective abortions, this approach has triggered ethical controversy.

Dental Management

1. Dental treatment should be carried out 2 to 3 hours after the medication to gain the maximum effect of the medicine.
2. Because of the tremors, the dentist may be obliged to resort to sedation procedures.
3. Patients should be raised uprightly only cautiously and carefully assisted out the dental chair, since Parkinsonism, L-dopa and some other agents may cause hypotension.
4. Epinephrine may interact with COMT inhibitors, to cause tachycardia, dysrhythmias and hypertension and, therefore, local analgesics without epinephrine should be used in these patients. Minimize the amount of epinephrine use in the patient on COMT inhibitors and use local anesthetics with 1: 200,000 epinephrine or without epinephrine, maximum 2 capsules.

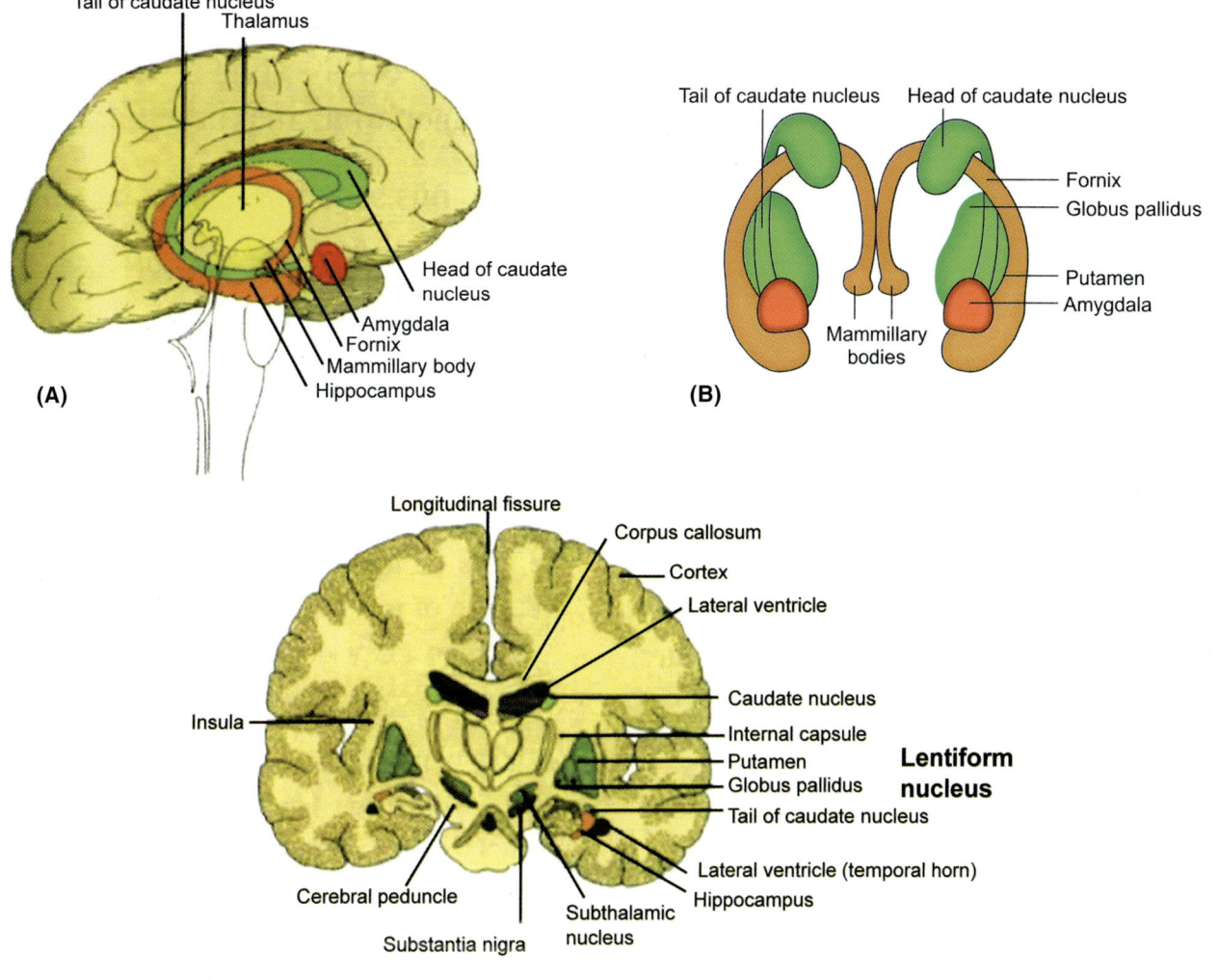

Fig. 12.19: Basal ganglia. **(A)** Section through the brain showing the parts of the basal ganglia (green). **(B)** Structures that make up the basal ganglia. **(C)** Frontal view. The structures of the basal ganglia shown in these drawings include the head and tail of the caudate nucleus, globus pallidus, putamen, lentiform nucleus, subthalamic nucleus, and substantia niagra *(Donna VW, 1995)*

5. Conscious sedation should be safe.

6. Pethidine should be used with caution in patients receiving monoamine oxidase inhibitors (MAOIs), to avoid acute hypertensive episodes.

7. Drooling of saliva may be troublesome. Orofacial involuntary movements (dyskinesia) such as "fly catcher tongue" and lip pursing are side effects of levodopas and may make the use of rotating dental instruments hazardous. Levodopa may cause taste disturbances and reddish saliva.

8. Anticholinergics are among the drugs used to manage Parkinson's disease, often results in xerostomia and nausea. If the patient is experi- encing xerostomia, then dysphagia and poor denture retention are likely. Salivary substitutes are beneficial in alleviating the symptoms. Topical fluoride should be considered for use in dentate patients with xerostomia to prevent root caries.

9. Mechanical tooth brushes should be advised to maintain adequate oral hygiene. Avoid clarithro- mycin, tetracycline, doxycycline, and azole antifungals with dopamine antagonist drugs.

About 40% of Parkinson's disease patients also develop dementia. The major symptoms of dementia are illustrated in Chapter 15-"D".

13

Hormonal Upsets

Introduction
    Functions of Major Endocrine Glands
    Hormone Interactions
    Biochemistry of Hormones
Adaptation Syndrome "Stress Response"
- **Pregnancy**
    Physiology
    Treatment considerations
- **Breastfeeding**
    Prolactin
    Drugs Contraindicated and Alternatives
      in Lactating Mothers

- **The Menopause**
- **Osteoporosis**
    Etiology
    Signs and Symptoms
    Localized Osteoporosis
    Treatment
    Suggested Dental Guidelines
    Osteopenia
- **Depression**
    Addictive Drugs and Mood Disorders
    Pineal Gland
    Treatment

HORMONAL UPSETS

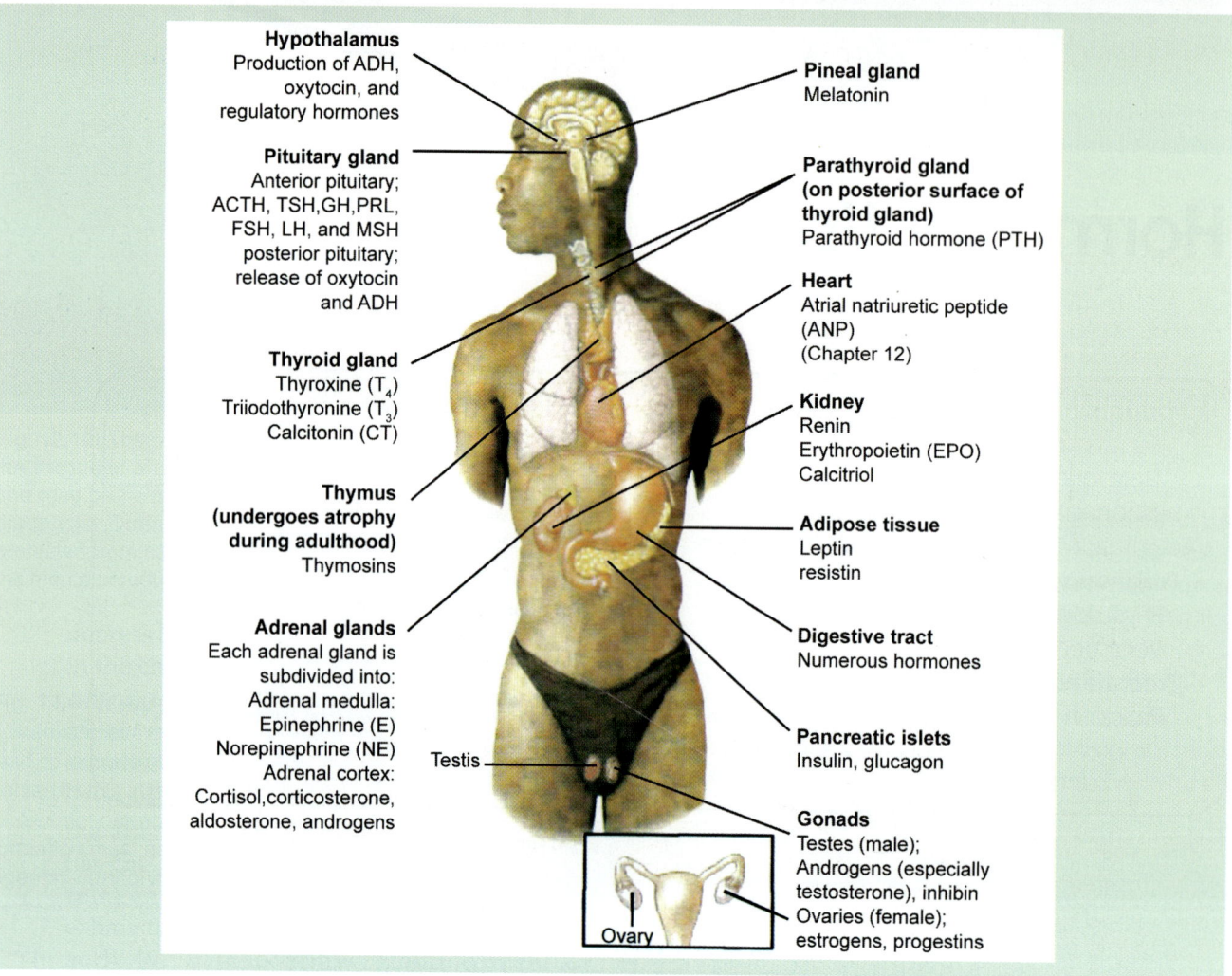

Hypothalamus
Production of ADH, oxytocin, and regulatory hormones

Pituitary gland
Anterior pituitary;
ACTH, TSH,GH,PRL, FSH, LH, and MSH posterior pituitary;
release of oxytocin and ADH

Thyroid gland
Thyroxine (T_4)
Triiodothyronine (T_3)
Calcitonin (CT)

Thymus (undergoes atrophy during adulthood)
Thymosins

Adrenal glands
Each adrenal gland is subdivided into:
Adrenal medulla:
Epinephrine (E)
Norepinephrine (NE)
Adrenal cortex:
Cortisol,corticosterone, aldosterone, androgens

Testis

Pineal gland
Melatonin

Parathyroid gland (on posterior surface of thyroid gland)
Parathyroid hormone (PTH)

Heart
Atrial natriuretic peptide (ANP)
(Chapter 12)

Kidney
Renin
Erythropoietin (EPO)
Calcitriol

Adipose tissue
Leptin
resistin

Digestive tract
Numerous hormones

Pancreatic islets
Insulin, glucagon

Gonads
Testes (male);
Androgens (especially testosterone), inhibin
Ovaries (female);
estrogens, progestins

Ovary

Plate (XVIII) An overview of the endocrine system *(Martine et al, 2008)*

Introduction

The term endocrine is derived from the Greek words *endo* and *krino* meaning within and to separate. The word implies that a secretion is produced within endocrine glands but the secretion has an effect at a location that is away from, or separate from the endocrine gland. The secretions of endocrine glands are transported in the blood to tissues some distance from the glands. The principal organs of the endocrine system "endocrine glands" are the pituitary gland, pineal gland, thyroid gland, parathyroid glands, thymus, adrenal glands, pancreas, testes, and ovaries (Plate XVIII). In contrast, exocrine glands secrete their products into ducts, which exit the glands and carry the secretory products to an external or internal surface such as the skin or digestive tract. Examples of exocrine glands are the sweat and the salivary glands. The endocrine system consists of all the endocrine glands of the body.

The endocrine system includes also scattered cells in other organs. Endocrine glands and specific cells lose their contact with the surface and have no ducts "ductless". They, however, have a high density of blood capillaries and secrete their products directly into the blood. In contrast, the secretions of exocrine glands such as sweat and salivary glands, empty directly into ducts that transport them to specific locations.

Chemical signals secreted by endocrine glands are called hormones, a term derived from the Greek word *harmon* meaning to set into motion, because hormones set responses by cells into motion. Traditionally, a hormone is defined as a substance that is produced in minute amounts by a collection of cells, is secreted into the circulatory system to be transported some distance, and acts on tissues at another site in the body to influence their activity in a specific way. The hormone is a specialized chemical substance and functions as chemical messengers to stimulate cells elsewhere in the body.

Hormones are distributed in the blood to all parts of the body, but only certain target tissues respond to each type of hormone. A target tissue for a hormone is made up of cells that have receptors for the hormone (Fig. 13.1). Each hormone can bind only to its receptors and cannot influence the function of cells that do not have receptors for the hormone (Fig. 13.2), i.e. hormones are effective only at specific target cells with compatible receptors on the surface of the plasma membrane or within the cytoplasm or nucleus, i.e. hormone receptors are located either on the cell membrane or inside the cell.

Function of the Endocrine System

Hormones help regulate the rate of biochemical reactions. Like enzymes, hormones are not changed by the reactions they regulate. The secretion rate of hormones varies from one gland to another and also for each gland, depending on physiological conditions. For example, the hormone epinephrine (commonly called adrenaline) is secreted by the adrenal glands in response to an emergency that calls for an immediate increase of blood flow to the muscles. In contrast, ovarian hormones are secreted cyclically over extended periods of time to regulate the ongoing menstrual cycle.

The principal function of the endocrine system is achievement of internal chemical communication and coordination of the different systems (Table 13.1). The endocrine system is a control system that is concerned mainly with three functions:

1. It helps maintain homeostasis by regulating activities such as the concentration of chemicals in body fluids and the metabolism of proteins, lipids, and carbohydrates.

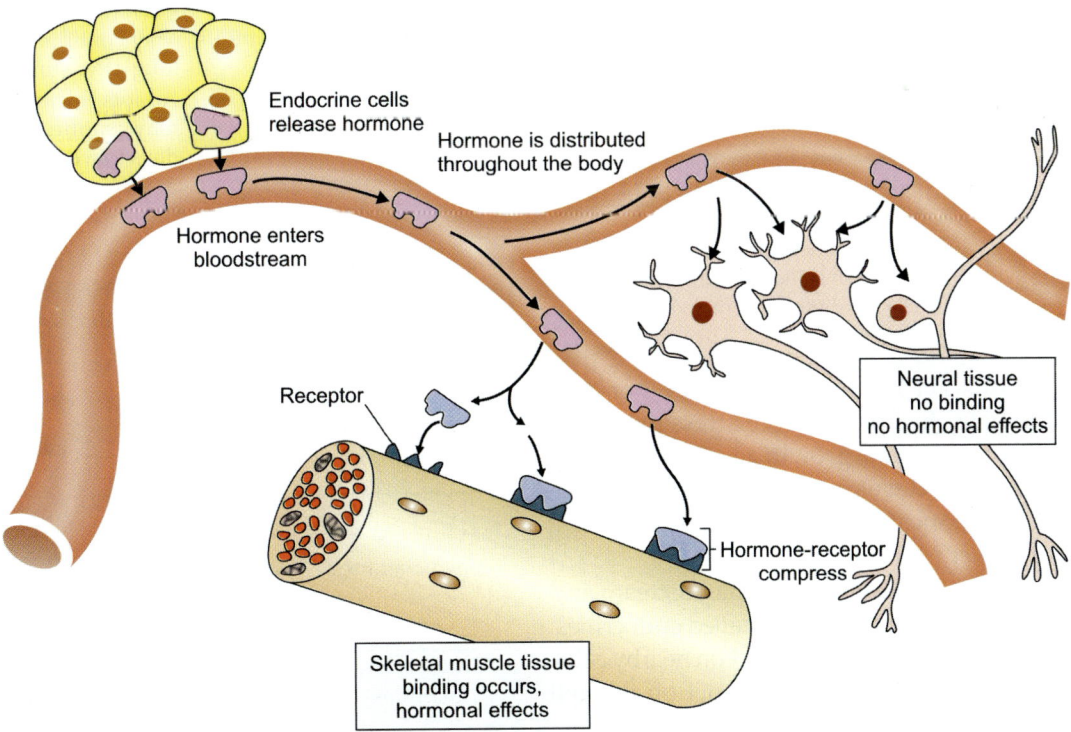

Fig. 13.1: The role of target cell receptors in hormone action. For a hormone to affect a target cell, that cell must have receptors that can bind that hormone and initiate a change in cellular activity. The hormone in this illustration affects skeletal muscle tissue but not neural tissue because only the muscle tissue has the appropriate receptors *(Martini et al, 2008)*

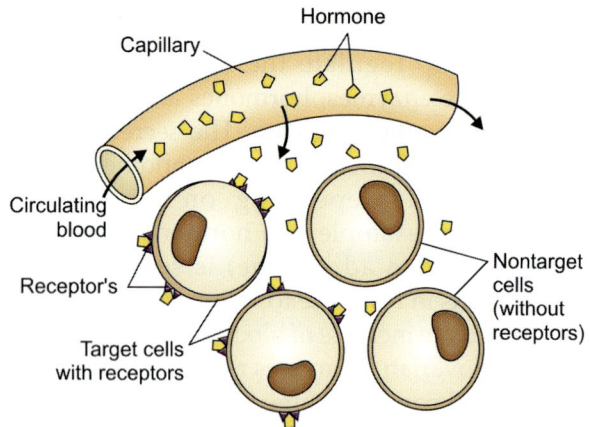

Fig. 13.2: Target cell response to hormones. Hormones are secreted into the blood and distributed throughout the body, where they diffuse from the blood into the interstitial fluid. Only target cells have receptors to which hormones can bind. Therefore, even though a hormone is distributed throughout the body, only target cells for that hormone can respond to it. *(Seeley et al 1996)*

Table 13.1: Functions of major endocrine glands

Structure	Main function
Hypothalamus	Regulates anterior pituitary hormones
Pineal gland	May affect sleep
Pituitary gland	Regulates growth and various metabolic activities of other endocrine glands
Thyroid gland	Controls rate of metabolism
Parathyroid glands	Regulates level of calcium and phosphate
Thymus	Processes developing T and B cells
Adrenal gland	Affects metabolism, blood pressure, sodium and potassium levels
Pancreas	Regulates blood glucose levels
Ovaries	Produces ova and female sex hormones
Testes	Produces sperm and male sex hormones

2. Its secretions act in concert with the nervous system to help the body react to stress properly.
3. It is a major regulator of growth and development, including sexual development and reproduction.

Generally, hormones may be classified according to the cells they act upon:

• Hormones that are released into the bloodstream and interact with distinct target cells are called endocrines.
• Paracrines are local hormones that act on nearby cells.
• Autocrines are local hormones that act on the cell that released them.

Comparison of the biological influence of endocrine system and nervous system is shown in Table 13.2 and Fig. 13.3.

Biochemistry of Hormones

Hormones are either: (1) lipid-soluble steroids, (2) derivatives of amino acids (biogenic amines) (3) water-soluble proteins and peptides, or (4) eicosanoids (prostaglandins and leukotrines). The type of secretion depends on the embryonic origin of the gland. Glands derived from endoderm secrete proteins, glands derived from ectoderm secrete biogenic amines, and glands derived from mesoderm secrete steroids (Table 13.3).

Hormones are synthetized from raw materials in the cell and secreted into the extracellular spaces,

Table 13.2: Comparison of the nervous and endocrine systems.

Nervous system	Endocrine system
Communicates by means of electrical impulses and neurotransmitters.	Communicates by means of hormone.
Release neurotransmitters at synapses at specific target cells.	Release hormones into bloodstream for general distribution throughout body.
Usually has relatively local, specific effects	Sometimes has very general, widespread effects.
Reacts quickly to stimuli, usually within 1 to 10 msec.	Reacts more slowly to stimuli, often taking seconds to days.
Stops quickly when stimulus stops.	May continue responding long after stimuli stops.
Adapts relatively quickly to continual stimulation.	Adapts relatively slowly; may continue responding for days to weeks of stimulation.

Table 13.3: Chemical classes of hormones

Chemical class	Representative examples	Source
Steroids	Estrogens, Progesterone, Testosterone, Aldosterone, Cortisol	Ovaries, Testes, Adrenal cortex
Biogenic amines	Thyroxine, Triiodothyronine	Thyroid gland
	Catecholamines, (epinephrine, Norepinephrine)	Adrenal medulla
Proteins and peptides	Insuline	Pancreas
	Oxytocin	Posterior pituitary
	Growth hormone	Anterior pituitary
Ecosanoids	Prostaglandins, Leukotrienes, Thromboxanes	Mast cells

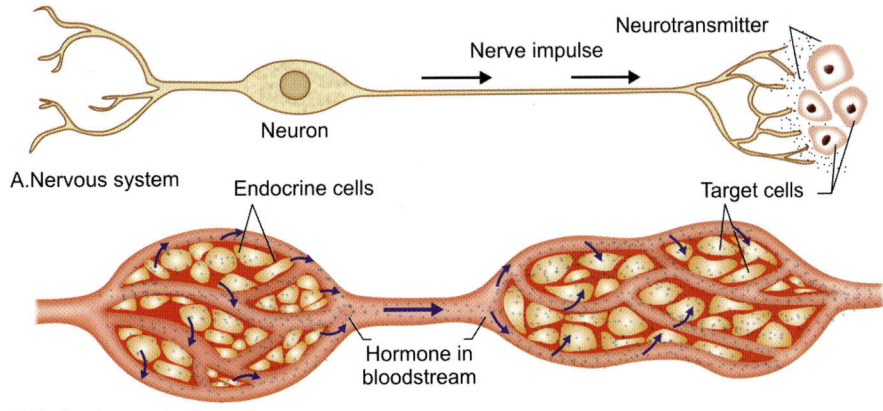

Fig. 13.3: Communication by the nervous and endocrine systems. **(A)** A neuron has a long fiber that delivers its neurotransmitter to the immediate vicinity of its target cells. **(B)** Endocrine cells secrete a hormone into the bloodstream. The hormone binds to target cells at places often remote from the gland cells *(Saladin, 2003)*

usually entering the bloodstream by way of capillaries that flow between the cells of the gland. Steroid hormones, being lipid-soluble, are probably soluble in the water portion of plasma and are transported in the blood in combination with plasma proteins. Some peptide hormones (thyroid hormones) also require carrier proteins to transport them to their target cells. Because protein hormones are water-soluble, many are transported freely in the circulating blood.

Hormone Interactions

There are many hormones in the blood and tissue fluid. The cells do not respond to all these hormones at the same time. Cells ignore the majority of them because they have no receptors for them, but most cells are sensitive to more than one. When more than a hormone acts within the cell, their effects are either synergistic, permissive, or antagonistic.

1. *Synergistic effects,* in which two or more hormones act together to produce an effect that is greater than the sum of their separate effects. Neither follicle stimulating hormone (FSH)*, secreted by the anterior lobe of the pituitary gland, nor testosterone alone, for example, can stimulate significant sperm production. When they act together, however, the testes produce some 300,000 sperm per minute.

2. *Permissive effects, in* which one hormone enhances the target organ's response to a second hormone that is secreted later. Estrogen** stimulates the up regulation of progesterone receptors in the uterus. The uterus would respond poorly to progesterone, if at all, had it not been primed by the first hormone. Estrogen thus has a permissive effect on progesterone action.

3. *Antagonistic effects,* in which one hormone opposes the action of another. For example, insulin lowers blood glucose level and glucagon raises it. During pregnancy, estrogen from the placenta inhibits the mammary glands from responding to prolactin***; thus milk is not secreted until the placenta is shed at birth.

The circulating concentrations of hormones are very low compared to other blood substances: in the order of nanograms per deciliter. Blood glucose, for example, is about 100 million times this concentrated. Only a few molecules of a hormone may be enough to produce a dramatic response in a target cell. Hormonal signals, like nervous signals, must be turned off when they have served their purpose. Most hormones are taken up and degraded by the liver and kidneys and then excreted in the bile or urine. Some are degraded by their target cells.

The following are examples of hormonal upsets.

---

* FSH: Follicle-stimulating hormone: Secreted by the anterior pituitary gland . The target organs are ovaries, and testes. Its principal effects in female is : growth of ovarian follicles and secretion of estrogen and in male: sperm production.

** Estrogen & androgen : Secreted by the adrenal cortex. Its target tissues are bone, muscle, integument and many other tissues.

*** PRL: Prolactin : (pro =-favoring, lact = milk) Secreted by the anterior pituitary gland. Its target organs are mammary glands and testes. Its principal effects in female is milk synthesis, in male it increases LH**** sensitivity and testosterone secretion.

ADAPTATION SYNDROME
"Stress Response"

Stress affects us all from time to time and we react to it in ways that are mediated mainly by the endocrine and sympathetic nervous systems. **Stress** is defined as any situation that upsets homeostasis and threatens one's physical or emotional well-being. *Physical causes* of stress *(stressors)* include injury, surgery, hemorrhage, infection, intense exercise, temperature extremes, pain, and malnutrition. *Emotional causes* include anger, grief, depression, anxiety and guilt. *Metabolic,* such as acute starvation. Whatever the cause, the body reacts to stress in a fairly consistent way called the stress response or general adaptation syndrome (GAS).

All stress-causing factors produce the same basic pattern of hormonal and physiological adjustments. The response typically involves elevated levels of epinephrine and glucocorticoids, especially cortisol; some physiologists now define stress as any situation that raises the Cortisol level. A pioneering researcher on stress physiology, Canadian biochemist Hans Selye, showed in 1936 that the GAS typically occurs in three stages, which he called the *alarm reaction,* the *stage of resistance* and the *stage of exhaustion* (Fig. 13.4).

THE ALARM REACTION

The initial response to stress is an **alarm reaction** mediated mainly by norepinephrine from the sympathetic nervous system and epinephrine from the adrenal medulla. These catecholamines prepare the body to take action such as fighting or escaping danger. One of their effects, the consumption of stored glycogen, is particularly important to the transition to the next stage of the stress response. Aldosterone and angiotensin levels also rise during the alarm reaction. Angiotensin helps to raise the blood pressure, and aldosterone promotes sodium and water conservation, which helps to offset possible losses by sweating and bleeding.

The temporary adjustments of the alarm phase remove or overcome the stress. But some stresses, including starvation, acute illness, or severe anxiety, can persist for hours, days, or even weeks. If stress lasts longer than a few hours, the individual enters the resistance phase of the GAS.

ALARM PHASE (fight or flight)
Immediate short-term response to crises

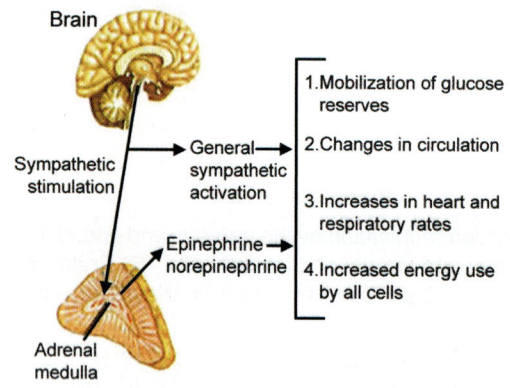

1. Mobilization of glucose reserves
2. Changes in circulation
3. Increases in heart and respiratory rates
4. Increased energy use by all cells

RESISTANCE PHASE
Long-term metabolic adjustments

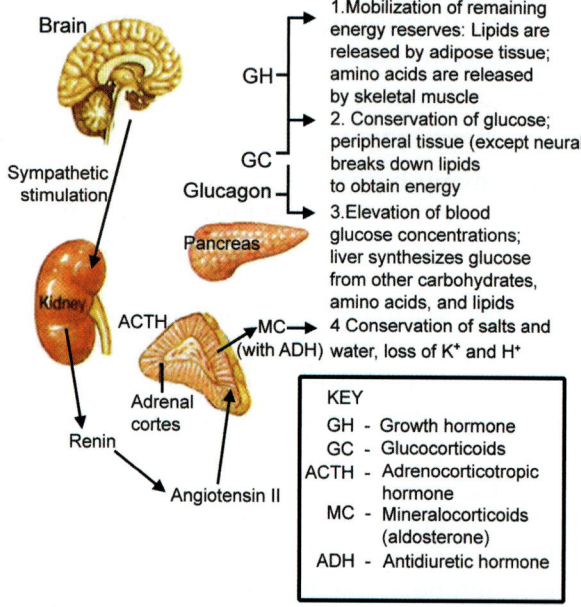

1. Mobilization of remaining energy reserves: Lipids are released by adipose tissue; amino acids are released by skeletal muscle
2. Conservation of glucose; peripheral tissue (except neural) breaks down lipids to obtain energy
3. Elevation of blood glucose concentrations; liver synthesizes glucose from other carbohydrates, amino acids, and lipids
4. Conservation of salts and water, loss of K^+ and H^+

KEY
GH - Growth hormone
GC - Glucocorticoids
ACTH - Adrenocorticotropic hormone
MC - Mineralocorticoids (aldosterone)
ADH - Antidiuretic hormone

EXHAUSTION PHASE
Collapse of vital system

Causes may include:
Exhaustion of lipid reserves
Inability to produce glucocorticoids
Failure of electrolyte balance
Cumulative structural or functional damage to vital organs

Fig. 13.4: Gradual adaptation syndrome (GAS) *(Martini et al, 2008)*

THE STAGE OF RESISTANCE

After a few hours, the body's glycogen reserves are exhausted, and yet the nervous system continues to demand glucose. If a stressful situation is not resolved before the glycogen is gone, the body enters the **stage of resistance,** in which the first priority is to provide alternative fuels for metabolism. This stage is dominated by cortisol (Fig. 13.5). The hypothalamus secretes corticotrophin releasing hormone (CRH), the pituitary responds by secreting adrenocorticotropic hormone (ACTH) and this, in turn, stimulates the adrenal cortex to secrete cortisol and other glucocorticoids. Cortisol promotes the breakdown of fat and protein into glycerol, fatty acids and amino acids, providing the liver with raw material for gluconeogenesis (glucose synthesis). Like epinephrine, cortisol inhibits glucose uptake by most organs and thus has a glucose-sparing effect. It also inhibits protein synthesis, leaving the free amino acids available for gluconeogenesis.

The immune system, which depends heavily on the synthesis of antibodies and other proteins, is depressed by term cortisol exposure. Lymphoid tissues atrophy, antibody levels drop, the number of circulating leukocytes declines, and inflammatory cells such as *mast cells* release less histamine and other inflammatory chemicals. Wounds heal poorly and a person in chronic stress becomes more susceptible to infections and some forms of cancer. Cortisol stimulates gastric secretion, which may account for the ulcers that occur in chronic stress, but it suppresses the secretion of sex hormones such as estrogen, testosterone and luteinizing hormone, causing disturbances of fertility and sexual function.

THE STAGE OF EXHAUSTION

When the resistance phase ends, the homeostatic regulatory mechanisms breakdown and the exhaustion phase begins. The body's fat reserves can carry it through months of stress, but when fat is depleted, stress overwhelms homeostasis. The **stage of exhaustion** sets in, often marked by rapid decline and death. With its fat stores gone, the body now relies primarily on protein breakdown to meet its energy needs. Thus, there is a progressive wasting away of the muscles and weakening of the body. After prolonged stimulation, the adrenal cortex may stop producing glucocorticoids, making it all the more difficult to maintain glucose homeostasis. Aldosterone sometimes promotes so much water retention that it creates a state of hypertension; and while it conserves sodium, it hastens the elimination of potassium and hydrogen ions. This creates a state of hypokalemia (potassium deficiency in the blood) and alkalosis (excessively high blood pH), resulting in nervous and muscular system dysfunctions. Death frequently results from heart failure, kidney failure, or overwhelming infection.

PREGNANCY

A pregnant patient, although not "medically compromised" per se, requires a management considerations by the dentist. Therapeutic dental care must be rendered to the mother, without adversely affecting the developing fetus. Pregnancy is a special event in a woman's life and as such, is emotionally charged. Therefore, establishment of a good patient–dentist relationship that encourages openness, honesty and trust is an integral part of successful management.

Physiology

Normal pregnancy lasts approximately 40 weeks. During the first three months (trimester), formation of organs and systems occurs, thus the fetus is most susceptible to malformation during this period. The uterus weighs about 50 g when a woman is not pregnant and about 900 g by the end of pregnancy (Fig. 13.6). Its growth is monitored by palpating the fundus, which eventually reaches almost to the xiphoid process. Table 13.4 shows how the weight gained in pregnancy is distributed.

Most developmental defects are of unknown etiology but, in addition to hereditary influences, infections and drugs, such as alcohol and smoking, can be implicated in some cases. The only safe course of action is, therefore, to protect the patient as far as

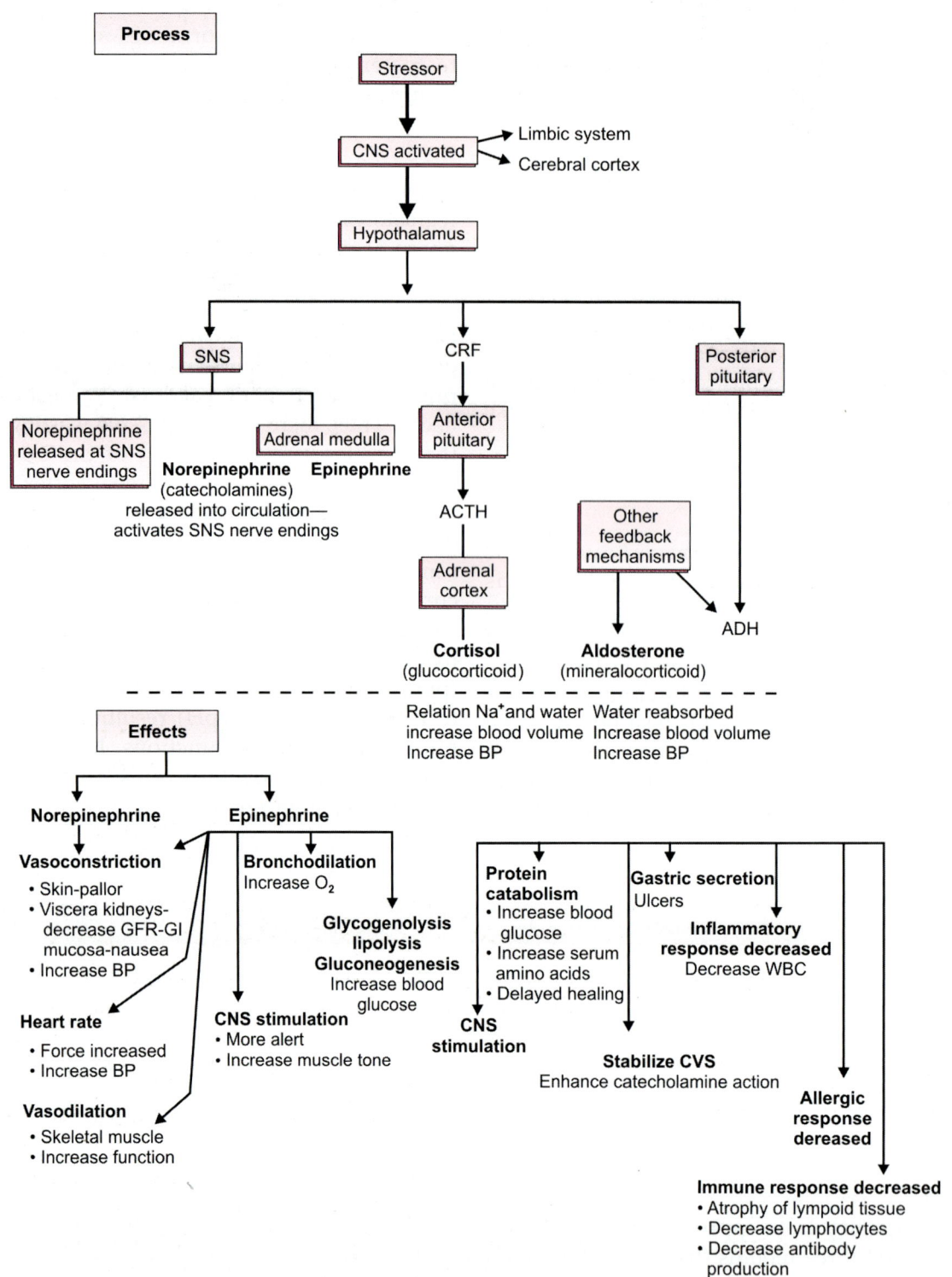

Fig. 13.5: The stress response. CNS, central nervous system, SNS, sympathetic nervous system, CRF, corticotropin-releasing factor, ACTH, adrenocorticotropic hormone. ADH,, antidiuretic hormone, GFR, glomerular filterate rate, GI, gastrointestinal, BP, blood pressure, WBC, white blood corpuscles, CVS, cardiovascular system. *(Gould 2006).* Possible complications include: Tension headache, insomnia, diabetes mellitus, infection, heart failure, peptic ulcer, fatigue

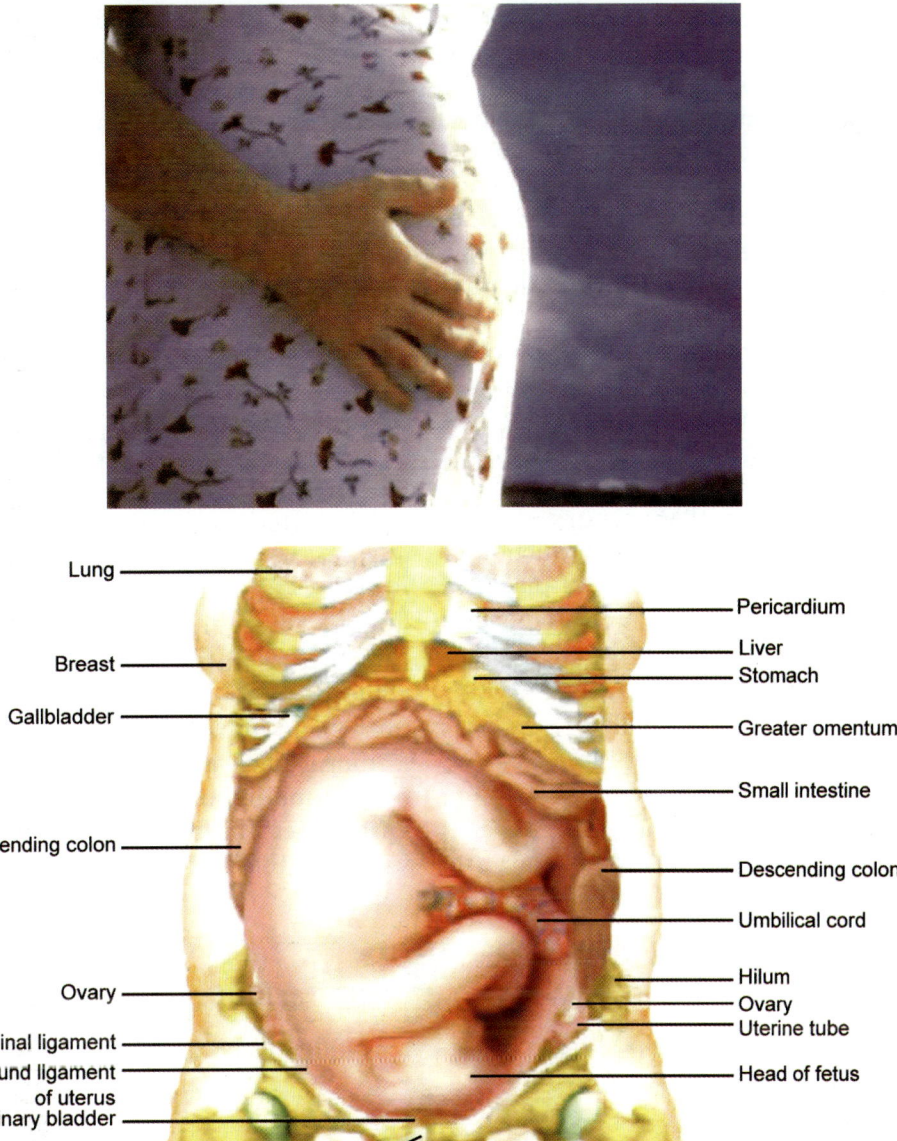

Lung
Breast
Gallbladder
Ascending colon
Ovary
Inguinal ligament
Round ligament
of uterus
Urinary bladder
Pubic symphysis

Pericardium
Liver
Stomach
Greater omentum
Small intestine
Descending colon
Umbilical cord
Hilum
Ovary
Uterine tube
Head of fetus

Anterior view

Fig. 13.6: The full-term fetus in vertex position

Table 13.4: Distribution of weight gain in pregnancy

Fetus	3kg (7 lb)
Placenta, total membranes, and amniotic fluid	1.8 kg (4 lb)
Blood and tissue fluid	2.7 kg (6 lb)
Fat	1.4 kg (3 lb)
Uterus	0.9 kg (2 lb)
Breast	0.9 kg (2 lb)
Total	**11 kg (24 lb)**

possible from infections and to avoid the use of drugs, particularly general anesthetics, and radiography during the first trimester. In contrast, it is now recognized that folic acid supplements are an important way of minimizing the risk of neural tube defects such as spina bifida and of facial clefts.

After the first trimester, the majority of formation has been completed and the remainder of fetal development is devoted primarily to growth and maturation. Thus the chances of malformation are markedly diminished after the first trimester. A notable exception to this is the fetal dentition, which is susceptible to dental staining caused by the administration of tetracycline during later pregnancy.

Another consideration relating to fetal growth is spontaneous abortion (miscarriage). Spontaneous abortion—the natural termination of pregnancy before the twentieth week of gestation—occurs in more than 15% of all pregnancies, the majority of which are caused by intrinsic fetal abnormalities.

It must be kept in mind that the fetus has a limited ability to metabolize drugs, because of its immature liver and immature enzyme system; therefore, any pharmacologic challenge of the fetus is to be avoided when possible.

The hormonal changes that occurs during pregnancy include an increase in the production of maternal hormones and the production of placental hormones. When operating on a gravid patient particular attention should be payed for alternations occurring in the cardiovascular, pulmonary, hematologic and gastrointestinal systems.

Cardiovascular System

Cardiovascular changes are varied. There is commonly a slight decrease in blood pressure, especially diastolic. Blood volume will increase 40 to 55% and the cardiac output increases 30%. The increased cardiac output is associated with tachycardia. These changes occur by the second trimester and then appear to remain constant. Corresponding to these volume changes are tachycardia and heart murmurs. A systolic murmur will develop in 90% of pregnant women but disappears shortly after delivery. A murmur of this type would be considered physiologic or functional. There may be dyspnea at rest that is aggravated by a supine position.

During late pregnancy, a phenomenon known as 'supine hypotension syndrome' may occur-manifested by an abrupt fall in blood pressure, bradycardia, sweating, nausea, weakness and air hunger (dyspnea) when the patient is in a supine position. Varicositis may develop (Fig. 13.7). Varicose (varix = dilated vein). This syndrome is due to impaired venous return to the heart and reduction of the cardiac output by 25 to 30%. This is due to compression of the inferior vena cava by the gravid uterus and impedes venous return to the heart and leading to decreased blood pressure, decreased cardiac output and impairment or loss of consciousness. In varicosities, the veins are dilated and tortuous. The valves in these veins have become non-functional

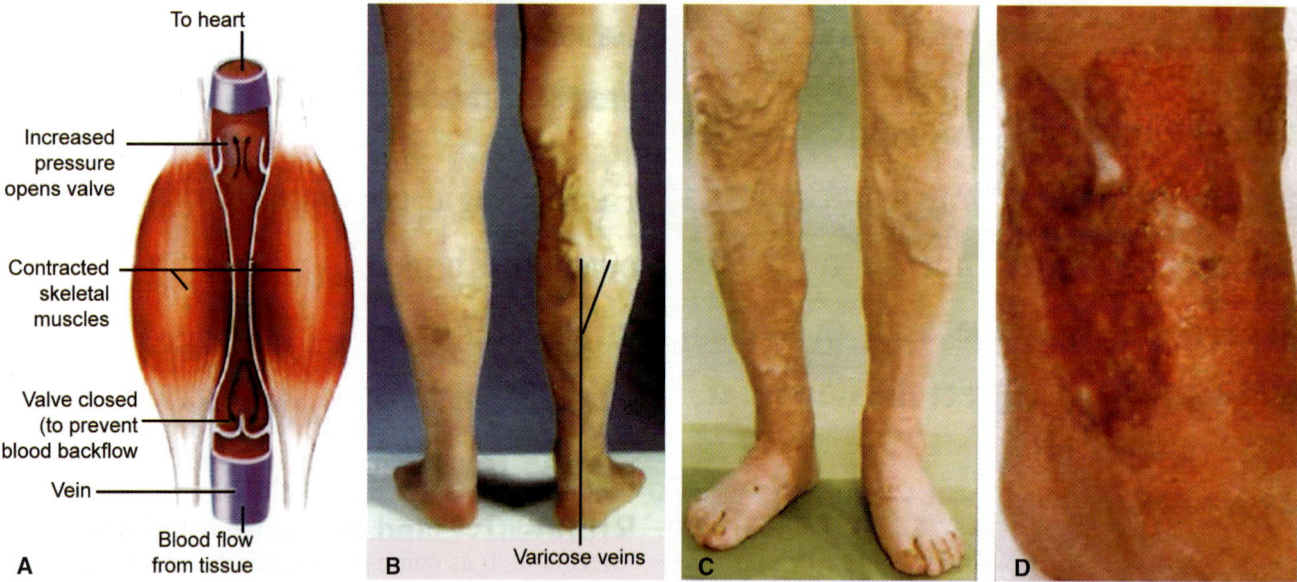

Fig. 13.7: (A) Valves in veins. Valves are one-way flaps that prevent pooling and backflow of venous blood to ensure that blood flows toward the heart, particularly in the lower limbs. **(B)** The contraction of the skeletal muscles squeezes the veins passing between muscles and forces blood toward the heart. **(C)** Varicose veins are a risk factor for deep vein thrombosis and may result from it *(Mckliney & O'Loughlin, 2006)*. **(D)** Varicose ulceration of the leg is usually a long-term complication of deep vein thrombosis. These ulcers can be extensive and indolent

causing blood to pool in one area and the vein to swell and bulge. Varicose veins are most common in the superficial vein of the lower limbs.

The fetus may also be compromised because of decrease arterial oxygenation. The remedy for the problem is to roll the patient over on to her left side, which lifts the uterus of the vena cava, with the right buttock and hip tipped upward approximately 15°, she should rapidly return to normal. *So the pregnant patient should not be placed in the supine position after the first trimester.*

Venoarterial pressure decreases early in pregnancy and usually by the second half of gestation, blood pressure continues to increase approaching normal values. Dyspnea, a prominent third heart sound, and peripheral edema.

An important complication of pregnancy is hypertension, which leads to increased morbidity and mortality in both fetus and mother. Hypertension may be asymptomatic but, when associated with edema and proteinuria (pre-eclampsia), may culminate in eclampsia (hypertension, edema, proteinuria and convulsions) which may be fatal. The fetus is at risk because of possible placental separation or damage leading to prematurity, fetal lung damage or intrauterine death. *Hypertensive pregnant patients should, therefore, rest as much as possible and have antihypertensive treatment.*

Respiratory System

One of the most important changes of the respiratory system is a 20% reduction of functional residual capacity, occurring by the fifth month of pregnancy, as a result of the diaphragm being displaced upward 3 to 5 cm (Fig. 13.8). This, together with a concomitant 15% increase in oxygen consumption, places the mother at increased risk of developing hypoxia during periods of apnea or hypoventilation. Dyspnea is also a common complaint in 60 to 70% of pregnant patients. This does not appear to be the result of mechanical or anatomical changes of pregnancy but rather of the hyperventilation associated with gestation.

Blood plasma and red cell volumes increase during nominal gestation, the former 2600 to 3650 cc and the latter from approximately 1350 cc in the nonpregnant patient to values near 1650 cc late in pregnancy. The increment in plasma volume is greater than that of the red cell mass and, therefore, a decrease in both hematocrit and hemoglobin concentration to values

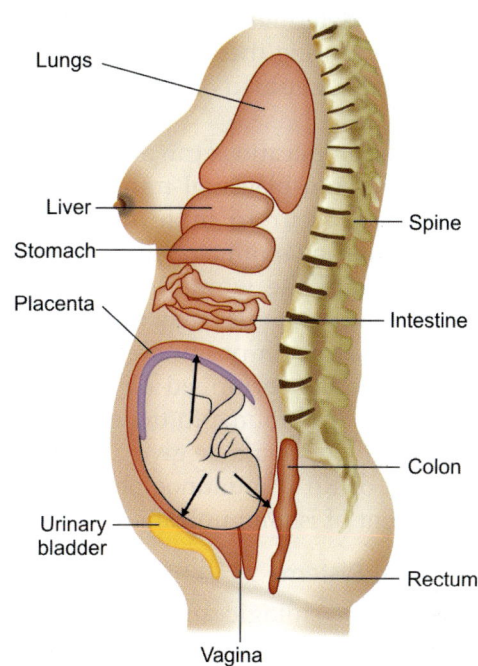

Fig. 13.8: Sagittal section of a pregnant woman demonstrating the effects of the expending uterus *(Gould, 2006)*

as low as 31 to 33% and 10.5 to 11 g/dL by the 34th gestational week may occur.

Pregnancy sometimes predisposes to an increased appetite for unusual foods. As a result, the diet may not be nutritious or balanced and may be high in sugars, which can adversely affect the dentition.

Blood changes in pregnancy include anemia and decreased hematocrit. Because of the increased blood volume, there is marked need for additional iron. There is also an increased white blood cell count due to a neutrophilia; changes in platelets are usually insignificant.

Several blood clotting factors are increased especially fibrinogen, and factors VII, VIII, IX and X and diminished fibrinolytic activity. These factors can augment the response of coagulation, making the pregnant patient hypercoagulable, not just because clotting occurs more readily, but because of reduced ability to lyse a formed clot. Hemostasis in the lower limbs and a rise in venous pressure in late pregnancy also increase the possibility of hypercoagulability and thromboembolism. This factor again emphasizes the importance of avoiding the supine position and using support stockings and pneumatic devices to improve lower extremity circulation and blood flow in the gravid patient. Low dose of heparin should also be considered to reduce the risk of venous thromboembolism. Platelet count should be determined before heparin therapy and periodically during therapy because of unusual occurrence with heparin associated thrombocytopenia.

Hematologic complications can also occur with Rh incompatibility. Transplacental transfer of fetal red blood cells can occur to maternal circulation, particularly in uterine trauma or surgery. If the fetus is Rh positive and the woman Rh negative, the production of IgG antibodies may be stimulated and adversely affect future Rh-positive fetuses. Therefore, when an operation is performed on an Rh-negative pregnant patient and trauma to the gravid uterus is likely, consideration should be given to the maternal administration of Rh D-immunoglobulin to prevent the development of isoimmunization.

Gastrointestinal System

Several of the physiologic and anatomic changes occurring during pregnancy may lead to an increase in gastric acidity and a delay in gastric emptying. Progesterone inhibits gastric and intestinal mobility and relaxes the gastroesophageal sphincter. Such alternations could likely explain the increased incidence of reflux esophagitis and heartburn in the gravid woman. The mechanical effect caused by the gravid uterus pushing the abdominal contents upward against the diaphragm may further compromise the competence of the gastroesophageal sphincter.

The temporary nausea called morning sickness may begin about the seventh week, however, some women become nauseated and vomit during early pregnancy. It may be caused by hormonal changes, especially the increased secretion of human chorionic gonadotropin, and it may also be related to the change in carbohydrate metabolism. Both factors are probably involved.

Pregnancy Gingivitis

In some pregnant women, gingivitis is aggravated (pregnancy gingivitis) or may even result in a pyogenic granuloma at the gingival margin (pregnancy epulis (Fig. 13.9). These conditions typically arise after the second month and resolve on parturition. In a few women subject to recurrent aphthae ulcers may stop (or occasionally become more severe) during pregnancy.

Treatment Considerations

1. If there is any doubt about the possibility of pregnancy, the surgery should be delayed until pregnancy is confirmed.

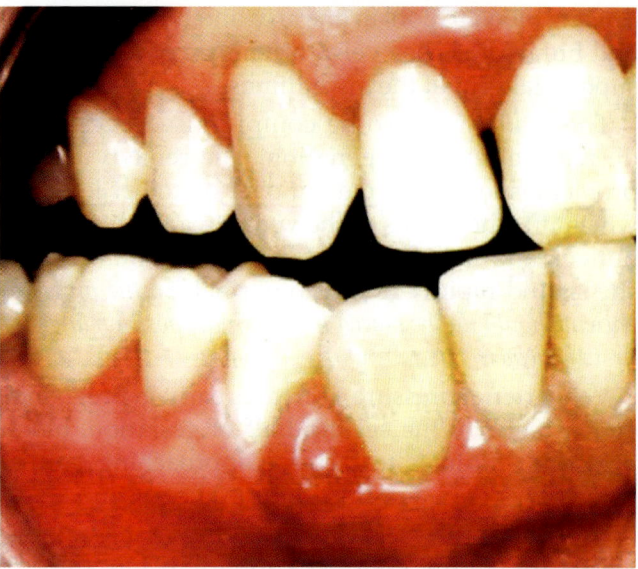

Fig. 13.9: Pyogenic granuloma —"pregnancy tumor" occurring during pregnancy.

2. Elective dental care is best avoided during the first trimester because of the potential underability of the fetus. **The second trimester is the safest period in which to provide routine dental care.**

3. Extensive reconstruction or significant surgical procedures are best postponed until after delivery; it should be borne in mind that pregnancy is a temporary condition.

4. *The early part of the third trimester is still a good time to provide routine dental care;* but after the middle of the third trimester, elective dental care is best postponed.

5. *Prolonged chair time should be avoided*, to prevent the complication of supine hypotensive syndrome (Box 13.1). If treatment becomes necessary during this period, the problems can be minimized by scheduling short appointments, allowing the patient to assume a semireclining position, or the patient is positioned in the chair about 10 to 15° on the left side and encouraging **frequent changes of position** in order to prevent the vena cava suppression syndrome.

6. It is most desirable not to have any irradiation during pregnancy, especially during the first trimester, because the developing fetus is particularly susceptible to radiation damage including developmental defects and growth retardation (Box 13.2). Of all aids, the most important for the pregnant patient is the

Box 13.1: Dental management considerations for patients who are pregnant

1. Evaluate patient; determine trimester and health status.
2. Confirm that medical prenatal care was provided, or facilitate entry into medical care.
3. Provide periodontal therapy and oral hygiene instructions.
4. Educate the patient: Discuss the importance and benefits of good plaque control and fluoride.
5. Minimize radiographic exposure.
6. Minimize drug use. Drug selection should be based on safety profile, risk to mother and fetus, potential for interactions and adverse effects.
7. Avoid prolonged appointment time in the dental chair (i.e. risk of supine hypotension).
8. The safest time for provision of dental treatment is the second trimester.

Box 13.2: Oral surgical considerations in pregnancy

Risk to mother
1. *Increased gingivitis and epulis formation*
2. *Risk of hypotension if supine*
3. *Risk of hypertension*
4. *Vomiting especially with general anesthesia*
5. *Aspirin may cause neonatal hemorrhage*

Risk to fetus
1. *Radiography hazardous*
2. *Respiratory depression with sedatives tooth staining with tetracyclines*
3. *Prilocaine rarely causes methemoglobinemia; some drugs are tetragenic*

Box 13.3: Drugs contraindicated and alternatives in pregnancy

	To be avoided	*Preferable*
Analgesics	Aspirin Mefenamic-acid NSAIDs Dextropropoxyphene Pentazocine Diamorphine	Paracetamol
Antimicrobials	Tetracyclines Fluconazole Aminoglycosides Co-trimoxazole Sulphonamides Rifampicin Metronidazole Ganciclovir	Penicillins Erythromycin Cephalosporins
Premedication	Long- acting benzodiazepines (e.g. diazepam) Opioids Atropine	Temazepam Benzodizepines (low dose)
Anesthesia	Barbiturates Prilocaine	Nitrous oxide Halothane
Others	Retinoids Antidepressants Beta-blockers Carbamazepine Corticosteroids Povidone-iodine Thalidomide Colchicine	Corticosteroids (low dose).

protective lead apron. The dentist must keep the facts of radiation biology. Animal and human data clearly support the conclusion that no increase in congenital anomalies or intrauterine growth retardation occurs as a result of exposures during pregnancy totaling less than 5 to 10 cGy, (one centgray 'cGy' is the unit of absorbed radiation equivalent to a rad (roentgen, R). For comparing purposes, the following can be considered: a medical chest radiograph results in an estimated fetal or embryonic dose of 0.008 cGy, a skull radiograph results in 0.004 cGy and a full mouth series of dental radiographs with a lead apron results in 0.00001 cGy. From these figures, it is evident that with use of lead apron, **one or two intraoral films are truly of no significance in terms of radiation effects to the developing fetus.** Studies in both animals and human indicate that no increase in gross congenital anomalies or intrauterine growth retardation occurs as a result of exposure below 5 to 10 rads. Fortunately, most diagnostic procedures result in fetal exposure less than one-tenth of this amount.

7. Drugs may be teratogenic (Box 13.3). A drug may cross the placenta and be toxic or tetragenic. Drug treatment should, therefore, be avoided where possible, especially in the first trimester (*see* table). Because of the risk of coincidental mishaps, it is wise to **avoid giving any drugs, possibly even local anesthetics** and postponing as much treatment as possible until after parturition in those with a history of abortions and those who have at last achieved pregnancy after years of failure. Many women are unaware of being pregnant in the early part of the first trimester and, therefore, it is preferable to avoid giving any

drugs to women of childbearing age, unless absolutely essential.

When drug treatment is unavoidable, penicillin, cephalosporins and erythromycin are probably safe antimicrobials, while paracetamol and codeine are probably safe analgesics (Box 13.3).

NSAIDs may cause closure of the ductus arteriosus in utero, and fetal pulmonary hypertension, as well as delaying or prolonging labour. Aspirin, in addition, causes a platelet defect. Corticosteroids can suppress the fetal adrenals and if given, a steroid cover is needed for labor. It is best to avoid metronidazole, or use a low dose, and to avoid azole antifungals, opioids and povidone-iodine. Tetracyclines may cause tooth discoloration. General anesthesia and possibly sedation with diazepam or midazolam are particular hazards and must be avoided in the first trimester and in the last month of pregnancy. Another *hazard* is an increased tendency to vomiting during induction in the third trimester.

During pregnancy, the application of local anesthetics is not without problems, since permeability of the placenta to the preparation must be considered. In principle, only local anesthetics not bound to proteins can enter the fetal circulation. **Therefore, compounds with high protein binding are more advantageous.** The ratio of the local anesthetic in the umbilical cord to that of the maternal blood is a good estimate of the permeability of the placenta to that compound. **All local anesthetics cross the placenta to some degree.** Highest concentrations in the fetal circulation follow injection of prilocaine and the lowest follow bupivacaine, with lignocaine in between. **Bupivacaine, however, is the most cardiotoxic of local anesthetics and is contraindicated in pregnancy.** In selection of the vasoconstrictor, it should be noted that systemically resorbed epinephrine can lead to constriction of the uterine vessels. Felypressin which is a derivative of vasopressin and related to oxytocin, has the potential to cause uterine contractions, although this would be extremely unlikely at the low concentration in local anesthetic; however, it is best avoided during pregnancy.

The local anesthetic of choice during pregnancy is lignocaine with adrenaline. Lidocaine as a local anesthetic agent appears to be safe in pregnant patient, with few reported findings of anomalies.

8. Many women are convinced that pregnancy causes tooth loss (a tooth for every pregnancy) or that calcium is withdrawn from the maternal dentition to supply fetal requirements (soft teeth). Calcium is present in the teeth in a stable crystalline form and as such, is not available to the systemic circulation to supply a calcium demand. However, calcium is readily mobilized from bone to supply these demands. Therefore, although calcium supplementation for the purpose of preventing tooth loss or soft teeth is unwarranted, the physician may prescribe calcium for general nutritional requirements of mother and infant.

9. A final dental finding is tooth mobility, which may be generalized. This sign is probably related to the degree of gingival disease and disturbance of the attachment apparatus as well as to some mineral changes in the lamina dura. The condition is reversible after delivery.

10. Abscesses should be drained immediately, and infected teeth should be extracted as quickly as possible or treated through more conservative measures. The use of appropriate and safe antibiotics based on culture and sensitivity principles aid in the treatment of these patients. Impacted teeth that are symptomatic can be removed in the pregnant use of conservative measures such as local irrigations.

BREASTFEEDING

The suckling of the child stimulates the many touch receptors around the mother's nipple, and afferent neurons carry an impulse to the hypothalamus. Neurosecretory cells in the hypothalamus cause the posterior pituitary gland to release oxytocin into the blood (Fig. 13.10). The oxytocin stimulates the release of milk from the breast.

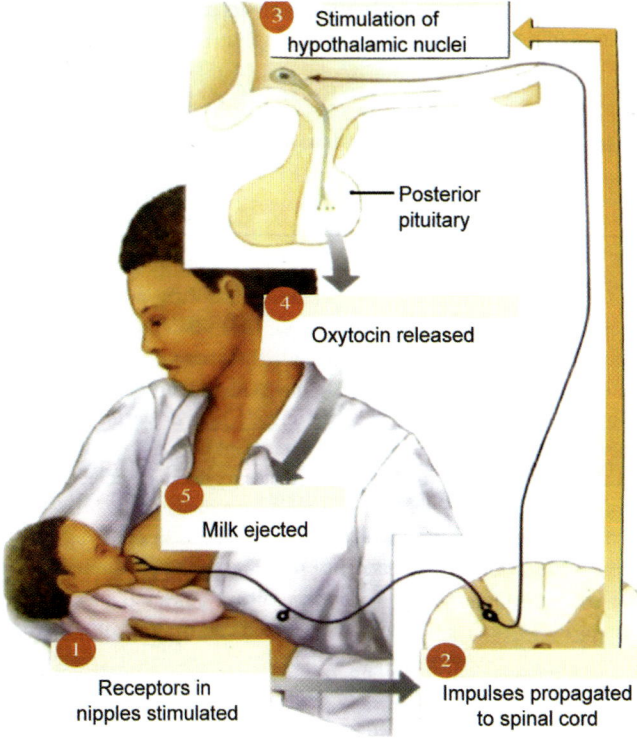

Fig. 13.10: The milk let-down reflex *(Martini et al, 2008)*

OXYTOCIN (OT)

(oxy =sharp, quick ; toc = childbirth)

During labor, oxytocin triggers a positive feedback cycle. Uterine stretching sends a nerve signal to the brain that stimulates oxytocin (OT) release. OT stimulates uterine contractions, which push the infant downward. This stretches lower end of the uterus some more, which results in a nerve signal that stimulates still more OT release. This positive feedback cycle continues until the infant is born.

Oxytocin is a hormone released by the posterior lobe of the pituitary gland has various reproductive roles. In childbirth, it stimulates smooth muscle of the uterus to contract, thus contributing to the labor contractions that expel the infant. In lactating mothers, it stimulates muscle-like cells of the mammary glands to squeeze on the glandular acini and force milk *to flow down the ducts to the nipple,* contractions that expel the infant. The infant does not receive any milk for about a minute after it starts suckling, but once oxytocin is secreted, the contraction of the myoepithelial cells that surround the ducts of the breast, begins and milk flows from the nipple. Although oxytocin stimulates milk ejection, the actual production of milk is stimulated by prolactin, a pituitary hormone. In both sexes, OT secretion surges during sexual arousal and orgasm. It may play a role in the propulsion of semen through the male reproductive tract, in uterine contractions that help transport sperm up the female reproductive tract, and in feelings of sexual satisfaction and emotional bonding.

Pregnant women are at risk of transmitting HIV to their newborns, with approximately 25% of exposed infants becoming infected unless intervention occurs. The exact timing of HIV transmission from mother to infant is unknown. The best estimate is that in developed countries approximately one-third of the infections occur in utero whereas two-thirds occur intrapartum. Risk factors for increased mother to infant transmission include women with low CD4+ lymphocyte counts, high HIV RNA loads, the presence of active sexually transmitted disease, rupture of amniotic membranes beyond 4 hours and prematurity of birth. Of all risk factors, plasma HIV RNA load is most important in determining the risk for mother to infant transmission.

Women can also transmit HIV through their breast milk, and such transmission accounts for one-third of all infant infections in developing countries, where a majority of HIV-infected women breastfeed their infants. In developing countries, the benefits of exclusive breastfeeding are believed by some experts to outweigh the risk of transmission of HIV through milk (estimated to be 5% within the first 6 months to 24 months). The claim by some investigators that exclusive breastfeeding decreases the risk of transmission from an infected mother to her infant is yet to be supported through a prospective clinical trial. Therefore, most experts believe that substitute feeding should be used whenever possible to prevent mother-to-infant transmission of HIV. HIV-infected women in developed countries should be strongly discouraged from breastfeeding their newborns.

Prolactin

Prolactin (lactogenic hormone) has two functions: (1) Together with the female sex hormone estrogen, it stimulates the development of the duct system in the mammary glands during pregnancy. (2) It stimulates milk production from the mammary tissue after childbirth. (Re-call that oxytocin stimulates milk ejection from the mammary glands during breastfeeding, but not milk production) (Fig. 13.10).

Because a woman is not pregnant most of the time, the secretion of prolactin is usually inhibited. Inhibition is accomplished by the secretion of prolactin-inhibiting hormone (PIH) "which is dopamine" by the hypothalamus. The inhibition of prolactin secretion diminishes during pregnancy and by the time the baby is born and the placenta is expelled from the uterus, most of the inhibitory effects are involved. In addition, the process of nursing a baby apparently causes the hypothalamus to secrete a prolactin-releasing hormone (PRH) which stimulates the secretion of prolactin.

Pregnancy and lactation put women at risk of hypocalcemia because of the calcium demanded by ossification of the fetal skeleton and synthesis of milk. The leading cause of hypocalcemic tetany is accidental removal of the parathyroid glands during thyroid surgery. Without hormone replacement therapy, the lack of parathyroid glands can lead to fatal tetany within 4 days.

Human milk is a suspension of fat and protein in a carbohydrate–mineral solution. The major proteins are casein and lactalbumin. Drug excretion into milk may be accomplished by binding to the proteins or on to the surface of the milk fat globule. Other methods of transport include lipid binding and solubility in the fat globule. If a mother needs medication, she should consider not nursing for a period of time. Also, scheduling doses just after a nursing period may have less of an effect on the child.

A drug administered to a nursing mother will find its way into the breast milk and be transferred to the nursing infant (Box 13.4). It is thought that placental transfer of maternal substances to the fetus is established at about the fifth week of fetal life.

Box 13.4: Drugs contraindicated and alternatives in lactating mothers

	Contraindicated	May be used instead
Analgesics	Aspirin (high dose) Dextropropoxyphene Diflunisal	Aspirin (low dose) Codeine Diclofenac Mefenamic acid Paracetamol
Antimicrobials	Tetracylines, Co-trimoxazole Metronidazole Sulphonamides Aminoglycosides Fluconazole Ganciclovir	Penicillins Erthromycin Rifampicin Rifampicin Cephalosporins
Premedication	Atropine Chloral hydrate	Benzodiazepines (low dose) Phenothiazines (low dose)
Others	Beta-blockers Antidepressants, Barbiturates Etretinate Carbamazepine Povidone-iodine Corticosteroids (high dose)	Corticosteroids (low dose)

- *A significant fact is that the amount of drug excreted in the breast milk is usually not more than 1 to 2% of the maternal dose; therefore, it is highly unlikely that most drugs are of any pharmacologic significance to the infant.*
- *Cephalexin is a useful antimicrobial as it is not excreted in the milk.*

THE MENOPAUSE
(CEASING THE MONTHLY)
(GR. MENESIS, MONTH + PAUSING, CESSATION)

Women between 45 and 55 years usually stop producing and releasing ova and the monthly menstrual cycle stops. The cessation of menstrual periods is called the menopause and it signals the end of reproductive ability. The average age for menopause is currently 52 and is increasing, probably because of nutrition. Menopause is not an abrupt change, it usually takes about 2 years of irregular menstrual periods before menstruation and ova production stop permanently.

The menopause, or climacteric, is a normal physiological phase in a woman's life and is primarily associated with regressive changes in the ovaries. The majority of women pass through it with a minimum

discomfort, but a small proportion complain of frequent hot flushes, intense headache, vertigo, insomnia, palpitation and depression, and may have a most distressing time.

The degree of discomfort experienced, apart from any menstrual disturbance, depends in large measure on the woman's temperament and outlook. Some women, especially those with large families who are haunted by the fear and anxiety of further child-bearing or those who suffer from intense menstrual discomfort, welcome the relief which the menopause brings. Generally such women have little trouble or discomfort. Others, however, who have longed for marriage of motherhood realize the significance of the advantaging years and view the climacteric with considerable fear and apprehension. Again, women of an interospective disposition dread the possibility of an increase in weight, the loss of attractiveness or a decline in sexual responsiveness.

The terms *'change of life'* and 'critical age' which have been, and unfortunately still are, employed to describe this phase, suggests to them something mysterious and foreboding. Such women may experience considerable distress and discomfort.

The importance of a well-regulated diet, adequate exercise, attention to personal appearance and the acquisition of new interests should be emphasized, as many women at the climacteric tend to relax, overeat, lose some muscle tone, may develop a few hairs on the chin or upper lip, and lose interest in their appearance. Hot flushes, when the patient feels a wave of heat passing over the body, are, however, common. Flushes may be momentary or last several minutes and their frequency is very variable. The decrease of estrogen that accompanies menopause is thought to be the cause of hot flashes of the skin, which results from changes in the vasomotor system that dilate blood vessels and increase blood flow.

Psychological disorders are not uncommon in the menopause. They are usually mild and include dizziness and insomnia, but depression or paranoia may develop. They should be advised that sexual desire does not diminish when menstruation ceases, but sometimes increases and may continue for many years. Severe menopausal symptoms, such as frequent hot flushes, intense headache, vertigo, dyspnea, and emotional instability mimic those of any systemic disease. As organic lesions related to the heart, blood vessels, kidneys, and pelvic organs are prone to become manifest during this phase of life, it is important that organic disease should be excluded before assuming that the symptoms are climacteric in origin.

Atypical facial pain and oral dysesthesias are most common but there is little evidence of benefit from steroid sex hormones. Dryness of mouth and so-called desquamative gingivitis are not hormonal in origin. Sjogren's syndrome, lichen planus and mucous membrane pemphigoid are all common in the middleaged or older and particularly in females.

Prompt control of symptoms by the administration of adequate amounts of estrogen has a beneficial psychological effect and as a rule changes the patient's whole outlook. Replacement of reduced estrogen secretion after menopause orally or implanted slows the development of osteoporosis and reduces the risk of osteoporotic fractures, as well as reducing overall mortality.

Although males usually experience a gradual decrease in testosterone secretion after they reach 40 or 50, they do not experience as drastic hormonal changes as women do at that age. The most likely cause of psychological problems during this period is not hormonal, but rather the fear of impotency and old age. Despite the decrease in testosterone, normal males may retain sexual potency in old age.

OSTEOPOROSIS

The World Health Organization (WHO) has defined osteoporosis based on bone density:

1. Normal bone is greater than 833 mg/cm^2.
2. Osteopenia, or decreased bone mass, is 833 to 648 mg/cm^2.
3. Osteoporosis is less than 648 mg/cm^2.

In osteoporosis, the following points should be considered:

- *It is very common, especially in women.*
- *Osteoporosis means thin bone that may break more easily.*
- *It is not painful except when a bone is broken or a vertebra is compressed.*
- *Often there is no particular cause.*
- *We can stop bones getting thinner with treatment.*
- *Following the treatment regularly will stop this from happening.*

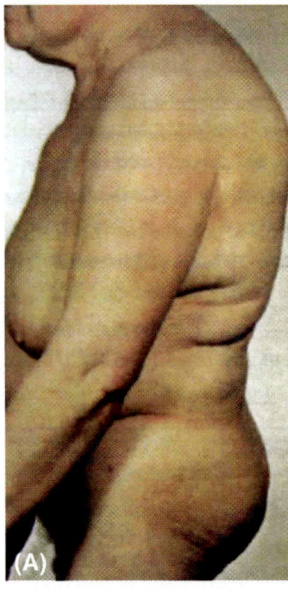 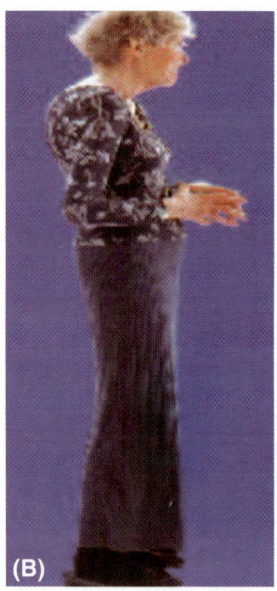

Fig. 13.11: (A) Osteoporosis results in loss of height and vertebral collapse is associated with chronic backache, bouts of severe backpain and kyphosis (Downger's hump). Creases often appear in the skin, and the ribs may rub on the iliac crest. **(B)** Woman with osteoporosis. Note the abnormal curvature (kyphosis) of the upper thoracic spine. This results from compression fractures of the weakened vertebrae. There is loss of weight and sudden pain on weightlifting *(Saladin 2003)*. *(Forbes and Jackson, 2003)*

Osteoporosis is defined as a disease characterized by low bone mass and microarchitectural deterioration of bone tissue, leading to enhanced bone fragility and an increased fracture risk. The disease can be: (1) generalized, involving major portions of the axial skeleton, or (2) regional, involving one segment of the appendicular skeleton.

Throughout a lifetime, old bone is removed (resorption) and new bone is added (formation) to the skeleton. During childhood and teenage years, new bone is added faster than old bone is removed. Consequently bones become larger, heavier and

denser. Bone formation continues at a pace faster than resorption until peak bone mass, or maximum bone density and strength, is reached, around age 30, after which bone resorption slowly exceeds bone formation. Bone mass, therefore, depends on peak mass attained and on the rate of loss later in life (Fig. 13.12).

Skeletal homeostasis depends on a very narrow range of plasma calcium and phosphate concentrations, which are maintained by the endocrine system. Therefore, endocrine dysfunction ultimately can cause metabolic bone disease. In addition to declining levels of sex steroids, the hormones most commonly associated with osteoporosis are parathyroid hormone, cortisol, thyroid hormone and growth hormone. Excessive intake of caffeine, alcohol and nicotine along with low body fat have been considered risk factors.

ETIOLOGY (BOX 13.5)

Osteoporosis is a complex, multifactorial chronic disease often progresses silently for decades until fracture occur. It is the most common disease that affects bone. It is not necessarily a consequence of the aging process because some older adults retains strong, relatively dense bones. In osteoporosis, the old bone is being reabsorbed faster than new bone is being made, causing the bones to lose density, becoming thinner and more porous. A progressive loss of bone mass may continue until the skeleton is no longer strong enough to support life. As bone becomes more fragile, falls, or bumps that would not have caused fracture previously at that point do cause a fracture. Poor nutrition and significant intake or malabsorption of dietary minerals, particularly calcium are factors in the development of osteoporosis. Calcium absorption from the intestine decreases with age. Deficiencies of vitamins, particularly vitamin C and D, also contribute to bone loss.

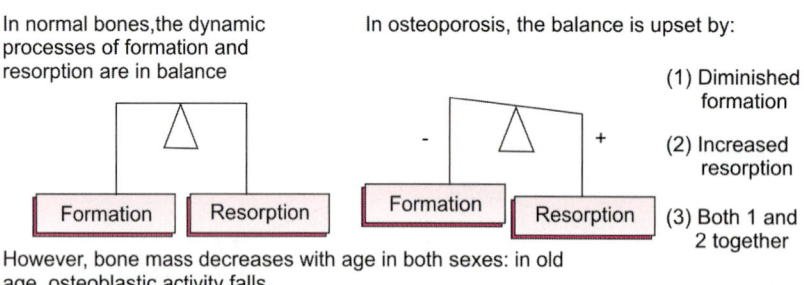

Fig. 13.12: In osteoporosis, the balance of bone formation and bone resorption is unequilibrated

Postmenopausal Osteoporosis

Sex hormones are important in maintain normal rates of bone deposition.

In women, bone loss is most rapid in the first years after menopause but persists throughout the postmenopausal years. Bone loss in women begins before menopause. Postmenopausal osteoporosis which occurs in middle-aged and older women is probably caused by changes in insulin-like growth factor (IGF), a combination of inadequate dietary calcium intake and lack of vitamin D, possibly decreased magnesium, lack of exercise, decreased levels of estrogen, and family history. IGF is known to help in fracture healing and collagen synthesis and improves conditions for bone mineralization. IGF levels significantly decline by age 60. Excessive phosphorus intake, chiefly through the intake of sodas and junk foods interferes with calcium-phosphorus balance, resulting in an increased risk of brittle bones. The highest incidence of osteoporosis is among elderly white women, where it is closely linked to age and menopause. Osteoporosis also affects men (white males somewhat more than black), although less severely than it does women. It rarely affects black women. In women, the changes are more pronounced and develop more rapidly, over the course of menopause (Fig. 13.13). The ovarian follicles are used up, gametogenesis ceases, and the ovaries stop producing sex steroids. This may result in vaginal dryness, genital atrophy, and reduced libido and make sex less enjoyable. With the loss of ovarian steroids, a postmenopausal woman has an elevated risk of osteoporosis and atherosclerosis. Ironically, osteoporosis also occurs among young female runners and dancers in spite of their vigorous exercise.

Their percentage of body fat is so low that they stop ovulating and the ovaries secrete unusually low levels of estrogen. When estrogen levels drop after menopause, it appears that circulating androgens become significant effectors on bone metabolism. In clinical studies of women, data have suggested that serum androgens influence bone density in pre-, peri- and postmenopausal women (Brown, 2008; Fogele et al, 2007). Androgens (i.e. testosterone and dihydro-testosterone) have long been recognized to stimulate bone formation. Increasing age in men and women is associated with declining levels of estrogen.

Secondary Osteoporosis

Secondary osteoporosis sometimes develops temporarily in individuals receiving large doses of heparin, perhaps because heparin promotes bone resorption by decreasing collagen synthesis or by increasing collagen breakdown. Osteoporosis caused by heparin therapy usually resolves when therapy ceases. Treatment with other medications may lead to development of osteoporosis, such as the use of glucocorticoid treatment for rheumatoid arthritis. Other medications increasing risk of osteoporosis include lithium, methotrexate, anticonvulsants, cyclophosphamide, and cyclosporine.

One form, transient osteoporosis of the hip, is associated with the third trimester of pregnancy or the immediate postpartum period. However, most transient osteoporosis is a typically self-limiting syndrome affecting the lower extremity joints of middle-aged men. The etiology is unknown and although most cases spontaneously resolve, some occurrences of bone demineralization may be related to osteonecrosis.

Localized osteoporosis is commonly due to disuse and is seen as a complication of other disorders, e.g. local immobilization following fracture, limb paralysis, and adjacent to severe joint disease with limitation of movement. This process can be acute with osteoclasis, but when function is resumed, normal bone structure is often restored.

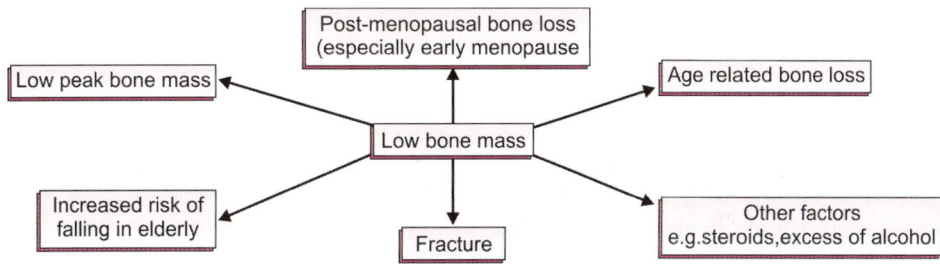

Fig. 13.13: Sex hormones, especially estrogen and testosterone, are significant in premenopausal bone maintenance

The most probable causes and risk factors of osteoporosis are categorized in Box 13.5.

Box 13.5: Causes and risk factors for osteoporosis

Physiological	Pathological
1. Ageing	1. Corticosteroid drugs, Cushing's syndrome.
2. Female sex	2. Low dietary calcium and vitamin D.
3. Early menopause	3. Rare causes
4. Immobility	a. Multiple myeloma.
5. Sedentary occupation	b. Diabetes mellitus.
6. Underweight	c. Hypogonadism.
7. Childhood maturation failure.	d. Thyrotoxicosis.
	e. Alcohol consumption.
	f. Smoking.
	g. High caffeine intake.
	h. Thyroid.
	i. Heparin.
	j. Cyclosporine.
	k. Methotrexate.
	l. Dilantin.
	m. Hyperparathyroidism.
	n. Rheumatoid arthritis.
	O. Renal insufficiency, hypocalciuria.

Signs and Symptoms

Osteoporosis literally means *"porous bones"*. It is characterized by:

1. Low bone mass.
2. Loss of both organic matrix and minerals,
3. Microarchitectural deterioration of bone, with
4. An increase in bone fragility, brittelness (Figs 13.14 and 13.15) and susceptibility to fracture. It affects spongy bone in particular, since this is the most metabolically active type.

Fractures are the most serious consequence of osteoporosis. They occur especially in the hip, wrist, humerus (Fig. 13.16), femur (Fig. 13.17), metacarpal bones (Fig. 13.18), vertebral column, abnormal curvature (kyphosis) of the upper thoracic spine (Figs 13.19 to 13.22) and mandible (Fig. 13.23). Fracture of osteoporotic bone may develop under stresses as slight as sitting down too quickly or after chewing hard food.

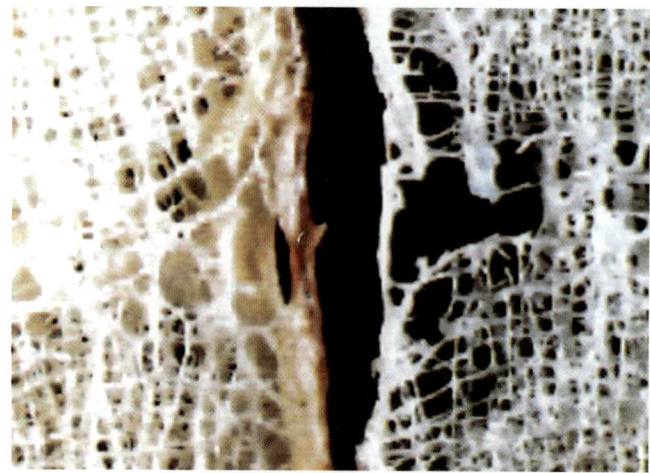

Fig. 13.14: Osteoporosis. The *left* side of the photo is a section through a healthy lumbar vertebra. The *right* side shows a lumbar vertebra in which much of the spongy bone has been lost to osteoporosis. *(Saladin: 2003)*

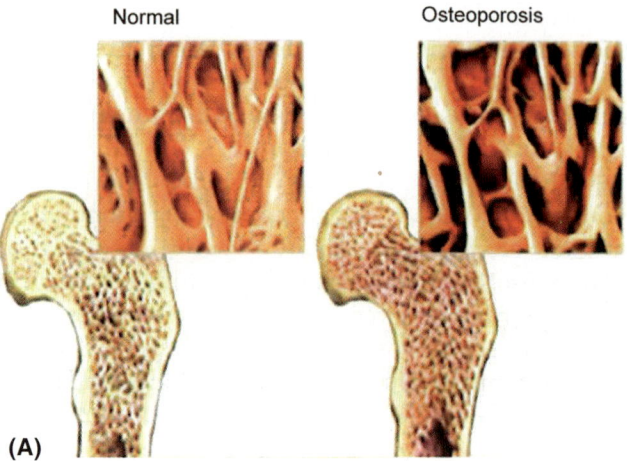

Normal   Osteoporosis

(A)

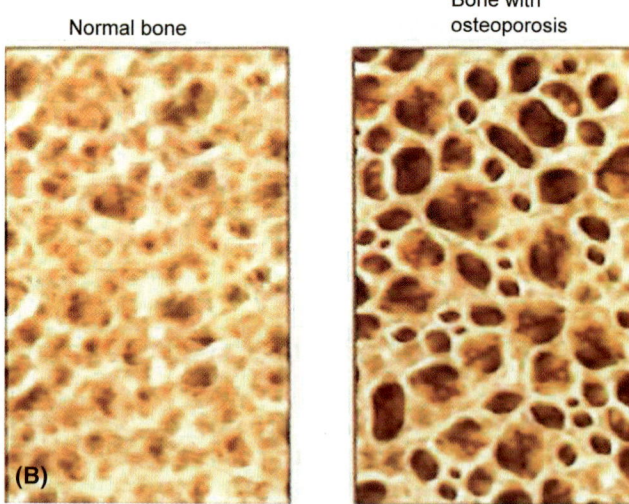

Normal bone   Bone with osteoporosis

(B)

Fig. 13.15: (A) Normal and osteoporotic femur bone. **(B)** Microscopic view

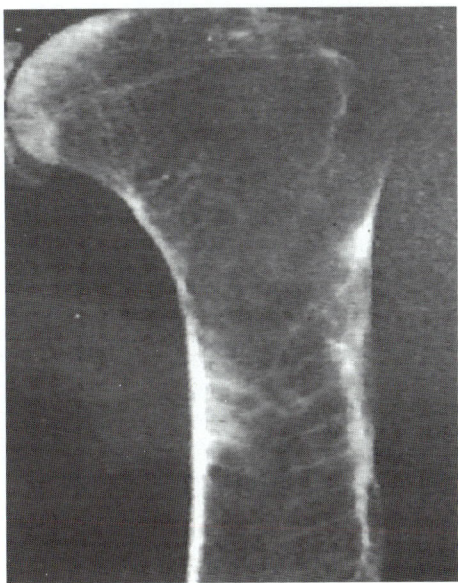

Fig. 13.16: Osteoporosis has caused a loss of cortical thickness and an opening up of the trabecular pattern in this radiograph of the humerus *(Forbes and Jackson, 2003)*

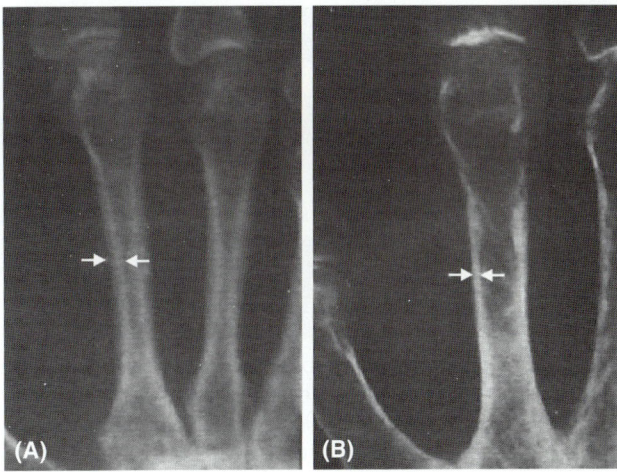

Fig. 13.18: (A) Normal metacarpal bone. **(B)** Osteoporotic metacarpal bone. *(From Helms CA: Fundamentals of Skeletal Radiology, 3rd ed. Philadelphia, WB Saunders, 2005)*

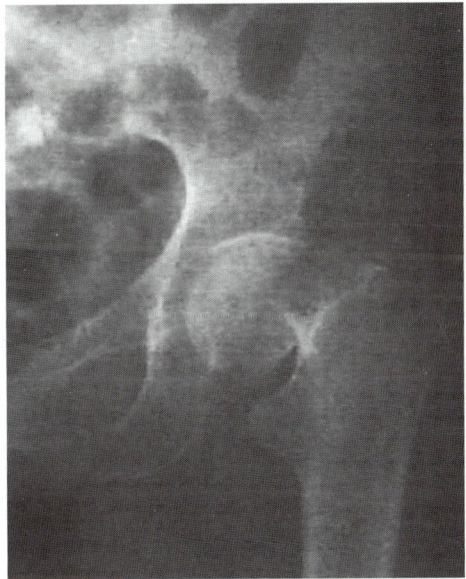

Fig. 13.17: Osteoporosis is the usual underlying disorder in fracture of the neck of the femur in the elderly. This patient has a subcapital fracture which may lead to osteonecrosis of the femoral head

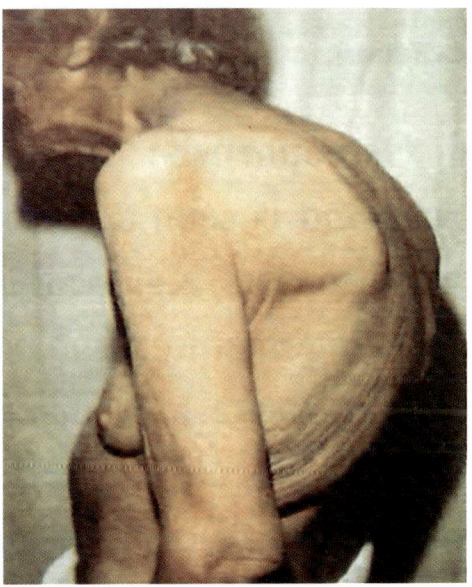

Fig. 13.19: Kyphosis. This older adult woman's condition was caused by a combination of spinal osteoporotic vertebral collapse and chronic degenerative changes in the vertebral column *(Kamal A, Brocklehurst JC: Color Atlas of Geriatric Medicine, 2nd ed., St Louis, 1992, Mosby)*

- *Early menopause:* Cessation of ovarian function at 45 years old.
- Previous osteoporotic fracture.

Diagnosis

Diagnosis of osteoporosis is from history, bone densitometry and biochemistry.

Generally, osteoporosis is detected radiographically as increased radiolucency of bone. By the time

The cases shown in the coming figures are of patients who are either be currently on treatment, or have it documented that they have been offered it:

- *Corticosteroid users:* Prednisolone 7.5 mg, if likely to be on this for 3 months and 50 years old (or 15 mg, if 50 years old).

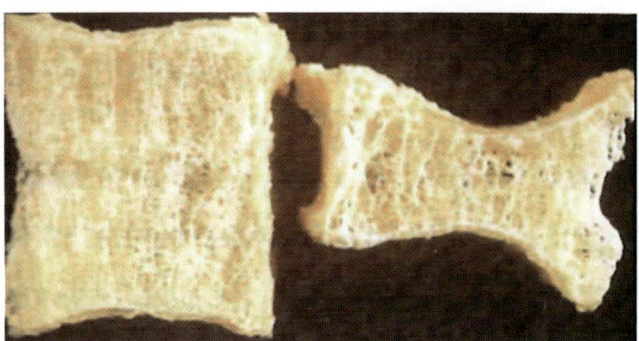

Fig. 13.20: Osteoporotic vertebral body (right) shortened by compression fractures, compared with normal vertebral body (left), *(From Kumar V, Abbas AK, Fausto M: Robbins and Cotran: Pathologic Basis of Disease, 7th ed. Philadelphia, WB Saunders, 2005)*

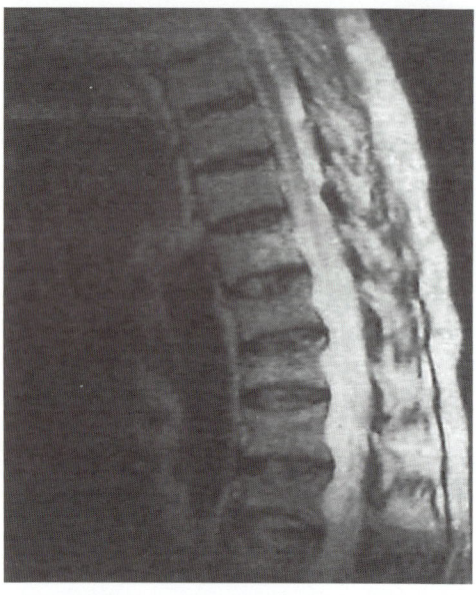

Fig. 13.22: Vertebral thining and collapse in osteoporosis demonstrated by MRI. The wedging and collapse is similar to that seen in Fig. 13.13. The patient experienced repeated episodes of severe back pain, radiating anteriorly on occasions as a result of nerve root compression *(Forbes and Jackson, 2003)*

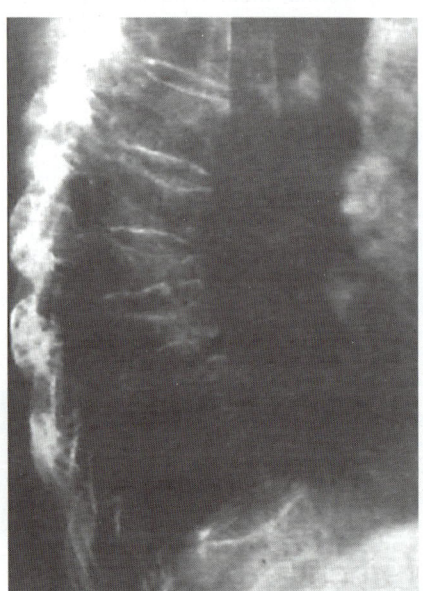

Fig. 13.21: Osteoporosis leads to vertebral collapse. This radiograph shows wedge-shaped flattening of the vertebral bodies in the midthoracic region *(Forbes and Jackson, 2003)*

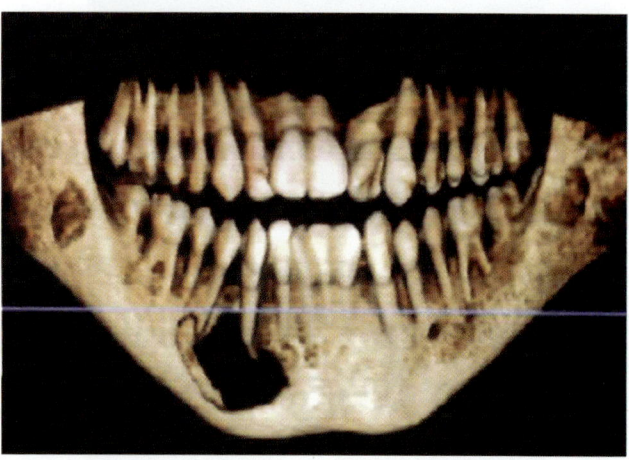

Fig. 13.23: The mandible, as the other bones, is involved in the osteoporotic process. The figure shows osteoporotic mandible of 22-year-old girl who was subjected to renal dialysis since 10 years

abnormalities are detected by X-ray examination, as much as 25 to 30% of bone tissue may have been lost. At present, DXA is the current examination of choice for diagnosis. Unfortunately, DXA does not provide information about bone strength or fracture risk. Type of radiologic examination includes single- or dual photon absorptiometry (SXA, DXA) and computed tomography (CT) scans. Because osteoporosis is asymptomatic unless fracture occurs, diagnosis is often delayed.

Densitometry is a radiographic technique that gives accurate and precise measurements of the amount of bone (not the quality), termed "bone mineral density

"(BDM). World Health Organization reported the osteoporosis is considered when the bone density is less than 648 mg/cm^2.

Poor bone mineral density and raised serum alkaline phosphatase are risk markers. The routine serum tests, particularly the calcium levels, are within the normal range. There is often no biochemical abnormalities but there may be raised alkaline phosphate levels and urinary loss of calcium and hydroxyproline. In women who lose bone particularly fast, urinary tests can be informative. Bone biopsy is neither practical nor necessary.

The diseases which are associated with osteoporosis are shown in Box 13.6.

Box. 13.6: Diseases associated with osteoporosis

Multiple myeloma	Chronic renal failure
Thyrotoxicosis	Hypogonadism
Gushing's syndrome	Hypopituitarism
Osteogenesis imperfecta	Post-gastrectomy

Treatment

The goals of treatment are to slow down the rate of calcium and bone loss and to stop the disease before it progresses too far. As is so often true, an ounce of prevention is worth a pound of cure. The time to minimize the risk for osteoporosis is between the ages of 25 and 40, when the skeleton is building to its maximum mass. The more bone mass a person has going into middle age, the less he or she will be affected by osteoporosis later. Treatments for osteoporosis are aimed at slowing the net rate of bone resorption. These include estrogen replacement, drugs to enhance estrogen sensitivity, and drugs that inhibit osteoclasts.

The Hormone Replacement Therapy (HRT)

It is effective in postmenopausal women and may also help to relieve other symptoms such as flushing, but oestrogen can cause vaginal bleeding and there is a slightly greater risk of breast cancer. HRT needs to be used lifelong for sustained benefit in bone. Estrogen replacement during menopause protects bone mass and lessens the risk of osteoporotic fractures.

Therapies to stimulate bone deposition, such as calcitonin nasal spray and small intermittent doses of parathyroid hormone, are still under investigation. Calcitonin—a hormone naturally produced in the thyroid and a powerful inhibitor of osteoclastic activity, produces modest improvements in bone mass. Combination therapy of calcium with vitamin D is necessary in the elderly, particularly those in residential care.

Controversial is the role of *calcium intake* to prevent and treat osteoporosis. It is well accepted that oral calcium intake sufficient to maintain normal calcium balance is necessary during adolescence to ensure development of peak bone mass and that calcium-deficient diets can aggravate bone loss associated with menopause and aging. Although recommendations have been established for young women of 1000 mg of calcium daily and for postmenopausal women of 1500 mg daily (with vitamin D) if receiving sex hormone replacement therapy, it has been difficult to translate these recommendations into clear-cut clinical outcomes.

Milk and other calcium sources and moderate exercise can also slow the progress of osteoporosis, but only slightly. The main sources of calcium are dairy products and green vegetables. Additional vitamin D is helpful. The main sources of vitamin D are sun exposure, margarine, breakfast cereals, oily fish, eggs and meat. Ample exercise and calcium intake (850–1,000 mg/day) are the best preventive measures.

Magnesium (Mg^{++}), another mineral important for skeletal development, is an essential mineral in many biochemical and physiologic functions, including activation of enzymes, involvement in adenosine triphosphate (ATP) synthesis, protein synthesis, regulation of membrane channels, and muscle contraction. New evidence suggests that large fluxes of magnesium can cross the cell plasma membrane in either direction following a variety of stimuli, resulting in a modification of activity for several cellular enzymes. Mg^{++} is important to bone quality because it controls hydroxyapatite crystal growth and thereby prevents formation of brittle bones. It seems reasonable that Mg^{++} is required for normal calcium (Ca^{++}) absorption because magnesium deficiency results in hypocalcemia.

Weight-bearing exercise. Regular, moderate weight bearing exercise can slow down the bone loss and in some cases, reverse demineralization because the mechanical stress of exercise stimulates bone formation. Weight bearing exercises such as walking, running, jogging, and dancing are recommended. Vitamin D and Mg^{++} also may be recommended. The best management of osteoporosis is to avoid falls and injuries and to consider use of hip protectors.

Biphosphonates, such as alendronate and risedornate, are adsorbed on to hydroxyapatite and can prevent or significantly slow the normal osteoclastic activity responsible for the resorption of bone and can lead to a 50% reduction in fractures compared with women taking calcium alone.

Suggested Dental Guidelines

Osteoporosis is a systemic skeletal disease characterized by low bone mass and microarchitectural deterioration of bone tissue with a consequent increase in bone fragility and susceptibility to fracture. Osteoporosis may lead to edentulism and markedly desorbed residual alveolar ridges that are unsuitable for construction of conventional dentures and are inadequate sites for dental implants. Besides it may lead to mandibular fracture during extraction procedures.

Concerning the dental aspects, patients with osteoporosis may have any of the problems of the elderly. They may be at risk during general anesthesia. If there has been vertebral collapse and chest deformities. There seems to be no correlation between osteoporosis and excessive alveolar bone loss in the elderly. Jaw osteoporosis is particularly a problem in women. Systemic treatment of osteoporosis may improve jaw bone density.

1. Temporary stop the biphosphonate therapy, as alendronate may induce oral ulceration and osteomyelitis.
2. Avoid any further dentoalveolar trauma.
3. Use oral antibiotic plus rinses and allow time for healing. Systemic and topical antibiotic therapy with oral penicillin or amoxicillin is suggested along with the use of 0.12% chlorhexidine gluconate oral rinses. This regimen is quite effective in controlling the pain associated with biphosphonate-related osteonecrosis (BRONJ). It is important to remember that there is no resolution of the lesion with this regimen.
4. Dental gingival flap placement may help stimulate healing.
5. Hyperbaric oxygen may need to be used in some cases to counteract osteonecrosis.

Osteopenia

The difference between the normal osteopenia of aging and the clinical condition of osteoporosis is a matter of degree.

Bones become thinner and relatively weaker as a normal part of the aging process. Inadequate ossification is called osteopenia, and all of us become slightly osteopenic as we age. The reduction in bone mass begins between the ages of 30 and 40, as osteoblast activity begins to decline while osteoclast activity continues at normal levels. Once the reduction begins, women lose roughly 8% of their skeletal mass every decade, whereas men's skeletons deteriorate at about 3% per decade. Not all parts of the skeleton are equally affected. Epiphysis, vertebrae and the jaws lose more than their fair share, which results in fragile limbs, a reduction in height, and loss of teeth.

DEPRESSION

Depression is a condition where a patient feels sad, hopeless, and/or disinterested in life in general. Depression is an illness that affects the way a person thinks, feels, behaves, and functions.

Depression should be suspected in patients who show depressed mood or loss of interest in everyday activities and four or more of the following symptoms for a period of 2 weeks or more. Feeling of worthlessness and guilt, impaired concentration, loss of energy and fatigue, thoughts of suicide, change in apatite and weight, insomnia, agitation, or retardation (Fig. 13.24).

ADDICTIVE DRUGS AND MOOD DISORDERS

Some individuals are unable to experience pleasure without the drug. Addictive drugs such as amphe-

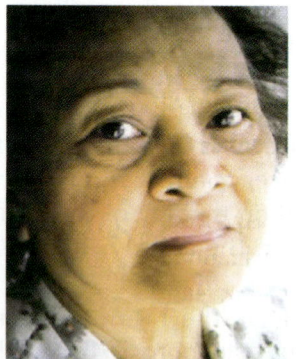

Fig. 13.24: Depressed lady with a feeling of worthlessness and guilt.

tamines and cocaine achieve elevation of the normal mood.

Amphetamines ("speed") chemically resemble norepinephrine and dopamine, two neurotransmitters associated with elevated mood.

- Dopamine is especially important in sensations of pleasure.
- Cocaine blocks dopamine reuptake and thus produces a brief rush of good feelings.

But when dopamine is not reabsorbed by the neurons, it diffuses out of the synaptic cleft and is degraded elsewhere. Cocaine thus depletes the neurons of dopamine faster than they can synthesize it, so that finally there is no longer an adequate supply to maintain normal mood.

The postsynaptic neurons make new dopamine as if "searching" for the neurotransmitter—all of which leads ultimately to anxiety, depression, and the inability to experience pleasure without the drug.

Pineal Gland

Pineal gland is a pine cone-shaped body located in the roof of the diencephalon deep within the cerebral hemispheres of the brain, at the posterior end of the third ventricle (Plate XVIII, Fig. 13.25). The pineal gland contains neurons, glial cells and secretory cells that synthesize the hormone melatonin. Branches of the axons of neurons that make up the visual pathways enter the pineal gland and affect the rate of melatonin production, which is lowest during daylight hours and highest at night.

Several functions have been suggested for melatonin in humans:

1. *Inhibition of reproductive function:* In some mammals, melatonin slows the maturation of sperm, ova, and reproductive organs. The significance of this effect remains unclear, but circumstantial evidence suggests that melatonin may play a role in the timing of human sexual maturation. Melatonin levels in the blood decline at puberty and pineal tumors eliminate melatonin production cause premature puberty in young children.

2. *Antioxidant activity:* Melatonin is very effective antioxidant that may protect CNS neurons from free radicals, such as nitric oxide (NO) or hydrogen peroxide (H_2O_2) that may be generated in active neural tissue. (Free radicals are highly

reactive atoms or molecules that contain unpaired electrons in their outer electron shell).

3. *Establishment of day-night cycles of activity:* Because of the cyclical nature of its rate of secretion, pineal gland may also be involved in maintaining basic circadian rhythms—daily changes in physiological processes that follow a regular day-night pattern. Increased melatonin secretion in darkness has been suggested as a primary cause of seasonal affective disorder (SAD). This condition, characterized by changes in mood, eating habits and sleeping patterns, can develop during the winter in high latitudes, where sunshine is scarce or lacking.

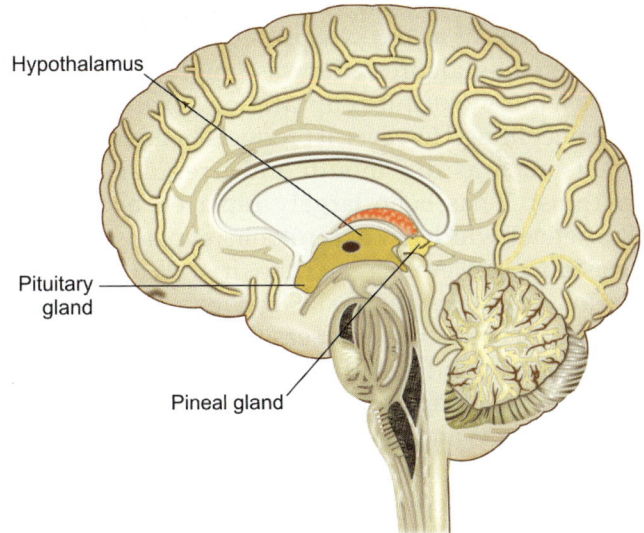

Fig. 13.25: Anatomic location of the pineal gland

The pineal gland has been called a "neuroendocrine transducer"—a system that converts a signal received through the nervous system (dark and light, for instance) into an endocrine signal (shifting concentrations of hormone secretion). Information about daily cycles of light and dark is detected by the eyes and conveyed via the optic nerve to the hypothalamus.

From there, sympathetic nerves convey the signal to the pineal gland.

Several chemicals that have hormonal activity have been isolated from the pineal gland. It produces serotonin by day and melatonin at night. The pineal gland regulates the timing of puberty. The pineal gland produces steady secretions of melatonin throughout the night; light inhibits the production of melatonin. It has been observed that melatonin causes mood disorders, including depression and sleep disturbances.

Some people experience a mood dysfunction called *seasonal affective disorder (SAD),* especially in winter when the days are shorter and they get less exposure to sunlight and in extreme northern and southern latitudes where sunlight may be dim to non-existent for months at a time. The symptoms—which include depression, sleepiness and irritability can be relieved by 2 or 3 hours of exposure to bright light each day *(phototherapy).*

Premenstrual syndrome (PMS) is similar to SAD and is also relieved by phototherapy.

Deficiencies of the monoamine neurotransmitter: Some cases of depression result from deficiencies of the monoamine neurotransmitters. Thus, they yield to drugs that prolong the effects of the monoamines already present at the synapses. One of the earliest discovered antidepressants was imipramine, which blocks the synaptic reuptake of serotonin and norepinephrine. However, it produces undesirable side effects such as dry mouth and irregular cardiac rhythms; it has been largely replaced by Prozac (fluoxetine), which blocks serotonin reuptake and pro-longs its mood-elevating effect; thus it is called a *selective serotonin reuptake inhibitor (SSRI).* Prozac is also used to treat fear of rejection, excess sensitivity to criticism, lack of self-esteem, and inability to experience pleasure, all of which were long handled only through counseling, group therapy, and psychoanalysis.

After monoamines are taken up from the synapse, they are degraded by monoamine oxidase (MAO). Drugs called *MAO inhibitors* interfere with the breakdown of monoamine neurotransmitters and provide another pharmacological approach to depression.

Treatment

It is not the professional responsibility of the dental surgeons to diagnose depression or prescribe accordingly. There are several classes of antidepressant drugs in clinical use:

1. Tricyclic antidepressants (TCAs), e.g. amytriptyline (elavil), imperamine (tofranil, norpramine, nortriptyline (aventyl) and doxepin (sinequan).
2. Monoaminooxidase inhibitors (MAOIs), e.g. phenelzine (nardil), isocarboxazid (marplan), and tranylcypromine (parnate).
3. Selective serotonin reuptake inhibitors (SSRIs), and serotonin-noradrenaline reuptake inhibitors (SNRIs), e.g. paroxetin (paxil), fluoxetine (prozac), sertraline (zoloft) and citalopram (celexa).

As far as dentistry is concerned, it is important to know that treatment for depression may alter the patient's behavior. The symptoms and their treatment may have effect on patient management.

Poor personal and oral hygiene, decreased salivary flow, increased dental caries, increased periodontal disease and facial pain syndromes are common in patients suffering from depression.

Patients suffering from anxiety or depression often experience aphthous ulcerations, ulcerative gingivitis, TMJ problems, lichen planus, geographic tongue and myofacial pain. These conditions must also be addressed in the dental setting.

Always show empathy toward the patient and try to clearly understand the patient's problems.

Both TCAs and MAOIs may cause **postural hypotension.** As much dentistry is carried out in the supine position, care must be taken to upright the patient slowly and ensure no ataxia when ambulant and before discharge.

Both TCAs and MAOIs have atropine-like action, which may cause **xerostomia.** This in turn, can increase the risk of caries and periodontal disease and may adversely affect denture retention. It may also predispose to oral candidiasis. Xerostomia is actually a genuine concern in patients taking all kinds of antipsychiatric medications.

Both TCAs and MAOIs increase risk of **arrhythmias and hypotension** with general anesthetic agents; the use of opioids either pre- or post-surgically may cause hypo- or hypertension (especially pethidine). **There is no clinical evidence of significant interaction with local anesthetics containing epinephrine leading to hypertension in either TCA or MAOI groups.**

Sedatives and narcotic analgesics with MAOIs are strictly contraindicated.

However, even in patients not suffering from depressive illness, there is an analgesic effect which some antidepressant drugs exert that may be of value in atypical or chronic facial pain syndromes and in some non-responsive patients with temporomandibular disorders (dysfunction). This property may be related to enhancing monoaminergic nerve transmission, which inhibits pain afferents or as a direct antidepressant effect. It may take several weeks to achieve relief of symptoms and treatment may extend over several months or longer according to the individual patient's need. These drugs also cause some muscle relaxation which may be beneficial in chronic orofacial pain syndrome.

14

Hemorrhage and Bleeding Disorders

HEMORRHAGE
Classification of Hemorrhage
Physiologically Induced Hemorrhage
Hemostasis

    I. Vascular Phase

    II. Platelet Phase

    III. Coagulation Phase

    IV. Fibrinolysis

BLEEDING DISORDERS
  1. Diseases due to a Defect in Coagulation
    A. Hemophilia
      i. Hemophilia A
      ii. Hemophilia B (Christmas Disease)
      iii. Pseudohemophilia C (von Willebrand's
        Disease)
    Dental Extraction in a Hemophiliac on
      Outpatient Basis

Dental Extraction in a Hemophiliac in the
    Hospital
    B. Hypoprothrombinemia
  2. Diseases due to Thrombocytopenia:
    i. Idiopathic Thrombocytopenic Purpura
    ii. Secondary Thrombocytopenia
  3. Diseases due to Abnormality of Capillaries.

DRUGS INDUCED HEMORRHAGE (ANTICOAGULANTS)
Indications of Anticoagulants
Types of anticoagulants
    A. Heparin
    B. Coumarin
    C. Aspirin
    D. Nonsteroidal Anti-inflammatory Drugs (NSAIDs)
Management of Patients on Anticoagulant
    Therapy
Local Methods for Control of Hemorrhage
Systemic Methods for Control of Hemorrhage

HEMORRHAGE AND BLEEDING DISORDERS

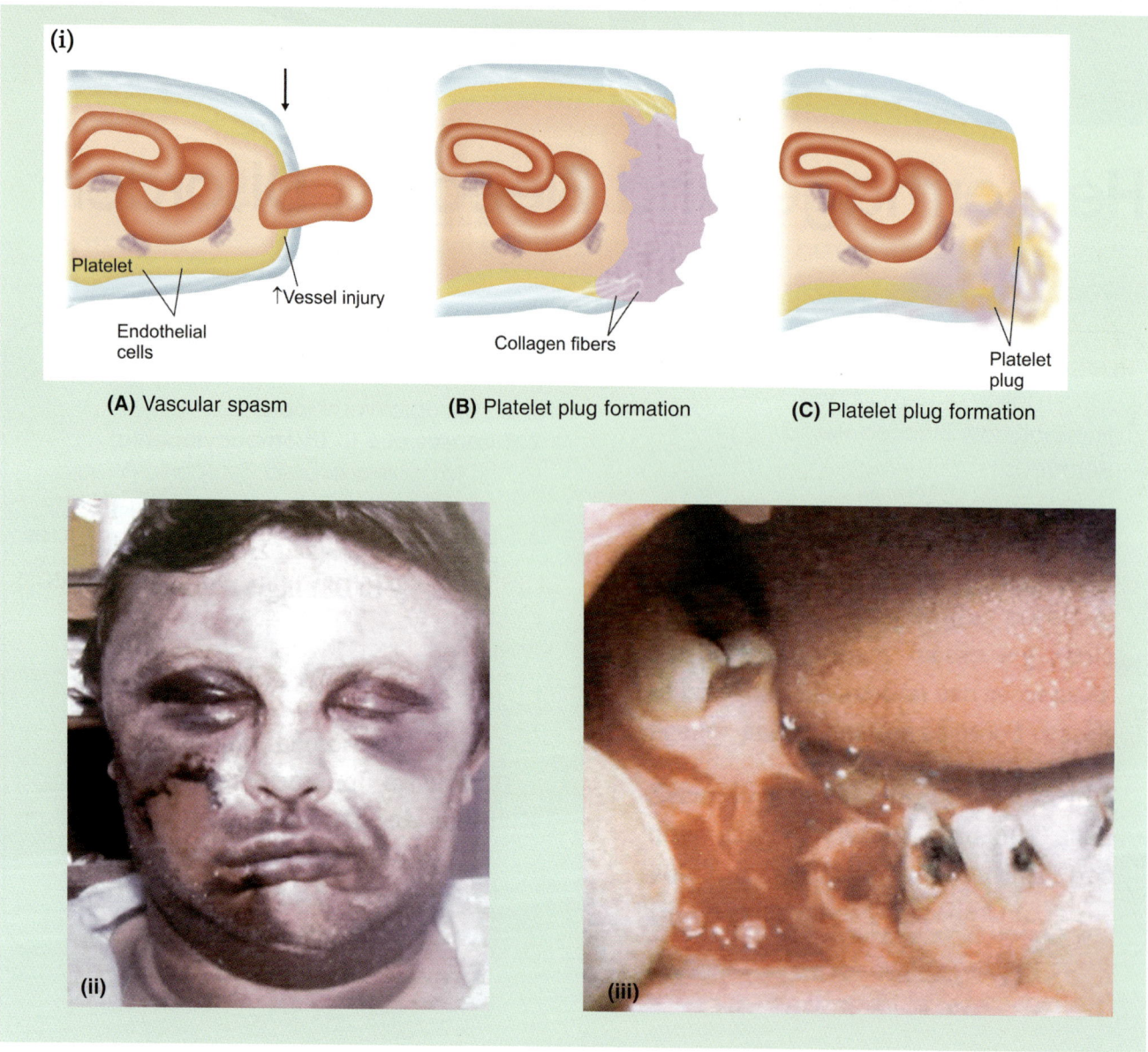

(A) Vascular spasm   **(B)** Platelet plug formation   **(C)** Platelet plug formation

Plate (XIX)

(i) Hemostasis. **(A)** Vasoconstriction of a broken vessel reduces bleeding. **(B)** A platelet plug forms as platelet adhere to exposed collagen fibers of the vessel wall. The platelet plug temporarily seals the break. **(C)** A blood clot forms as platelets and erythrocytes become enmeshed in fibrin threads. This forms a longer lasting seal and gives the vessel a chance to repair itself (*Saladin*: Anatomy & Physiology: The Unity of Form and Function. 3rd ed. McGraw-Hill Co. 2003)

(ii) Hemophilia. This was a mild and unsuspected hemophiliac who had never had any pervious serious bleeding episodes. This enormous hematoma developed after a submucous injection for extirpation of an incisor pulp. (Cawson R A, Odel E W: Cawson's Essentials of Oral Pathology and Oral Medicine 7th ed., Churchil-Livingstone 2002).

(iii) Severe hemorrhage after dental extraction is often the first due to more minor degrees of coagulation disorder and is a common presentation in hemophilia, Christmas disease and von Willebrand's disease.

HEMORRHAGE

By virtue of the coagulation or clotting cascade, blood and blood vessels are a self-limiting system and, therefore, have an inherent ability to provide hemostasis.

Hemorrhage is defined as an acute loss of circulating blood. The blood volume is approximately 7% of the adult ideal body weight. A 70 kg male has approximately 5 L of circulating blood volume. The blood volume usually does not increase significantly in obese patients, and in children, the blood volume is usually between 8% and 9% of body weight (80 to 90 mL/kg).

CLASSIFICATION

The classification of hemorrhage is based on three criteria: time of occurrence, nature of blood vessel involved and deficiency in clotting factor involved. Accordingly, hemorrhage is referred to as *primary*, *intermediate* and *secondary*, *arterial*, *venous* and *capillary*, *extravascular* and *intravascular*. All classifications are significant and have both clinical implications and applications.

Time of Hemorrhage

Based on the time of occurrence, hemorrhage can be classified as primary, intermediate and secondary.

Primary hemorrhage occurs during the time of surgery and is attributed to cutting the blood vessels. Under normal conditions, the application of pressure along with the retraction and contraction of blood vessels is sufficient to promote arrest. Frequently, when infiltration analgesia is used, the vasoconstrictor agent involved also helps to promote the arrest of hemorrhage.

Intermediate hemorrhage refers to bleeding which occurs within 24 hours of surgery. The likelihood of this occurring is attributable to many factors, e.g. removal of pressure, dissipation of vasoconstrictor agents and relaxation of blood vessels.

Secondary hemorrhage occurs 24 hours after surgery and is frequently attributable to many factors, e.g. intrinsic trauma (loose bone chips), infection, etc.

Type of Blood Vessels

Hemorrhage can be classified according to the nature of the vessels from where the blood escapes: *arterial*, *venous* or *capillary*.

Arterial hemorrhage is bright red in color and is pumped out of the wound; the flow can be described as pulsating.

Capillary hemorrhage is also red but always oozes out of the wound.

Venous hemorrhage is dark red in color and slowly oozes or well out of the wound.

Intra- and Extravascular Hemorrhage

Intravascular Hemorrhage

Intravascular hemorrhage also known as disseminated intravascular coagulation (DIG) and consumption coagulation, is a condition, often life-threatening, that involves both excessive bleeding and excessive clotting occurs. Disseminated intravascular coagulation (DIG) is a major complication where a stimulus results in a widespread deposition of fibrin-platelet thrombi in the arterial and venous tree. There is inappropriate extensive coagulation, often in fundamentally normal blood vessels. It occurs as a complication of numerous primary problems, which activate the clotting process in the microcirculation throughout the body (Figs 14.1 and 14.2). In disseminated intravascular coagulation, the coagulation system is activated, but the consumption of platelets and clotting factors which follows leads to paradoxical bleeding tendency.

Patients suffering from acute DIG present with a dramatic illness with hemorrhagic manifestations. They are usually severely ill, with fever, acidosis and hypoxoia and hypotension caused by severe blood loss. There may be extensive petechiae or frank bleeding into the skin, especially at site of trauma, for example, wounds, venipuncture sites, or under blood pressure cuff. There may also be bleeding in the eyes, and alimentary, respiratory, genital or renal tracts. On occasions, thrombosis may dominate the initial picture and there may be gangrene of skin and digits with signs of ischemia of heart, brain, kidneys and lungs.

Clotting may be induced by the release of tissue thromboplastin or by injury of the endothelial cells, causing platelet adhesion. The process causes multiple thrombosis and infarctions but also consumes the available clotting factors and platelets and stimulates

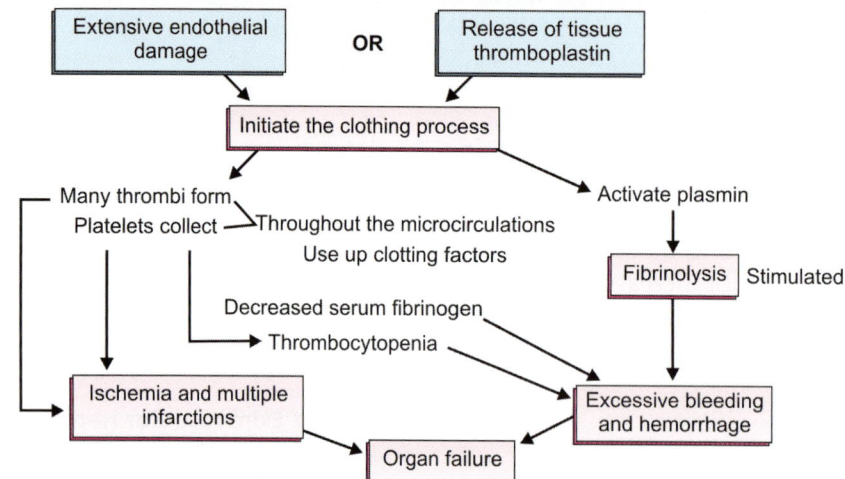

Fig. 14.1: Disseminated intravascular coagulation (DIC) *(Gould, 2006)*

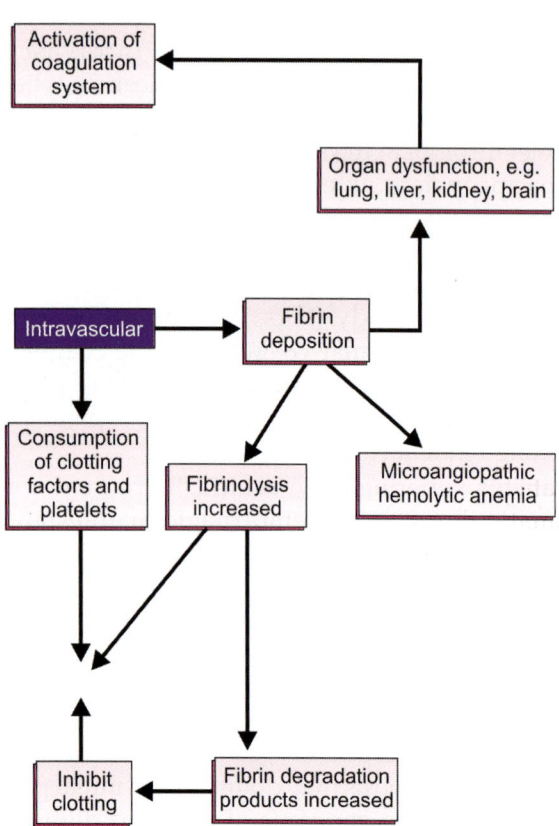

Fig. 14.2: A routine blood film may show fragmentation of red cells that results from cell damage by strands of fibrin thrombus. Simple screening tests for DIC include the platelet count (which is reduced), the APPT (which is prolonged), and the presence of fibrinogen-fibrin degradation products (FDPs) that have resulted from fibrin digestion

the fibrinolytic process. This consumption of the clotting factors and fibrinolysis then leads to hemorrhage and eventually to hypotension and shock. A variety of disorders can initiate DIG. It may result from an obstetric complication such as toxemia or amniotic fluid embolus. Infection, gram-negative infection, leads to endotoxins that cause endothelial damage or stimulate the release of thromboplastin from monocytes. Many carcinomas release substances that trigger coagulation. Major trauma, such as burns or crush injuries and widespread deposits of antigen-antibody complexes result in endothelial damage, releasing thromboplastin and initiating the process. Investigations show consumption of fibrinogen and platelets. DIG may develop following massive blood transfusion, intravascular hemolysis, cardiopulmonary bypass, artificial heart and dialysis.

Treatment

- Identification of the underlying cause
- Intensive support of the patient
- Restoration and maintenance of the peripheral circulation.
- Replacement therapy with plasma, plasma products, clotting factors, or platelets.

Control of the thrombotic component with heparin is rarely useful, and is complicated by the effects of some heparin on platelets.

Extravascular Hemorrhage

Extravascular hemorrhage is the escape of the blood outside the body.

Extravascular factors are the most common cause of hemorrhage. The reasons for such relate directly to the nature of the wound, the location of the wound, the prevalence of infection and surgical trauma.

1. *Nature of the wound:* The post-extraction wound basically, consists of two types of tissues: hard and soft. The hard tissue component; bone, constitutes the greater part of the wound, whereas the soft tissue makes up the smallest part of the wound. Hemorrhage thus can occur from either one of the components.

   Hemorrhage from bone can be difficult to control because unlike a soft tissue wound, the walls cannot be collapsed and approximated to apply the pressure required to collapse the lumen of the vessels and provide the relaxation required to promote retraction and contraction of the vessels. Sometimes the existence of certain anatomical peculiarities can augment or aggravate the problem. The presence of prominent nutrient blood vessels can lead to a profuse arterial type hemorrhage. Additionally, bone is fractured during extraction, subsequent to which there is irritation, inflammation, infection and secondary hemorrhage.

2. *Location of the wound:* An intraoral wound, by virtue of its location, is highly exposed and susceptible to trauma and infection, secondary to which there can be inflammatory hyperemia and extensive bleeding.

3. *Presence of infection:* Perhaps the most common cause of hemorrhage is due to the presence of infection, periodontal and periapical. Whenever there is infection frequently inflammatory proliferation (granulation tissue) and inflammatory hyperemia occur. Thus there is an increase in the number of blood vessels along with hyperemia.

4. *Surgical trauma:* All too frequently in the hands of the unskilled oral surgeon the following mishaps can occur: tissue is torn and bone is fractured, both of which induce bleeding due to laceration of blood vessels, inflammation and infection seen secondary to trauma.

PHYSIOLOGICALLY INDUCED HEMORRHAGE

1. *Endocrine imbalance:* We have long been aware that endocrine imbalance in the female will have a tendency to prolong the bleeding time and create coagulation problem on a prior grounds alone. There seems to be a tendency among women who have prolonged menstruation or who suffer from such disorders as menorrhage to have a tendency toward prolonged post-operative bleeding. Patients of this type are particularly prone to secondary hemorrhage starting two or three days following the surgery.

2. *Pregnancy:* Pregnancy generally is no contra-indication to a surgical procedure from a bleeding point of view; however, there is often considerable oozing in pregnant patients that would otherwise not be present.

3. *Hypertension:* Patients with severe hypertension pose potential bleeding problems in that the hydrostatic pressure within the vessel itself creates a simple mechanical problem. The fibrin clot that acts as a plug in the capillary or arterial opening is more easily dislodged. The effect of blood pressure is often particularly apparent on a patient who is under a general anesthetic. A clinician should be considerably more prudent in the observation of a patient who has a severe hypertension for the spontaneous recurrence of bleeding in the immediate postoperative period of routine surgery such as dental extraction or dentoalveolar surgery.

4. *Infection:* The presence of infection brings large quantities of blood to an area. The increased vascular bed will produce an increased bleeding at the time of surgery that should not alter the mechanism of clotting except from the standpoint of quantity alone. Certain complications may arise following streptococcal infections and certain malignancies, resulting in a hypofibrinogenemia. Suitable laboratory procedures for the fibrinogen determination can be conducted. The diagnosis once established will necessitate immediate therapy to prevent circulatory collapse.

5. *Trauma:* If there has been severe trauma in the recent past so that there is a large enough area of ecchymosis or hematoma in the tissues involved in surgery, the bleeding response will be prolonged and the amount of blood loss will be considerably increased.

6. *Tumor:* When there is a tumor it is fed by various vessels that normally would not be present. The surgeon may well encounter abnormal bleeding with any areas of this field of operation which

would necessitate more careful dissection and considerably more detailed attention to the tributary arteries and veins.

7. *Certain pathologic entities:* There are a large number of pathologic entities involving blood vessels as blood tumors (e.g. cavernous hemangioma, aneurysm) which obviously require careful evaluation prior to surgical intervention because bleeding from these can be extremely serious and at times fatal.

Diseases of the liver, biliary system, gastrointestinal tract, bone marrow and spleen may profoundly influence Hemostasis. For example, the liver whose function is compromised by advanced cirrhosis fails to produce adequate amounts of prothrombin and other essential plasma factors. Diseases causing bone marrow and spleen disturbances affect a depression or destruction of megakaryoctes which are the precursors of indispensable platelet.

8. *Hematoma formation:* Postoperative hematoma formation is due to a combination of inadequate postoperative hemostasis or lack of drainage where this is appropriate. All potential dead spaces should be drained and pressure dressing applied to their flaps to discourage capillary ooze and the consequent accumulation of blood. In intraoral surgery, lack of drainage may be due to overtight suturing of the wound. It may result in a considerable facial swelling which is tender to palpation. The condition is usually present on the first postoperative day and should be treated by:

a. Removal of one or more sutures.

b. Evacuation of the hematoma possibly by aspiration with a sterile wide bore needle.

c. In the mouth, it is usually sufficient to institute an intensive regime of hot saline mouth baths.

d. These effusions of blood often become infected and if the patient has a pyrexia, suitable antibiotic therapy should be instituted. An infected hematoma inevitably leads to breakdown of the suture line and protracted healing of the wound.

e. The use of fibrinolytic agents.

There are some agents which could be used to dissolve a blood clot that has been formed either *within* a vessel or extravascularly within various special areas throughout the body. The lytic enzyme fibrinolysin is believed to be responsible for the resolution which is spontaneously carried out throughout the body whenever any blood has extravasated from a vessel into a tissue space. There are many enzymes, streptokinase and streptodornase (varidase) and proteolytic enzymes (ananse, papase, trypsin) which have varying degrees of clot liquefying effectiveness. Fibrinolytic therapy is discussed in Chapter 15, Page 445,"F".

HEMOSTASIS

- Hemostasis is the arrest of blood loss from damaged vessels and the formation of a fibrin-reinforced blood clot.
- Four distinct stages can be identified: vessel wall contraction; platelet aggregation, blood coagulation, andfibrinolysis.
- Vessel wall contraction is of short duration (5–20 min), but can be prolonged by epinephrine (adrenaline).
- Platelets adhere to the exposed collagen of cut blood vessels and release ADP and thromboxane A2.
- Thromboxane A2 is powerful inducer of platelet aggregation, which facilitates the formation of the platelet plug.
- The platelet plug is reinforced with fibrin, which is formed during the clotting cascade.
- Vitamin K is essential for the formation of the clotting factors II, VII, IX, and X.
- Fibrinolysis is the final stage of hemostasis and involves the breakdown of the clot by plasmin.

The four phases of hemostasis for controlling bleeding are:

i. Vascular

ii. Platelet adhesion and aggregation

iii. Coagulation, and

iv. Fibrinolysis

I. VASCULAR PHASE (THE VESSEL WALL CONTRACTION)

The most immediate consequence of injury to a blood vessel is a vascular contraction of a varying degree, depending upon the size and nature of the vessel that has been severed or injured. Retraction of arteries that have been cut, and the build up of extravascular pressure by blood loss from cut vessels aids in collapsing the adjacent capillaries and veins in the area of injury. Vasoconstriction is mediated both as a local reflex and by a number of mediators that are released mainly from activated platelets. The vascular phase is responsible for maintenance of vasoconstriction. Vasoconstriction is maintained by platelet secretion of serotonin, prostaglandin and thromboxane. This vasoconstriction is only of short duration (usually

5–20 minutes) but can be prolonged by topical or local infiltration of epinephrine (adrenaline).

Thus, although coagulation, as measured by clotting time, takes around 8 min to occur, haemorrhage is reduced and arrested sooner. Exposure of vessel wall subendothelial tissues, collagen, and basement membrane through chemical or traumatic injury serves as a tissue factor (old term was tissue thromboplastin) and initiate coagulation via extrinsic pathway (Fig. 14.3). An inducible endothelial cell prothrombin activator may directly generate thrombin. Vascular wall integrity is important for maintaining the fluidity of blood. The smooth endothelial lining consists of non-wettable surface that, under normal conditions, does not activate platelet adhesion or coagulation.

II. PLATELET PHASE (PLATELET ADHESION AND AGGREGATION)

The platelet phase is responsible for the formation of soft plug. Both the vascular and the platelet phases are short lived. If flow is allowed *to increase, the soft plug could* be sheared from the injured surface, possibly creating emboli.

Platelets are cellular fragments from the cytoplasm of megakaryocytes that last 8 to 12 days in the circulation. Platelets do not have a nucleus. Aged or nonviable platelets are removed and destroyed by the spleen and liver.

Functions of platelets include maintenance of vascular integrity, formation of platelet plug to aid in initial control of bleeding and stabilization of platelet plug through involvement in the coagulation process.

Within seconds after injury, the platelets begin to adhere to the surface of the injured vessel *(adhesion)* and to one another **(aggregation)**.

Throughout vascular contraction, a cement-like substance is liberated from the mesenchymal supporting tissues of the vessel and from the ruptured endothelial lining of the vessel wall. This plays an important role in the formation of the platelet plug.

So contraction of the severed vessel not only tends to slow down and restrict the flow of blood from the vessel but also sets up a turbulence which causes the platelets to form a platelet plug.

Subendothelial tissues are exposed at the site of injury and, through contact activation, cause the platelets to become sticky and adhere to subendothelial tissues.

Following injury:

1. Injured endothelial cells result in the release of adenosine diphosphate (ADP) which initiate platelet adhesion.
2. The exposures of subendothelial tissues to a plasma factor known as von Willebrand factor (vWF). Thus the injured endothelial cells promote platelet adhesion and thrombus formation.

Platelets aggregation is initiated by:

1. Adenosine diphosphate (ADP) released by damaged endothelial cells (primary wave).
2. A product of platelets, thromboxane. When platelets release their secretion, a second wave of aggregation occurs, and this results in binding with fibrinogen which is converted to fibrin

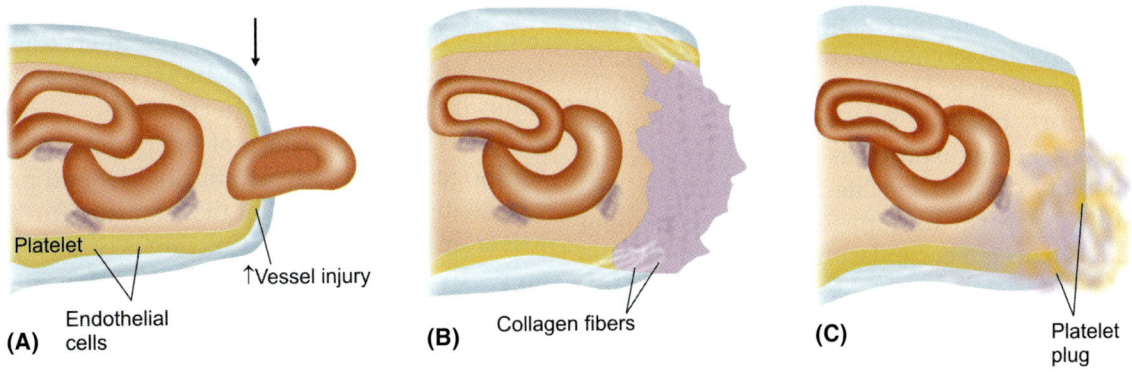

(A) Platelet / Endothelial cells / ↑Vessel injury   (B) Collagen fibers   (C) Platelet plug

Fig. 14.3: Hemostasis. **(A)** Vasoconstriction of a broken vessel reduces bleeding. **(B)** A platelet plug forms as platelet adhere to exposed collagen fibers of the vessel wall. The platelet plug temporarily seals the break. **(C)** A blood clot forms as platelets and erythrocytes become enmeshed in fibrin threads. This forms a longer lasting seal and gives the vessel a chance to repair itself *(Saladin: Anatomy and Physiology: The Unity of Form and Function. 3rd ed. McGraw-Hill Co. 2003)*

stabilizes the platelet plug. The result of the preceding processes is a clot of platelets and fibrin attached (Fig. 14.4).

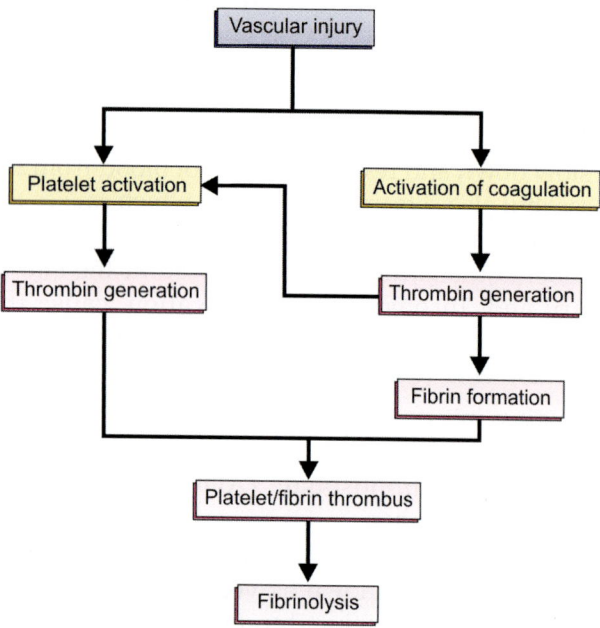

Fig. 14.4: Vascular injury triggers activation of the coagulation system and activates platelet aggregation. These two systems lead to a platelet/fibrin clot or thrombus. Once the clot has served its role in the control of bleeding, plasminogen converted to plasmin promotes degradation of the clot. When thrombus formation must be inhibited, antithrombotic drugs (antiplatelet agents, fibrinolytic agents, and anticoagulants) are used. *(Hoflman R et al, 2005)*

The enzyme cyclooxygenase is essential in the process of generation of thromboxane. Endothelial cells, through a similar process, generate prostacycline, which inhibits platelet aggregation. Aspirin acts as an inhibitor of cyclooxygenase and this causes irreversible damage to the platelets. However, endothelial cells can, after a short period, recover and synthetise cyclooxygenase, thus aspirin has only a short effect on the availability of prostacycline from these cells. The net result of aspirin therapy is to inhibit platelet aggregation. This effect can last for up to 9 days (time needed for old platelets to be cleared from the blood).

The processes of platelet adhesion and aggregation are complex and utilize a poorly defined plasma factor (vW factor) which is lacking in von Willebrand's disease and ADP derived from injured tissues, including erythrocytes, and the platelets themselves.

Adhesion occurs because glycoproteins on the platelet surface adhere to a sticky von Willebrand factor (vWf), which is bound to the exposed subendothelium. Platelets collect across the injured surface. These platelets are then activated by contact with collagen. Collagen-activated platelets form pseudopodes which stretch out to cover the injured surface and bridge exposed fibers. The collagen activated platelet membranes expose receptors which bind circulating fibrinogen to their surfaces. Fibrinogen has many platelet binding sites. An aggregation of platelets and fibrinogen build up to form a soft plug. Platelet aggregation occurs about 20 seconds after injury.

III. COAGULATION PHASE

Blood coagulation is the process by which fluid blood is converted into a coagulum or a clot. The process of fibrin forming system is called coagulation. The overall time involved from injury to a fibrin-stabilized clot is about 9 to 18 minutes. This process involves the interaction of various poorly defined trace plasma proteins "the coagulation factors". This is done in essentially four parts: (a)The activation of thromboplastin, (b) The conversion of prothrombin to thrombin, (c) The conversion of fibrinogen to fibrin and (d) The contraction of the fibrin clot.

The nomenclature of the coagulation factors has now been standardized by designating each with a Roman numeral (Table 14.1). The coagulation factors are proenzymes which are normally inert, but when activated, they are transformed into proteolytic enzymes, each sequentially activating the proenzyme next in line (the cascade or waterfall hypothesis) that is one factor becomes activated and it, in turn, activates another and so on in an ordered sequence and finally create a fibrin clot. Platelets, blood proteins, lipids and ions are involved in the process. Thrombin is generated on the surface of the platelets and bound fibrinogen is converted to fibrin. The end product of coagulation is a fibrin clot that can stop further blood loss from injured tissues. Calcium is essential for most steps in the coagulation process. Several of the coagulation factors are utilized or consumed during in vitro coagulation (factors V, VIII, XIII, fibrinogen and prothrombin), whereas the remainder are found in the serum.

- All clotting factors, with the exception of factor VIII, are manufactured in the liver.

Table 14.1: List of coagulation factors

	Synonyms	Function	Deficiency Synonym
I	Fibrinogen	Precursor of fibrin	Hypofibrinogenemia Afibrinogenemia
II	Prothrombin	Precursor of thrombin (enzyme which converts fibrinogen to fibrin)	Hypoprothrombinemia
III	Thromboplastin	Activates factor VII.	
IV	Calcium	Necessary for several intermediate reactions	
V	Labile factor Proaccelerin	Required for activation of tissue thromboplastin	Parahemophilia
VI	No activity assigned this number		
VII	Stable factor Proconvertin	Required for activation of tissue thromboplastin	Hypoproconvertinemia
VIII	Antihemophilic globulin (AHG)	Component of intrinsic thromboplastin generating system	Classic hemophilia Hemophilia A
IX	Plasma thromboplastin component (PTC) Christmas factor	Component of intrinsic thromboplastin generating system	Christmas disease Hemophilia B
X	Stuart factor Prower factor	Required for activation of tissue thromboplastin	
XI	Plasma thromboplastin antecedent (PTA)	Component of intrinsic thromboplastin generating system	Hemophilia C
XII	Hageman factor Glass factor	Component of intrinsic thromboplastin generating system	Hageman trait
XIII	Fibrin stabilizing factor (FSF) Fibrinase	Catalyzes normal polymerization of fibrin	

- Factor VIII and vWF are manufactured in the endothelial cells of the blood vessels.
- Factors II, VII, IX and X are vitamin K-dependent clotting factors and they participate in the intrinsic and extrinsic clotting cascades.

The coagulation cascade consists of two routes that run in parallel—the intrinsic pathway and the extrinsic pathway. Both are common pathways to form the end product fibrin. Figs 14.5 and 14.6 show these coagulation pathways.

The extrinsic pathway (faster): Tissue factor released from the injured vasculature immediately activates factor VII in the extrinsic system. The activated factor VII in turn, activates factor X, where the common pathway starts. Tissue factor (TF) is expressed on the surface of the subendothelial tissue that is exposed when endothelium is damaged.

In the past, the trigger for initiating the extrinsic pathway was referred to as a tissue thromboplastin. The term extrinsic pathway continues to be used today, despite the fact that it is somewhat outdated. Ionized calcium is a crucial cofactor for many of the clotting factors and deficiency has an important effect on coagulation.

Intrinsic pathway: This is the more intricate portion of the coagulation cascade. Essentially contact with injured tissue results in activation of factor XII, which in turn activates factor XI. In this intrinsic system, coagulation is believed to be initiated when Hageman factor (factor XII) is converted from its inert preactive form. The activated Hageman factor reacts with plasma thromboplastin antecedent (factor XI), which in turn activates factor IX (Christmas factor), which in turn activates factor VIII (antihemophilic factor). The antihemophilic factor activates factor X or the

Stewart factor, which activates factor V (proaccelerin) which in turn cascades to the common pathway as shown in Fig. 14.5.

Common pathway: This is the common end point of the intrinsic and extrinsic pathways. It begins with

activation of factor X and via other steps shown in Fig. 14.5, results in the formation of cross-linked fibrin (Box 14.1).

Again the coagulation phase is done in essentially four parts:

A. The activation of thromboplastin.

B. The conversion of prothrombin to thrombin.

C. The conversion of fibrinogen to fibrin.

D. The contraction of the fibrin clot.

Box 14.1

Factor X (intrinsic and extrinsic)	Factor V Factor VII Ionic calcium	Prothrombinase (thromboplastin)

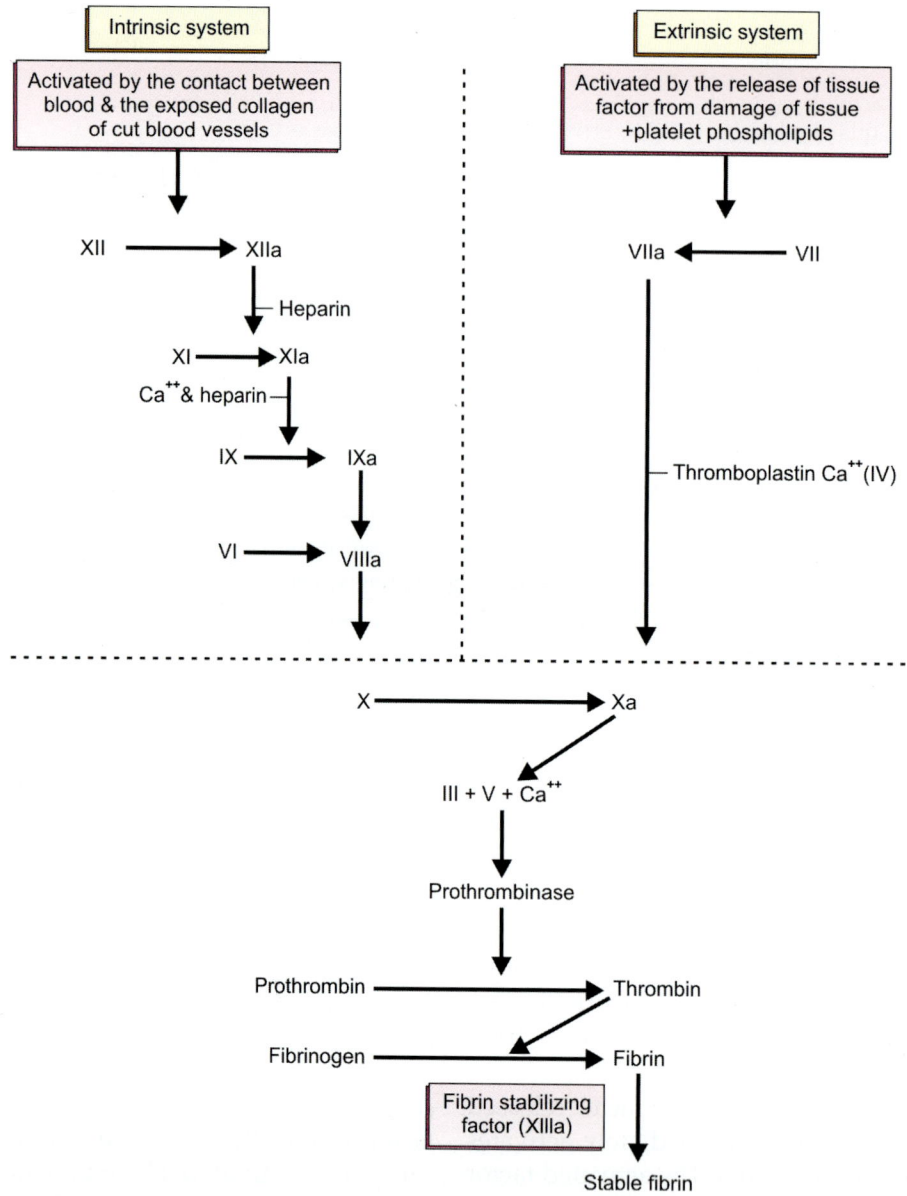

Fig. 14.5: The coagulation cascade showing the numbered factors (a, activated form). The factors involved in the intrinsic system, beginning with the activation of factor XII and ending with the activation of factor X are all present in the circulating plasma. The extrinsic system consists of tissue thromboplastin and includes factor VII, not involved in the intrinsic system. Activated factor X along with factor V initiates the final steps, culminating in the conversion of fibrinogen to fibrin by thrombin

A. The Activation of Thromboplastin

Prothrombinase (thromboplastin) can be produced by the aforementioned sequence of reactions beginning with contact activation and involving factors XII, XI, IX and VIII. This is termed the *intrinsic* pathway. The production of prothrombinase by means of this pathway is relatively slow but requires neither tissue thromboplastin nor factor VII (Fig. 14.6).

A functionally identical prothrombinase can be produced in a matter of seconds by tissue thromboplastin. This involves a sequence of reaction termed the extrinsic pathway which, in addition to factors X and V requires only factor VII. Consequently, this pathway bypasses the steps initiated by contact activation involving factors XII, XI, IX and VIII. Thus, blood coagulation is initiated by only two processes, i.e. contact activation and tissue thromboplastin, it

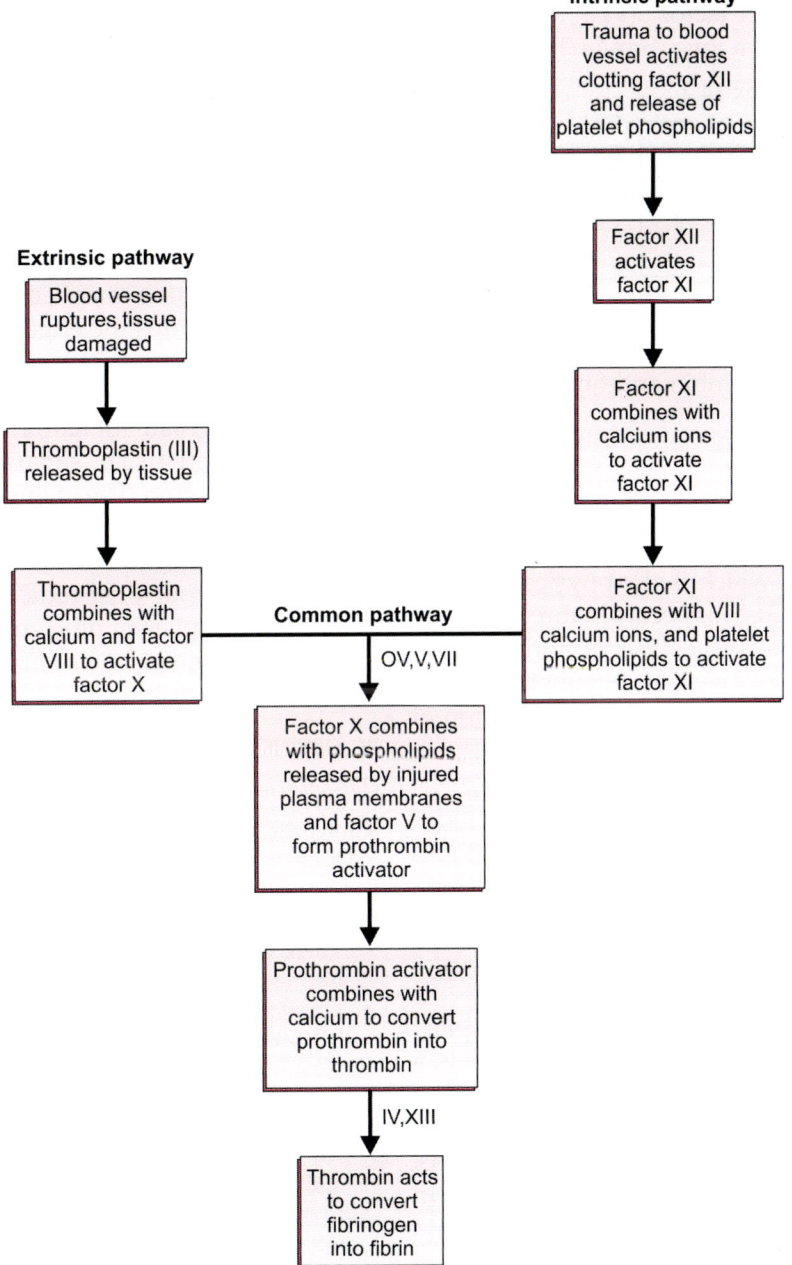

Fig. 14.6: Extrinsic and intrinsic pathways of blood clotting. Note how the two pathways combine to form the common pathway. Factor VIII is often absent in hemophiliacs

proceeds initially via two separate pathways, i.e. the tissue activated extrinsic pathway and the contact activated intrinsic pathway.

B. The Conversion of Prothrombin to Thrombin

Thrombin is generated from prothrombin by the action of thromboplastin now called prothrombinase. Prothrombin is, therefore, a pro-enzyme. Prothrombinase is generated by the combination of factor Xa (which results from the activation of factor X) with the phospholipid platelet factor 3(PF3) and factor V in the presence of calcium ions (Box 14.2).

Box 14.2

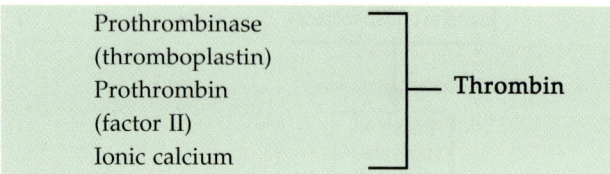

Prothrombinase (thromboplastin)
Prothrombin (factor II) — **Thrombin**
Ionic calcium

Later steps leading to the formation of fibrin proceed via a common pathway, requiring factors X, V, phospholipids, prothrombin and fibrinogen.

C. The Conversion of Fibrinogen to Fibrin (Thrombin–fibrinogen Action)

The final step in the coagulation phase, the thrombin–fibrinogen reaction. It involves the transformation of fibrinogen into fibrin, which is the physical basis of all blood clots (Box 14.3). This occurs in three separate steps, via the enzymatic proteolysis of fibrinogen by thrombin, the formation of a visible but unstable fibrin polymer (soluble fibrin) and finally the formation of a stable.

Box 14.3

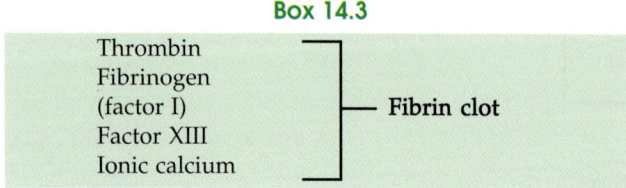

Thrombin
Fibrinogen (factor I) — **Fibrin clot**
Factor XIII
Ionic calcium

Fibrinogen is a glycoprotein composed of three pairs of polypeptide chain, A, B and X. Thrombin is a proteolytic enzyme which remove first of all 19 amino acids from one end of both A chains and then more slowly 14 amino acids from one end of both B chains. The remainder of the molecules forms the fibrin monomer which polymerizes end to end to form a soluble polymer, fibrin Ia. Insoluble fibrin is precipitated by factor XIIIa which results from the action of thrombin on factor XIII.

D. The Contraction of the Fibrin Clot

After a clot has formed, spinous pseudopods of the platelets adhere to strands of fibrin and contract. This pulls on the fibrin threads and draws the edges of the broken vessel together. Through this process of **clot retraction,** the clot becomes more compact within about 30 minutes. Platelets and endothelial cells secrete a mitotic stimulant named *platelet-derived growth factor (PDGF)*. PDGF stimulates fibroblasts and smooth muscle cells to multiply and repair the damaged blood vessel. Fibroblasts also invade the clot and produce fibrous connective tissue, which helps to strengthen and seal the vessel while the repairs take place. Clot retraction is the result of the mechanical shrinkage of fibrin strands within a clot. The platelets supply both the energy (ATP) and the contractile apparatus required for this process (thrombathenin, a protein which functions like actomyosin of muscle). The clot retraction may constitute a physiologic ligature which pulls the edge of a wound together.

Clot retraction test: This is a very simple test for a laboratory to run. It involves essentially the observation of a clot in waterbath for half, 1, 2, 3, 4, and 24 hours for signs of retraction, i.e. separation of the clot with expression of serum. The inability of a clot to retract or change in size indicates a possible hemostatic problem and may be indicative of a rather annoying bleeding difficulty. It, of course, is predicated upon the formation of an adequate platelet plug and the availability of the elements that the platelets supply in the formation of the clotting mechanism.

IV. FIBRINOLYSIS

(Dissolution of Clot)

Clot prevention is important, but so clot destruction, or fibrinolysis "fibrin clotting". Small blood clots form continually in blood vessels throughout the body. If they are not removed promptly, the blood vessels become clogged.

- There are systems that can either promote or inhibit fibrinolysis.
- Fibrinolytic agents include streptokinase, urokinase and t-PA; they all enhance the conversion of plasminogen to plasmin.
- Fibrinolytic drugs are used in the management of acute thromboembolic disorders such as myocardial infarction.
- Antifibrinolytic agents include epsilone-aminocaproic acid and tranexamic acid. These drugs encourage stabilization of thrombin and are useful in the management of postextraction hemorrhage.

Now that a clot is formed and the vessel has healed and re-endothelialized, there must be a mechanism that will inhibit the further formation of a clot so as not to continue to develop thromboembolic episodes that would run rampant throughout the entire circulatory system.

The fibrin lysing system (fibrinolytic) is needed to prevent coagulation of intravascular blood away from the site of injury and to dissolve the clot, once it has served its function in hemostasis. This system involves plasminogen, a proenxyme for the enzyme plasmin, which is produced in the liver and various plasminogen activators and inhibitors of plasmin.

The system of the dissolution of a clot (fibrinolysis) is achieved by a small cascade of reactions with a positive feedback component. In addition to promoting clotting, factor XII catalyzes the formation of a plasma enzyme called **kallikrein.** Kallikrein, in turn, converts the inactive protein *plasminogen* into **plasmin,** a fibrin-dissolving enzyme that breaks up the clot. Thrombin also activates plasmin and plasmin indirectly promotes the formation of more kallikrein, thus completing a positive feedback loop (Fig. 14.7).

The effect of plasmin on fibrin and fibrinogen is to split off large pieces that are broken up into smaller and smaller fragments which is degraded to soluble fibrin degradation products (FDPs) (Fig. 14.8). Antiplasmin factors present in circulating blood rapidly destroy free plasmin but are relatively ineffective against plasmin that is bound to fibrin. Thus, under normal conditions, once an injury has occurred, coagulation proceeds to the formation of fibrin. At the same time, bound plasminogen and free plasminogen become activated to plasmin. Free plasmin is rapidly destroyed and does not interfere with the fomation of a clot. Bound plasmin is not activated, and is free to dispose of the fibrin clot after its function in homeostasis has been fulfilled. In a sense, the clot is programmed at the time of its formation to self-destruct.

One drug that digests that the fibrin threads of a clot **streptokinase,** which is released by certain streptococcal bacteria. Strptokinase activates plasminogen to speed up fibrinolysis (clot destruction). It is used to dissolve blood clot (thrombi) in veins and arteries. Streptokinase also helps disolve to fibrin threads in a blood clot by converting plasminogen into plasmin, the fibrin destroying enzyme.

Fibrinolysis maintains vessel patency and helps to prevent overpropagation of clot. Not surprisingly, there are also inhibitors of plasmin and plasminogen activators. Levels of fibrinogen and FDPs can be measured and provide helpful diagnostic clues.

Euglobulin clot lysis time. This test is becoming very important to indicate an imbalance in the fibrinolytic activity. The euglobulin clot is normally lysed more rapidly than the whole blood clot. If this euglobulin clot will dissolve in less than 90 minutes, it indicates an increase in the fibrrinolytic activity which could lead to a bleeding problem.

Physiologic Prevention of Inappropriate Clotting

Small blood clots form continually in blood vessels throughout the body. If they are not removed promptly, the blood vessels become clogged. In the process of fibrinolysis, a blood protein called plasminogen is activated into an enzyme called plasmin. The plasmin digests the threads of fibrin by first making them soluble and then breaking them into small fragments. The fragments are removed from the bloodstream by phagocytic white blood cells and macrophages.

To prevent inappropriate clotting in normal blood vessels, physiological systems act to counteract those that stimulate blood clotting. The mechanisms that

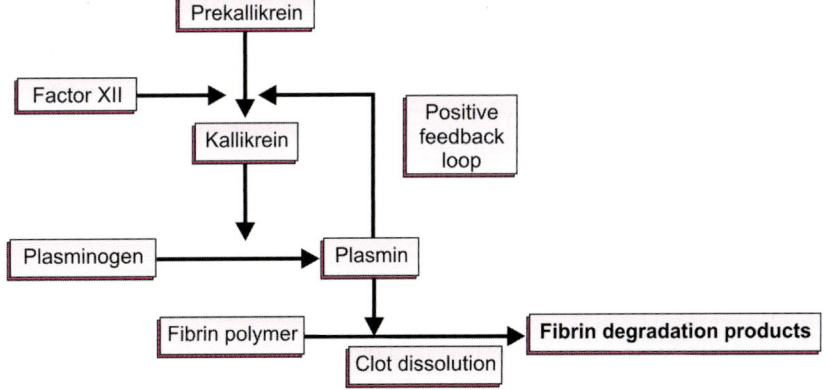

Fig. 14.7: Factors involved in fibrinolysis

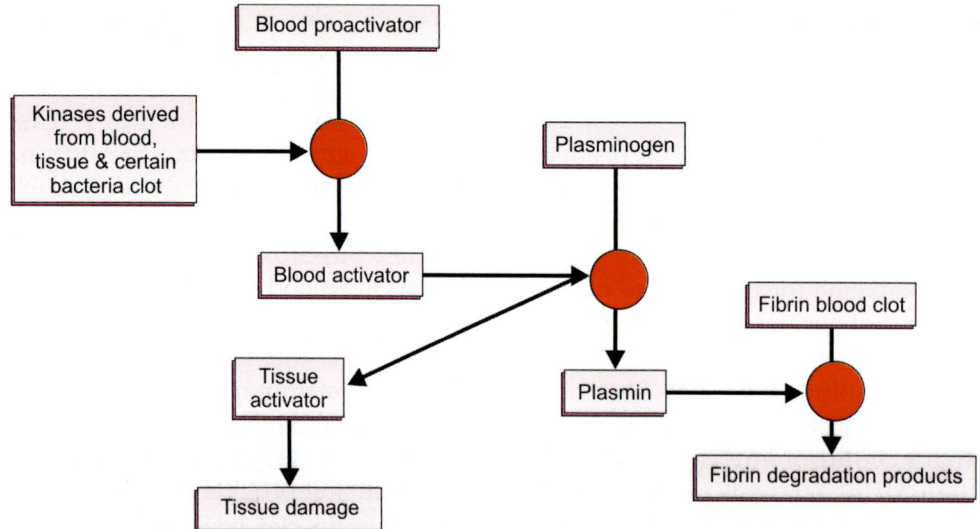

Fig. 14.8: Schematic representation of the stages involved in fibrinolysis

prevent blood from clotting in normal blood vessels can be divided into structural and chemical:

1. *Structural prevention mechanisms:* The smooth lining of the blood vessel provided by the endothelium does not express surface proteins that stimulate platelet adhesion as has been described above. Rough or damaged endothelium (e.g. atherosclerotic plaques) not only allows platelets to come into contact with proteins that they adhere to but results in turbulent blood flow, which also predisposes to blood clotting.
2. *Chemical mediators:* Normal vascular endothelium produces the prostaglandin, prostacycline (PGI 2). This opposes the action of T × A 2, causing vaso-dilation and opposing platelet activation and aggregation.

Fibrinogenolysis

Primary fibrinogenolysis may develop, if active plasmin is generated in the circulation at a time when the clotting cascade is not in operation. It can occur in patients with liver disease, cancer of the lung, cancer of the prostate, or heat stroke. Severe bleeding result from the depletion of fibrinogen (split by plasmin) and the formation of fibrin-split products (with their anti-coagulant properties) from fibrinogen. Fibrinogenolysis can be treated with epsilon-aminocaproic acid (EACA) or tranexamic acid, which inhibits both plasmin and plasmin activators.

Causes of Clotting Factor Deficiency

The following cause clotting factor deficiency:
1. Hemophilia A (factor VIII deficiency).

2. Hemophilia B (factor IX deficiency).
3. Some cases of von Willebrand's disease (vWD) can present with factor VIII deficiency.
4. Anticoagulants heparin (affects the intrinsic pathway) and coumadin (affects the extrinsic pathway).

BLOOD COAGULATION TESTS (CLOTTING FACTOR TESTS PT/ INR AND PTT)

Several tests are used to determine blood clotting time. The more popular ones are platelet count, bleeding time, clotting time and clotting time tests as **PT/ INR and PTT** (Table 14.2).

The blood platelet count must be greater than 150,000 per cubic millimeter in order for normal coagulation to take place. Also if platelet function is not normal, normal coagulation may not occur. A pierced fingertip or earlobe usually bleeds for 3 to 6 min. A longer bleeding time for this wound generally (but not always) indicates a platelet deficiency.

Clotting Time

It is determined by placing blood in a test tube and tipping it back and forth every 30 sec or until it clots. This usually occurs in 5 to 8 min. Because the condition and size of test tubes vary, standerization is necessary to obtain accurate results.

Prothrombin Time (PT)/International Normalized Ratio (INR)

The test for prothrombin time (PT) indicates the amount of prothrombin in the blood. Immediately after blood is removed, oxalate is added to prevent

Test	Defect
Bleeding time	A defect in platelet function or, rarely, afibrinogenemia
Prothrombin time (normal 10–14s)	Deficiency or inhibition of factors V, VII, X, II, fibrinogen indicates defect in extrinsic or common pathway
Activated partial thromboplastin time (normal 30–40s)	Deficiency or inhibition of factors XII, IX, VIII, X, V, II and fibrinogen Indicates defect in intrinsic and/or common pathways, particularly, sensitive for deficiencies in factors VII and IX
Thrombin clotting time (normal 14–16s)	A lack of fibrinogen or an inhibitor of thrombin. Useful in differential diagnosis of disseminated intravascular coagulation.

The PT/INR measures the extrinsic pathway, and the normal range of PT is 10–12 sec.

the prothrombin from being converted into thrombin. When calcium ions and tissue extract containing thromboplastin are added to the blood sample, the calcium offsets the effect of the oxalate and the tissue extract activates the conversion of prothrombin. The time usually required for blood to clot, referred to as the prothrombin time, is about 12 sec. (A longer prothrombin time may also mean a decreased quantity of some factors other than prothrombin.)

The International Normalized Ratio (INR)

The INR is a universal test that is used to effectively monitor the effect of warfarin (coumadin). INR is the prothrombin time (PT) ratio obtained using the international reference thromboplastin reagent (*see the equation*) (Box 14.4). The normal INR range is 0.9–1.2; the average is 1. Only the PT/INR is affected by therapeutic doses of warfarin (coumadin).

The Partial Thromboplastin Time (PTT)

The PTT measures the intrinsic pathway. The normal PTT range is 25–38 sec. PTT is affected by IV heparin and high doses of coumadin. When the patient is anticoagulated with IV heparin, the PTT is maintained at 1.5–2.5 times normal. PTT is not affected by low molecular weight heparins (LMWHs).

Box 14.4: International normalized ratio calculation equation

$$INR = \frac{Patient's\ PT}{Control\ PT} \bullet ISI$$

PT: Prothrombin time;
ISI: International Sensitivity Index.

BLEEDING DISORDERS

The natural hemostatic mechanism is an interlocking mechanism of three processes: vascular contraction, aggregation and fibrin formation. Immediately after vascular injury, the platelets adhere to the damaged tissue and to each other to build up a hemostatic plug which in case of very small vessels is sufficient to stop bleeding, but in larger vessels must be reinforced by fibrin in order to withstand the blood pressure. Vascular contraction is important as it reduces the diameter of the vessel and so helps to consolidate the hemostatic plug. The mechanism of vascular contraction is imperfectly understood but it may occur as a result of the direct effect of trauma on the muscle of the vessel wall or to nervous impulses, but it is also due to the vasoactive substance, e.g. 5-hydroxytryptamine (5HT), released by the platelets and to

substances formed in the blood as a result of clotting. Platelet aggregation is probably due to adenosine diphosphate; a powerful platelet agglutinin which is known to be released in areas of damage and also by the platelets themselves when they are exposed to foreign surfaces or the action of thrombin.

Bleeding disorders are conditions that alter the ability of blood vessels, platelets, and coagulation factors to maintain hemostasis (Box 14.5).

Bleeding and clotting disorders may be either inherited or acquired. In the majority of cases such disorders are known to the patient. Inherited bleeding disorders are genetically transmitted. Acquired bleeding disorders occur as a result of diseases that affect vascular wall integrity, platelets, coagulation factors, drugs, radiation or chemotherapy for cancer. The hemorrhagic diseases can be divided into three main groups:

1. Diseases due to a defect in coagulation:
   A. Hemophilia
   B. Hypoprothrombinemia.
2. Diseases due to thrombocytopenia:
   A. Idiopathic.
   B. Secondary.
3. Diseases due to abnormality of capillaries.

1. DISEASES DUE TO A DEFECT IN COAGULATION

A. Hemophilia

The basic process of clotting mechanism may be summarized as follows (Fig. 14.9).

Hemophilia, in general term, refers to a severe, life long tendency toward excessive bleeding. Hemophilia has been recognized for thousands of years. The Talmud states that a male infant should not be circumcised, if two or more of his brothers died from post-circumcision bleeding.

Hemophilia is classified into hemophilia A or the classical hemophilia (factor VIII deficiency) and hemophilia B or Christmas disease (factor IX deficiency) and hemophilia C, or Rosenthal's syndrome (factor XI deficiency).

Hemophilia A, hemophilia B and von Willebrand's disease are the three most common inherited in males and follow an X-linked pattern. Patients may born with a deficiency of one of the factors needed for blood coagulation, for example, factor VIII deficiency (hemophilia A) or factor IX deficiency (hemophilia B or Christmas disease). Factor VIII has a half-life activity of 8–12 hr. Factor IX has a half-life activity of 12–24 hr.

Hemophilia Severity Classification

Hemophilia can be of mild, moderate or severe intensity:

1. **Mild hemophilia:** The specific factor (VIII or IX) level is 5–30% of normal. The mild hemophilia bleeds minimally bleeding is usually associated with surgery, and the past history reveal bleeding after dental extraction.
2. **Moderate hemophilia:** The specific factor (VIII or IX) level is 1–5% of normal. A moderate hemophiliac bleeds after minor injury and requires immediate attention.
3. **Severe hemophilia:** The specific factor (VIII or IX) level is less than 1% of normal. A serve hemophiliac bleeds very often, with or without provocation.

i. Hemophilia A

Hemophilia has an incidence of 1 or 2 per 100,000 of the population and it is caused by a deficiency of antihemophilic globulin (AGH) or factor VIII in the plasma. It is inherited as a sex-linked recessive character appearing only in males and is transmitted to them by clinically normal female carriers. Females, who always have two X chromosomes, almost always have one normal gene to balance the hemophilic gene. All sons of hemophiliacs are free from the hemophiliac gene and all daughters are carriers. When the female marries a normal man half the sons are hemophiliacs and half the daughters are carriers (Fig. 14.10). If a hemophiliac carrier marries a hemophiliac, it is possible for their daughter to be a hemophiliac.

Normal plasma contains 1 unit of factor VIII per mL, a level defined as 100%. The defective gene on the X chromosome causes a deficiency of factor VIII which can be complete or partial. If the level is 25–50% of normal, the patient has no trouble unless he

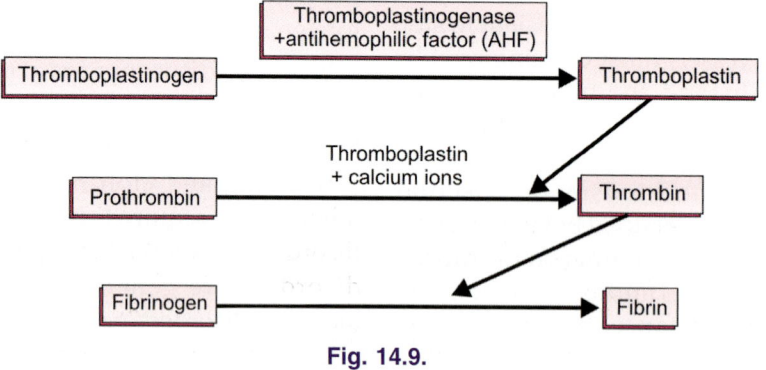

Fig. 14.9.

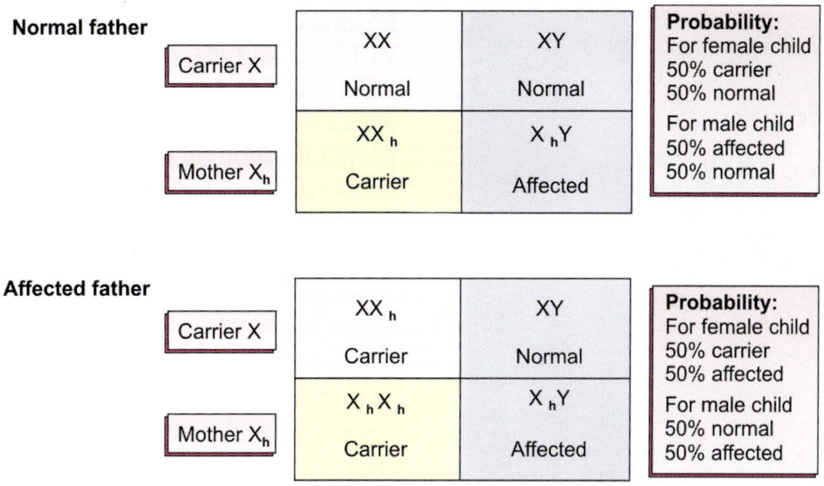

	Normal father			
Carrier X		XX Normal	XY Normal	**Probability:** For female child 50% carrier 50% normal
Mother X$_h$		XX$_h$ Carrier	X$_h$Y Affected	For male child 50% affected 50% normal

	Affected father			
Carrier X		XX$_h$ Carrier	XY Normal	**Probability:** For female child 50% carrier 50% affected
Mother X$_h$		X$_h$X$_h$ Carrier	X$_h$Y Affected	For male child 50% normal 50% affected

Fig. 14.10: Hemophilia is inherited as a sex-linked recessive character

suffers from major trauma. Minor injuries do not bleed normally owing to the fact that the hemostatic function is quantitative and what is enough for minor injuries is insufficient for major trauma (Fig. 14.11). At levels of 10–25% more serious bleeding occurs after minor injuries and below 10% bleeding into muscles and joint occurs (Figs 14.12 and 14.13). The blood coagulation time is normal with factor VIII levels above 1–2%, but the severe hemophiliac usually has 0% factor VIII.

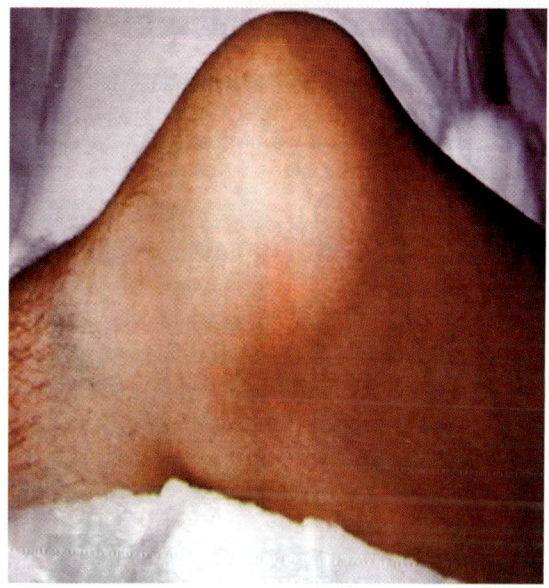

Fig. 14.12: Acute hemarthrosis of the knee is a common complication of hemophilia. It may be confused with acute infection unless the patient's coagulation disorder is known, because the knee is hot, red, swollen and painful

The Investigation of a Hemophiliac Requiring Oral Surgery

The investigation of a suspected case of hemophilia requires the services of a skilled hematologist and once the missing factor in the coagulating mechanism has been identified and the patient can be rendered fit for surgery by injecting the missing factor intravenously. The clotting time in hemophilia is not prolonged until the level of AHG falls below 1% and a relatively normal reading could prove most deceptive to the surgeon (Table 14.3). The only safe test for hemophilia

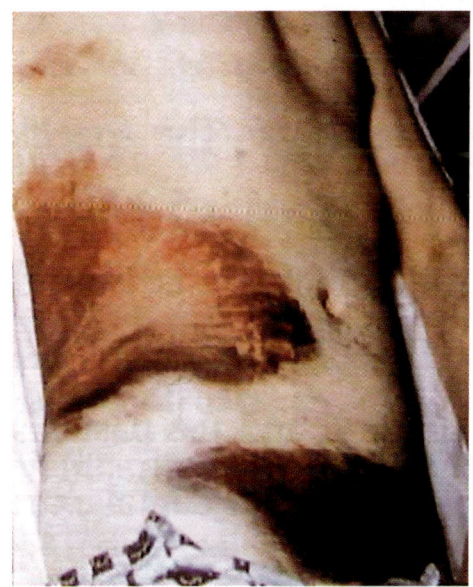

Fig. 14.11: Massive hematomas in a patient with hemophilia. In the absence of major trauma, hematomas of this size always indicate a severe coagulation abnormality. Possible causes include hemophilia, Christmas disease, von Willebrand's disease and uncontrolled anticoagulant therapy. Internal bleeding is a common accompaniment and patients require urgent investigation and treatment

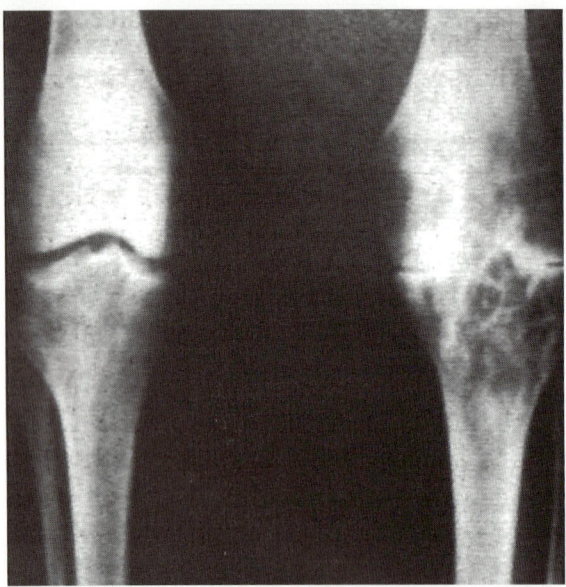

Fig. 14.13. X-ray of the knees in a patient with hemophilia. The left knee has been severely damaged by recurrent hemarthrosis. Note the narrowing of the joint space, the presence of irregular erosions and the evidence of cyst formation in the tibial head

is to estimate the AHG level in the patient and this requires the services of a specially equipped laboratory.

It should be remembered that unless the patient has a 0% concentration of AHG, coagulation could eventually occur and if, for example, the coagulation time is half an hour, gentle pressure for just over half an hour will eventually succeed in staunching the flow. Normally, the missing factor will of course have been replaced by the intravenous route shortly before operation and so coagulation can be confidentially expected in a comparatively short time. It is generally observed that a level of 20% factor VIII falling to 5% is adequate for minor injuries and single tooth extraction (i.e. use of plasma). More serious trauma such as multiple extractions require 40% falling to 10% which can be achieved with human AHG. Major

trauma or surgery will probably require a 100% factor VIII level and, therefore, animal AHG will have to be used. It should be stressed, however, that most patients become resistant to treatment with the particular animal AHG within 7–10 days of starting treatment and their factor VIII response after transfusion of the dose gradually diminishes.

ii. *Hemophilia B (Christmas Disease)*

Christmas disease has the same inheritance and clinical features as hemophilis, but is about one-tenth as common as hemophilia A and female carriers often have a bleeding tendency and the Christmas factor (factor IX) is much more stable than antihemophiliac globulin and stored blood can be used in its treatment. Cryoprecipitate does not contain factor IX and is not appropriate in the treatment of Christmas disease. Fresh frozen plasma or, if they are available, Factor IX concentrates are used.

The earlier comments on dental management in hemophilia A apply equally to patients with hemophilia B but factor IX replacement is needed before surgery. Human dried factor IX concentrate is supplied as a powder to be reconstituted with distilled water for intravenous administration. A dose of 20 units factor IX per kg body weight is used intravenously one hour preoperatively.

Absorbable hemostatic agents such as oxidized regenerated cellulose (Surgicel) or microcrystalline collagen (Avitene) may be put in the socket to assist clotting.

Antifibrinolytics significantly reduce factor VIII requirements. Tranexamic acid (cyclocaprone) is used in a dose of Ig (30 mg/kg) orally, four times daily starting 24 hours preoperatively. Tranexamic acid used topically significantly reduces the bleeding. Ten ml of 5% solution used as a mouth rinse for 2 minutes, four times daily is recommended. The solution can be made up by diluting 10% tranexamic acid solution for injection, with sterile water.

Table 14.3

Diagnosis	Platelet	BT	PT	PTT
Idopathic thrombocytopenic purpura	Decreased	Prolonged	Normal	Normal
Salicylates	Normal	Prolonged	Normal	Normal
Factor VIII deficiency	Normal	Normal	Abnormal	Normal
Hemophilia classical (IX) Christmas disease	Normal	Normal	Normal	Abnormal
Liver disease	Normal	Normal	Abnormal	Abnormal
Coumarin	Normal	Normal	Abnormal	Abnormal
Heparin	Normal	Normal	Abnormal	Abnormal

Suturing (though theoretically unnecessary) is desirable to stabilize gum flaps and to prevent postoperative disturbance of wound by eating. Nonresorbable sutures are preferred and should be removed at 4–7 days.

Prevention of infection: Antimicrobials such as oral penicillin V 250 mg four times daily should be given postoperatively for a full course of 7 days to reduce the risk of secondary hemorrhage. Infection also appears to induce fibrinolysis.

Postoperatively, care should be taken to watch for hematoma formation which may manifest itself by swelling, dysphagia, or hoarseness. The patent airway must always be ensured.

Intramuscular injections should be avoided unless replacement therapy is being given, as they can cause large hematomas. Oral alternatives are in many cases satisfactory.

iii. *Pseudohemophilia (von Willebrand's Disease)*

The diagnosis of von Willebrand's disease is based on the findings of a prolonged bleeding time clinically, a decreased platelet adhesiveness and a decreased titre of antihemophilic factor. The primary defect in this disease is related to the adhesiveness of the platelet that is, a disturbance at the enzymatic level which renders the platelet inefficient in the very early phase of plugging off the severed or injured vessel.

The disease affects both males and females; approximately one-third have a positive family history of prolonged bleeding. Bleeding evidences itself in the mucous membranes, as skin ecchymosis, joints and menorrhagia and occurs after trauma. Pregnancy frequently offers remission until term. Transfusion of fresh plasma helps to correct the defect and in some cases adrenocorticosteroids have been found to provide significant temporary improvement.

Dental Extraction in a Hemophiliac on Outpatient Basis

The management of the hemophiliac is essentially a hematological problem which consists of an exact diagnosis of the condition followed by replacement of the missing factor. There are, however, certain additional steps which should be taken by the oral surgeon. The most likely operation to be performed is of course the extraction of a tooth or teeth for no one would advocate more major surgery unless it was absolutely vital (Plate XIX-iii).

Every effort should be made to conserve teeth and no more extractions should be carried out than are absolutely essential. The following scheme is of value to be considered when a dental procedure is carried out (Box 14.6):

1. Transfusing the patient with a deficient factor level up to 20% on the day of the surgery.
2. The tooth is extracted as soon as possible after this infusion.
3. Antibiotics are routinely given prophylactically.
4. The local anesthetic is administered by periradicular infiltration (periodontal injection) in the four quadrants around the root.

   Mandibular block injections are contraindicated, the difficulty is that when a local anesthetic is given, the needle can grip invisible vessels deep in the tissues.

   Persistent hemorrhage into the parapharyngeal tissues may occur. Death following a mandibular block injection has been reported. Local infiltration causes bleeding at each point where the needle is inserted (Plate XIX-ii) and the only absolute safe site for injection is down the periodontal membrane. This is painful and infection could be introduced, by the needle, but it gives good analgesia and the area is to be disrupted by the forceps beaks any way.

5. The tooth to be removed should be extracted as atraumatically as possible, without using mucoperiosteal flap, after which the sides of the socket are gently squeezed together gently.
6. The socket should not be sutured for not only would the needle wounds bleed but blood which could not escape into the mouth would merely be directed down the facial planes of the neck. If the patient does bleed postoperatively, it is preferable for the blood to flow into the mouth where it can be seen and be treated.
7. After removal, a piece of Surgicel or gelfoam, dusted with powdered bovine thrombin, is placed in the apical portion of the root socket. Also a small pledget of folded gauze sponge saturated with topical epinephrine or other local hemostatic agent should be placed over the socket. Sutures are not used unless it is necessary to mobilize a flap for the removal of the tooth.
8. An initial dose of epsilon-aminocaproic acid (EACA) is given immediately after the

Box 14.6: Dental management of the patient with hemophilia*

Postoperative	Operative	Dental	Preoperative
• Advice the patient to consume cold liquids and soft foods until bleeding stops and avoid using a straw because it promotes sucking and consequent clot displacement	• Use good surgical technique	• There is no contraindication to any local . anesthetics	• Hematology consult Confirmation of diagnosis and severity of disease Presence of inhibitors (antibodies to factor VIII)
• Prescribe amicar or cyclocapron orally or as mouthwash, to minimize postoperative factor transfusion.	• Use reabsorbable sutures because they retain less plaque and, therefore, cause less inflammation at the surgical site.	• Treat any acute oral infection.	• Patients with mild to moderate hemophilia are usually treated in the dental setting
• Depending on the procedures done and the gravity of the hemophilia, factor replacement is necessary. Factor VIII is given q 12 h and factor IX is given q 24 h.	• Use pressure packs (mild cases)	• Establish good oral hygiene.	• Patients with severe hemophilia and those with inhibitors are usually treated in the hospital
• Patients treated in the dental office may require second dose of DDAVP or replacement factor	• Use Gelfoam with thrombin to control bleeding and/or other agents	• Construct splints for patients with moderate to severe hemophilia who are having multiple extractions	• The more invasive the procedure, the more likely the patient will be treated in the hospital – Confirm with the hematologist, if preoperative DDAVP (stimate) use will suffice.
• Hospitalized patients will require additional doses of DDAVP, factor VIII, or other agents. Patients given factor VIII replacement must be examined for signs of allergy.	• Place palatal splints (moderate and severe cases)	• Factor VIII levels must be raised to 50% of normal for block anesthesia.	– Confirm route and time of administration for preoperative use. Surgery will begin in 30–60 min with IV use, in 60–90 min with intranasal use, and in 0.9–1.5 hr with oral use. DDAVP can minimize Factor VIII use in some patients.
• Examine patient 24–48 hours after surgery for the following: – Signs of infection—treat, if present – Bleeding—Use local measures to control; if not effective, use other systemic measures as indicated – Healing	• Hematologist will monitor treatment of hospitalized patients		– Confirm with the hematologist when the factor replacement should be done. It is usually done 15 min prior to most surgical procedures.
• Avoid aspirin, aspirin-containing compounds and NSAIDs			• Management recommendation – DDAVP 0.3 µg/kg (maximal dose, 20 to 24 µg), given parenterally, 1 hour before the procedure
• Acetaminophen with or without codeine is suggested for most patients			– EACA 6 g every 6 hours, orally, for 3 to 4 days
• Provide antibiotic coverage with penicillin 250–500 mg qid or clindamycin 150–300 mg tid/qid (in the presence of penicillin allergy) for 5 days.			– Factor VIII replacement-Loading, 0 or 30–40 U/kg, IV; maintenance, 10–40 U/kg, IV every 12 hours

APCC, Activated prothrombin complex concentration; DDAVP 1-desmino 8 D-arginine vasopressin; EACA, e-aminocaproic acid; IV, Intravenous; NSAIDs, nonsteroidal anti-inflammatory drugs; PCC, prothrombin complex concentrate.

extraction. This is used to prevent lysis of the initial clot. An initial dose of 5 mg for adults or 2.5 mg for children is used. Subsequent doses of half that amount are given every six hours around the clock for 10 days.

9. The postextraction diet is extremely important, and for the first 24 hours nothing is taken except a syrup containing the EACA. For the next 48 hours, limited amount of cold, clear liquids (no dairy products) are consumed. After 72 hours, for the next week, foods with the consistency of apple sauce or malted milk are allowed. Chewing of food is not permitted.

10. Daily contact with the patient is maintained. If bleeding persists, necessitating replacement therapy, then dietary control resumes with a clear liquid for an additional 10 days.

Dental Extraction in a Hemophiliac in the Hospital

In the hospital, the patient should be subjected to the following regime:

1. On the morning of operation, the patient is given a cryoprecipitate or lyophilized human AHG sufficient to raise his factor VIII level to 50% of the normal, this usually represents 30 to 40 units of factor VIII per kg/body weight.

2. At the same time the patient is given tranexamic acid IV, which is repeated 6 hourly by mouth for 7 to 10 days. Under these circumstances, clotting formation should be adequate.

3. The patient usually also is given oral penicillin six-hourly for 70–10 days to prevent infection.

4. *Anesthesia:* When the patient is receiving fresh plasma, local anesthesia may be safely used without fear of a hematoma developing. In some ways, local anesthesia is preferable to general anesthesia, for bleeding could occur at the back of the throat and the region of the glottis as a result of passing an endotracheal tube. When general anesthesia is contemplated, an oral-endotracheal tube is used instead of risking nasal trauma and bleeding with a nasoendotraheal tube.

5. Following extraction, there is usually no need to suture the socket, though, as with many other patients, the socket margins should be squeezed firmly together to approximate the socket margins as closely as possible.

6. The patient should be on absolute bed-rest and should be nursed in the sitting position, or the head of the bed is elevated to about 30°.

7. To prevent breakdown of the clot by muscular movement, the mandible hould be immobilized by applying a barrel bandage.

8. Warm liquid diet should be ordered.

9. The patient should not have hot drinks.

10. The patient should best be in a room on his own so that the bleeding is not started by excessive talking.

11. Visitors should be kept away for the same reason.

12. Atropine is indicated to reduce salivation and expectoration.

13. In order to endure this regime, the patient should be sedated with phenobarbitone 30 mg twice daily(b.d).

14. Factor VIII or cryoprecipitate is not given again unless clotting fails and the patient starts to bleed again. It has to emphasis that antihemophilic globulin is very labile, its half-life in circulation is said to be 10 to 12 hours.

15. Adrenocorticosteroids are of benefit and are used as an adjunct in the treatment of the hemophilic patient undergoing dental surgery. Beginning preoperatively and continuing for a period of 7 to 14 days, prednisone (20 mg 3 or 4 times per day) appears to enhance the postoperative retention of the original clot and reduce the length of hospital stay and the amount of transfusion necessary. It seems that adrenocorticosteroids modify the vascular bed and decrease revascularization and in this manner helps control bleeding in the hemophilic patient.

16. It needs hardly be added that such analgesics as aspirin are absolutely contraindicated in view of the danger of severe hematemesis and even in small doses aspirin is known to impair platelet aggregation and this added hemostatic defect in the hemophiliac can make him prone to bleed. As an alternative to aspirin as an analgesic, paracetamol or dihydrocodiene may prove effective.

Preparations Containing Factor VIII

The treatment of hemophilia is essentially a problem for the hematologist, first by, diagnosing the exact nature of the disorder and then by replacing the missing factor in the blood, it may be possible to render the patient relatively normal so far as the surgery is concerned. The blood level can be raised by the injection of various substances, but the effect is short lived. The preparations which contain factor VIII are:

1. Fresh whole blood.
2. Fresh or frozen plasma.
3. Cryoprecipitate prepared from human plasma.
4. Freeze-dried animal AHG (antihemophilic globulin).
5. Freeze-dried human AHG (antihemophilic globulin).

Fresh whole blood and plasma have low concentrations of factor VIII and as one can only give a certain volume without overloading the circulation, only a limited blood level can be attained. The policy, therefore, should be to give blood transfusions only to replace blood loss and not to use as a source of factor VIII. The best factor VIII level which can be attained with whole blood is 5–7% and with frozen or fresh plasma 15–20%. By using human AHG a, level of 50–60% can be obtained and a level of 60–100% can be attained by using animal AHG. There is a shortage of human AHG and the supplies are inadequate for the demand, but the animal AHG which is derived from ox or pig blood is readily available. Unfortunately, this material is a foreign protein and is antigenic and if the treatment with this agent is unduly protracted and the patient will develop resistance and there also be a loss of therapeutic effect and probably an allergy will develop. Animal AHG should, therefore, be reserved for emergencies.

Cryoprecipitate and fresh frozen plasma are the preparations usually used to cover exodontias. One of the two preparations, cryoprecipitate is the more concentrated (anything from 5–15 times more concentrated) so that higher blood levels of AHG are more easily obtained and there is less risk of overloading in the circulation, particularly in a child. Further cryoprecipitate can be given intravenously with a syringe, while fresh frozen plasma requires an intravenous infusion. Plastic bags containing 5–20 ml of plasma are in use and concentration are between 15 and 45 New Oxford units per ml. Each pack will, on average, increase the level of factor VIII in the blood of a 70 kg man by 3.5% so that about 8–10 packs may be needed preoperatively. While much AHG is lost in the preparation the technique is comparatively simple compared with the preparation of dried human AHG. The excess of fibrinogen does not normally matter.

The half-life of injected factor VIII in the body is about 12 hours and 24 hours after an injection it will be down to a quarter of its immediate post-injection level.

Cryoprecipitate is prepared by freezing fresh plasma at a sufficiently low temperature. Antihemophilic factor together with fibrinogen and other proteins come out of solution (precipitated) and can be separated from the rest of the plasma by centrifugation. The cryoprecipitate which has been separated in this way contains most of the antihemophilic factor and is collected in plastic bags and stored in a deep freeze at –20°C. This concentrate of anti-hemophilic factor has to be thawed at 37°C and reconstituted in sterile fashion before use and this is somewhat time consuming. The reconstituted cryoprecipitate can be given as a single injection or by an infusion through a drip set, depending on the volume required.

Human Antihemophilic Factor

It is a protein concencentrate rich in factor VIII which can be stored in a freeze-dried state in a refrigerator at–4°C for more than a year without significant loss of factor VIII activity. This preparation can be reconstituted immediately before use by adding sterile pyrogen-free distilled water. The advantages of freeze-dried human AHF over cryoprecipitate are that the factor VIII content of the material is known, the preparation can be reconstituted easily and rapidly, it is stable for long periods even in domestic refrigerator and finally it allows a relatively high concentration of factor VIII to be given in an injection of very small volume. The main disadvantage of purified human antihemophilic factor, apart from its enormous cost, is the fact that it is made from large pools of plasma and this has the risk of transmitting hepatitis.

B. Hypoprothrombinemia (Prothrombin Deficiency)

Liver Disease and Blood Clotting

Proper blood clotting depends on normal liver function for two reasons. First, the liver synthesizes most of the clotting factors. Therefore, diseases such as hepatitis, cirrhosis and cancer that degrade liver function result in a deficiency of clotting factors. Second, the synthesis of clotting factors II, VII, IX and X requires vitamin K. The absorption of vitamin K from the diet requires bile, a liver secretion. Gallstones can lead to a clotting deficiency by obstructing the bile duct and thus interfering with bile secretion and vitamin K absorption. Efficient blood clotting is especially important in childbirth, since both the mother and infant bleed from the trauma of birth. Therefore, pregnant women should take vitamin K supplements to ensure fast clotting, and newborn infants may be given vitamin K injections. The lack of factor VIII causes classical hemophilia (hemophilia A), which accounts for about 83% of cases and afflicts 1 in 5,000 males worldwide. Lack of factor IX causes hemophilia B, which accounts for 15% of cases and occurs in about 1 out of 30,000 males. Factors VIII and IX are, therefore, known as antihemophilic factors A and B. A rarer form called hemophilia C (factor XI deficiency) is autosomal, not sex-linked, so it occurs equally in both sexes.

The liver produces most of the protein coagulation factors thus, any patient with significant liver disease may have a bleeding problem. In addition to possible disorder in coagulation, the patient with liver disease who develops portal hypertension and hypersplenism may be thrombocytopenic as a result of splenic overactivity, which leads to increased sequestration of platelets in the spleen.

Prothrombin deficiencies are both congenital and acquired. The congenital variety does not respond to vitamin K. Acquired hypoprothrombinemias respond well to the therapeutic use of vitamin K. Vitamin K is not water-soluble and is available as an emulsion for intramuscular or intravenous use. The water-soluble preparations available today, such as Aquamephyton, Synkavite, and Hykinone, do not require bile salts for their absorption and utilization.

Any condition that so disrupts the intestinal flora that vitamin K is not produced in sufficient amounts will result in a decreased plasma level of the vitamin K-dependent coagulation factors. Vitamin K is needed by the liver to produce prothrombin (factor II) and factors VII, IX, and X. Prothrombin is produced in the liver and vitamin K (napthaquinone) is required for its synthesis. There are two sources of vitamin K—an exogenous source in the diet and an endogenous source from the intestine where it is synthesized by certain bacteria. Vitamin K is not properly absorbed in the absence of bile-salts. Biliary tract obstruction, malabsorption syndrome, and excessive use of broad-spectrum antibiotics can lead to low levels of prothrombin and factors VII, IX and X on this basis.

Clinical prothrombin deficiency is, therefore, seen in:

1. Newborn babies in whose intestines the vitamin-K forming organisms have not yet become established, i.e. hemorrhagic disease of newborn. This condition can be largely prevented by giving intramuscular vitamin K either to the mother before birth or to the baby as soon as it is borne.

2. Patients with obstructive jaundice who should also be given vitamin K analogues, if any surgical operation is contemplated, otherwise serious hemorrhage occurs.

3. Patients in whom the vitamin K-forming organisms have been greatly reduced as a result of protracted therapy with broad-spectrum antibiotics, or who are washed out through severe dysenteries. In these patients, vitamin K production may be inadequate and so again hemorrhage may occur. The conditions also can be corrected by administering water-soluble vitamin K analogues.

4. Patients with severe liver damage as a result of hepatitis, multiple metastasis, etc. in whom again there is a failure to produce prothrombin, but this condition is not wholly dependent on the lack of vitamin K and may be improved, but cannot be corrected by its administration.

5. Conditions of extreme malnutrition.

6. Patients receiving an oral anticoagulant.

7. Patients suffering from fatty diarrhea, e.g. celiac disease.

The main importance to the oral surgeon of all these conditions is that he should be aware of the possibility of severe hemorrhage following even minor surgery when working upon any of these categories of patients. Water-soluble vitamin-K analogues i.m. for three days preoperatively may be helpful in such cases.

Vitamin K promotes the formation of prothrombin by the liver. The use of vitamin K preparations orally or intravenously should be reserved for valid evidence that the prothrombin level is decreased or that there is some deficiency. The vitamin K deficiency can become significant only when the synthesis of the vitamin K by intestinal bacteria is markedly reduced by altered flora (antibiotics, etc.), or completely absent from the patient's intake. Severe liver disease may cause hypoprothrombinemia from the injury of the hepatic cells and may not respond to the administration of vitamin K. The use of vitamin K in patients under anticoagulant therapy must be done with consultation. The prophylactic use of vitamin K for patients with somewhat depressed prothrombin levels who are not on anticoagulant therapy is good practice.

DISEASES DUE TO THROMBOCYTOPENIA

Platelets (thrombocytes) are small formed elements in the circulating blood about one-fourth the size of a red blood corpuscles. They are formed in the reticuloendothelial system, primarily in bone marrow. Healthy platelets are essential to the effective coagulation of blood. They contain several factors which are integral parts of the coagulation system. Platelets are altered or modified by, many dietary hormonal, drug and mechanical or environmental stimuli. Any of these modifications in normal platelet function or availability would have an effect upon the coagulation system.

There is approximately one platelet to every twenty red cells in normal conditions. The normal platelet count is from 200,000 to 400,000. A real diminution of platelets with counts persistently under 100,000 constitutes thrombocytopenia.

Thrombocytopenia is a decrease in the number of circulating platelets. *A real increase in platelets with counts persistently above 500,000 constitutes* **thrombocythemia.** *Spontaneous bleeding may occur with platelet counts of less than 50,000. Severe bleeding may occur with platelet counts of less than 20,000.*

Bleeding manifestations do not usually occur until the count has fallen to less than 60,000 mm³. Thrombocytopenia may be subdivided into two broad categories—one in which the cause is unknown, idiopathic thrombocytopenia purpura and one in which the cause is known, e.g. secondary thrombocytopenia.

i. Idiopathic Thrombocytopenia

This is a rare disease of young adults characterized by episodes of skin purpura, epistaxis and alimentary and urinary hemorrhage. The disease, is based upon a depletion in the number of platelets, is frequently caused by the presence of circulating antiplatelet antibodies. The platelet count is low (below 40,000 per c mm) and the bleeding time is prolonged but the coagulation time is normal. Temporary remissions are obtained by treatment with corticosteroids. A majority of these patients are improved by splenectomy.

Bleeding in thrombocytopenia is excessive after even minor trauma so that tiny wounds such as needle punctures can bleed for prolonged periods, or give rise to a spreading hematoma. Widespread bruising and petechial hemorrhages are also characteristic of a platelet deficiency or abnormality rather than a clotting defect (Figs 14.14 to 14.18). There are also a number of diseases in which the platelets are normal in number but abnormal in function. Salicylates is among the drugs which may cause thrombocytopenia. If possible, oral surgery should be deferred

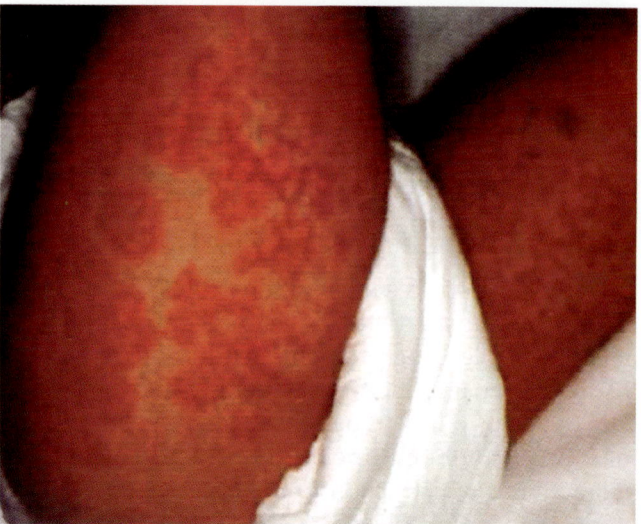

Fig. 14.14: Petechial subcutaneous bleeding is characteristic of thrombocytopenia

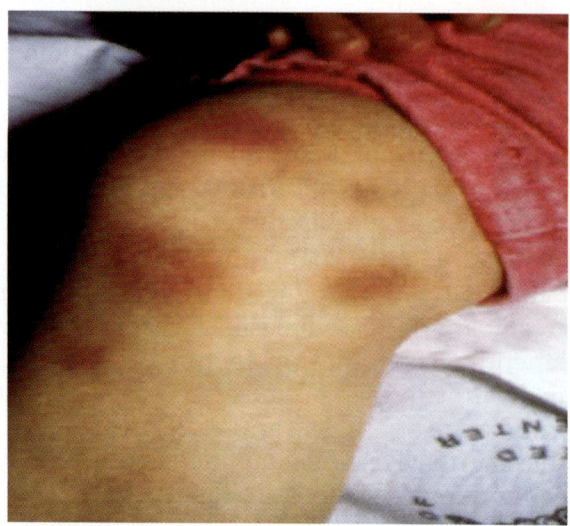

Fig. 14.15: Bruising around the knee joint due to platelet deficiency

until the platelet count can be improved with steroid therapy. Postoperative bleeding may require transfusions with fresh whole blood or transfusion of packed platelets.

ii. Secondary Thrombocytopenia

It may occur as a result of decreased marrow production (marrow infilteration, alcoholism, viral), decreased platelet survival as drugs (e.g. NSAIDs) (Box 14.7), increased platelet consumption (hemolytic uremic syndrome, meningococcus), platelet sequestration (hypersplenism, hypothermia) and platelet loss (hemorrhage). Collectively thrombo-

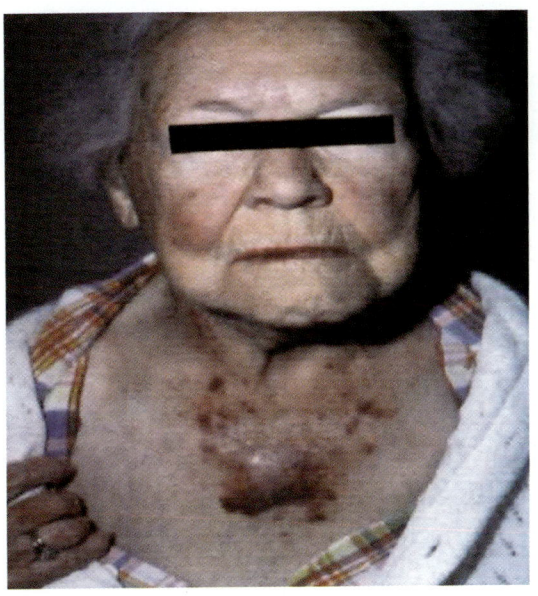

Fig. 14.16: Thrombocytopenic purpura and ecchymosis may involve any part of the body

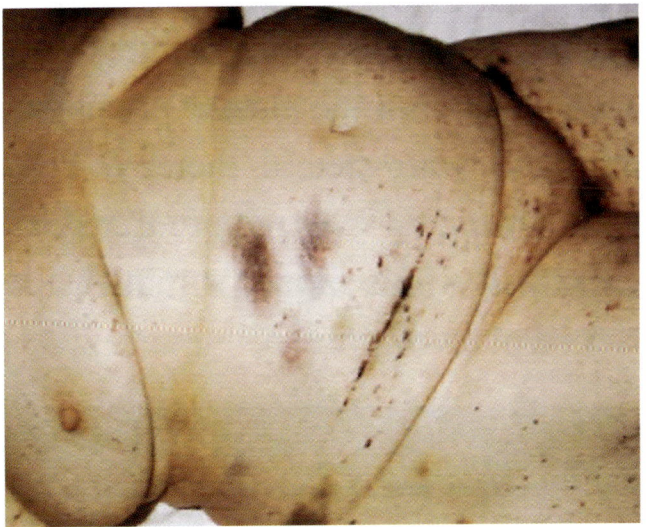

Fig. 14.17: Diffuse purpuric rash with areas of sheet hemorrhage (ecchymosis) in a patient with thrombocytopenia of unknown cause

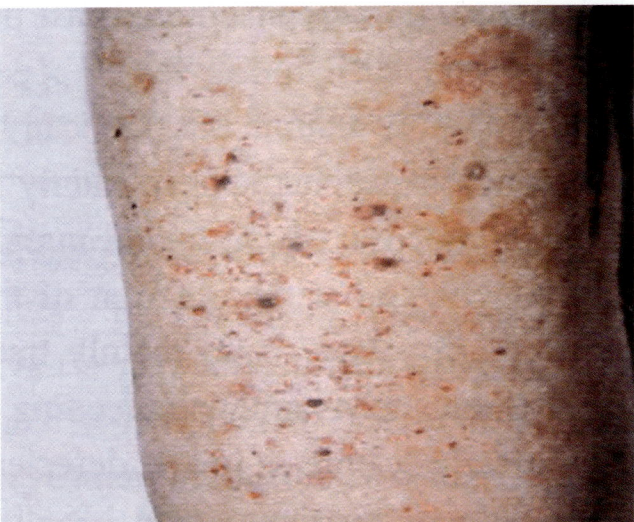

Fig. 14.18: Acute idiopathic thrombocytopenic purpura commonly manifests itself with purpuric lesions of this kind, though they may often be more widespread by the time the patient seeks medical attention. It is important to remember that purpura of identical appearance may result from many other causes

2. Leukemia, lymphoma, or bone marrow tumors.
3. HIV, mumps, rubella, or parvovirus infections.
4. Sequestration of the platelets by an enlarged spleen. Acute or chronic liver disease is the leading cause for an enlarged spleen.

Manifestations of Thrombocytopenia

Spontaneous gingival bleeding, oral petechiae and ecchymosis may appear, mainly at sites of trauma but they can be spontaneous. Petechiae appear mainly in the buccal mucosa, on the lateral margin of the tongue and at the junction of the hard and soft palates—sites mainly traumatied. Spontaneous gingival bleeding is often an early feature in platelet deficiencies or defects. Postextraction bleeding may be a problem, the, management of such cases in association with oral surgical and maxillofacial procedures is categorized in Box 14.9.

3. DISEASES DUE TO ABNORMALITY OF CAPILLARIES

Purpura may be seen in any of the acute fevers, especially meningococcal infections and can also occur as a result of drug sensitivity with agents such as heavy metals, sodium salicylate, isoniazid, thiouracil, cholopromazine, etc. Senile purpura occurs in elderly and purpura also occurs as a result of avitaminosis (scurvy).

cytopenia may result secondary to leukemia; cytotoxic drugs; or unwanted effects of drugs, notably aspirin and chloramphenicol. Remember that aspirin is the most common acquired cause, its effect being irreversible for 1 week.

Collectively, the following are causes of secondary thrombocytopenia:

1. Drugs as heparin, chemotherapeutic agents, alcohol.

Box 14.7: Causes of secondary thrombocytopenia

1. Drugs
   A. Myelosuppressive agents used in therapy of neoplastic disease. These drugs, when used in sufficient dosage, will cause thrombocytopenia in all patients.
   B. Drugs causing thrombocytopenia as a side effect on an individual patient-sensitivity basis, usually by inducing autoimmunity. Those drugs which might be used by the dentist which have been frequently implicated are sedatives (barbiturates), analgesics (phenylbutazone, salicylates), antimicrobials (sulfonamides), antihistamines (diphenhydramine hydrochloride) and tranquilizers (meprobamate).
2. Diseases
   A. Infections—viral, bacterial.
   B. Metabolic—uremia, megaloblastic anemias
   C. Neoplastic—carcinoma, leukemia, sarcoma, lymphoma.
   D. Bone marrow replacement or destruction other than neoplastic—myelofibrosis, radiation therapy

Box 14.8: Some drugs that may cause abnormal platelet function

Manifestations of thrombocytopenia and management of surgery	
Non-steroidal anti-inflammatory drugs	• Aspirin • Diclofenac • Ibuprofen
β-lactam antibiotics	• Ampicillin and derivatives • Methicillin • Penicillin G (benzyl penicillin) • Cephalosporins (some)
General anesthetic agents	• Halothane
Antihistaminics	• Some

Box 14.9: Manifestations of thrombocytopenia and management of surgery

Platelet count (×109/1)	Severity of thrombocytopenia	Manifestations	Management in relation to type of oral surgery	
			Dentoalveolar	Maxillofacial
100–150	Mild	• Mild purpura • Sometimes Slightly prolonged in postoperative bleeding	• No platelet transfusion • Local hemostatic measures • Observe	• Consider platelet transfusion • Local hemostatic measures • Observe
50–100	Moderate	• Purpura • Postoperative bleeding	• Platelets may be needed • Local hemostatic measures • Consider postoperative tranexamic acid mouthwash for 3 days.	• Platelets needed • Local hemostatic measures • Postoperative tranexamic acid mouthwash for 3 days.
30–50	Severe	• Purpura • Postoperative bleeding, even from vene puncture	• Platelets needed • Local hemostatic measures • Postoperative tranexamic acid mouthwash for 3 days	• Platelets needed • Local hemostatic measures • Avoid surgery where possible • Postoperative tranexamic acid mouthwash for 3 days.
<30	Life-threatening	• Purpura • Spontaneous bleeding	• Platelets needed • Local hemostatic measures • Avoid surgery where possible • Postoperative tranexamic acid mouthwash for 3 days.	• Platelets needed • Local hemostatic measures • Avoid surgery where possible • Postoperative tranexamic acid mouthwash for 3 days

Vitamin C is used to maintain capillary integrity. Being water-soluble, it is rapidly depleted, if the patient's diet is markedly altered, such as after the removal of four impacted third molars. While not dramatic in its effect, this substance will make noticeable differences in the oozing of the marginal patient. It has an effect upon the availability of the mesenchymal cementum substance and, therefore, alters hemostasis. A minimum of 500 mg per day of vitamin C should be prescribed. It is good to start the day before surgery and continue for five days after the procedure is finished or the oozing has terminated.

Capillary Fragility

The blood pressure cuff is inflated to half-way between the systolic and the diastolic pressure for 10 minutes. The forearm is examined 5 minutes after removal of the cuff for petechiae (Fig. 14.19). Normally, an area the size of a 25% piece on the volar surface of the forearm will show up to 20 petechiae. The other arm is used as a control and examined as well.

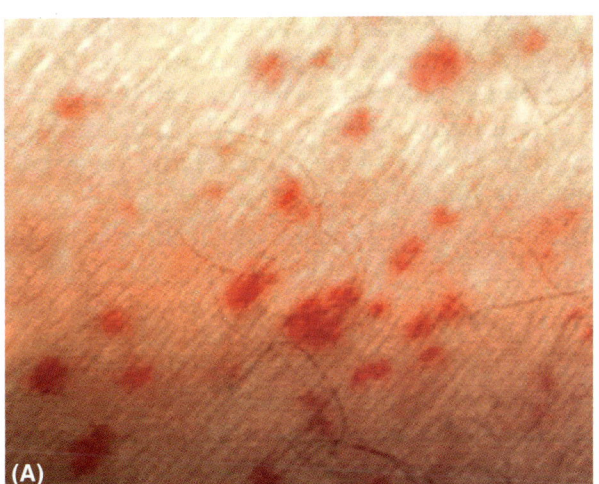 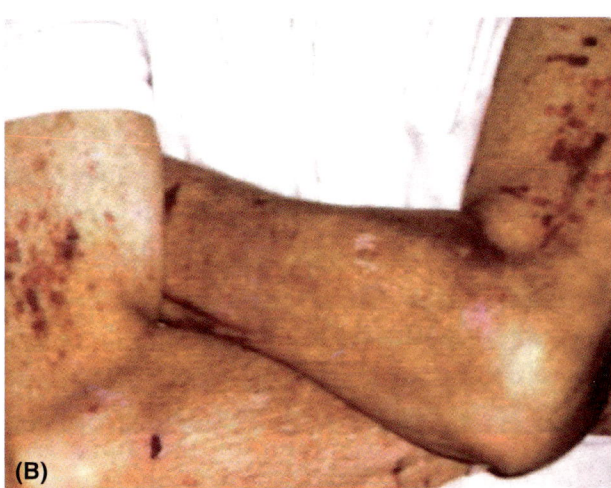

Fig. 14.19: Petechiae and ecchymosis in a patient that may signal a bleeding disorder

DRUGS INDUCED HEMORRHAGE (ANTICOAGULANTS)

- Heparin and warfarin are the main anticoagulants used in clinical practice.
- Heparin can only be given parenterally and acts by increasing the activity of antithrombin III.
- The onset of heparin-induced anticoagulation is rapid and the effects are reversed by protamine sulfate.
- Low molecular weight heparin (LMWHs) have less effect on thrombin than standard heparin and are associated with fewer unwanted effects.
- Warfarin is the main oral anticoagulant that inhibits the vitamin K-dependant factors (II, VII, IX and X).
- Warfarin has a long half-life (37–38 hours) and is extensively protein bound.
- Onset of anticoagulation with warfarin can take up to 16 hours due to the variable rate of synthesis of the clotting proteins.
- Anticoagulant effects of warfarin are assessed by the INR, which should be in the range of 2 to 4.
- The anticoagulant effects of warfarin are reversed by vitamin K, and excessive bleeding may also require the use of fresh frozen plasma.
- Warfarin is often implicated in drug interactions; especially those that involve displacement from the plasma-protein binding site, or that inhibit metabolism of the drug.

INDICATIONS OF ANTICOAGULANTS

Anticoagulant drugs are generally prescribed for the treatment of people suffering from thromboembolic disease, e.g.

1. Thrombophlebitis.
2. Embolic cerebral vascular accidents and transient ischemic attacks.
3. Prevention of mural thrombus formation

4. Atrial fibrillation to prevent clot formation in the atrial appendage.
5. Coronary artery bypass graft surgery.
6. Cardiac valve replacement.
7. Vascular reconstruction and microvascular surgery.
8. Hemodialysis for renal failure.
9. History of pulmonary emboli.
10. Congenital or acquired hypercoagulable states.

Consultation with the physician responsible for the anticoagulant therapy and extreme postoperative vigilance over this patient for a period of six to eight hours following surgery for any possible bleeding complications are absolutely essential.

TYPES OF ANTICOAGULANTS

Basically, anticoagulants come under two major categories: heparin and related drugs and those of the coumarin family.

A. Heparin

Heparin is naturally occurring in minute accounts in mast cells. It:

1. Blocks the conversion of fibrinogen to fibrin.
2. Retards the formation of thrombin from prothrombin by interfering with the activity of thromboplastin. Heparin acts as an antithrombotic factor to depress the formation of fibrin. Heparin interferes with blood coagulation at several stages of the cascade reaction, which is mediated through the plasma cofactor, resulting in a substance which inactivates thromboplastin. These reactions are due to the drug enhancing the activity of antithrombin III, which is a glycosated polypeptide synthetized in the liver. Antithrombin III neutralizes several of the activated clotting factors, namely factors IXa, Xa, XIa, and XIIa. It also inactivates prothrombin (II) by forming an irreversible complex with this clotting protein. Heparin facilitates the inhibitory action of antithrombin III by at least 1000-fold, thus acting as a catalyst template. The long-term use of heparin therapy is associated with a depletion of antithrombin III; this decreases the effect of subsequent heparin therapy.
3. *Decreases platelet adhesiveness:* Because it is highly ionized and is very poorly absorbed from the gut, heparin must be administered parenterally. It is metabolized in the liver by the enzyme heparinase

and the metabolites excreted via the kidney. Low doses of heparin can be given subcutaneously, but high doses should be given via a slow intravenous infusion. Intramuscular injections of heparin should be avoided because large hematomas can form at the site of injection.

After intravenous administration, heparin has an immediate onset of action and a half-life of between 1–5 hours. The higher the dose, the longer the half-life, since metabolism is readily saturated. Patients under dialysis treatment are kept on heparin therapy, if they wait until the day after dialysis, these patients can receive invasive dental treatment. Heparin is bound to a number of plasma proteins thereby decreasing its bioactivity. Heparin activity is assayed via partial thromboplastin time (PTT) or by clotting time. The action of heparin is rapidly reversed by protamine sulfate.

Heparin is used almost exclusively in a hospital setting. Given the indication for its use, it is likely that oral surgery to be performed on heparinized patients will be of an emergent nature. The degree of urgency of the procedure must be balanced against the risk of transiently discontinuing heparin therapy. Heparin should be discontinued only an hour or so before an intended procedure, if approved by the patient's physician. Patients requiring longer term anticoagulant therapy are switched to warfarin sodium.

Fragments of heparin with slightly different anticoagulant activity from the parent molecule are now available. They have lower molecular weights and are hence referred to as low molecular weight heparins (LMWHs). The synthetic drug is the only effective, direct acting anticoagulant immediately effective on fresh blood. The low molecular weight heparin has a less protein binding and thus greater bioavailability following subcutaneous injection than standard heparin.

Hemorrhage is the principle unwanted effect associated with heparin, usually occurring from the gastrointestinal or genitourinary tract. Hence heparin should not be given to any patient with a bleeding disorder or ulceration of the gastrointestinal tract.

A mild transient thrombocytopenia is reported in about 25% of patients receiving heparin. However, in a few, thrombocytopenia can be severe and deaths have occurred. Platelet counts should be carried out at regular intervals for all those on heparin therapy. Commercial preparations of heparin are obtained

D. Temporary withholding of the Anticoagulant Therapy

Surgeons who are in favor of withholding the anticoagulant therapy advise that when dental surgery is contemplated and the risk of thrombo-embolic complication appears minimal, the anticoagulant may be stopped and the patient's condition checked by determination of the prothrombin time and the international normalized ratio (INR). It usually takes at least 48 to 72 hours for the anticoagulant effect to be significantly diminished, and another 48 to 72 hours after therapy is reinstituted with Dicumarol products to achieve optimal anticoagulant effect.

The dentist may see patients who are treated on an outpatient basis with an low molecular weight heparin (LMWH), including patients with total hip or knee replacement and those being treated on an outpatient basis for deep thrombi or asymptomatic pulmonary embolism. Elective surgical procedures can be delayed until the patient is taken off the LMWH, which, in most cases, will occur within 3 to 6 months. If an invasive procedure must be performed, the dentist has several options. First, the dentist should consult with the patient's physician regarding the need for and the type of surgery. The half-life of the LMWHs is less than 1 day. **Thus, the physician could suggest that the drug be stopped and the surgery be performed within 1 to 2 days.** The other option is to go ahead with the surgery and deal with any bleeding complications on a local basis. It appears that these patients can undergo minor surgical procedures with little risk for any serious bleeding considerations. **Michael Wahl (1998)** cited that out of 542 documented cases of withdrawal of anticoagulants therapy for dental procedures, 5 patients had serious embolic complications including 4 deaths. Reviewing those 5 cases, however, show that the period of withdrawal of anticoagulants was either unknown or ranged from 5 days of discontinuation to 19 days discontinuation. This is quite an extended period of withdrawal and would in most patients normalize their coagulation status. One wonders, if these complications would have occurred, if the anticoagulation had been stopped for 2 to 3 days so that the international normalized ratio is not normalized, but below therapeutic range. It seems that these 5 cases of normalization of anticoagulation should not make the argument against reduction of anticoagulant therapy. A brief summary concerning the management of patient on anticoagulant therapy is mentioned in Chapter 15, Page 439, "C": Coagulopathy

Box 14.10 summarizes appropriate dental management of the patient who is taking warfarin, or coumadin.

Box 14.10: Dental management of the patient taking warfarin or coumadin for whom invasive procedure are planned

Preoperative
- Medical consult
- Confirmation of diagnosis
- Status of medical condition
- Type of surgery or invasive procedures planned
- Need for dosage reduction
- Based on level of anticoagulation
- Based on amount of expected bleeding
- Confirmation of INR level

Dental
- Free of acute infection—if infection is present, treat prior to providing elective dental care
- Good oral hygiene
- Level of anticoagulation and need to alter dosage to avoid excessive bleeding
- INR, 2.0–3.0—dosage does not have to be altered.
- INR, 3.0–3.5—dosage may be altered, usually will be altered for major oral surgery
- INR greater than 3.5—delay invasive procedure until dosage is decreased
- Decision is made to alter dosage of anticoagulation medication
- Physician will reduce patient's dosage
- Effect of reduced dosage takes 3–5 days
- Dental appointment must be scheduled within 2 days once desired reduction in INR has been confirmed

Operative
- Confirmation of status of INR on day of surgery
- Use of good surgical technique
- Control of bleeding by local means

Postoperative
- Avoid aspirin and NSAIDs
- Acetaminophen can be used with reduced dosage and can be combined with codeine.
- Tell patient to call, if bleeding occurs during first 24–48 hours
- See patient within 48–72 hours and observe for the following:
  – Healing
  – Infection—treat, if present
  – Bleeding—use local means to control, if present
- Patients whose anticoagulant dosage was reduced
  – If free of complications, call patient's physician and have patient returned to normal anticoagulation dosage
  – If not free of complications, treat and then call patient's physician to start normal dosage

INR, International Normalized Ratio; NSAIDs. nonsteroidal anti-inflammatory drugs.

CONTROL OF HEMORRHAGE FOLLOWING DENTAL PROCEDURES

Primarily, detection of the patient who is bleeder is of utmost importance (Box 14.11).

The patient is reassured and seated comfortably on the dental chair. A good source of illumination and suction should be available. Clean the mouth blood and blood debris by gentle irrigation with saline. Examine the area of the extracted tooth to detect the source of bleeding.

Box 14.11: Detection of the patient who is a bleeder

1. *History*
   a. Bleeding problems in relatives
   b. Bleeding problems after operations and tooth extractions
   c. Bleeding problems after trauma (cuts, etc.)
   d. Medications that may cause bleeding problems
      1. Aspirin
      2. Anticoagulants
      3. Long-term antibiotic therapy
      4. Certain herbal preparations
   e. Presence of illnesses that may have associated bleeding problems
      1. Leukemia
      2. Liver disease
      3. Hemophilia
      4. Congenital heart disease
      5. Renal disease—uremia
   f. Spontaneous bleeding from nose, mouth, ears, etc.
2. *Examination findings*
   a. Jaundice, pallor   b. Spider angiomas
   c. Ecchymoses   d. Petechiae
   e. Oral ulcers   f. Hyperplastic gingival tissues
   g. Hemarthrosis
3. *Screening laboratory tests*
   a. PT   b. aPTT
   c. TT   d. PFA-100
   e. Platelet count
4. *Surgical procedure:* Excessive bleeding after surgery may be first clue to underlying bleeding problem.

If bleeding is coming from a nutrient canal, the bleeding point is crushed with the tip of a hemostat in order to close the orifice of the canal. If the bleeding point originates from the socket walls, the socket is packed with one of the local hemostatic agents and the margins of the wound are compressed to allow the blood vessels to retract and contract. If bleeding is from soft tissue laceration, sutures should be applied to approximate the wound margins, thereby minimizing gapping and facilitate clotting.

Both local and systemic methods can be employed to control hemorrhage. Local methods must always be used. Seldom is there the need for systemic methods, but whenever there is an indication for systemic methods, they should be used in conjunction with local measures.

LOCAL METHODS FOR CONTROL OF HEMORRHAGE (BOX 14.12)

The local methods used can be arbitrary grouped as follows: prevention, pressure, cold, hemostatic agents (e.g. epinephrine, Monsel's solution, thrombin, Russel viper venom, tannic acid, gel foam, oxycel, surgical, micrifibrillar collagen—Avitene, bone wax) and tissue adhesives (e.g. fibrin sealant and platelet gel), electrocoagulation and ligation and suture of the injured or severed vessel.

Prevention

Methods to minimize, if not prevent, hemorrhage should be resorted to. Atraumatic surgery, elimination of chronic bleeding granulation tissue, removal of fractured bone spicules, removal of old necrotic clots are suggested measures well worth taking. Preventive therapy is perhaps the most effective form of therapy available to control hemorrhage.

Pressure

This method is perhaps the most effective method and consists of the following:
   a. Compressing the margins of the wound to relieve tension, thus permitting the blood vessels to retract and contract. Allowing the patient to bite on gauze for one hour to aid in collapsing blood vessels and promote blood coagulation.
   b. If hemorrhage is anticipated, it is advisable to fabricate acrylic plate prior to surgery that can be wired in place or worn by the patient over the surgical area. This will create pressure over the bleeding area and will stabilize tissues so that the inadvertent motions of eating and swallowing will not reactivate the bleeding in the capillary bed of the flap. An acrylic plate should be made to cover the wound, hold hemostatic agents and protect the clot. The plate should be comfortable and self-retaining and is more effective than using swabs and a barrel bandage.

Cold Application

Topical ice application, on five minutes and off five minutes for the first four hours, sometimes will help reduce bleeding. However, some tests have shown this

Box 14.12: Topical Hemostatic agents used to control bleeding*

Product	Company	Description	Indications and features
Gauze		2" × 2" sterile gauze pads; place over the wound and have the patient put pressure on it by closing or finger pressure.	Bleeding immediately following extractions or minor surgical procedures.
Gelfoam	Upjohn	Absorbable gelatin sponge made from purified gelatin solution; absorbs for 3–5 days.	Useful for most patients taking an anti-thrombotic agent; helpful to place topical thrombin on Gelfoam; for extensive or invasive surgery, should consider placing inside a splint
Instat	Johnson & Johnson	Absorbable collagen made from purified and lyophilized bovine dermal collagen; can be cut or shaped; adheres to bleeding surfaces when wet, but does not stick to instruments, gloves, or gauze sponges.	Mild to moderate bleeding is usually controlled in 2–5 minutes; more expensive than Gelfoam.
Surgicel	Johnson & Johnson	Oxidized regenerated cellulose; exerts physical effect rather than physiologic.	After 24–48 hours, it becomes gelatinous; can be left in place or removed; useful to control bleeding when other agents are ineffective.
Oxycel	Becton-Dickinson	Swells upon contact with blood with resultant pressure adding to hemostasis; thrombin ineffective with these agents because of inactivation as a result of pH factors	
Avitene	MedChem	Microfibrillar collagen hemostat; dry, sterile, fibrous, water-insoluble HCL acid salt	Thrombin ineffective with these agents because of inactivation as a result of pH factors; use for moderate to severe bleeding.
Helistat	Marion Merrell Dow	Purified bovine corium collagen; MCH attracts platelets and triggers aggregation in fibrous mass	
Colla-cote Tape, Plug	Colla-tec, Inc Marion	Absorbable collagen dressings from bovine; can be sutured into place, used under stents, dentures, or alone; fully resorbed in 10–14 days	Shaped according to intended use; Cote ¾" × 1.5" ; tape 1" × 3", plug 3/8" × 3/4" all are superior hemostats for moderate to severe bleeding.
Thrombostat	Pake Medical	Topical thrombin; directly converts fibrinogen to fibrin; derived from bovine sources	One 5000-U vial dissolved in 5 mL saline can clot equal amount of blood in less than 1 second; useful in severe bleeding
Thrombinar Thrombogen	Jones Medical J & J/Merck		
Cyklokapron	Kabi Vitrum	Tranexamic acid; works as a competitive inhibitor of plasminogen activation.	Useful over short term for preventing hemorrhage after dental extractions.
Amicar	Wyeth-Ayerst	ε-Amino caproic acid; works as a competitive inhibitor of plasminogen activation; used as a rinse.	Useful over short term to prevent bleeding.
Beriplast	Behringwerke	Fibrin/tissue glue.	Not available in United States at this time.

Little JW, Falace DA, Miller CS, Rhodus naRhodus NL, Dental Management of the Medically Compromised Patient. Mosby Inc., 2008; p 423.

to be totally ineffective. Thermocouple implant studies in skin have shown the insulation properties of skin to be extremely efficient. Patients with ice applications of long duration showed no applicable change in temperature of the subdermal layers owing to the network of capillaries just below the skin. Tests have shown that ice applied to a local area will increase bleeding time considerably. The flow may be reduced somewhat but the bleeding duration is increased.

Epinephrine

Epinephrine, 1:1000 concentration, applied locally with a piece of cotton or gauze, or injected locally in a concentration of 1:50,000 for hemostasis, is quite effective, but its action is reversible. This technique should not be used on patients with severe hypertension or previous existing cardiovascular disease. Severe toxic effects can be elicited by the topical use of 1:1,000 concentration solution of epinephrine, particularly over wide areas of the mouth. The rationale for its use lies in the temporary arresting bleeding long enough for a mechanical plug to clot or occlude the vessel. When the vasoconstrictor effect wears off, the patient must be watched carefully for further recurrence of the bleeding, as the plug may become dislodged again.

Moist Tea Bag

Some literature shows that biting down on a moist tea bag for 10–30 min can decrease bleeding because the tannic acid present in the tea.

Monsel's Solution

Monsel's solution of ferric subsulfate may be used topically or on an area of capillary bleeding to precipitate the protein. It is relatively harmless to tissues and is quite applicable and effective for the postextraction bleeding in medullary bone. It should not be applied over large areas. It should be used via a pack.

Thrombin

Thrombin is a commercially available hemostatic agent of bovine or human origin. It acts as a precipitating agent for the fibrin clot, if there is fibrinogen present in the plasma. The topical (it must never be injected) use of thrombin is favored by many because of its physiologic compatibility to normal processes. It is very kind to tissues and can be quite effective.

Russell Viper Venom

Russell viper venom (Stypven), a dry powder constituted with water, made in 5 ml ampules, is a preparation of thromboplastin that can be used similarly in a socket or topically over an area of bleeding to precipitate blood clot formation.

Tannic Acid

The tannic acid in a tea bag will help precipitate protein and cause clot formation. It is best applied by having the patient bite down on the folded tea bag, dry or very slightly moist, for five minutes, repeating if necessary, three times. The tea bag may well be used in conjunction with the folded dry sponge to apply adequate pressure when the mouth is edentulous.

Many hemostatics are a mixture of tannic acid, alum and chlorobutanol. It is quite effective when applied on either Surgicel or iodoform for the control of a troublesome, oozing type of bleeding.

Gelfoam (Absorbable Gelatin Sponge)

The gelatin sponge is an absorbable material created from purified gelatin solution (porcine gelatin) through which nitrogen has been bubbled in order to produce a porous product. This method was first introduced by Correll and Wise in 1945. The sponge has no intrinsic hemostatic action but induces hemostasis through its intensity porous structure, which enables it to absorb 45 times its weight in blood. As it fills with blood the platelets come into close contact and begin to collide initiating the clotting cascade. It is absorbed in four to six weeks.

Oxycel

Oxidized cellulose is a fabric material that is obtained by the oxidation of cotton, gauze, or other cellulose fabric using nitrous oxide to achieve oxidation. The process was first described by Yackel and Kenyon of Eastman Kodak Laboratories in 1942. This reaction converts certain of the hydroxyl radicals to carboxyl groups and makes the material soluble at physiologic conditions. Oxidized cellulose releases cellulosic acid which has caustic properties that lead to hemostasis via the initial denaturation of blood proteins.

Surgicel

Oxidized regenerated cellulose (Surgicel) offers some improvement over Oxycel in that the gauze pad has more tenacity and resistance and the poly- and hydroglutonic acids resulting from this product do not inhibit epithelialization. It can, therefore, be used on surface dressings where epithelium is involved. Surgicel swells immediately on contact with blood and forms a stick mass. On doing so, it presses down on the bleeding site causing hemostasis. Unlike most of the other preparations, it works very efficiently and as it is absorbable it can be safely buried in the tissues. Surgicel partially dissolves to form acid products which coagulate plasma proteins together with hemoglobulin so as to form a black sticky clot. The pH of the mass remains acidic and may theoretically interfere with normal clotting locally. However, this is not a practical disadvantage since the surgicel clot is not formed by the normal physiological mechanism. Nevertheless, because of the low pH, thrombin solutions should not be used with the gauze because the activity of the thrombin will be rapidly destroyed. It is available as bulk ribbon or individually packaged for single application in sealed glass bottles. The bulk from can be cut to any size desired, and is very economical.

Bone Wax

Bone wax (Horsley's) is a purely mechanically acting hemostatic agent. It consists of bees wax (yellow) 7 parts by weight, olive oil 2 parts, phenol 1 part. This substance is packed into bleeding bone ends to control the hemorrhage. Some operators still use this substance, but it should not be used with any frequency as appreciable quantities can result in the formation of wax granuloma.

Microfillar Collagen (Avitene)

It is water-insoluble hemostatic agent prepared from purified bovine dermal collagen. With its micro-fibrillar structure, Avitene attracts and aggregates platelets, enhancing the clotting process. Unlike other agents, it does not require thrombin to enhance its efficiency. It is provided in sheet and flour forms. It is active, absorbable, 100% collagen, soft, pliable fabric, easy to handle. It does not swell after application. It requires no preparation or soaking in any solution.

Fibrin Glue (Fibrin Sealants, Tissue Adhesives) Contain Fibrinogen and Thrombin

Treatment of bleeding disorders in hemophilia A and B and patients suffering from von Willebrand disease or other types of coagulation factor deficiencies (e.g. XI or VIII) is based on substitutive therapy by intravenous infusion of plasma—derived or, when available, recombinant coagulation factor products. Another category of hemostatic products produced from human blood/plasma are proving to be helpful topical agents to stop or control bleeding in the those patients, including those who developed an inhibitor, at least in some surgical situations. Fibrin sealant, also called fibrin glue, may reduce or eliminate the need to infuse coagulation factor concentrates during some surgical procedures.

Fibrin sealants are prepared in clinical practice by mixing, at the time of use, two plasma-derived protein fractions: (a) fibrinogen-rich concentrate and (b) a thrombin concentrate. Mixing fibrinogen and thrombin mimics the last step of the blood coagulation cascade, resulting in the formation of a semi-rigid to rigid fibrin clot that consolidates and adheres to the application site and acts as a fluid-tight sealing agent able to stop bleeding and hold tissues and materials in a desired configuration. Fibrin sealants have hemostatic sealing and healing properties. Their advantages over synthetic surgical glues include bio-compatibility, biodegradability, and the absence of induction of the inflammatory reactions or tissue necrosis. Readsorption of the fibrin clot is achieved within days to weeks following application, depending upon the type of surgery, the amount of product used, or the proteolytic activity of the site treated. In general clinical practices, the plasma donations used as starting material can be obtained from the patient (autologous use) or from another plasma donor (homologous).

Immediately after extraction of a tooth, the socket is curetted and then suctioned to keep the site as dry as possible. Surgicel is placed in the apical third of the socket. Fibrin glue is applied to the socket walls followed by suturing the wound edges. A final application of glue is then placed over the socket to seal any gingival bleeding.

Platelet Gel

This newly introduced biomaterial is obtained by combining a platelet-rich blood fraction, such as platelet concentrate or platelet-rich plasma, with calcified thrombin. This mimics the same physiological reaction as that of fibrin sealant and results in the formation of a soft, gel-like biomaterial. The platelet concentrate can be obtained from a blood bank and is produced by standard whole blood centrifugation or by platelet aphoresis. For patients not suffering from bleeding disorders, a small amount of their own blood

(50 ml) may be collected prior to clinical need and processed using special devices to isolate a platelet rich fraction. Platelet fractions are then mixed, prior to clinical application, with thrombin. The mixture results, in 5 to 20 seconds, in the formation of a fibrin enriched gel that contains platelet-derived cell growth promoting factors.

Platelet Glue

As the fibrinogen content in the platelet concentrate is less than that used for fibrin sealant, the strength of the resulting gel is significantly less and the product cannot be used as efficiently to stop bleeding. The platelet-rich blood fraction can possibly be premixed with cryoprecipitate which, upon mixing with thrombin, produces a product often referred to as 'platelet glue' with better adhesive properties and higher resistance to body fluid and pressure than platelet gel.

Cyanoacrylate Glue (Histoacryl Glue)

The cyanoacylate (CA) glues are biodegradable and bacteriostatic agents formed from the chemical reaction between formaldehyde and a cyanoacrylate ester. The cyanoacrylates have long been used experimentally and clinically as tissue adhesives, and as hemostatic or embolic agent (El-Balasyetal, 2003).

Following extraction, the wound edges are approximated by interrupted resorbable sutures. The surgical region is thoroughly cleaned and dried. Topical application of the histoacryl is carried out by applying gentle pressure on the histoacryl glue syringe where a fine continuous streaks of the glue is flowed along the wound edges. This is left undisturbed until the glue becomes opaque. The glue is applied in three consecutive layers.

Electrocautery Heat

It is used to cause the ends of the cut vessels to fuse closed (thermal coagulation). Heat is usually applied through an electrical current that the surgeon concentrate on the bleeding vessel by holding the vessel with a metal instrument such as a hemostat, or by touching the vessel directly with an electrocautery tip. There are many instances when bleeding of some size can be controlled by electrocautery through two modalities:

  a. After securing a moderate sized vessel with a hemostat, the cautery can be touched to the hemostat, creating a precipitation of the protein

elements in the end of the wound and sealing off the vessel through a contact with the occluded vessel.

  b. A common use is to apply the cautery directly to small vessels that are oozing or bleeding. This will coagulate the blood and the protein in the area, and will arrest bleeding from extremely vascular and troublesome sites. It is not prudent to expect electrocautery to replace ligation of a large vessel, but, used when indicated. Electrocautery is a convenient and effective way of controlling hemorrhage. Three conditions must be created for proper use of thermal coagulation.

    1. First, the patient must be grounded to allow the current to enter the body.

    2. Second, the cautery tip and any metal instrument the cautery tip contacts cannot touch the patient at any point other than the site of the bleeding vessel, otherwise, the current may flow on undesirable path and create a burn.

    3. The third necessity for thermal coagulation is the removal of any blood or fluid that has accumulated around the vessel to be cauterized. Fluid acts as an energy sump and thus prevents a sufficient amount of heat from reaching the vessel to cause closure.

Ligation and Sutures

The use of absorbable gut for deep ties to ligate large vessels, and of silk or nylon sutures for surface constriction of a bleeding or oozing area, is good surgical practice. However, unless there has been sufficient mobilization of flap or bone removal to allow tight and adequate tissue approximation, sutures in the alveolar crest area only provide additional sites of bleeding. It is important to use atraumatic needles whenever possible to prevent additional bleeding sites.

If a sizable vessel is already severed, each end is grasped with a hemostat. The surgeon then ties a non-absorbable suture around the vessel. If a vessel can be dissected free of the surrounding connective tissue before it is cut, two hemostats can be placed on the vessel, with enough space left between them to cut the vessel, once the vessel is severed, sutures are tied around each end and the hemostats removed.

SYSTEMIC METHODS FOR CONTROL OF HEMORRHAGE

Occasionally, the systemic administration of drugs and fluids is required. The following represents a list of the most commonly used.

a. Vitamin K may be effective, if there is some problem relating to prothrombin. The effects, of any occur, will not be immediate. Effective within 24 hours, if given orally and within 6 hours, if given intravenously.

b. Plasma

c. Whole blood

d. Parenteral fluids

e. Vitamin K

f. Vitamin C

g. Other drugs as:

  i. Premarin, adrenosem, kutapressin and koagamin

  ii. Adrenosem, kutapressin and koagamin

  iii. Desmopressin

  iv. Antifibrinolytic, e.g. epsilone aminocaproic acid (EACA) epsicapron and tranexamic acid (cyclokaprone).

Premarin

The female hormone has been used quite effectively in women, sometimes with dramatic response to control capillary or mechanical bleeding. It has no effect on deficiency diseases. Sometimes these compounds are used in the management of epistaxis and bleeding from gastrointestinal causes. There is evidence to indicate that intravenous estrogens can produce prompt increase of circulating prothrombin and accelerated globulin and a decrease in the antithrombin activity of the blood. Theoretically these changes tend to enhance the coagulability of blood, thereby providing a rationale for the current, popular short-term use of the estrogens in spontaneous hemorrhage. A single dose of 20 mg of the conjugated estrogen (premarin) given intravenously is reputed to have a remarkable effect. Therapy should not be continued beyond one dose. Premarin has been favorably employed to control both troublesome oozing over a large area and frank venous bleeding of a rather large magnitude.

Adrenosem, Kutapressin and Koagamin

These drugs occasionally are used to control capillary bleeding. Adrenosem acts by decreasing capillary permeability or increasing capillary resistance. Kutapressin is only effective for capillary oozing. Koagamin is oxalic and malonic acid and has a tendency to release prothrombin for the formation of thrombin. These drugs are of questionable value and are reported by many to be entirely ineffective. One should not expect these drugs to have dramatic results. They will be most effective, if started the day before surgery and continued for three to five days when capillary oozing problems are anticipated in the patient.

Desmopressin

A synthetic version of a naturally occurring hormone. It is given as an intravenous infusion (0.5 mg/kg, repeated 12 hourly, if necessary) temporarily corrects the hemostatic defect in mild hemophilia by releasing factor VIIIC (endogenous procoagulant) and von Willebrand factor into the blood. Desmopressin may be useful for patients with factor VIII inhibitors. It is increasingly widely used for the management of mild hemophiliacs for extractions. As desmopressin also causes release of plasminogen activator, tranexamic acid should be given. The dosages of DDAVP are as follows:

1. *DDAVP IV dose:* Give 0.3 µ/kg DDAVP in 50 cc saline slowly over 15–30 min. Levels peak in 30–60 min.
2. *DDAVP intranasal dose:* Available as 1.5 mg/ml spray. Each spray pumps 0.1 ml, giving a 150 µ/g dose. Levels peak in 60–90 mins. Dose lasts for 5–21 h.

  Adult intranasal dose: 300 µg

  Child intranasal dose: 150 µg

3. *DDAVP oral dose:*

  Rx: DDAVP, 0.1 or 0.2 mg/tablet

  Sig: 0.05 mg twice daily

  Total daily dose: 0.1–1.2 mg

Antifibrinolytics

The clotting mechanism, which depends ultimately on the formation of fibrin, protects the body against loss of blood from the system. On the other hand, it is obviously undesirable that fibrin should be deposited within the vessels. The fibrinolytic system can, therefore, be regarded as operating parallel with the clotting mechanism. This system inhibits further formation of a clot so as not to continue to develop thromboembolic episodes that would run rampant throughout the entire circulatory system.

Plasminogen is present in the plasma and the tissues, particularly apparently in the alveolar bone, and when activated forms plasmin, a proteolytic enzyme which causes fibrinolysis. In the normal state, there is a balance between these two processes which maintains the patency of the vessels. Excessive fibrinolytic activity can itself cause severe hemorrhage and on rare occasions dental hemorrhage from this cause has been described. Fibrinolysis alone is nevertheless a very common cause of excessive hemorrhage, but in cases where the clotting mechanism is defective, as in hemophilia, fibrinolysis even of minimal degree exacerbates the problem by dissolving such little clot as can form.

Antifibrinolytics are synthetic antifibrinolytic agents which act as inhibitors of plasminogen activation. They significantly reduce factor VIII requirements. Antifibrinolytics include epsilon-aminocaproic acid (EACA) also known as Epsikapron (amicar) and tranexamic acid (cyclocapron). Tranexamic acid is a more potent analogue of EACA with fewer side effects. EACA alone has been used successfully for control of hemorrhage after dental extractions in hemophiliacs, but is not itself adequate for the management of more severe cases where antihemophiliac factor must also be given. In many centers, therefore, tranexamic acid is used in conjunction with antihemophilic factor for dental extraction in hemophilic patients to reduce the amount of cryoprecipitate or factor VIII that has to be given.

Before prescribing these drugs always confirm that the patient has no prior history of moderate to severe headaches, acute vision problems, transient ischemic attacks, cardiovascular accidents (strokes), blood clots, or any other indicators for thrombosis. Confirm that the liver and kidneys are optimally functioning.

The antifibrinolytic drugs can be ingested by mouth (PO), used as a mouth wash, or injected IV. Always advise the patient to discontinue the oral or IV antifibrinolytic drugs and proceed to the nearest emergency center, should symptoms and signs of thrombosis develop. Sudden severe headaches, acute vision loss, sudden severe pains in the chest, calves, or abdomen, or sudden motor/sensory deficits in the extremities should be the cause for immediate action and attention.

Tranexamic acid (cyklocapron) is used in a dose of 1 g (30 mg/kg) orally, four times daily starting 24 hours preoperatively. Tranexamic acid when used topically it significantly reduces bleeding. Ten ml of a 5% solution used as a mouth rinse for 2 minutes, four times daily for 7 days is recommended. This solution can be made up by diluting 10% tranexamic acid solution for injection, with sterile water.

Epsilon-Aminocaproic Acid (Amicar) Oral (PO) and Mouthwash Prescriptions

The following prescriptions are of value:

1. R_x: Epsilon-aminocaproic acid (amicar), 500 mg/tablet.
   Sig: First dose: 5g (10 tablets) orally, 1 hour post-surgery, followed by 2 g (4 tablets) q6h, postoperatively till the bleeding stops, or prescribe for 5–7 days.
   Maximum dose: 30 g/day.
2. R_x: Amicar syrup 250 mg/mL or 1.25 g/tsp(5 ml).
   Sig: 5–10 mL qid x 5–7 days, starting 6 hrs prior to surgery, if needed. Use as mouthwash for 2 minutes and expectorate.

The mouth wash decreases recurrent bleeding and the need for factor replacement after surgery. Amicar prevents clot breakdown by the enzymes in the saliva. This allows healing of the tissues beneath the clot. Disp: 240 mL/480 mL bottle.

Tranexamic Acid/ Cyclocapron Oral (PO) and Mouthwash Prescriptions

1. R_x: Tranexamic acid (cyclocapron), 500 mg/ tablet.
   Sig: 25 mg/kg orally tid/qid × 2–8 days, starting one day prior to surgery.
2. R_x: 4.8% cyclocapron oral rinse solution.
   Sig: Use 10 mL as mouthwash for 2 min. and expectorate, qid x 5–7 days.
   Disp: 280 ml.

Cyclocapron is 10 times more potent than amicar and it has a longer half-life. The cyclocapron oral rinse is not PDA-approved. It is important to remember that the saliva and the oral mucosa contain plasminogen activators that can trigger fibrinolysis. Use of amicar or cyclocapron mouthwash is, therefore, very beneficial to prevent clot lysis.

Excessive postsurgical oozing can additionally be controlled by sustained pressure and the use of local hemostatic materials.

Replacement of Blood Loss

Blood Transfusion

The ABO blood group is based on the presence (or absence) of two major protein antigens on red blood cell membranes—antigen A, and antigen B (Fig. 14.20). A person's erythrocytes have on their surfaces one of four antigen combinations: only A, only B, both A and B, or neither A nor B. The resulting ABO blood type, because it reflects a protein combination, is inherited.

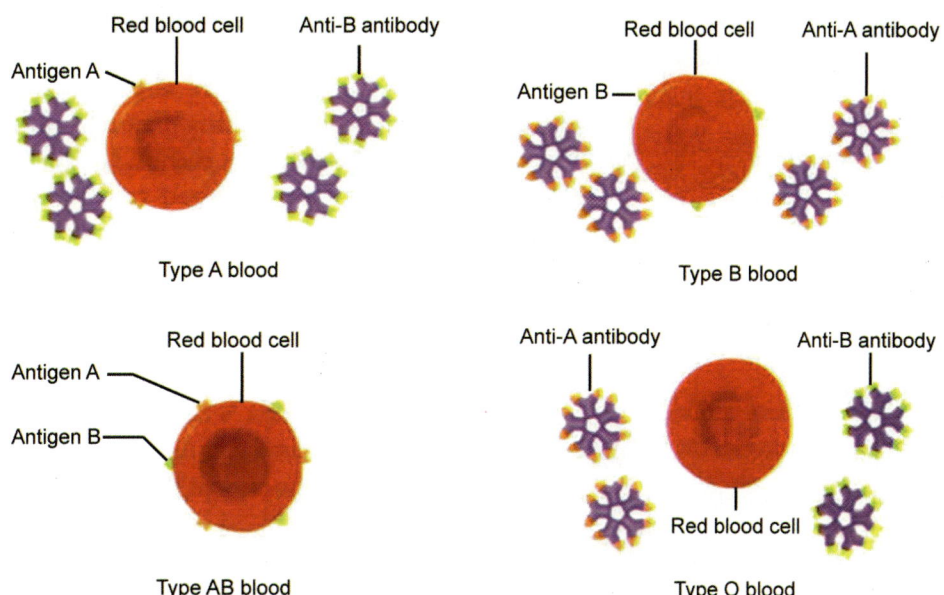

Fig. 14.20: Different combinations of antigens and antibodies distinguish blood types (cells and antibodies not drawn to scale).
(Shier D, Butler J, Lewis R: Hole's Essential of Human Anatomy and Physiology 10th ed, McGraw-Hill– Higher education, 2009)

After referring to the immune system, we now know that our immune system ignores the surface antigens —also called agglutinogens—on our own RBCs. However, our plasma contains antibodies, or agglutinins, that will attack surface antigens on RBCs of a different blood-type (Fig. 14.21 A). Thus, the plasma of individuals with type A blood contains circulating anti-B antibodies, which will attack type B surface antigens and the plasma of type-B individuals contains anti-A antibodies, which will attack type A surface antigens. Similarly, type AB individuals lack antibodies against either A or B surface antigens, whereas the plasma of individuals with type O blood contains both anti-A and anti-B antibodies (Fig. 14.21 A).

The presence of these antibodies is why, before blood is transfused, the blood types of donor and recipient are identified. If an individual receives blood of a different blood type, antibodies in the recepient's plasma meet their specific antigen on the donated RBCs, and a cross-reaction occurs (Fig. 14.21B). Initially, the binding of antigens and antibodies causes

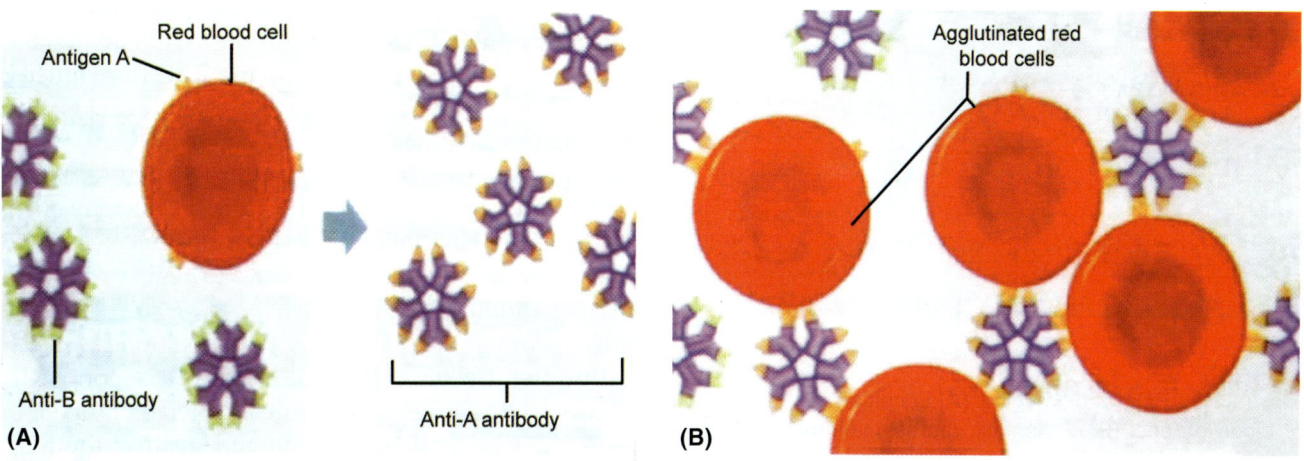

Fig. 14.21: Agglutination. **(A)** If red blood cells with antigen A are added to blood containing anti-A antibody. **(B)** The antibody reacts with the antigens, causing clumping (agglutination). *(Shier D, Butler J & Lewis R: Hole's Essential of Human Anatomy and Physiology, 10th ed, McGraw-Hill-higher education, 2009)*

the foreign RBCs to clump together—a process called agglutination. Subsequently, the RBCs may break up, or hemolyze (Fig. 14.22). Clumps and fragments of RBCs under attack from antibodies form drifting masses that can plug small vessels in the kidneys, lungs, heart, or brain, damaging or destroying tissues. Such cross-reactions, or transfusion reactions, can be avoided by ensuring that the blood types of donor and recipient are compatible.

In practice, the surface antigens on the donor's cells are more important in determining compatibility than are the antibodies in the donor's plasma. Unless large volumes of whole blood or plasma are transferred, cross-reactions between the donor's plasma and the recepient's blood cells will fail to produce significant agglutination. Packed RBCs, with a minimal amount of plasma, are commonly transfused. Even when whole blood is transfused, the plasma is diluted through mixing with the recepient's relatively large plasma volume.

Unlike the case for type A and type B individuals, the plasma of an Rh-negative individual does not normally contain anti-Rh antibodies. These antibodies are present only if the individual has been sensitized by previous exposure to Rh-positive RBCs. Such exposure can occur accidentally, during a transfusion, but it can also occur in a normal pregnancy when an Rh-negative mother carries an Rh-positive fetus.

Rh Blood Group

The Rh blood group was named after the rhesus monkey in which it was first studied. In humans, this group includes several Rh antigens (factors). The most prevalent of these is antigen D. If the Rh antigen is present on the red blood cell membranes, the blood is said to be Rh-positive. Conversely, if the red blood cells lack Rh antigen, the blood is called Rh-negative. As in the case of antigens A and B, the presence (or absence) of Rh antigen is an inherited trait. But unlike anti-A and anti-B, antibodies that react with Rh antigen (anti-Rh antibodies) do not appear spontaneously. Instead, they form only in Rh-negative persons in response to special stimulation.

If an Rh-negative person receives a transfusion of Rh-positive blood, the Rh antigen stimulates the recipient to begin producing anti-Rh antibodies. Generally, this initial transfusion has no serious consequences, but if the Rh-negative person—who is now sensitized to Rh-positive blood—receives another transfusion of Rh-positive blood some months later, the donated red cells are likely to agglutinate.

A related condition may occur when an Rh-negative woman is pregnant with an Rh-positive fetus for the first time. Such a pregnancy may be uneventful; however, at birth (or if a miscarriage occurs), the placental membranes that separated the maternal blood from the fetal blood during the pregnancy tear, and some of the infant's Rh-positive blood cells may enter the maternal circulation. These Rh-positive cells may then stimulate the maternal tissues to begin producing anti-Rh antibodies (Fig. 14.23).

If a woman who has already developed anti-Rh antibodies becomes pregnant with a second Rh-positive fetus, these antibodies, called hemolysins, cross the placental membrane and destroy the fetal red blood cells (Fig. 14.23). The fetus then develops a condition called hemolytic disease of the fetus and newborn (erythroblastosis fetalis).

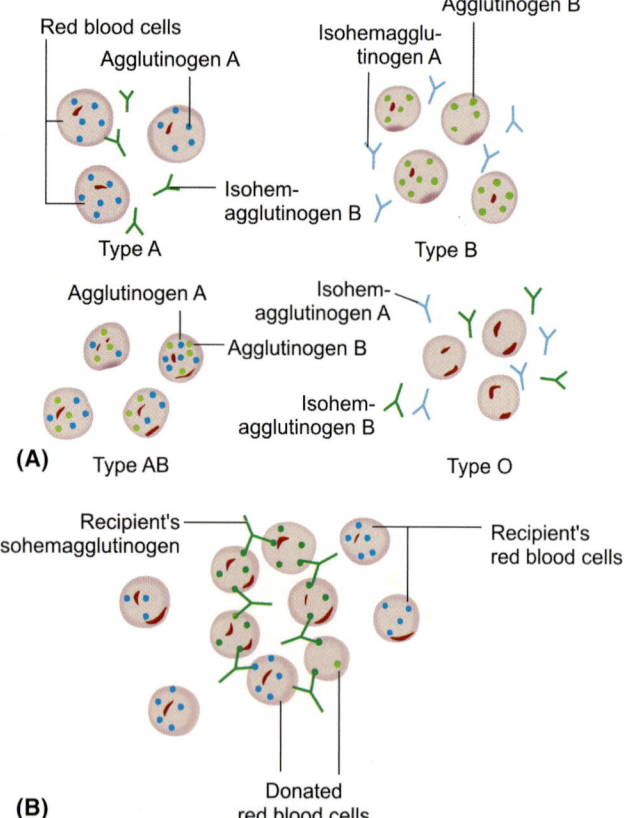

Fig. 14.22: ABO blood grouping. **(A)** Schematic representation of blood groups. **(B)** Schematic representation of antibody–antigen complex formed when type B red blood cells are transfused into a recipient with type A blood. The agglutinins of the donated blood have little or no effect on the red blood cells of the recipient *(Donna et al, 1995)*

Clinical Note

- In order to prevent a hemolytic transfusion reaction, blood must be tested for compatibility between the donor and the recipient.
- Blood products are tested for the major antigens (AB and Rh). In addition, they are tested for minor antigen compatibility.
- The analysis and selection of blood products for transfusion is a time-consuming typing and cross-matching.
- In a critical emergency, there may not be time to wait for blood typing and cross-matching. In these situations, type O-negative (O⁻) blood can be safely administered. Type O⁻ blood does not contain the A, B or Rh antigen. Thus, it will not induce a hemolytic reaction in a patient with a different blood type. Because of this, persons with type O blood are referred to as universal donors.
- Persons who have type AB blood are referred to as universal recepients. They have both the A and B antigens on their RBCs and thus lack circulating antibodies against both A and B. In an emergency, they can receive any type of blood, as they already have the antibodies.

In an emergency setting, if time permits, it is preferred to wait until the blood is fully typed and cross-matched. If there is no adequate time for this, the patient can be given type specific blood. Type specific blood has been tested for the major (ABO and Rh) antigens. It has been tested for the minor antigens.

Finally, as described above, in critical situations, the patient may be given uncross-matched type O blood until typing and cross-matching have been completed.

Platelets do not contain any minor blood antigens. Platelets should be of the same ABO and Rh type. They are rapidly destroyed by the body and must be frequently administered.

II. BLOOD PRODUCTS

Blood is a precious commodity and must be utilized so that it can provide the most benefit for the greatest number of people. A unit of whole blood consists of approximately 450 milliliters of blood with about 65 grams of hemoglobin. In current medical practice, it is uncommon to administer whole blood. Instead, the blood is separated into its various elements and those elements are administered as needed. Elements

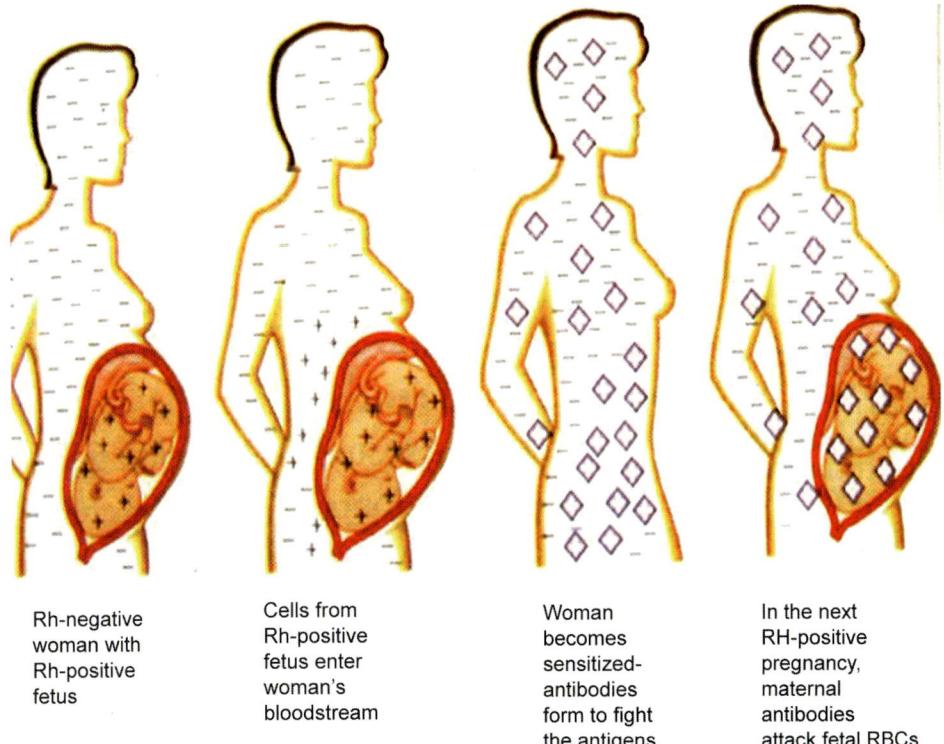

| Rh-negative woman with Rh-positive fetus | Cells from Rh-positive fetus enter woman's bloodstream | Woman becomes sensitized-antibodies form to fight the antigens | In the next RH-positive pregnancy, maternal antibodies attack fetal RBCs |

Fig. 14.23: Rh incompatibility. If a man how is Rh-positive and a woman how is Rh-negative conceive a child how is Rh-positive, the woman's body may manufacture antibody that attack future Rh-positive offspring *(Shier D, Butler J, Lewis R: Hole's essential of human anatomy and physiology 10th ed,McGraw-Hill-Higher education, 2009)*

derived from whole blood include the red blood cells (packed red blood cells), platelets, granulocytes and plasma (fresh frozen plasma). Patients receive only the blood elements that they need. A patient who has sustained hemorrhage, for instance, will receive packed RBCs and crystalloid fluids, while a patient with a platelet disorder will receive platelet transfusion.

Blood is commonly fractionated into its constituent parts, which are used for specific indications. This ensures more efficient use of each unit of donated blood. The range of blood products available is listed in Box 14.13 and are discussed below.

> **Box 14.13:** Blood products
>
> a. *Red blood cells concentrate*
> b. *Platelets*
> c. *Fresh frozen plasma*
> d. *Cryoprecipitate*
> e. *Factor concentrates*
> f. *Albumin solution*
> g. *Other*

a. *Red cell concentrate (RCC)*

RCC is used for transfusion in patients with anemia and in those suffering acute blood loss, but it has a reduced oxygen-carrying capacity. It must be blood group ABO- and Rhesus factor compatible. One unit of RCC is derived from one donation. The shelf life is 35 days at 4°C. The volume varies by unit, but is approximately 400 mL.

Red cells are extracted and suspended in a near optimum solution containing glucose, adenine, mannitol, sodium chloride and citrate (the last prevents clotting). Cell lysis during storage means that each unit contains a high concentration of extracellular potassium. RCC has a hematocrit of 65–75% and hence has poor flow characteristics. Simultaneous crystalloid infusion reduces the hematocrit and provides volume repletion.

b. *Platelets*

Infused platelets are suspended in plasma (and, therefore, infusions contain some clotting factors). Full cross-match is not necessary before transfusion. One unit is obtained from 4–6 blood donations. The shelf life is 5 days at room temperature and the volume is 300 mL. No viral inactivation procedures are used in processing. Platelets are used perioperatively in patients with thrombocytopenia.

c. *Fresh frozen plasma (FFP)*

This is pure plasma that is separated and frozen shortly after donation. It contains all the plasma derived clotting factors, but has relatively low levels of factor VIII and fibrinogen. The shelf life is one year at –30 °C and its volume is 150–300 mL per unit. FFP is used for correcting factor deficiencies.

d. *Cryoprecipitate*

It contains high levels of factor VIII and fibrinogen. Again the shelf ife is one year at –30°C . Each unit is approximately 10–20 mL and the standard dose is 10 units.

e. *Factor concentrates*

Multiples are available and are either derived from plasma or are manufactured using recombinant DNA technology.

f. *Albumin solution*

This is derived from whole blood after removal of cells and factors. Shelf life is 3–5 years. It is used to expand intravascular volume, although it has now been largely superseded by synthetic gelatin solutions such as gelofusin and haemacel. It is also used for fluid replacement after burns and during plasmapheresis.

g. *Other*

There are multiple other blood products available for treatment of more unusual conditions, including specific immunoglobulins.

COMPLICATIONS

The complications of blood transfusion can be immunological, infective or due to miscellaneous causes (Box 14.14).

> **Box 14.14:** Complications of blood transfusions
>
> a. *Immunological*
>   1. *Immediate hemolytic*
>   2. *Non-hemolytic*
>   3. *Delayed hemolytic*
> b. *Infective*
> c. *Miscellaneous*
>   1. *Fluid overload*
>   2. *Hyperkalemia*
>   3. *Coagulation disorder*
>   4. *Hemosiderosis*
>   5. *Hypothermia*

A. Immunological Complications

1. Immediate Hemolytic Complications

This can result from mismatched blood cell antigens between donor and recipient. The most important antigens are those of the ABO system. These reactions are severe and sudden and most often result from human error, for example, if wrong unit of blood is given to the wrong patient because of a labeling, handling or patient identification error. Activation of the complement system occurs when the recipient possesses antibodies to an antigen on the donated red blood cells and hemolytic (breakdown of red blood cells) ensues.

Clinically, the patient rapidly becomes unwell with fever, hypotension and difficult breathing. Activation of coagulation can occur, leading to DIG. The hemoglobin released from the hemolysis, along with hypotension, can cause acute renal failure. Treatment involves preventing further reaction by stopping the transfusion immediately. The patient might require life saving resuscitation, including measures to maintain oxygenation and blood pressure.

Intensive care might be appropriate. Where a reaction occurs, the unit of blood must be returned to the laboratory, along with a cross-match sample from the patient.

2. Non-hemolytic Complications

Febrile, allergic and anaphylactic reactions can occur and will necessitate immediate cessation of the transfusion and possibly medical resuscitation, depending on the severity. Allergic and anaphylactic reactions might require immediate treatment with adrenaline (epinephrine), antihistamine or corticosteroids.

3. Delayed Hemolytic Complications

These result from incompatibility of blood with regards to less important antigens. They occur in patients who have previously been sensitized to the antigens. Examples include Rhesus antibodies and rare antibodies to minor antigens such asd Kell and Duffy. Hemolysis occurs several days after the transfusion. The patient is not generally acutely unwell and might develop jaundice and anemia several days after the transfusion.

B. Infective Complications

The donated blood should be routinely screened for HIV, syphilis, hepatitis B and hepatitis C. However, a number of these diseases have a latent period before their detection is possible and so transmission of infection can still occur. Before screening for certain diseases was introduced, many blood recipients were infected with hepatitis C and people with hemophilia contracted HIV.

The risk of transmission of infection is related to how many donors the blood product was derived from and to the pretransfusion treatment the product has received.

C. Miscellaneous Complications

1. Fluid Overload

The volume load of the transfusion might precipitate heart failure in the elderly or those with a history of heart disease, particularly as a unit of blood has to be transfused in less than 4 hours. Prophylactic diuretic therapy is often given with a transfusion to prevent this.

2. Hyperkalemia

Stored blood has a high concentration of potassium and when multiple units are given, the recepient's serum potassium level can rise to dangerous levels. Electrolyte levels must, therefore, be monitored.

3. Coagulation Disorder

This was considered above.

4. Hemosiderosis

Patients who receive regular or multiple blood transfusions can suffer from iron overload. Excess iron is deposited in vital organs such as the pancreas, myocardium, or liver, causing them to dysfunction. This is reduced by using an iron chelator such as desferrioxamine.

5. Hypothermia

Blood is stored cooled to 4°C. If large volumes of unwarmed blood are transfused, the patient will suffer hypothermia. The role of blood warmers is particularly important in trauma cases.

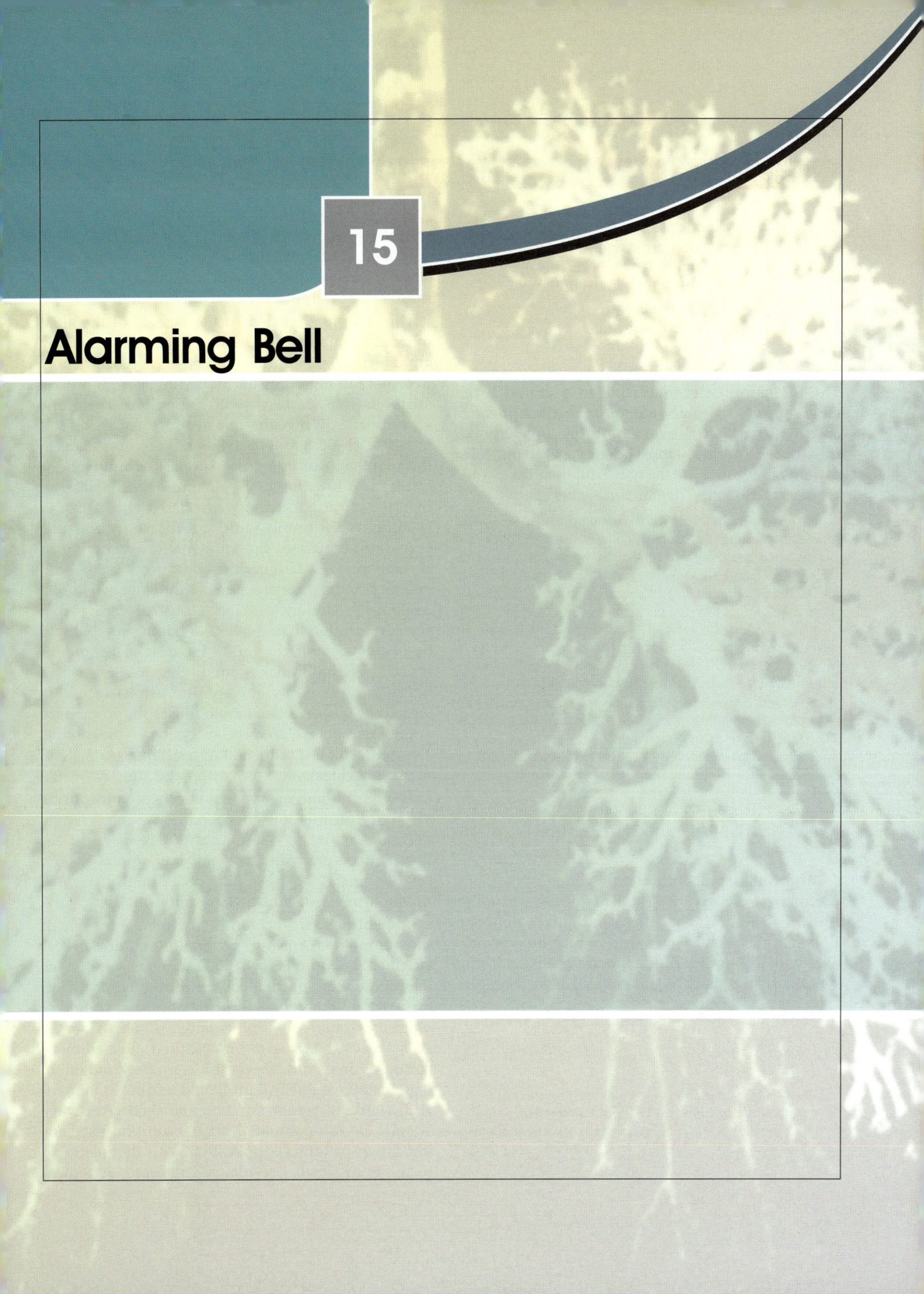

15

Alarming Bell

ALARMING BELL

A	• Adrenergic drug (adrenaline) • Analgesics and NSAIDs • Antibiotics • Anticholinergic • Anticonvulsants

ADRENERGIC DRUG (ADRENALINE)

The inclusion of epinephrine in a dental office emergency kit is mandatory for the treatment of cardiac arrest and overwhelming anaphylaxis (Box 15.1). However, it must be emphasized that these extreme conditions are the only situations that would require its use in the dental office emergency.

There are a few clinicians who maintain the mistaken belief that epinephrine is the drug of choice in shock or shock-like states. There are three principal reasons for disrupting this belief: First of all, in shock from almost any cause there is decreased venous return to the heart because of peripheral venous pooling. Since the peripheral action of epinephrine is primarily on the arterial side, there is little gain in promoting peripheral vasoconstriction, which is already present because of the massive release of endogenous catecholamines (epinephrine and norepinephrine).

The second possible deleterious effect is an increase in selective ischemia that takes place in certain viscera such as the kidney. Here, as in peripheral vessels, the blood supply is constricted in a compensatory effort to increase blood flow to the more vital brain and heart tissues. Perpetuation of this condition could be undesirable.

A third important factor is the possible precipitation of ventricular fibrillation in the ischemic and irritable myocardium.

Adrenaline (epinephrine hydrochloride) is the most useful and perhaps the best example of a drug that initiates the activity of sympathetic discharge. Epinephrine has its major effects on the myocardium and smooth muscles of the blood vessels and lung. The heart is considered to contain beta receptors;

therefore, epinephrine acts as a direct cardiac stimulant. Both small and large doses of epinephrine cause an increase in strength of contraction, cardiac rate, cardiac output, and oxygen utilization.

The receptors located in the vessels of the skin, mucous membranes and kidney are predominantly alpha so that epinephrine will cause vasoconstriction. Receptors in those vessels located in skeletal muscle are for the most part, beta with some alpha. Therefore, epinephrine will cause vasodilation in skeletal muscles. These two responses are very important in the regulation of blood pressure. Slow intravenous infusion of low doses of epinephrine will cause an increase in cardiac activity associated with a rise in systolic pressure but with a decrease in diastolic pressure because of the vasodilation occurring in skeletal muscles. Larger doses produce a rise in both systolic and diastolic pressures, as the cutaneous alpha response predominates. Since alpha response is of a shorter duration than the beta, a fall in pressure will be observed after the initial increase. The smooth muscles of the bronchi contain beta receptors and hence are relaxed by epinephrine. Alpha receptors located in the vascular smooth muscle of pulmonary arterioles respond with vasoconstriction to epinephrine. The net result is a reduction in resistance to air flow, which provides relief from asthmatic attacks.

The central nervous system effects of epinephrine are more prominent when accidental intravenous injections occur or when excessive doses are used. These effects are manifest by anxiety, apprehension, restlessness, weakness and occasionally tremor. Epinephrine also stimulates metabolism.

Epinephrine hydrochloride is available for use in the commercial form of adrenaline chloride. It is supplied in ampoules of 1; 1000 aqueous solution for injection either subcutaneously, intramuscularly, or, for extreme emergencies, intravenously. The most often used route of administration is subcutaneous. This allows the drug to be absorbed over a longer period of time with less central nervous stimulation. If given intravenously, 1 ml should be diluted to 10 ml with sterile water for injection and then given very slowly. Do not confuse the 1;100 dilution used for inhalation or topical application with the injectable form, as disastrous results might occur. A topical

Box 15.1: Primary reasons for using epinephrine

In cases of cardiac arrest	Anaphylaxis
↓	↓
Direct (beta) stimulation of the myocardium	Antagonist to the results of histamine release, e.g. bronchiolar constriction, which leads to decreased oxygen consumption

solution 1;1000, I also available for use as a hemostatic on bleeding gingival or pulpal tissues. All epinephrine should be stored in the original dark containers, as light will also decompose the solution. The presence of a brownish color is indicative of an epinephrine solution that has lost its potency and should be discarded.

Uses

1. Epinephrine is the drug of choice for acute asthmatic and allergic reactions. It may be injected subcutaneously, intramuscularly or intravenously in doses of 0.2 to 0.5 ml of the 1;1000 aqueous solution.
2. The drug is employed as a vasoconstrictor in local anesthetics.
3. It is employed as a cardiac stimulant in cardiac arrest where fibrillation is absent. Because the drug is a direct cardiac stimulant, it could cause ventricular fibrillation in certain cardiac emergencies. For this reason, its use in hemorrhagic, traumatic, or cardiogenic shock is not recommended.

ANALGESICS AND NSAIDs

Analgesics and NSAIDs are discussed in Table 15.1

ANTIBIOTICS

All infections do not require antibiotic therapy. Unfortunately, there is no simple rule that can be employed to give an immediate yes or no answer in regard to the need for antibiotics. The basic question is " Does this particular patient need the assistance of antibacterial agents to resolve this particular infection"? The decision to use or not to use, can be made only after considering all those factors that would tend to indicate a need against those that tend to obviate a need. The following should be evaluated.

1. *The patient:* One should never lose sight of the fact that the best "antibiotic: known is neutrophil. Properly functioning defense mechanisms in the healthy patient are of primary importance. The lack of these defenses, as may occur in conditions previously mentioned, must receive close attention. The presence or absence of fever, malaise and lymphoadenopathy are indicators as to how well the patient is doing on his own.

2. *The infection:* The virulence and invasiveness of the etiologic microorganisms are important in determining the acuteness, severity and spreading tendency of the infection. Obviously, the acute, severe, rapidly spreading infection should generally be treated with antibacterial agents. The other end of the spectrum is the mild localizing infection where drainage can be established. Most cases lie somewhere between these extremes. In these cases, the decision can only be based on the clinician's capability to balance all pertinent factors as to the patient's need for pharmacologic assistance.

Prophylactic Indications

A definitive indication for prophylactic antibiotic coverage exists when patients with rheumatic or congenital heart disease or those with heart prostheses

Table 15.1: Analgesics and NSAIDs

Analgesics (in order of potency)		
Advice that they be taken, if needed. Maximum doses are indicated here		
Paracetamol	500–1000 mg	6 hourly
Paracetamol with codeine	1–2 tablets	6 hourly
Paracetamol with dihydrocodeine	1–2 tablets	every 6–8 hours
Dihydrocodeine	30–60 mg	every 6–8 hours
Non-steroidal anti-inflammatory drugs (NSAIDs)		
Always to be taken with food. Use slow-release preparations in inflammatory conditions or if more regular pain control is needed. Examples:		
Ibuprofen	200–400 mg	Every 6–8 hours
Ibuprofen slow release	600–800 mg	Every 1–3 days
Diclofenac	25–50 mg	8 hourly
Diclofenac slow release	75–100 mg	1–2 daily
Celecoxib	200 mg	1–2 daily

are to undergo procedures that may precipitate a bacteremia. This prophylaxis is against bacterial endocarditis. Other prophylactic uses of antibacterial agents in dental practice are not so definitive. Some clinicians employ antibiotic coverage for surgical patients in an attempt to avert post-surgical infection, enhance the surgical results, and reduce post-surgical discomfort. This philosophy can be summarized as follows: although parallel dental studies are not available, the failure of prophylactic antibiotic coverage to prevent post-surgical infections is well documented in the medical literature.

Most patients who undergo periodontal surgery are not going to develop a postoperative infection. Infections that do evolve might have been prevented by prophylactic antibiotics, if the invading organisms were susceptible to the particular drug selected. It is apparent from medical literature that some individuals who would not have developed a postoperative infection may do so if prophylactic antibiotics are used. The mechanism of this may be related to alternations in the normal flora which were induced by the antibiotic. Thus, in the final analysis, one must balance the infections he prevents with antibiotics against the infections he causes with antibiotics.

Bactericidal Versus Bacteriostatic Antibiotics

The following discussion of antibacterial drugs refers to the various agents as being bactericidal or bacteriostatic. It is of clinical importance that one is familiar with this distinction. Bactericidal drugs kill bacteria; bacteriostatic drugs retard the growth of bacteria, leaving final elimination to body defensive mechanisms. It is apparent that bacteriostatic agents are relatively ineffective in the patient whose defense mechanisms are severly impaired. Drugs that may be only bacteriostatic at low concentrations against some microorganisms, may be bactericidal at higher concentrations against the same or other microorganisms. Thus, the labeling of a drug as bactericidal or bacteriostatic is far from absolute.

ANTICHOLINERGIC (ATROPINE, SCOPOLAMINE)

The parasympatholytics or anticholinergic drugs of a large group of natural and synthetic drugs that prevent the action of acetylcholine at postganglionic parasympathetic endings. Acetylcholine release is not prevented, but its interaction with the receptor is blocked. Thus, the anticholinergic drugs effectively block the action of acetylcholine on smooth muscle, glandular tissues, and the heart. In the therapeutic dosage used by dentists, little or no effect will be observed at the ganglia and neuromuscular junction. The principal drugs in this category are the naturally occurring belladonna alkaloids atropine and scopolamine. These two drugs are useful in dentistry as agents to control salivary secretion and as preanesthetic medication.

Atropine in the usual dose employed in dentistry does not show a central nervous system response although in larger doses stimulation may occur.

Atropine and scopolamine are used:

a. To reduce salivary flow
b. Prevention of cardiac slowing during general anesthesia. Both drugs block the cardiac slowing effect of the vagus nerve with a resultant tachycardia.
c. In the therapy and examination of the eye. These drugs produce dilation (mydriasis) and paralysis of accommodation for distal vision and light (cycloplegia).
d. Functional gastrointestinal disorders and pepticulcer.
e. To control the secretion of common cold and in some cases asthma.
f. Parkinsonism and motion sickness.

Specific contraindications to the use of anticholinergic drugs include glaucoma, prostate hypertrophy (may cause urinary retention), and in intestinal obstruction. Since these drugs affect the cardiovascular system, caution should be observed when using them in patients with severe cardiovascular problems. **The side effects** include: blurring of vision, tachycardia, urinary retention, constipation, decreased salivation, sweating and dry skin.

Atropine sulfate may be used either orally or by injection to reduce salivary flow. **Doses for adults range from 0.3 to 1 mg and should be given at least 1 to 2 hours prior to dental procedure. Nursing mothers excrete atropine in their milk; therefore, one must consider the real need for reduction of salivation in these patients.**

ANTICONVULSANTS

Epilepsy is a disease that encompasses frank convulsions in its most serious aspects to brief periods of unconsciousness in one of its more mild forms. The seizure is believed to be initiated by an ectopic focus in the brain that fires for an unknown reason and his excitation spreads throughout the brain until excessive impulses are sent to the skeletal muscles, resulting in convulsion.

- The anticonvulsants or antiepileptics are not prescribed, as such, by dentists. The dentist should know, if his patient is susceptible to seizures and if he is taking medication for this disease. The seizure could occur almost anytime, such as when the patient is in a dental office.

- One should be aware of the fact that pain, anxiety, or excitement or all three may participate a seizure in an epileptic who is not well controlled. Consequently, the dentist should be prepared to respond to an epileptic seizure in his office. He should also discuss the epileptic patient with his physician prior to treatment in order to determine the: (1) state of control, (2) need for increased medication, (3) other considerations that the physician may be aware of that would facilitate effective and safe dental treatment.

- It should be emphasized that in the majority of cases convulsive episodes are usually self-limiting and require only supportive care in the form of protection of the patient from physical harm and, in some cases, administration of positive pressure oxygen. This is especially true of convulsion secondary to decreased cardiac output and cerebral hypoxia. In this instance, barbiturates are contraindicated and corrective measures should be directed toward tissue oxygenation.

- The most likely cause of a convulsive episode in the dental office is a toxic reaction to local anesthetic from overdose or idiosyncrasy. Here the problem is primarily one of central depression. Although the initial phase of the reaction may be manifested by stimulation in various forms, including convulsion, in dealing with lidocaine the stimulation is actually caused by depression of central inhibitory centers. The eventual or, in some cases, initial response is respiratory and ciculatory depression. It is logical, therefore, to be conservative in the use of anticonvulsant drugs, which may enhance this central depression.

- Convulsion may occasionally be severe enough to be life-threatening in the form of respiratory embarrassment and require drug intervention. Each must decide for himself, before the occasion arises, when to intervene chemically and what drug to use.

- The dentist has a choice of several drugs for use in the event of a serious convulsion occurring in his office. Some of these include pentobarbital sodium (nembutal), thiopental sodium (pentothal sodium), and succinylcholine (anectine). The drug or drugs selected for an emergency kit will depend upon the experience of the person dealing with the emergency.

In most, the most practical anticonvulsant is probably pentobarbital sodium (nembutal). It has the advantage of versatility in the route of administration in that it may be administered intramuscularly or intravenously. The disadvantage of this drug is that it is longer than thiopental sodium or succinylcholine. However, the latter drugs must be administered intravenously. This may be difficult in the convulsive patient.

The ultrashort action of thiopental sodium (pentothal sodium) is advantageous in that there will be less danger of prolonging or enhancing the central depression that follows a convulsion. However, an extravascular injection of thiopental sodium, which is highly alkaline, may result in tissue necrosis and slough. Additionally, inadvertent intra-arterial injection may result in the loss of an extremity. Despite these potential dangers, the dentist familiar with the use of thiopental sodium will probably consider this the drug of choice in the convulsing dental patient in that it can be more accurately titrated for the desired effect with less risk of prolonged depression. The possibility of laryngospasm occurring with the use of thiopental sodium needs no elaboration to the clinician familiar with its use.

The neuromuscular blocking agents, such as succinylcholine (anectine), are potent anticonvulsants, but their use requires special skill and equipment concerned with support of respiration in the paralyzed patient. They are, therefore, recommended for use in the dental office.

| **B** | • Bacterial Endocarditis
• Botulism |

BACTERIAL ENDOCARDITIS

Patients with rheumatic or congenital heart disease who undergo dental or surgical procedures are more prone to develop bacterial endocarditis. This statement provides the physician and the dentist with guidelines and specific regimens for preventing bacterial endocarditis during these procedures.

Bacterial endocarditis is one of the most serious complications of congenital heart disease and rheumatic and other acquired forms of valvular heart disease. It has a high mortality and its sequelae can be crippling. Therefore, its prevention is one of the most important tasks of those caring for patients with these forms of heart disease—physician and dentists alike.

Dental or surgical procedures may be associated with transitory bacteremia. Bacteria in the bloodstream may lodge on damaged or abnormal valves or endocardium, such as are found in rheumatic or congenital heart disease and cause bacterial endocarditis. It is impossible to predict the specific patients in whom this will occur.

Although no data are available from controlled clinical trials on the prevention of bacterial endocarditis, prophylaxis is recommended in those situations most likely to be associated with bacteremia since it is known that bacterial endocarditis cannot occur without a preceding bacteremia. In choosing antibiotics for prophylaxis, one should consider the organisms that are likely to be seeded into the bloodstream from any given site and among these organisms those most likely to cause bacterial endocarditis (Table 15.2). Patients with the forms of heart disease mentioned above should maintain the highest level of oral health to eliminate or minimize potential sources of bacterial seeding, because dental caries, periodontal and periapical disease.

Patients with natural teeth are not free from the risk of bacterial endocarditis even in the absence of dental procedures. The incidence of bacteremia following dental procedures varies with the extent of the procedure, the traumatization of the gingivae and the presence of infection. Ulcers produced by ill-fitting dentures should be promptly cared for, since they may be the source of bacteremia. Prophylaxis is recommended with all dental procedures that are likely to cause bleeding. Since viridans streptococci are the organisms most commonly implicated in bacterial endocarditis following these procedures, prophylaxis is directed specifically against them.

BOTULISM

Botulism results from ingestion of the endotoxin of *Clostridium botulinum* or, in some cases, from the release of endotoxins by surviving ingested organisms in the gut. This is usually caused by bacterial or spore contamination of improperly canned or preserved meat and meat products, which allows growth of the organism and toxin production. Rarely, wounds may be infected with *C. botulinum*. The toxin interferes with

Table 15.2: Antibiotic regimens for a dental procedure for the prevention of infective endocarditis

Situation	Agent	Regimen single dose 30–60 minutes before procedure	
		Adults	Children
Oral	Amoxicillin	2g	50 mg/kg
Unable to take oral medication	Ampicillin or Cafezolin or	2 g IM or IV	50 mg/kg IM or IV
	Ceftriaxone	1 g IM or IV	50 mg/kg IM or IV
Allergic to penicillins or ampicillin	Cephalexin* Clindamycin	2g	50 mg/kg
		600 mg	20 mg/kg
	Azithromycin or	500 mg	15 mg/kg
Allergic to penicillins or ampicillin (oral)	Cafezolin or Ceftriaxone	1g IM or IV	50 mg/kg
and unable to take oral medicine		600 mg IM or IV	20 mg/kg IM or IV

* Or other first- or second-generation oral cephalosporin in equivalent adult or pediatric dosage
Prevention of infective endocarditis. A guideline from the American Heart Association Rheumatic Fever, Endocarditis, and Kawasaki Disease Committee, Council on Cardiovascular Disease in the Young, and the Council on Clinical Cardiology, Council on Cardiovascular Surgery and Anesthesia, and the Quality of Care and Outcomes Research Interdisciplinary Working Group. (2007), American Heart Association, Inc. IM, intramuscularly; IV, intravenously.

the release of acetylcholine at the neuromuscular junction and, as a result progressive descending muscle paralysis dominates the clinical picture with diplopia, laryngeal and pharyngeal palsy and generalized symmetrical paralysis of muscles, especially those of the cranial and respiratory systems. Loss of papillary reflex is an early sign.

Botulinum toxin is the most toxic material known to man and it is estimated that 1 gram has the potential to kill one million people. The toxin has potential uses in biological warfare and terrorism, and its distribution as an aerosol or in deliberately contaminated food are the most likely methods, as it is rapidly inactivated by standard water treatment processes.

The diagnosis of botulism is confirmed by finding toxin in the food, gastric contents or feces by specialized laboratory testing, which takes days to complete; so clinical diagnosis on the basis of symptoms and signs is necessary. Airway support with assisted ventilation is the keystone of treatment. Antitoxin is of value and antibiotics may have a role, if organisms survive in the gut. Mortality is about 50%. Public health measures are aimed at prevention during food preparation for preservation, especially when this done at home. A trivalent antitoxin is available for prophylaxis after exposure and also for those presenting with early symptoms. It neutralizes the toxins of *C. botulinum* types A, B and E. Contraindications to its use are a history of hay fever, asthma or other allergy.

C	• Coagulopathy • Anticoagulant Therapy

COAGULOPATHY

Box. 15.2: Management of patient: Who is therapeutically anticoagulated

I. *Patients receiving aspirin or other platelet-inhibiting drugs*
1. Consult physician to determine the safety of stopping the anticoagulant drug for several days.
2. Defer surgery until the platelet-inhibiting drugs have been stopped for 5 days.
3. Take extra measures during and after surgery to help promote clot formation and retention.
4. Restart drug therapy on the day after surgery, if no bleeding is present.

II. *Patients receiving warfarin (coumadin)*
1. Consult the patient's physician to determine the safety of allowing the PT to fall to 1.5 INR for a few days.
2. Obtain the baseline PT,
3. (a) If the PT is 1 to 1.5 INR, proceed with surgery and skip to step 6 (b) If the PT is more than 1.5 INR, go to step 4.
4. Stop warfarin approximately 2 days before surgery.
5. Check the PT daily and proceed with surgery on the day when the PT falls to 1.5 INR.
6. Take extra measures during and after surgery, to help promote clot formation and retention.
7. Restart warfarin on the day of surgery.

III. *Patients receiving heparin*
1. Consult the patient's physician to determine the safety of stopping heparin for the perioperative period.
2. Defer surgery until at least 6 hours after the heparin is stopped or reverse heparin with protamine.
3. Restart heparin once a good clot has formed.

If the patient's physician believes it is unsafe to allow the PT to fall, the patient must be hospitalized for conversion from warfarin to heparin anticoagulation during the perioperative period. INR, International Normalization Ratio, PT prothrombin time.

ANTICOAGULANT THERAPY

Box 15.3: Management of Patient with a coagulopathy*

- Defer surgery until a hematologist is consulted about the patient's management.
- Obtain baseline coagulation tests as indicated (prothrombin time, partial thromboplastine time, Ivy bleeding time, platelet count) and a hepatitis screen.
- Schedule the patient in a manner that allows surgery soon after any coagulation-correcting measures have been taken (after platelet transfusion, factor replacement or aminocaproic acid administration).
- Augment clotting during surgery with the use of topical coagulation—promoting substances, sutures and well-placed pressure packs.
- Monitor the wound for 2 hours to ensure that a good initial clot forms.
- Instruct the patient in ways to prevent dislodgment of the clot and in what to do if bleeding restart.
- Avoid prescribing non-steroidal anti-inflammatory drugs (NSAIDs).
- Take hepatitis precautions during surgery.

* Patients with severe coagulopathies who require major surgery should be hospitalized.

D	• Dementia • Diabetes • Drug Interactions

DEMENTIA

Dementia is an acquired global impairment of intellect, memory and personality, but without impairment of consciousness. There is often an associated deterioration in emotional control, social behavior and motivation. Long- and short-term memories showed deficits. In the early stages of dementia, the memory lapses may be similar to those that we all experience from time to time—forgetting the name of someone we know casually, our own phone number, or what we went into the next room to get. Most of us eventually remember what we temporarily forgot, rather spontaneously or by tricks that jog our memories. The difference with dementia is that memory does not return spontaneously and may not respond to reminders or other memory cues.

Dementia is Characterized by the Permanent Loss of Basic Cognitive Functions*

Memory impairment, including impaired ability to learn new information or to recall previously learned information.

- Aphasia (language disturbance)
- Apraxia (inability to carry out motor activities despite intact motor function)
- Agnosia (failure to recognize or identify objects despite intact sensory functioning
- Disturbance in excutive functioning (such as planning, organizing, sequencing and abstracting information).

People in the early stages of dementia may repeat questions because they do not remember asking them moments ago, or they do not remember getting answers. They misplace items such as keys frequently. Long-term memory also becomes impaired. People with dementia will forget the order of major events in their lives, such as graduation from college, marriage and the birth of their children.

People with dementia will have tremendous difficulty producing the names of objects or people and may often use terms such as "thing" or vague references to "them" to hide their inability to produce names. There is deterioration of language known as "aphasia". If asked to identify a cup, for example, they may say that it is a thing for drinking but unable to name it as a cup.

People with dementia have an impaired ability to excute common actions, such as saying good-bye or putting on a shirt. This deficit is not caused by problems in motor functioning (such as moving an arm), in sensory functioning, or in comprehending what action is required. The following is a case which represent the typical behaviors of dementia patient as reported by Spitzer et al, 1981.

Aside from sustaining head injury of uncertain significance while a young man in the service, Mr. Abbot B. Carrington had no medical or psychiatric problems until the age of 56. At that time, employed as an officer of a bank, he began to be forgetful. For example, he would forget to bring his briefcase to work or he would misplace his eyeglasses. His efficiency at work declined. He failed to follow through assignments. Reports that he prepared were in complete.

Although still friendly and sociable, Mr. Carrington began to lose interest in many of his usual activities. He ignored his coin collection. He no longer thoroughly perused The Wall Street Journal each day. When he discussed economics, it was without his previous grasp of the subject. After about a year of these difficulties, he was gradually eased out of his responsible position at the bank and eventually retired permanently. At home, he tended to withdraw into himself. He would arise early each morning and go for a long walk, occasionally losing his way if he reached an unfamiliar neighborhood. He needed to be reminded constantly of the time of the day, of upcoming events and of his son's progress in college. He tried to use electric appliances without first plugging them in the socket. He shaved with the wrong side of the razor. Mostly, he remained a quiet pleasant and tractable person, but sometimes particularly at night, he became exceptionally confused and at these times he might be some what irritable, loud and difficult to control.

Approximately 2 years following the onset of these symptoms, he was seen by a neurologist, who conducted a detailed examination of his mental status. The examiner noted that Mr. Carrington was neatly dressed, polite and cooperative. He sat passively in the office as his wife described his problems to the doctor. He himself offered very little information. In fact, at one point, apparently bored by the procedures, he unceremoniously got up from the chair and left the room to wander in the corridor. He did not know the correct date or the name and location of the hospital. In which he was being examined. Mr. Carrington was then told the name and place,

---

* *The diagnostic and statistical manual of mental disorders, fourth edition. American psychiatric association, 2000.*

but 10 minutes later he had forgotten his information. Although a presidential election was then in progress, he did not know the names of the candidates. Despite his background in banking and economics, he could not give any relevant information concerning inflation, unemployment, or the prime lending rate. When questioned about the events of his own life, Mr. Carrington was also frequently in error. He confused recent and remote events. For example he thought his father had recently died, but in fact this had occurred many years earlier. He could not provide a good description of his occupation.

The patient's speech was fluent and well articulated, but vague and imprecise. He used long, roundabout, cliché-filled phrases to express rather simple ideas. Sometimes he would use the wrong word, as he substituted prescribe for subscribe. Despite his past facility with figures, he was unable to do simple calculations. With pencil and paper, he could not copy two dimensional figure or cube. When instructed to draw a house, he drew successions on attached square. Asked to give a single word that would define the similarity between an apple and an orange he replied "round". He interrupted the proverb, "people who live in glass houses shouldn't throw stones "to mean that" people don't want their windows broken. He seemed to have little insight into his problems. He appeared apathetic rather than anxious or depressed. Mr. Carrington was slowly loosing his ability to remember the most fundamental facts of his life, to express himself through language and to carry out the basic activities of everyday life. This is the picture of **dementia,** *the most common cognitive disorders.*

Dementia most commonly occurs in late life. The estimated prevalence of the most common type of dementia that due to Alzheimer's disease, is 2 to 5% in people over 65 years of age. The prevalence of most types of dementia increases with age, with an estimated prevalence of 20% in people over 85 years of age. Notice, however, that the vast majority of older people do not suffer from dementia. Severe cognitive decline is not an inevitable part of old age.

In addition to Alzheimer's disease, a wide range of other conditions may cause dementia (Box 15.4). Some are treatable, so investigation is important in younger patients with dementia. Tests may include CT scanning, MRI or SPECT scanning and may also involve full blood count (including serum B_{12} and folate), renal, liver and thyroid function tests, blood sugar and calcium. Serology for syphilis and HIV, chest and skull X-rays, EEG, CSF examination and heavy metal screening may be appropriate in selected cases.

Box 15.4: Causes of dementia

Unknown	Alzheimer's disease. Multiple sclerosis Parkinson's disease.
	Vascular Uremia
	Liver failure
	Hypothyroidism
	Vitamin B_{12} deficiency.
	Other vitamin B deficiency
	Hypoparathyroidism
	Hypoglycemia
Physical	Space-occupying lesions (tumor, hematoma)
	Post-head injury, especially in subdural hematoma.
Genetic	Huntington's chorea
	Down's syndrome
Infections	HIV infection
	Tuberculosis
	Toxoplasmosis
	Syphilis
Toxic	Poisoning with mercury, manganese, carbon monoxide, alcohol, cupper
Other	Pseudodementia (depression)

Management of Dementia

Treating the disorder that is the cognitive problem (if possible).

- Controlling the symptom or behavior pattern.
- Controlling the resultant disability.
- Providing help for the carers at a social, nursing and medical level; this includes especially home care, day care and long-term residential care.

The amount of news coverage on dementia has increased substantially in recent years, and at times it seems that here is an epidemic of this disorder. Three factors probably contributed to the increase public attention to dementia. First, there have been substantial advances in our understanding of some types of dementia in the past decade, which have made the news. Second, in previous generations, people died of heart disease, cancer, and infectious diseases at younger ages and, therefore, did not reach the age at which dementia often has onset. These days, however, people are living long enough for dementia to develop and affect their functioning. Third, as the baby-boomer generation ages, the number of people who reach the age at which dementia typically occurs is increasing. Indeed, the number of people with dementia is expected to double in the next 50 years, due to the aging of the general population.

DIABETES

Box 15.5: Dental management of the patient with diabetes

1. Non-insulin-dependent patient:
   - If diabetes is well-controlled, all dental procedures can be performed without special precaution.
2. Insulin-controlled patient:
   - If diabetes is well-controlled, all dental procedures can be performed without special precaution.
   - Morning appointments are usually best.
   - Patient advised to take usual insulin dosage and normal meals on day of dental appointment; information confirmed when patient comes for appointment.
   - Advise patient to inform dentist or staff, if symptoms of insulin reaction occur during dental visit.
   - Glucose source (orange juice, soda, glucola) should be available and given to the patient, if symptoms of insulin reaction occur.
3. If extensive surgery is needed:
   - Consult with patient's physician concerning dietary needs during postoperative period.
   - Antibiotic prophylaxis can be considered for patients with brittle diabetes and those taking high doses of insulin who also have chronic states of oral infection.

   If not well-controlled (i.e. does not meet ANY of above criteria: fasting blood glucose <70 mg/dL or >200 mg/dL and ANY complications [post MI, renal disease, congestive heart failure, symptomatic angina, old age cardiac dysrhythmia, cerebrovascular accident], and blood pressure >180/110 mmHg, or functional capacity <4 metabolic equivalents):
   - Provide appropriate emergency care only.
   - Request referral for medical evaluation, management, and risk factor modification
   - If symptomatic, seek immediate referral.
   - If asymptomatic, request routine referral.

Dental management of patient with diabetes and acute oral infection

1. Non-insulin-controlled patients may require insulin; consultation with physician required
2. Insulin-controlled patients usually require increased dosage of insulin; consultation with physician required
3. Patient with brittle diabetes or receiving high insulin dosage should have culture(s) taken from the infected area for antibiotic sensitivity testing
   a. Culture sent for testing
   b. Antibiotic therapy initiated
   c. In cases of poor clinical responses to the first antibiotic, a more effective antibiotic is selected according to sensitivity test results
4. Infection should be treated with the use of standard methods
   a. Warm intraoral rinses
   b. Incision and drainage
   c. Pulpotomy, pulpectomy, extractions, etc.
   d. Antibiotics

DRUG INTERACTIONS

Drug interactions usually result in undesired drug effects. This phenomenon is defined as the action of an administered drug upon the effectiveness or toxicity of another drug administered earlier, simultaneously, or later. It is a problem of growing concern to the health professions and is directly related to the increased incidence of multiple drug therapy. One study has shown that hospitalized patients received an average of 14 different medications during confinement (Cluff et al, 1964). Another study has observed that the incidence of drug interactions ranged from 4 to 5% when two drugs were used to 45% when more than two were used (Stuart, 1968).

Dentistry has more than just an academic interest in this drug problem. Much of the population receiving dental treatment is receiving concurrent drug therapy in the form of prescribed medication or as over-the-counter self-medication. Every dentist should be aware that medications prescribed by him may interact with other drugs to produce undesired effects in his patient. Taking a complete medical history and familiarity with the pharmacologic actions, thertapeutic uses and side effects of individual drugs are both often sufficient for the dentist to predict the consequences of drug therapy. Often, however, unexpected drug interactions may occur to the surprise of the prescriber. Therefore, a review of the current status of drug interactions in dentistry is necessary. The table mentioned here (Table 15.3) serves as a guide in preventing drug interactions.

Table 15.3: Selected interactions of drugs used in dental practice

Primary drug	Action	Interactants
Acetaminophen	enhances	coumarine anticoagulant
Aspirin	antagonizes	probenecid
Aspirin	antagonized by	phenylbutazone
Atropine	enhances	phenothiazines, isoniazid
Barbiturates	enhanced by	MAO inhibitors
Chloral hydrate	antagonizes	coumarine anticoagulants
Codeine	enhances	secobarbital
Codeine	enhanced by	aspirin
Coumarins	enhanced by	chloramphenicol, penicillins, Sulfonamides, tetracyclines
Diphenhydramine	enhanced by	imipramine, amphetamine,
Meperidine	enhanced by	diazepam, MAO inhibitors, Neostigmine, phenothiazines
Morphine	enhanced by	phenothiazines, propranolol
Penicillins	enhanced by	Salicylates, sulfonamides
Phenobarbital	antagonizes	coumarine anticoagulants,
Pyridoxine (vit. B$_6$)	antagonizes	L-dopa.
Salicylates	enhance	coumarine anticoagulants
Salicylates	enhanced by	corticosteroids
Sulfonamides	enhance	coumarine anticoagulants, penicillins
Tetracyclines	antagonized	penicillins
Tetracyclines	antagonized by	antacids, ferrous sulfate.

E Emergency	• Steps for Assessment in Emergency • Dental Office Emergency

STEPS FOR ASSESSMENT IN EMERGENCIES

Box 15.6: Steps for assessment in emergencies

1. **Level of consciousness**
   • What is the level of responsiveness of the patient to questions and to painful stimuli (drowsy, confused, stupor)?
   • When unconscious, is the patient totally unresponsive but breathing?
   • Should the position of the patient be adjusted?

2. **Airway**
   • Is it unobstructed?

3. **Breathing**
   • Is the patient breathing?
   • What are the characteristics of the patients breathing (rate, labored, noisy)?
   • If breathing is not present, should CPR be performed?

4. **Circulation**
   • Is there a pulse?
   • What are the characteristics if there is a pulse (rate, regular, weak)?
   • Measure blood pressure, if possible.
   • What are the characteristics of the blood pressure?

5. **Patients appearance**
   • Skin color?
   • Temperature?
   • Sweating?
   • Eyes and pupils? Responsive?
   • Movements coordinated? Are there spasms?

6. **Is there bleeding or obvious injury?**

7. **Is there a precipitating factor?**

8. **Obvious diagnosis, such as seizure?**
   Specific emergency responses for selected disorders are listed in the appropriate chapter.

DENTAL OFFICE EMERGENCY

Box 15.7: Dental office emergency

Diagnosis	Signs and Symptoms	Treatment
Syncope	1. Pulse weak and slow 2. Skin pale, cold, calmmy 3. Dizziness or loss of conciousness	1. Supine position 2. 100% oxygen 3. Ammonia crush ampoule
	1. Loss of central inhibitory centers	
	a. Apprehension, restlessness b. Increase in blood pressure and respiratory rates, tachycardia c. Convulsion	1. Supine position 2. Positive pressure oxygen 3. Anticonvulsant of choice in severe case
	2. Signs of central depression	
Toxic reaction to local anesthetic	a. Decreased level of consciousness b. Decreased blood pressure and respiratory rate, bradycardia	1. Continue to support respiration as necessary 2. IV infusion of 5% dextrose in water 3. Phenylephrine, 1 ml IV, if severe or prolonged
Cardiac arrest	1. Sudden collapse 2. Absence of carotid pulse 3. Dilated pupils 4. Cold, pale extremities or cyanosis	1. Sharp blow to precorium; repeat, if necessary 2. External cardiac massage 3. Positive pressure oxygen 4. Epinephrine, 0.5 ml IV; repeat as needed 3 to 8 minutes 5. IV infusion of 5% dextrose in water 6. Sodium bicarbonate, 10 ml per 5 minutes of arrest 7. Hydrocortisone, 2 ml IV (slowly)
Allergic reaction 1. Mild 2. Anaphylactic	1. Urticaria 2. Pruritus 3. Tightness in chest 4. Sudden collapse 5. Fall in blood pressure, tachycardia 6. Cardiac arrest	1. Diphenhydramine, 5 ml IV or IM 2. Epinephrine, 0.5 ml IV 3. External cardiac massage and positive pressure oxygen as needed 4. IV infusion of 5% dextrose in water 5. Hydrocortisone, 2 ml IV (slowly)
Angina pectoris	1. Sudden severe chest pain; may radiate to left arm, neck, or mandible 2. Extreme apprehension 3. Increased blood pressure, tachycardia	1. Sitting position 2. Oxygen 3. Nitroglycerine, 0.6 mg tablet sublingually 4. Reassurance
Myocardial infarction	1. Similar to angina but prolonged and no response 2. Arrhythmia	1. Sitting position 2. Oxygen 3. Morphine, 1 ml IM
Acute adrenal insufficiency	1. History of long-term steroid therapy 2. Weakness, syncope 3. Decreased blood pressure, tachycardia	1. Supine position 2. Oxygen 3. Hydrocortisone, 2 ml IV (slowly)
Extrapyramidal reaction (phenothiazines)	1. Restlessness 2. Eyes rolled back 3. Spasm of neck or back muscles (head extended) 4. Trismus 5. Difficulty in swallowing 6. Parkinsonian symptoms	1. Diphenhydramine, 5 ml IV
Respiratory depression (narcotics or sedatives)	1. Shallow, slowed respirations 2. Tachycardia 3. Coma	1. Narcotics—nalorphine, 1 to 2 ml IV or IM 2. Sedatives—methylphenidate 20 to 30 mg IV or IM

| **F** | • Fibrinolytic Therapy |

FIBRINOLYTIC THERAPY

For the preservation of an intact vascular system, it is not only necessary that the blood should not clot, but also that there should be a mechanism for removing blood clot when it has served its purpose of stopping a vascular leak, and repair of the blood vessel and its endothelial lining has occurred. The coagulation and fibrinolytic systems may be in a state of dynamic equilibrium.

The therapeutic potentialities of fibrinolytic substances are obvious. Anticoagulants may prevent thrombosis, fibrinolytics can remove formed thrombi and emboli. Any substance that dissolves clot or inactivates coagulation factors must also carry danger of hemorrhage by preventing clotting, so that laboratory control of this sort of therapy is likely to be needed.

The mechanism of fibrinolysis depends upon infusion of a plasminogen activator, e.g. streptokinase or urokinase. This converts plasminogen (an inert gamma globulin) in the blood into plasmin (fibrinolysin). Plasmin is a proteolytic enzyme, that dissolves fibrin and other proteins, including some coagulation factors (II, V, VIII). The infusion is given as near the clot or embolus as possible, for about 1 to 3 days. Angiograms are invaluable for detecting just where the infusion should be placed. The principal risk is hemorrhage and an antiplasmin (antifibrinolytic), e.g. aminocaproic acid (epsikapron) or tranexamic acid (cyclocapron) should be kept at hand.

Obviously therapy with fibrinolytics (streptokinase, urokinase) is likely to be most important in arterial occlusion by thrombosis or embolism and in those situations where tissue death distal to the block is slowest, giving time to institute therapy before permanent damage is done and where the ideal site for infusion is anatomically accessible. The prospects are thus better for thrombosis or embolism in a limb rather than in the brain or heart.

Fibrinoltyic therapy makes use of the normal body supply of plasminogen and to prevent spontaneous thrombosis after therapy, heparin (initially) and a coumarin are given for 7 days to cover the period of restoration of plasminogen and physiological fibrinolytic function.

The antiplasmins (antifibrinolytics) (aminocaproic acid and tranexamic acid) can be used in hyperplasminemic states that occur due to disease, e.g.

trauma, surgical or accidental, when tissues rich in plasminogen activator, e.g. lung, have been handled or damaged, or in some obstetric disorsers (retained dead fetus, accidental hemorrhage), menorrhagia or in hepatic cirrhosis. Attempts to use antiplasmins to encourage clotting in hemophilia have shown some promise, particularly in dental extraction.

Streptokinase-streptodornase mixtures (varidase) are obtained by growing a special medium. They are used locally to liquefy clotted blood or pus, e.g. in empyemas and fistulae. They do not dissolve living cells, but local inflammation is usual. They also cause fever, leukocytosis and anaphylaxis; albumin and casts may appear in the urine. They should not be used, if there has been recent hemorrhage at the site of application.

| **G** | • Graves' Disease
• Goiter |

GRAVES' DISEASE

Graves' disease is a type of hyperthyroidism results from excessive production of thyroid hormone (TH). It is characterized by increased metabolic rate, weight loss, hyperactivity and heat intolerance. In this particular form of hyperthyroidism, there is a peculiar change in the eyes known as exophthalmos (protruding and bulging eyeballs) (Fig. 15.1). Hyperthyroidism is treated by removing the thyroid gland, either by surgery or intravenous injections of radioactive iodine. In the latter procedure, the thyroid literally "cooks itself as it sequesters the radioactive iodine, but other organs are not damaged because they do not store iodine as does the thyroid (patients whose thyroid glands have been removed must take hormone supplements on a daily basis).

Management of Patient with Hyperthyroidism

1. Defer surgery until thyroid dysfunction is well controlled.
2. Monitor pulse and blood pressure before, during and after surgery.
3. Limit amount of epinephrine used.

GOITER (HYPOTHYROIDISM)

Goiter refers to enlargement of the thyroid gland, typically due to an insufficient amount of the dietary iodine needed to produce TH (Fig. 15.2). Although the pituitary releases more TSH in an effort to

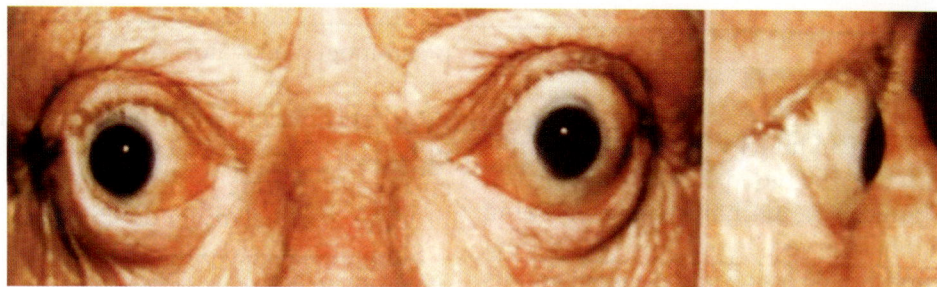

Fig. 15.1: Individuals with Graves' disease (hyperthyroidism) exhibit exophthalmos (bulging and protruding eyeballs) *(McKliney and Loughlin, 2006)*

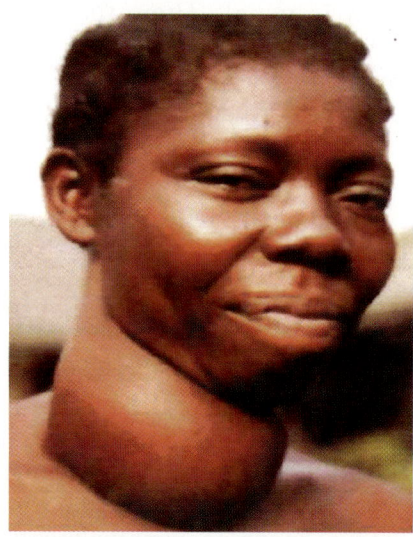

Fig. 15.2: Endemic goiter is caused by dietary iodine deficiency. *(McKliney and Loughlin, 2006)*

stimulate the thyroid, the lack of dietary iodine prevents the thyroid from producing the needed TH. The long-term consequence of the excessive TSH stimulation is overgrowth of the thyroid itself. Unfortunately, goiters do not readily regress once iodine is restored to the diet, and surgical removal is often required.

H	• Angina Pectoris • Heart Failure

ANGINA PECTORIS

Box 15.8: Dental management considerations for patients with unstable angina or recent myocardial infarction within the past 30 days.

- Avoid elective care.
- If treatment is necessary, consult with physician and limit treatment to pain relief, treatment of acute infection, or control of bleeding.

- Consider including the following:
  o Prophylactic nitroglycerin
  o Placement of intravenous line
  o Sedation
  o Oxygen
  o Continuous electrocardiographic monitoring
  o Pulse oximeter
  o Frequent monitoring of blood pressure
  o Cautious use of epinephrine in local anesthetic, combined with above measures.

Box 15.9: Dental management considerations for patients with stable angina or past history of myocardial infarction*

- Morning appointments.
- Short appointments.
- Comfortable chair position.
- Pretreatment vital signs.
- Nitroglycerin readily available.
- Stress-reduction measures:
  o Good communication.
  o Oral sedation (e.g. triazolam 0.125 to 0.25 mg on the night before and 1 hour before the appointment).
  o Intraoperative N_2O/O_2
  o Excellent local anesthesia.
- Limited use of vasoconstrictor (maximum 0.036 mg epinephrine, 0.20 mg levonordefrine); also applicable if patient is taking a nonselective beta blocker.
- Avoidance of epinephrine-impregnated retraction cord.
- Antibiotic prophylaxis *not* recommended for patients with coronary artery stents.
- Antibiotic prophylaxis *not* recommended for history of coronary artery bypass graft (CABG).
- Avoidance of anticholinergics (e.g. scopolamine, and atropine)
- Adequate postoperative pain control.

Defined as longer than 1 month since myocardial infarction (MI), with no ischemic symptoms. It is recommended that at least 4 to 6 weeks should elapse after an uncomplicated Ml before elective procedures are performed.

HEART FAILURE

Box 15.10: Dental management of the patient with heart failure

- Evaluate patient for history, signs, or symptoms of heart failure (HF).
- For patients with symptoms of untreated or uncontrolled HF, defer elective dental care and refer to physician.
- For patients diagnosed and treated for HF:
  o Confirm status with patient or physician
  o New York Heart Association (NYHA) class 1 patients (asymptomatic)—provide routine care.
  o NYHA class II (and some class III patients)—obtain consultation with physician for medical clearance and provide routine care.
  o NYHA (some class III and class IV) patients—obtain consultation with physician; consider treatment in a special care or hospital setting.
  o Identify underlying cardiovascular disease (i.e. coronary artery disease, hypertension, cardiomyopathy, valvular disease) and manage appropriately.
- Drug considerations:
  o For patients taking digitalis, avoid epinephrine; if considered essential, use cautiously (maximum 0.036 mg epinephrine or 0.20 mg levonordefrin); avoid gag reflex; avoid erythromycin and clarithromycin, which may increase the absorption of digitalis and lead to toxicity.
  o For patients with NYHA class III and IV congestive heart failure, avoid use of vasoconstrictors; if use is considered essential, discuss with physician.
  o Avoid epinephrine-impregnated retraction cord.
- See Table 6.1 for drug considerations and adverse effects.
- Schedule short, stress-free appointments.
- Use semisupine or upright chair position.
- Watch for orthostatic hypotension, make position or chair changes slowly and assist patient into and out of chair.
- Avoid the use of nonsteroidal anti-inflammatory drugs (NSAIDs).
- Watch for signs of digitalis toxicity (i.e. tachycardia, hypersalivation, visual disturbances, etc.).
- Nitrous oxide/oxygen sedation may be used with a minimum of 30% oxygen.

I	• Adrenal Insufficiency • Adrenal Medulla

ADRENAL INSUFFICIENCY

Box 15.11: Dental management of the patient with possible adrenal insufficiency

1. Patient past history of systemic corticosteroid use
   a. Evaluate the patient.
   b. Determine whether systemic corticosteroid was taken within the past 2 weeks and the reason for discontinuing usage.
   c. Determine type, dose and duration of systemic corticosteroid used.
   d. Identify signs and symptoms of possible adrenal insufficiency.
   e. If major invasive oral procedure is planned and corticosteroid was taken within the past 2 weeks, consult with the physician regarding status and stability (adrenocorticotropic hormone [ACTH] or perform corticotropin-releasing hormone [CRH] test performed). If adrenal insufficient, implement steroid supplementation protocol*. Note that risk of medical complications increases when major surgical procedures are performed on persons who have low adrenal reserve.

2. Patient currently taking systemic corticosteroids
   a. Evaluate the patient.
   b. Determine dose and duration of systemic corticosteroid used.
   c. Identify signs and symptoms of possible adrenal insufficiency.
   d. For diagnostic and minimally invasive procedures, have patient take the usual daily dose, and perform oral procedure in the morning, shortly after the corticosteroid is taken. Stress reduction measures should be implemented, blood pressure recorded during the procedure.
   e. For major invasive oral procedures, consult with the physician regarding status and stability (ACTH or CRH test performed). Implement the steroid supplementation protocol as discussed below.

3. Patient not taking systemic corticosteroids, or have adrenal insufficiency
   a. Evaluate the patient for historical findings, associated with risk for adrenal insufficiency.
   b. Identify signs and symptoms of adrenal insufficiency.
   c. Refer to the physician for ACTH testing.
   d. If the patient is found to be adrenally insufficient defer dental treatment until stabilized with corticosteroid treatment. Then, follow the steroid supplementation protocol as defined below.

Steroid supplementation protocol for major surgical procedure

- Discontinue drugs that decrease cortisol levels (e.g. ketoconazole) at least 24 hours before surgery with the consent of the patient's physician.
- Have patient take usual morning dose (or the parenteral equivalent as a preoperative dose), and provide supplemental hydrocortisone preoperatively and intraoperatively to achieve 100 mg within first hour of surgery. Give hydrocortisone 25 mg every 8 hours subsequent to surgery for 24 to 48 hours. Perform in hospital environment.
- Provide adequate operative and postoperative analgesia.

– Use barbiturates with caution and knowledge of the potential for adverse effects on plasma cortisol levels.

– Monitor blood pressure (BP) and blood loss throughout the procedure, if BP drops to below 100/60 mm Hg and the patient is unresponsive to fluid replacement.

– Vasopressive measures, administer supplemental steroids.

– Communicate with the patient at the end of the appointment and within 4 hours postoperatively to determine whether features of week pulse, hypotension, dyspnea, myalgias, arthralgia, ileus, and fever are present. Signs and symptoms of adrenal crisis dictate transport to a hospital for emergency care.

ADRENAL MEDULLA

The principal hormone released from the adrenal medulla is **epinephrine, or adrenaline** but small amounts of **norepinephrine** are also released. Epinephrine and norepinephrine are released in response to stimulation by the sympathetic nervous system, which becomes most active when a person is excited or physically active (Fig. 15.3). Stress and low blood glucose levels can also result in increased sympathetic stimulation of the adrenal medulla. Epinephrine and norepinephrine are referred to as the fight-or-flight hormones because of their role in preparing the body for vigorous physical activity.

Some of the major effects of the hormones released from the adrenal medulla are:

1. Stimulation of smooth muscle in the walls of arteries supplying the internal organs and the skin, but not those supplying skeletal muscle. The resulting constriction of the blood vessels causes the blood pressure to increase and blood flow to internal organs and the skin to decrease. Blood flow through skeletal muscles increases.

2. Increase in the heart rate, which also causes the blood pressure to increase.

3. Increase in the metabolic rate of several tissues, especially skeletal muscle, cardiac muscle, and nervous tissue.

4. Dilation of the air passages called bronchiole.

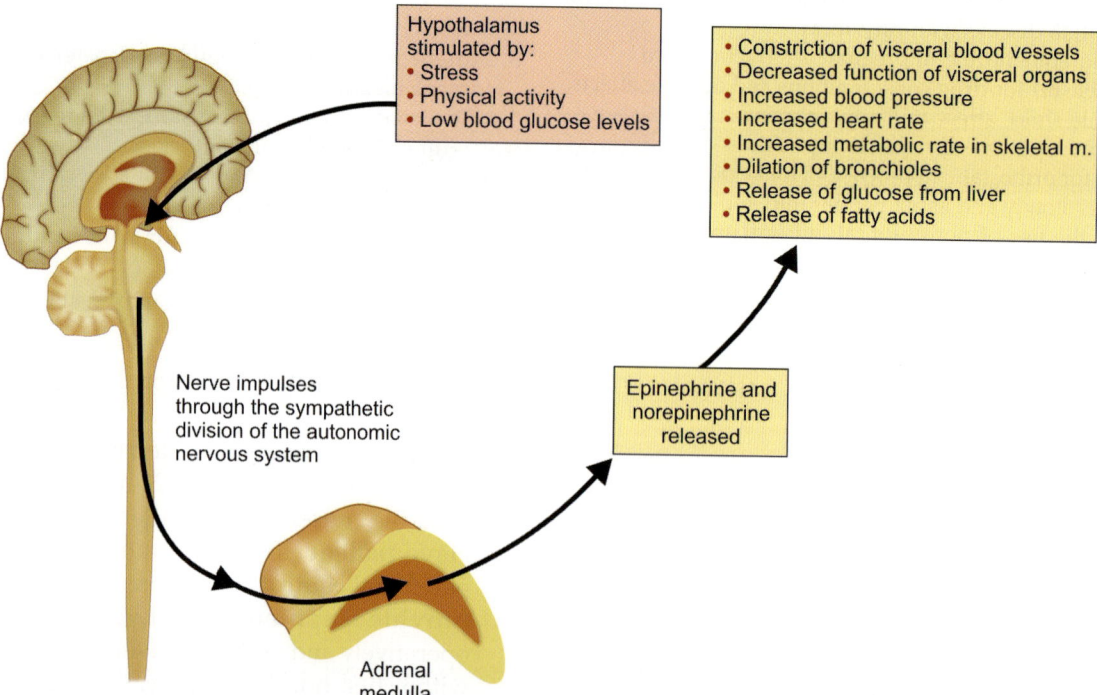

Fig. 15.3: Regulation of adrenal medullary secretions. Stimulation of the hypothalamus by stress, physical activity, or low blood glucose levels causes action potential to travels through the sympathetic nervous system to the adrenal medulla. In response, the adrenal medulla releases epinephrine and smaller amount of norepinephrine which has several effects on the body to prepare for physical activity *(Seeley et al)*

| **K** | • Kaposi's Sarcoma |

KAPOSI'S SARCOMA

Kaposi's sarcoma (KS) is a vascular malignancy with four different presentations:

1. In association with drug-induced immuno-suppressions, e.g. after kidney transplantation.
2. An endemic form in equatorial Africa.
3. A classic form presenting on the lower legs of older men.
4. In association with acquired immunodeficiency syndrome (AIDS).

Kaposi-associated herpes virus 8 is found in all four forms of KS and may be a common etiology for all types of KS through the development of an angiogenic-inflammatory state. Immunosuppression allows for opportunistic infections and malignancy. Proliferation of the tumor depends on the presence of platelet-derived and other growth factors.

The human immunodeficiency virus (HIV) and CMV have been proposed as cofactors in the development of KS. The endothelial cell is thought to be the progenitor of KS but the specific origin is elusive. The lesions emerge as purplish brown macules and develop into plaques and nodules. They tend to be multifocal rather then spreading by metastasis. The lesions initially appear over the lower extremities in the classic form. The rapidly progressive form associated with AIDS tends to spread symmetrically over the upper body, particularly the face and oral mucosa (Fig. 15.4). The lesions are often pruritic and painful. About 75% of individuals with epidemic KS have involvement of lymph nodes, particularly in the gastrointestinal tract and lungs. Organ involvement is much less common in the classic form. The rapidly progressive form has a poor prognosis and shorter survival rates than the classic form.

Diagnosis is by skin biopsy, with a high index of suspicion for those with immunodeficiency. The disease is incurable. Local lesions can be excised. Multiple disseminated lesions may be treated with a combination of immunomodulator, cytotoxic and antiviral drugs. The new, highly active antiretroviral therapy (HAART) for AIDS treatment is decreasing the incidence of KS.

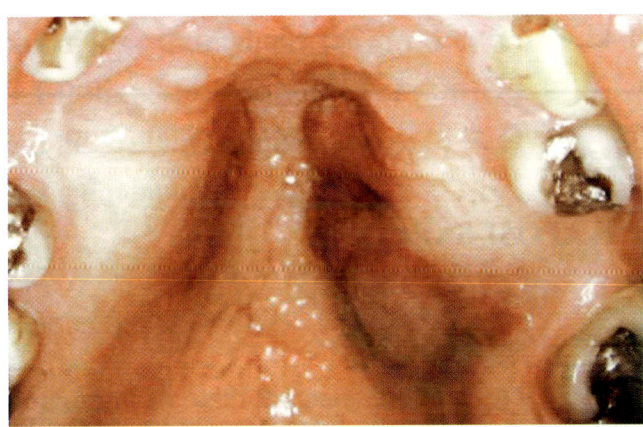 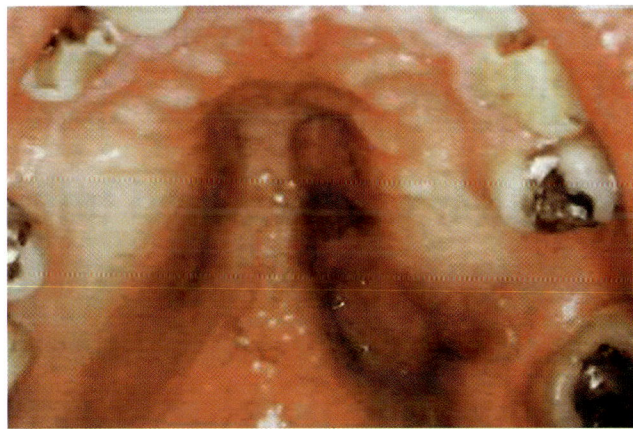

Fig. 15.4: Advanced stage of Kaposi's sarcoma of the palate. Kaposi's sarcoma is typically observed bilaterally, as is the case here, following the course of the palatal vessels. On the left side, the lesions have already progressed into the tumorous stage. Treatment consists of intralesional injection of cytostatics or intraoral irradiation. All types of therapy are only palliative

| **L** | • Liver Disease |

LIVER DISEASE

Table 15.4: Drugs contraindicated and alternatives in patients with liver disease

Analgesics	Aspirin	Codeine
	Codeine	COX-2 inhibitors
	Indometacin	(celecoxib, rofecoxib)
	Mefenamic acid	Hydrocodone

	Meperidine* NSAIDs Opioids Paracetamol/ acetaminophen*	Oxycodone
Antimicrobials	Aminaglycosides Azithromycin Azole antifungals (miconazole, fluconazole, ketoconazole, itraconazole) Clarithromycin* Clindamycin* Co-amoxiclav* Co-trimoxazole Doxycycline Erythromycin estolate Metronidazole* Roxithromycin Talampicillin	Amoxicillin Ampicillin Cephalosporins Erythromycin stearate Imipenem Minocycline Nystatin Penicillins Tetracycline
Antidepressants	Monoamine oxidase inhibitors	SSRIs Tricyclics*
Muscle relaxants	Suxamethonium	Atracurium Cisatracurium Pancuronium Vecuronium
Local anesthetics		Articaine Prilocaine
Anesthetics	Halothane Methohexitone Thiopentone	Desflurane Isoflurane Sevoflurane
Central nervous system depressants	Barbiturates Diazepam* Midazolam* Phenothiazines Propofol*	Lorazepam* Oxazepam* Pethidine*
Corticosteroids	Prednisone	Prednisolone
Others	Anticoagulants Anticonvulsants Biguanides Diuretics Liquid paraffin Lomotil Methyldopa Oral contraceptives	

or given in lower doses than normal

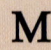

M | • The Use of Local Anesthesia in Medically Compromised Patients
• Metabolic Rate

THE USE OF LOCAL ANESTHESIA IN MEDICALLY COMPROMISED PATIENTS

Box 15.12 is of value for the dental surgeon who is hesitated to administer local anesthesia or carry out the dental procedure under general anesthesia when dealing with a medically compromised patient.

METABOLIC RATE

Metabolic rate means the amount of energy liberated in the body per unit of time, expressed in such terms as kcal/hr or kcal/day. Metabolic rate can be measured directly by putting a person in a

Box 15.12: Local anesthesia in medically compromised patients

Condition	Clinical problem and tissue	Avoiding action
Cardiovascular		
Ischemic heart disease, e.g. angina, myocardial infarction, coronary artery bypass grafts	Arrhythmias Further ischemia General anesthetic risk	Control pain and anxiety Local anesthetic preferred Consider hospital treatment
Heart failure	Orthopnoea	Sit patient up Local anesthetic preferred
Thromboembolic disease	Deep vein thrombosis Pulmonary embolus	Local anesthetic preferred Avoid general anesthetic
Respiratory		
Asthma	Acute asthmatic attack	Local anesthetic preferred
Chronic bronchitis Emphysema	General anesthetic risk-obstructed airways Postoperative chest infection	Use local anesthetic
Nervous		
Cerebrovascular accident (stroke)	Further cerebrovascular accident Potential general anesthetic risk	Use local anesthetic
Multiple sclerosis	Exacerbation of multiple sclerosis	Use local anesthetic
Gastrointestinal		
Liver failure	Hemorrhage Impaired drug metabolism	Reduce dosage Local anesthetic preferred
Inflammatory bowel disease Malabsorption conditions	Steroid therapy (steroid crisis) Anemia (potential general anesthetic risk)	Give steroid cover Local anesthetic preferred
Hematological		
Clotting/platelet disorder (factor VIII) Anticoagulant therapy	Excessive bleeding	Consult with physician Give factor replacement therapy/reduce anticoagulant therapy Caution with inferior dental block (danger of parapharyngeal hematoma—restriction of airway)
Anemia, special sickle cell	**General anesthetic risk**	**Use local anesthetic**
Endocrine		
Diabetes mellitus Hyperthyroidism	Hyper-hypoglycemia Arrhythmias Thyroid crisis	Use local anesthetic Avoid adrenaline in local anesthesia Avoid general anesthetic
Hypothyroidism Pregnancy	**Slow drug metabolism** Teratogenicity Premature labor	**Local anesthetic preferred** Avoid elective procedures Local anesthetic preferred (lignocaine and adrenaline)

calorimeter, a closed chamber with water-filled walls that absorb the heat given off by the body. The rates of energy release is measured from the termperature change of the water. Metabolic rate can also be measured indirectly with a spirometer, an apparatus that can be used to measure the amount of oxygen a person consumes. For every liter of oxygen, approximetely 4.82 kcal of energy is released from organic nutrients. This is only an estimate, because the number of kilocalories per liter of oxygen varies slightly time of measurement.

Metabolic rate depends on physical activity, mental state, absorptive or postabsorptive status, thyroid hormone and other hormones and other factors.

N	• Narcotics–Morphine

NARCOTICS–MORPHINE

Narcotics are drugs that produce narcosis (stupor). Narcotics are important in dental practice against pain that cannot be controlled by the less potent non-narcotic drugs. The narcotics are classified as opium alkaloids (morphine, codeine), semisynthetic derivative of morphine (heroin, dicodeine, oxycodone) and synthetic narcotics (demerol, leritine, dolophine, levodromoran).

Morphine provides effective analgesia against severe pain. The greater potency over non-narcotic analgesics is related to the fact that in addition to raising the pain threshold the narcotics also affect the cerebral cortex to depress the reaction to pain. Sedation is also produced by analgesic doses.

Morphine sharply depresses the respiratory center in the medulla. Respiratory depression is the cause of death in overdose. Although the usual adult doses of morphine have minimal effects on respiration in healthy patients, even therapeutic doses may dangerously decrease pulmonary ventilation in elderly or debilitated patients and those with severe pulmonary diseases. Morphine and other narcotics have been said to be contraindicated in cases of myxedema, Addison's disease and cirrhosis of the liver because small doses may cause respiratory failure. Special care is also indicated in patients with other respiratory limitations such as those in shock or those suffering from severe asthma or chronic lung disease. The use of narcotics in pregnant women should also be avoided when possible to preclude possible anoxia to the fetus. The practitioner should also reduce the dosage of morphine for patients who are taking other drugs that also depress respiration, such as barbiturates.

Morphine causes cerebral vasodilation, which appears to be secondary to respiratory depression. This results in an increase in intracranial and spinal fluid pressure. Consequently, morphine should not be used in patients with head injuries or where intracranial pressure may already be present.

The usual adult dose (as the sulfate salt) is used parenterally against severe pain. The usual adult dose of 10 to 15 mg subcutaneously should cover severe dental pain for about 6 hours. For children, the dose is 0.1 to 0.2 mg/kg/dose, with the maximal dose being 15 mg. Close observation should follow the use of morphine in a child. Parenteral solutions of morphine sulfate that contain 8, 10, 15 and 30 mg/ml are available.

O	• Oxyhemoglobin • Methemoglobinemia • Carbon Monoxide Poisoning

OXYHEMOGLOBIN

The concentration of oxygen in arterial blood, by volume, is about 20 mL/dL. About 98.5% of this is bound to hemoglobin and 1.5% is dissolved in the blood plasma. Hemoglobin consists of four protein (globin) chains, each with one heme group (Fig. 15.5). Each heme group can bind 1 O_2 to the ferrousion at its center; thus, one hemoglobin molecule can carry up to 4 O_2. If even one molecule of O_2 is bound to hemoglobin, the compound is called **oxyhemoglobin (HbO$_2$),** whereas hemoglobin with no oxygen bound to it is **deoxyhemoglobin (HHb).** When hemoglobin is 100% saturated, every molecule of it carries 4 O_2; if it is 75% saturated, there is an average of 3 O_2 per hemoglobin molecule; if it is 50% saturated, there is an average of 2 O_2 per hemoglobin; and so forth. The poisonous effect of carbon monoxide stems from its competition for the O_2 binding site).

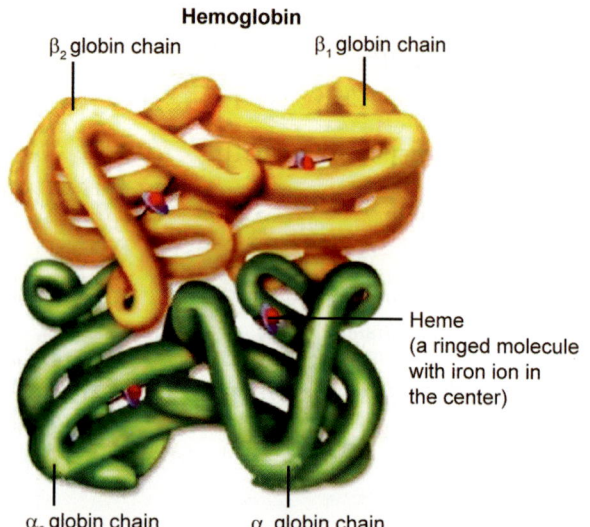

Fig. 15.5: Molecular structure of hemoglobin. A single molecule of hemoglobin is composed of four protein subunits, called globins, each containing a heme group that holds a single iron ion in its center. Each hemoglobin molecule transports four oxygen molecules that are weakly attracted to the iron ions *(McKliney & O'loughlin, 2006)*

METHEMOGLOBINEMIA

Oxyhemoglobin (HbO$_2$), the oxygen-saturated form of hemoglobin, transports oxygen from the lungs to tissues, where the oxygen is released. HbO$_2$ becomes reduced hemoglobin (Hb). While oxygen-saturated hemoglobin is bright red, reduced hemoglobin is bluish red, accounting for the difference in the color of the blood in arteries and veins. Certain chemicals readily block the oxygen-transporting function of hemoglobin. For example, carbon monoxide (CO) rapidly replaces oxygen in HbO$_2$, resulting in the formation of the stable compound carboxyhemoglobin (HbCO). Nitrates and certain other chemicals oxidize the iron in Hb from the ferrous to the ferric state, resulting in the formation of methemoglobin (met-Hb). Methemoglobin contains oxygen bound tightly to ferric iron, as such, it is useless in respiration. Cyanosis, the dark blue coloration of skin associated with anoxia, becomes evident when the concentration of reduced hemoglobin exceeds 5 g/dL. Cyanosis may be rapidly reversed by oxygen, if the condition is caused only by a diminished oxygen supply. However, cyanosis caused by the intestinal absorption of nitrates or other toxins, a condition known as "enterogenous cyanosis", is due to the accumulation of stabilized methemoglobin and is not rapidly recersible by the administration of oxygen alone.

A reducing substance is needed to convert the methemoglobin (ferric iron) back to oxyhemoglobin (ferrous iron) whenever enough has formed seriously to impair the oxygen carrying capacity of the blood. Ascorbic acid is non-toxic, but is less effective than methylene blue. Both can be given orally, i.v. or i.m. Excessive doses of methylene blue can cause methemoglobinemia.

Methemoglobinemia may be drug-induced as phenacetin, sulfonamides, bismuth subnitrate, nitrites, nitrates (may occur in well water), primaquine, pyrimidium, acetanilide, phenazone and other drugs). In the rare instance of there being urgency, methylene blue 1–2 mg/kg i.v. benefits within 30 minutes. In the congenital form, methylene blue (3 to 6 mg/kg/day in divided doses) with or without ascorbic acid (0.5 g/day) gives benefit in days to weeks.

CARBON MONOXIDE POISONING

The lethal effect of carbon monoxide (CO) is well known. This colorless, odorless gas occurs in cigarette smoke, engine exhaust and fumes from furnaces and space heaters. It binds to the ferrous ion of hemoglobin to form *carboxyhemoglobin (HbCO)*. Thus, it competes with oxygen for the same binding site. Not only that, but it binds 210 times as tightly as oxygen. Thus, CO tends to tie up hemoglobin for a long time. Less than 1.5% of the hemoglobin is occupied by carbon monoxide in most nonsmokers, but this figure rises to as much as 3% in residents of heavily polluted cities and 10% in heavy smokers. An atmospheric concentration of 0.1% CO, as in a closed garage, is enough to bind 50% of a person's hemoglobin and an atmospheric concentration of 0.2% is quickly lethal.

P	• Body Planes
	• Pulmonary disease
	• Pregnancy

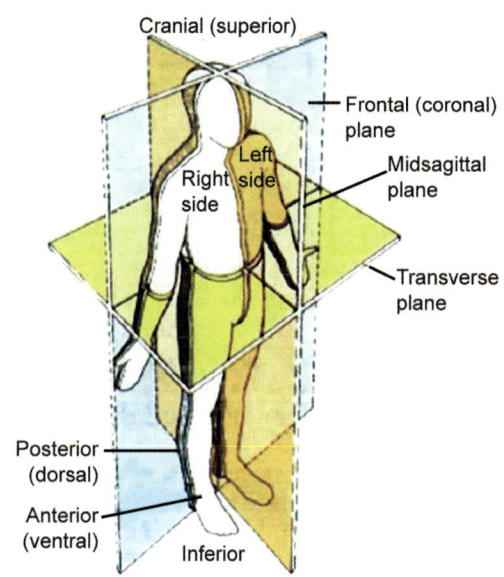

Fig. 15.6: The body planes

BODY PLANES

Body planes are:
- *Coronal:* A line from side to side, dividing the front and back halves of the body.
- *Midsagittal:* A line from superior to inferior along the midline, dividing the right and left halves of the body.
- *Sagittal:* A vertical line from superior to inferior at any point that divides the body into right and left parts.
- *Transverse:* A line dividing the upper and lower halves of the body.

- In a resting person, atrial systole lasts about 0.1 second; ventricular systole, 0.3 second; and the *quiescent period* (when all four chambers are in diastole), 0.4 second.

Q	• Quiescent Period

QUIESCENT PERIOD

Total duration of the cardiac cycle is, therefore, 0.8 second (800 msec) in a heart beating at 75 bpm.

R	• End-stage Renal Disease • Respiratory Stimulants

END-STAGE RENAL DISEASE

Box 15.13: Dental management of the patient with end-stage renal disease (including emergency dental care).

Under conservative care

- Consult with physician regarding physical status and level of control.
- Avoid dental treatment, if disease is unstable (poorly controlled or advanced).
- Screen for bleeding disorder before surgery (bleeding time, platelet count, hematocrit, hemoglobin).
- Monitor blood pressure closely.
- Pay meticulous attention to good surgical technique.
- Avoid nephrotoxic drugs (acetaminophen in high doses, acyclovir, aspirin, nonsteroidal anti-inflammatory drugs)
- Adjust dosage of drugs metabolized by the kidney (*see* Table 13.2).
- Aggressively manage orofacial infections with culture and sensitivity tests and antibiotics.
- Consider hospitalization for severe infection or major procedures.
- Consider corticosteroid supplementation as indicated.

Receiving hemodialysis

Same as conservative care recommendations.
Beware of concerns of arteriovenous shunt.
Consult with physician about risk for infective endarteritis or endocarditis.
Avoid blood pressure cuff and IV medications in arm with shunt.
Avoid dental care on day of treatment (especially within first 6 hours afterward); best to treat on day after.
Consider antimicrobial prophylaxis (based on guidelines [*see* Box 13.4]).
Consider corticosteroid supplementation as indicated.
Assess status of liver function and presence of opportunistic infection in these patients because of increased risk for carrier state of hepatitis B and C viruses and human immuno-deficiency virus (HIV).

Special precaution may be needed for patient with complications of diabetes, renal disease, heart disease.

RESPIRATORY STIMULANTS

Respiratory stimulants have some place in case of fainting (syncope) and in cases of acute respiratory failure due to: (A) Depression of respiratory center by poisons, e.g. barbiturates, as an emergency measure only, until mechanical respiration is available. (B) Pulmonary failure with hypercapnea, drowsiness and inability to cough, to stimulate respiratory and coughing, as a short-term measure only, e.g. "buy time" for chemotherapy to control infection.

Drugs used are general CNS stimulants and for most the effective respiratory stimulant does is close to that causing convulsions, preceded by restlessness and twitching (at first round the mouth), itching, vomiting and flushing; convulsions may occur though the patient remains unconscious.

Available drugs include, nikethamide (courmaine), doxapram (dopram), vandid and megimide. They are generally given i.v. Oral use is probably therapeutically worthless. Theophylline (e.g. aminophylline) is also a respiratory stimulant. Irritant vapours as inhaled ammonia, irritates trigeminal sensory endings with a resulting reflex stimulation of medullary respiratory and vasomotor centers.

S	• Sialorrhea

SIALORRHEA

Sialorrhea is defined as an excessive secretion of saliva or hypersalivation. The cause is an increase in saliva production or a decrease in salivary clearance. Hypersalivation, can be caused by medications (Table 15.5), hyperhydration, infant teething, the secretory phase of menstruation, idiopathic paroxysmal hypersalivation heavy metal poisoning, organophosphorus (acetylcholinestrase) poisoning, nausea, gastropharyngeal reflux disease, obstructive esophagitis, neurologic changes such as in a cerebral vascular accident (CVA), neuromuscular disease, neurologic diseases, and neurologic infections.

Minor hypersalivation may result from local irritations, such as aphthous ulcers or an ill-fitting oral-prosthesis.

Clinical Presentation

Hypersalivation can cause drooling, which produces social embarrassment, rejection and a severe impairment in the quality of a person's life. In severe cases, a partial or total blockage of the airway can occur, producing aspiration of oral contents and possibly aspiration pneumonia. Hypersalivation also causes perioral irritations and traumatic ulcerations that can become secondarily infected by fungal or bacterial organisms.

Table 15.5: Causes of hypersalivation and drooling

Medications
Pilocarpine
Cevimeline
Lithium
Bethanechol
Physostigmine
Clozapine
Resperidone
Nitrazapam
Neurologic disease
Parkinson's disease
Autism
Cerebral palsy
Down's syndrome
Heavy metals
Iron
Lead
Arsenic
Mercury
Thallium

Diagnosis

Since there is a multitude of etiologic causes of hypersalivation, it is essential to:

- Obtain the exact history of the hypersalivation as well as thorough and complete past medical history.
- A systemic oral evaluation should be performed, focusing on salivary gland enlargements, oral ulcerations, head/neck/oral masses, neuromuscular function and condition of removable intraoral prosthesis.
- A salivary flow rate should be determined. The normal rate of unstimulated salivary output from all glands is approximately 2.0 to 3.5 mL per 5 minutes. Collection of unstimulated whole saliva using a drooling technique into a preweighed container that results in more than 5.0 mL in 5 minutes suggests greater than normal production of saliva and can help differentiate between an overproduction of saliva versus a salivary clearance issue.
- Blood samples should also be obtained and evaluated for heavy metals and organophosphate pesticides.
- Premenopausal women should be evaluated for potential pregnancy and in postmenopausal or male patients, androgen levels should be determined to rule out androgen excreting tumor. If onset is acute, a CT scan of the brain should be obtained to rule out a CVA or a central nervous system mass.

Treatment

Depending on the etiology, there are two types of treatments: medications and surgery.

Medications

Drug-based treatments for hypersalivation are devised based upon etiology.

a. If the patient is experiencing hypersalivation secondary to a pharmaceutical treatment, alternate medications can be evaluated and if the therapeutic regimen cannot be altered, compatible xerostomic agents (scopolamine transdermal patch, propantheline, benztropine, atropine, glycopyrrolate, diphenylhydramine hydrochloride) should be considered.

b. Consultation should be made with the patient's physician to help prevent deleterious drug-drug interaction problems or polypharmacy-induced side effects.

c. Hypersalivation that occurs secondary to chronic nausea (e.g. during chemotherapy) can be treated with antiemetic medications.

d. Hypersalivation due to gastroesophageal reflux disorder (GERD) is a protective buffering response to acids encountered in the oral cavity. The GERD should be treated and under most circumstances, hypersalivation will resolve.

e. Neurologic and neuromuscular conditions (e.g. CVA, Down syndrome, central neurologic infections) can result in neuromuscular incompetence in swallowing function, resulting in salivary pooling in the anterior floor of the mouth and salivary spillage from the oral cavity (drooling). Xerostomic medications as shown above can be attempted for these conditions.

f. Based on open-label and controlled studies, intraglandular botulinum toxin injections can be used to improve sialorrhea in patients with Parkinson's disease, motor neuron disease and cerebral palsy. Botulinum toxin A (7.5–15 units) can be infiltrated, by trained individuals, into the body of the parotid gland. However, the response is only temporary and necessitates reinfiltration 2 to 3 months later. Possible side effects are xerostomia, pain at the injection site, and temporary facial nerve paralysis, if the injections are placed deep within the gland.

Surgery

A number of surgical techniques have been devised to treat hypersalivation particularly in patients with poor or deficient neuromuscular function.

a. Historically, redirection of the submandibular ducts and parotid ducts posteriorly to the tonsillar pillars has been performed with good success, although patients with poor salivary clearance will not benefit from this technique.

b. Bilateral tympanic neurectomy has been performed, but this leaves a permanent anesthesia to the anterior portion of the tongue and is not recommended.

c. Excision of sublingual glands.

d. Ligation of all major sunmandibular/sublingual ducts.

These techniques are successful in reduction of drooling approximately 80% of the time, with occasional postoperative complications such as ranula formation, pain and numbness. The advantage of duct ligation technique is that it involves an intraoral surgical approach, thereby reducing the risk of damaging the facial nerve.

e. A final strategy is excision of one or more major salivary glands.

T	• Trismus
	• Disorders of Taste

TRISMUS

The word *trismus* is derived from Greek word *Trismous* meaning gnashing or lock jaw. Up to seventeenth century, it was used almost exclusively when referring to tetanus.

Trismus term is boldly used for inability to open the mouth. *Trismus*, "A condition of spasm of the jaw muscles causing them to the rigid and preventing the opening of mouth either partially or totally, temporarily or permanently".

In 1973, Nally and Eggleston defined trismus simply and lucidly, "inability to open the mouth due to reflex muscle spasm".

But, probably best in all aspect, trismus is defined by Sir Norman L, Rowe in his famous William Guy lecture in 1981. *Trismus* is mediated by the " Servo feed back" of arthokinetic reflex arc from proprioceptive nerve endings in the periodontium, the muscle spindles and the mechanoreceptors of the joint capsule via the brainstem to the muscles, which activates the closure of the lower jaw. Once the existing stimulus is removed, the condition disappears.

The causes of trismus include:

1. Odontogenic—MPDS (myofacial pain dysfunction syndrome), malocclusion, erupting teeth.
2. Infection—periodontitis, pericoronitis, submasseteric, temporal, peritonsillar space infection, parotitis.
3. Traumatic—fracture of the mandible, fracture of the zygoma impinging the coronoid.
4. Neoplastic—tumors involving the jaw muscles, retromolar fossa, tonsillar fossa, nasopharynx (Trotter's syndrome).
5. Pharmacological—some phenothiazines.
6. Psychological—hysterical trismus.
7. Neurotoxic—tetanus.
8. Neurological—central and peripheral lesion.

Some analytical observation on clinical perspective:

1. Treatment of trismus is primarily based on etiological factors, clinical panaroma and degree of myospasm.
2. The antibiotics are most effective in trismus of odontogenic infection involving muscles of mastication directly, or via facial planes.
3. Surgical interference is mandatory according to necessity (removal of offending tooth or teeth, drainage of abscess).
4. Infraray therapy helps in localization abscess in earlier stage and in relieving spastic condition of muscle due to inflammatory process.
5. Muscle relaxant property of diazepam is widely used in practice.
6. Use of brisment force. Mechanical appliance (Fergusion's mouth gag, acrylic screw) is found to be helpful in relieving trismus in post-extraction cases.
7. Trismus is not always associated with pain.
8. Trismus is a reversible condition mostly and irreversible partly.

Ankylosis can be defined as stiffness or immobility of the joint due to fibrous adhesion or bony fusion within the joint or between two bones. The causes of ankylosis can be categorized as:

- *Extra-articular causes* as inflammation around the temporomandibular joint, e.g. oral submucous fibrosis, mucosal scaring (e.g. in epidermolysis bullosa) or fibrosis due to burn and irradiation
- *Intra-articular causes:* Congenital ankylosis, traumatic ankylosis, ankylosis following pyogenic arthritis, ankylosis following juvenile arthritis and neoplasms and other cause of enlargement of the condyle.

DISORDERS OF TASTE

The complex process of tasting begins when molecules stimulate special sensory cells in the nose, mouth, or throat. These gustatory or taste cells react to food and beverages. Another chemosensory mechanism, the common chemical sense, contributes to appreciation of food flavor, especially to sensation like the sting of ammonia, the coolness of menthol and the irritation of chili peppers. Human can commonly identify at least five different taste sensations: sweet, sour, bitter, salty and umami (the taste elicited by glutamate, found in chicken broth, meat extracts and some cheeses). Flavors are recognized mainly through the sense of smell.

Taste buds are present on the tongue mainly, but also on the soft palate, uvula, epiglottis, pharynx, larynx and esophagus. Taste perception can be tested with salt (NaCl), sweet (saccharin), acidic (citrus) and bitter (quinine), or by electrogustometry. Disorders of taste are fairly common and can have a wide range of causes (Table 15.6). Similar conditions to those that cause halitosis can cause a bad taste in the mouth (dysguesia). The sense of taste can also be temporarily disturbed by the use of chemicals such as chlorhexidine. Gymnemic acid abolishes the perception of sweet tastes while amiloride abolishes salt perception. Loss of taste can be due to medical disorders, or anesthesia of the nerves involved, particularly damage to chorda tympani (from herpes zoster oticus, otitis media, mastoiditis, or cholesteatoma). The most common taste complaint is of phantom taste perceptions. Additionally, testing may demonstrate a weakened ability to taste sweet, sour, bitter, salty and umami (ageusia). Rarely there is complete lack of taste perception (ageusia). Perceived loss usually reflects a smell loss, which is often confused with a taste loss. In order disorders of the chemical senses, the system may misread and/or distort an odor, a taste or a flavor. Alternatively, a person may detect a foul taste from a substance that is normally pleasant tasting.

Causes of Hypogeusia Include

Table 15.6 describes causes of hypogeusia.

1. Upper respiratory infections
2. Head injury
3. Chemicals such as insecticides
4. Some drugs
5. Oral health problems
6. Surgery with nerve damage (third molar extraction and middle ear surgery)
7. Radiation therapy
8. Diabetes
9. Hypertension
10. Malnutrition

Table 15.6: Causes of taste loss or change

Aging		
Local causes	Xerostomia	
	Irradiation of the oral cavity	
Drugs	Antihistamines	
	Antihypertensives	
	Antidepressants	
	Cytotoxic agents	
	Protease inhibitors	
Neurological causes	Alzheimer's disease	
	Chorda tympani damage	
	Facial palsy	
	Head trauma	
	Multiple sclerosis	
	Parkinson's disease	
	Riley-Day syndrome	
	Temporal lobe epilepsy	
Nutritional defects	Cancer	
	Zinc deficiency	
	Vitamin B deficiency	
Endocrinopathies	Addison's disease	
	Diabetes	
	Cushing's syndrome	
	Hypopituitarism	
	Hypothyroidism	
Metabolic disorders	Chronic renal failure	
	Hepatic disease	
Viral infections		

U	• Management of Unconscious Patient
	• Cardiopulmonary Resuscitation (CPR)

MANAGEMENT OF UNCONSCIOUS PATIENT

The loss of consciousness depresses many of the body's vital functions, including its protective reflexes-choking, coughing, sneezing and swallowing and the ability of the victim to maintain an open or patent airway. The following steps allow the rescuer to maintain these vital functions until the victim either recovers spontaneously or is transported to a hospital equipped with the resources for more definitive management.

1. Positioning of the Patient

The patient is placed in the supine position (horizontal) with the brain at the same level as the heart or the feet can be elevated slightly (a 10 to 15° angle). Rescuers should avoid (Trendelenburg) position because gravity pushes the abdominal viscera superiorly up into the diaphragm, restricting respiratory movement and diminishing the effectiveness of breathing.

2. Establishment of a Patent Airway

Opening of the airway and restoration of breathing are the most basic and important steps which can be performed without equipment or assistance as follows.

Head Tilt-Chin Lift Technique

The rescuer places the fingers of one hand under the bony symphysis region of the victims to lift the tip of the mandible up and bring the chin forward. Because the tongue is attached to the mandible, it is pulled forward and off the posterior pharyngeal wall. The tips of rescuer's fingers should be placed only on bone, not on the soft tissues of the chin. Compressing these soft tissues increases airway obstruction, pushing the tongue further upward into the oral cavity. The head tilt chin lift technique stretches the tissues between the larynx and mandible, lifting the base of the tongue and epiglottis from the posterior pharyngeal wall (Fig. 15.7).

Jaw Thrust Technique

Although head tilt is effective in re-establishing airway patency in most situations, occasionally an airway may remain obstructed. In most instances, additional

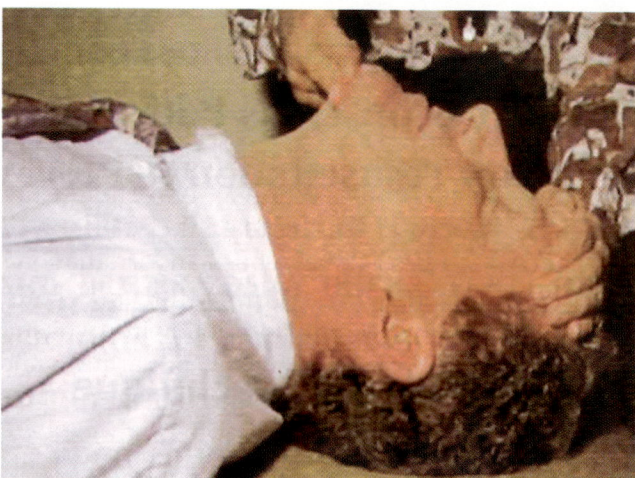

Fig. 15.7: The cardiac arrest patient should be placed flat on a hard surface. His head and neck should be extended by lifting the chin with one hand and pressing the forehead with another. The airway may be cleared digitally or with suction, if available at this time *(McKliney & O'loughlin, 2006)*

forward displacement of the mandible performed with the jaw thrust maneuver adequately removes this obstruction. To perform the technique, the rescuer's fingers are placed behind the posterior border of the ramus of the mandible; the rescuer displaces the mandible forward, while tilting the head backward.

3. Administration of Oxygen

Using the **look-listen-and-feel technique,** the rescuer then determines whether the victim is breathing. If no air can be felt or heard at the mouth or the nose and there is no evidence of chest or abdominal movement, a tentative diagnosis of respiratory arrest is made and artificial ventilation is started immediately.

The dental team must ventilate the victim so that adequate oxygen is available to the brain. The victim may receive artificial ventilation in one of three ways:
  A. Exhaled air ventilation.
  B. Atmospheric(ambient) air ventilation.
  C. Oxygen-enriched ventilation.

A. Exhaled Air Ventilation (Mouth-to-Mouth Breathing)

In this technique of artificial ventilation, the rescuer may deliver exhaled air to the victim's lungs as one source of oxygen. The air we breathe contains approximately 21% oxygen. The exhaled air ventilation contains 16 to 18% oxygen is adequate to sustain life. To adequately perform mouth-to-mouth ventilation, the rescuer uses the head-tilt or head tilt-chin lift position to maintain the patient's head in an optimal backward tilt. The rescuer's hand on the patient's forehead continues to help maintain a backward tilt while the doctor's thumb and index finger pinch the victim's nostrils closed (Figs 15.8 and 15.9). With mouth wide open, the doctor takes a deep breath, makes a tight seal around the patient's mouth and blows into the mouth. A rapid and deeply inhaled breath immediately before blowing delivers expired air with the lowest carbon dioxide content.

The first cycle of ventilation should consist of two full breaths, with the doctor allowing 1½ to 2 seconds per inspiration and taking a breath after each ventilation. Exhalation occurs passively when the doctor's mouth is removed from the patient's, allowing gravity to deflate the lungs. Artificial respiration in the adult must be repeated once every 5 to 6 seconds (20 times per minute) for as long as necessary. The rescuer can gauge the adequacy of ventilation effort by using the following two guides; Feeling air escape as the victim passively exhales. Seeing the rise and fall of the victim's chest.

B. Atmospheric Air Ventilation

The administration of increased concentrations of oxygen enhances any resuscitative effort. Devices are

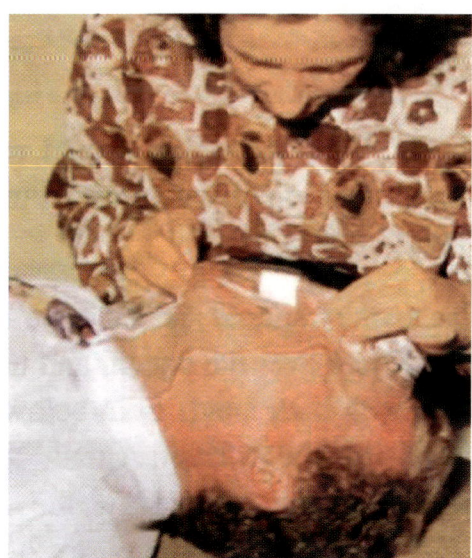

Fig. 15.8: Artificial respiration should be started using the mouth-to-mouth technique. The nose is occluded with the thumb and index finger, and the movement of the chest provides an index of the efficacy of ventilation. In this case, protection for the operator is provided by a simple plastic sheet with a small mesh-covered vent at the mouth (Laerdal) *(McKinley and Loughlin, 2006)*

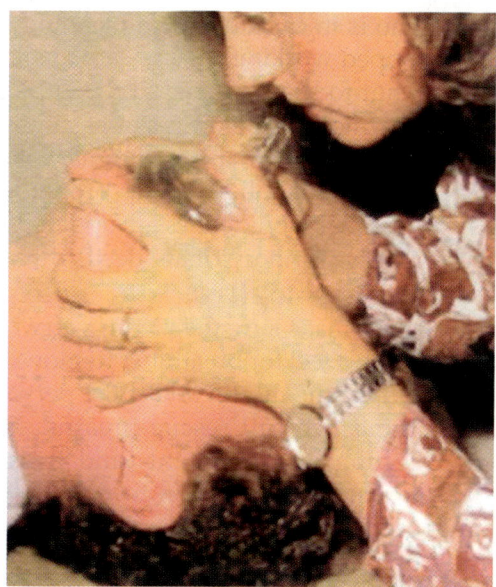

Fig. 15.9: A more efficient way to avoid mouth-to-mouth contact and to ensure adequate respiration with a Laerdal mask. These should be available in all hospital wards and carried by all members of the resuscitation team. Supplemental oxygen may be added to the inlet port *(McKinley and Loughlin, 2006)*

available that permit the rescuer to deliver atmospheric air to the victim's lungs. Bag-valve-mask(BVM) devices, such as the Ambubag usually provide less ventilatory volume than mouth-to-mouth ventilation because of the difficulty in maintaining an airtight seal.

C. Oxygen-Enriched Ventilation

Whenever possible, the rescuer should use artificial ventilation with supple mental oxygen. Exhaled air ventilation delivers 16 to 18% oxygen, whereas atmospheric air provides 21% oxygen. Because the object of basic life support is to provide the brain with oxygen, the use of supplemental oxygen (> 21%) is preferred. Sources of oxygen available in the dental office include portable cylinder with adjustable oxygen flow (10 to 15 L per minute) and a face mask.

Artificial Airways

Artificial airways (oropharyngeal, nasopharyngeal) may be used to assist in airway management but only by persons well-trained in their use.

CARDIOPULMONARY RESUSCITATION (CPR)

All adults should learn technique known as cardio-pulmonary resuscitation (CPR). CPR is a combination of rescue breathing and chest compressions given to an individual who is in cardiac arrest, meaning that the heart has stopped working. Classes are available for those who want to learn proper CPR techniques and obtain CPR certification. Below is a brief summary about CPR, but please note that this summary is not comprehensive and not a substitute for proper CPR certification. Further, CPR guidelines are updated and changed periodically, so individuals need to renew their certification on a yearly basis.

After dialing, first make sure the victim's airway is open. Look, listen and feel for breathing. Remove any foreign material from the mouth and if the person is not breathing, give two full rescue breaths. If no breathing, coughing or movement (and thus no normal signs of circulation) result in response to the two rescue breaths, chest compression should be performed. Abdominal thrust in an unconscious patient is preferred to be carried out while the patient lying flat on a hard surface. Kneel over the patient (Figs 15.10 to 15.12) and:

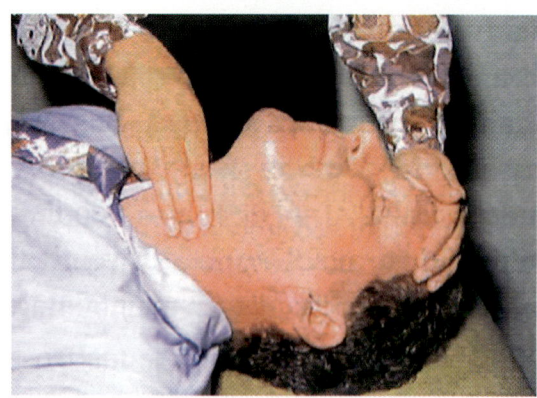

Fig. 15.10: Cardiac arrest. The diagnosis is established clinically by feeling of the carotid pulse. The head should be slightly extended, if possible and the neck should be palpated for evidence of a carotid pulse on one side of the thyroid cartilage for 10 seconds. An absent carotid pulse indicates probable cardiac arrest, but the peripheral pulselessness or the absence of heart sounds are unreliable signs *(McKinley and Loughlin. Human Anatomy)*

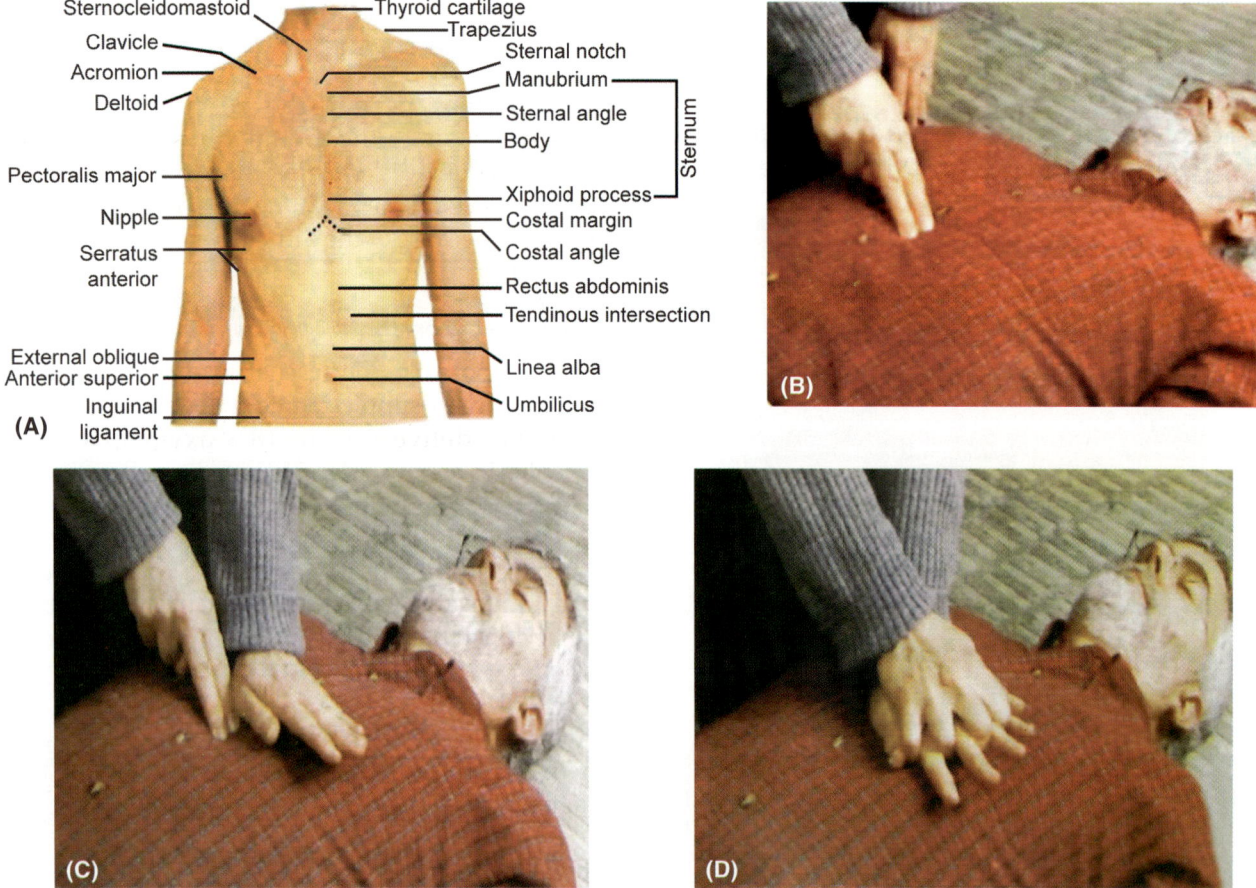

Fig. 15.11: Steps of cardiopulmonary resuscitation. **(A)** Figure male anterior view, anatomical identification of the xiphoid process. **(B)** palpate xiphoid process. **(C)** place hands on body of sternum. **(D)** start chest compression *(McKinley and Loughlin. Human Anatomy, 2006)*

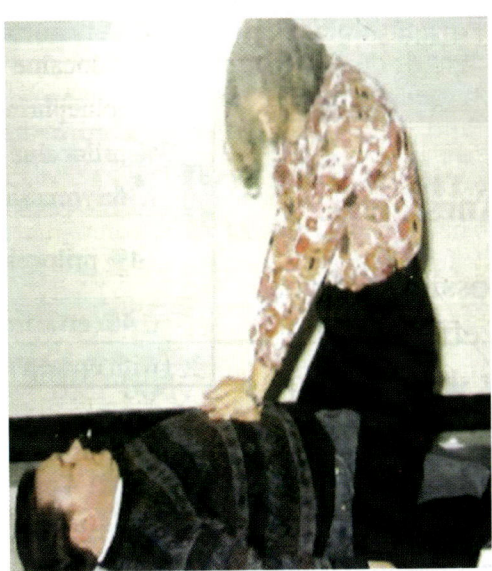

Fig. 15.12: Abdominal thrust is performed while kneeling over the patient *(McKinley and Loughlin. Human Anatomy, 2006)*

- Palpate the xiphoid process and placing two fingers there,
- Place the heel of the hand superior to the two fingers so that the hand rests on the body of the sternum; and
- Press down about 2 inches on the body of the sternum, the place where the heart will receive maximum benefit. This technique should result in a violent expulsion of air from the lungs.

Or the patient should lie flat on a hard surface. Kneel over the patient and thrust upwards with both hands from below the xiphisternum. The technique should result in a violent expulsion of air from the lungs and may be repeated. Any dislodged foreign body should be removed from the mouth or pharynx by a finger sweep.

Scientific ratios of chest compression to rescue breathing must be performed, depending upon whether the patient is child or adult. CPR classes provide instruction and further details about this procedure. Become CPR certified: Someone's life may depend on what you know.

V	• Vasoconstrictors

VASOCONSTRICTORS

Conditions in which vasoconstrictors should be avoided or used at minimum doses are given in Box 15.14.

Box 15.14: Conditions in which vasoconstrictors should be avoided or used at minimum doses

- Blood pressure greater than 200 mg Hg systolic or 115 mm Hg diastolic
- Myocardial infarction within 6 months.
- Cerebrovascular accident with 6 months
- Daily episodes of or unstable angina
- Coronary artery bypass surgery within 6 months
- Uncontrolled cardiac arrhythmias
- Uncontrolled congestive heart failure
- Uncontrolled hyperthyroidism
- Sulfite-sensitive asthma or true sulfite allergy.

Maximum Safe Doses of Anesthesia

Calculated on the basis of possible effects of the local anesthetic, the effects of the vasoconstrictor should not be ignored. For example, the addition of epinephrine to lidocaine raises the safe maximum dose by slowing its absorption into the circulation, but this 'slowing down' process may not be as significant as once thought (Tables 15.7 and 15.8).

Table 15.7: Maximum safe doses of different anesthetic agents as related to the patient's weight

Anesthetic agent	Dose
Lidocaine with epinephrine	4.4 mg/kg
Prilocaine	6 mg/kg
Articaine	7 mg/kg

These figures, when transferred into volumes of the local anesthetic solution for a fit, healthy patient of average weight, suggest the following (Table 15.8).

Table 15.8: The safest number of cartridges administered vauise with anesthetic agent and the vasoconstrictor content.

Anesthetic agent	Number of cartridges
2% lidocaine with epinephrine	6–7 cartrdiges of 2.2 ml
3% prilocaine with felypressin	5–6 cartridges of 2.2 ml.
4% prilocaine	4 cartridges of 2.2 ml
4% articaine (with epinephrine)	4 cartridges of 2.2 ml.

These maximum doses should be suitably reduced for: elderly people, children, debilitated, cardiac disease. Toxicity can be reduced for all patients by the following measures: use of an efficient aspirating technique, slow deposition of the solution. Controversy exists whether epinephrine-containing local anesthetics should be used for patients with known heart disease. Epinephrine has powerful effects on the cardiovascular system and may also reduce potassium levels in the bloodstream—potentially of importance in patients on diuretics therapy who may be potassium depleted. Use of epinephrine-free solutions will avoid these problems. However, some clinicians consider lidocaine with epinephrine achieves a more profound anesthesia and is, therefore, less likely to cause the release of endogenous epinephrine, which is evident when pain is felt during the operative procedure.

Intravascular Injection of Local Anesthesia

The intravascular injection of local anesthetics is a real danger to anyone and particularly to those patients with cardiovascular disease. Without special precautions, the concentration of local anesthetics and/or added vasoconstrictors may be inadvertently, built up and death or serious cardiovascular complications may result. Intra-arterial injections provoke distant anesthesia and blanching of the immediate area, while intravenous injection may cause central nervous system stimulation or depression and produce hypertensive crises or dangerous degrees of myocardial ischemia. The instruments sometimes used by dentists do not allow for preliminary aspiration. However, aspirating cartridge syringes, now on the market, provide increased safety for the patient with fewer anesthetic failures, as well as fewer anesthetic reactions.

Intravascular injection can be avoided, provided that the following precautions are observed:

1. Use a needle no smaller than 25 gauge. Smaller needles often prevent aspiration.
2. Prevent intravascular injection by aspirating before injection.
3. If the position of the needle is changed during injection, reaspirate before continuing the injection.
4. If blood is aspirated, the cartridge should be discarded and another cartridge used.

| **W** | • Body Weight and Energy Balance |

Weight is determined by the body's energy balance—if energy intake and output are equal, body weight is stable. We gain weight, if intake exceeds output and lose weight, if output exceeds intake. The subject of nutrition quickly brings to mind the subject of body weight and the popular desire to control it. From studies of identical twins and other people, it appears that about 30 to 50% of the variation in human weight is due to heredity and the rest to environmental factors such as eating and exercise habits.

APPETITE

The struggle for weight control often seems to be a struggle against the appetite, but despite decades of research, we are still far from a complete understanding of how appetite is regulated. In the 1940s, it was discovered that a region in the lateral area of the hypothalamus seems to trigger the desire for food. When this **feeding center** is destroyed in animals, they exhibit drastic **anorexia*** (loss of appetite) and starve to death, if not force-fed. It was recently discovered that, at least in rats, this area of the hypothalamus secretes a hormone named *orexin,* which rises during fasting and stimulates intense hunger. The ventromedial hypothalamus has a **satiety center;** damage here causes **hyperphagia**** (overeating) and extreme obesity.

Merely chewing and swallowing food briefly satisfies the appetite, even if the food is removed through an esophageal fistula (opening) before reaching the stomach. Inflating the stomach with a balloon inhibits hunger even in an animal that has not actually swallowed any food. Appetite is not merely a question of *how much* but also *what kind* of food is consumed. Even animals shift their diets from one kind of food to another, apparently because some foods provide nutrients that others do not. In humans, different neurotransmitters also seem to govern the appetite for different classes of nutrients. For example, norepinephrine stimulates the appetite for carbohydrates, galanin for fatty foods, and endorphins for protein.

OBESITY

Obesity is clinically defined as a weight more than 20% above the recommended norm for one's age, sex, and height (Fig. 15.13). To judge whether you are obese or not, you can calculate your *body mass index (BMI). The*

---

* *an–without; rexia–appetite*

** *hyper–excessive; phagia–eating*

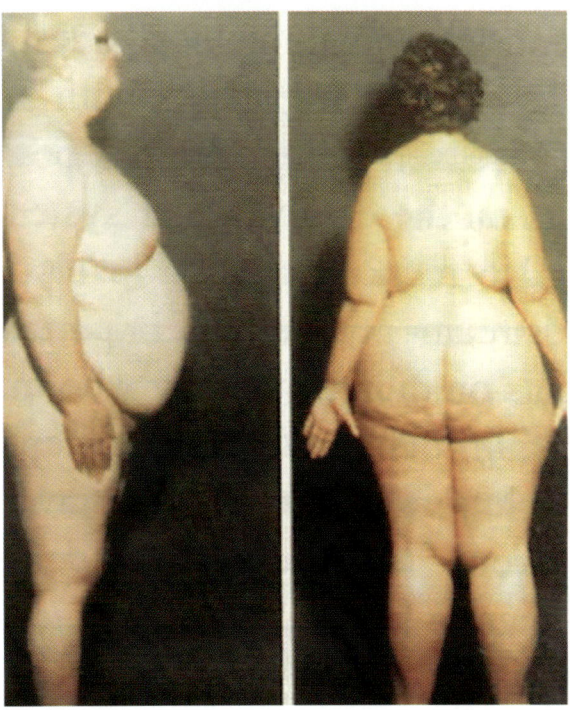

Fig. 15.13: Simple obesity in these women has led to excessive fat deposition in the upper arms, breasts, abdomen, buttocks and thighs. This distribution is typical *(Forbes & Jackson, 2003)*

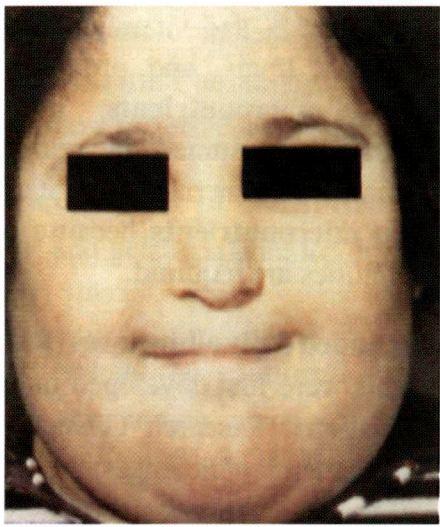

Fig. 15.14: Simple obesity may lead to gross roundness and fatness of the face. It is important to differentiate this appearance from that of Cushing's syndrome.

body mass index expressed as weight/height^2 (BMI; kg/m^2) is used to identify overweight and obesity in children and adolescents. If W is your weight in kilograms and H is your height in meters, BMI = W/H^2. (English-metric conversion factors can be found inside the back cover of this book.) A BMI of 20 to 25 kg/m^2 is considered to be optimal for most people. A BMI over 27 kg/m^2 is considered overweight and above 30 kg/m^2 is considered obese.

Causes of obesity are multivariable and multidimensional. Generally, the causes include: socioeconomic status, early childhood nutrition, level of physical activity and engagement of sedentary activities, such as watching television and computer use. Excess weight shortens life expectancy, gross roundness and fatness of the face (Fig. 15.14) and increases a person's risk of asthma, sleep apnea, atherosclerosis, hypertension, diabetes mellitus, joint pain and degeneration, kidney stones and gallstones; cancer of the breast, uterus and liver in women; and cancer of the colon, rectum and prostate gland in men. The excess thoracic fat in obese people interferes with breathing and results in increased blood PCO_2, sleepiness, and reduced vitality. Obesity is also a significant obstacle to successful surgery.

A predisposition to obesity is often established by overfeeding in infancy and childhood. During childhood, consumption of excess calories causes the adipocytes to increase in size and number—that is, adipose tissue grows by both hypertrophy and hyperplasia. In adulthood, adipocytes do not divide except in some extreme weight gains; their number remains constant while weight gains and losses result from changes in cell size.

CALORIES

One calorie is the amount of heat that will raise the temperature of 1g of water 1°C. One thousand calories is called a Calorie (capital C) in dietetics and a **kilocalorie** (kcal) in biochemistry. The relevance of calories to physiology is that they are a measure of the capacity to do biological work. Nearly all dietary calories come from carbohydrates, proteins, and fats. Carbohydrates and proteins yield about 4 kcal/g when they are completely oxidized and fats yield about 9 kcal/g. Some foods such as sugar and alcohol are said to provide "empty calories" because they provide nothing useful except for calories.

By suppressing the appetite but failing to provide other nutrients the body requires, they can contribute to malnutrition. In sound nutrition, the body's energy needs are met by more complex foods that simultaneously meet the need for proteins, lipids, vitamins, and other nutrients. When a chemical is described as **fuel** in this chapter, we mean it is oxidized solely or primarily to extract energy from it. The extracted energy is usually used to make adenosine triphosphate (ATP), which then transfers the energy to other physiological processes.

NUTRIENTS

A nutrient is any ingested chemical that is used for growth, repair, or maintenance of the body. Nutrients fall into six major classes: water, carbohydrates, lipids, proteins, minerals, and vitamins. Water, carbohydrates, lipids and proteins are considered **macronutrients** because they must be consumed in relatively large quantities. Minerals and vitamins are called **micronutrients** because only small quantities are required.

Recommended daily allowances (RDAs) of nutrients were first developed in 1943 by the National Research Council and National Academy of Sciences; they have been revised several times since. An RDA is a liberal but safe estimate of the daily intake that would meet the nutritional needs of most healthy people. Consuming less than the RDA of a nutrient does not necessarily mean you will be malnourished, but the probability of malnutrition increases in proportion to the amount of the deficit and how long it lasts. Many nutrients can be synthesized by the body when they are unavailable from the diet. The body is incapable, however, of synthesizing minerals, most vitamins, eight of the amino acids and one to three of the fatty acids. These are called **essential nutrients** because it is essential that they be included in the diet.

| X | • Xerostomia (Dry Mouth) |

XEROSTOMIA

Xerostomia is a symptom, not a diagnosis or disease. It is important to recognize that a patient complaining of dry mouth should not be assumed immediately to have salivary dysfunction. Although oral dryness is most commonly the result of reduced salivation, it may have other causes.

A dry mouth may result from the following disorders:

1. Local inflammation.
2. Dehydration states.
3. Drug therapy:
   a. Tranquilizers.
   b. Antihistamines
   c. Anticholinergics.

4. Infection and fibrosis of major salivary glands.
5. Autoimmune diseases
   a. Mikulicz's disease,
   b. Sjögren's syndrome.
6. Chemotherapy
7. Postradiation changes.
8. Alcoholism.

Clinically, the lips are often cracked, peeling and atrophic. The buccal mucosa may be pale and corrugated in appearance and the tongue may be smooth and reddened, with loss of papillation. Patients may report that their lips stick to the teeth, and oral mucosa may adhere to the dry enamel. There is often marked increase in erosion and caries, particularly decay on root surfaces and even cusp tip involvement. Candidiasis most commonly of the erythematous form, is frequent, appearing as red patches on the mucosa, rather than the more familiar white, cured-like mucocutaneous type (thrush). Angular cheilitis is also common.

Two additional indications of oral dryness that have been gleaned from clinical experience are the "lipstick" and "tongueblade" signs. In the former, the presence of lipstick or shed epithelial cells on the labial surfaces of the anterior maxillary teeth is indicative of reduced saliva (saliva would normally wet the mucosa and aid in cleansing the teeth). To test for the latter sign, the examiner can hold a tongue blade against the buccal mucosa; in a dry mouth, the tissue will adhere to the tongue blade as the blade is lifted away. Both signs suggest that the mucosa is not sufficiently moisturized by saliva.

The treatment may be divided into: symptomatic (palliative) and systemic salivary stimulation.

The symptomatic treatment includes water sipage. The patients should be encouraged to sip water throughout the day; this will help moisten the oral cavity, hydrate the mucosae and clear debris from the mouth. The use of water with meals can make chewing and forming the food bolus easier, will ease swallowing and will improve taste perception.

Use of sugar-free carbonated drinks is not recommended as the acidic content of many of these beverages is high and may increase tooth demineralization.

An increase in environmental humidity is exceedingly important. The use of room humidifiers, particularly at night, may lessen discomfort markedly. Apart from the normal diurnal variation, salivary flow drops almost to zero during rest.

There are number of oral rinses, mouthwashes and gels available for dry mouth patients.

Patients should be cautioned to avoid products containing alcohol, sugar, or strong flavoring that may irritate sensitive mucosa.

Moisturizing creams are important.

The frequent use of products containing vera or vitamin E should be encouraged.

There are many commercially available salivary substitutes as "artificial saliva". Chewing gum will stimulate salivary flow as will sour and sweet tastes.

Systemic stimulation: Systemic secretogogues are used for salivary flow stimulation. Examples mycolytic drugs as bromhexine, anetholtrithione significantly increase salivary flow. Pilocarpine HCl is EDA approved specifically for the relief of xerostomia following radiotherapy for head and neck cancers and for those with Sjögren's syndrome. After administration of pilocarpine, salivary output increases fairly rapidly, usually reaching a maximum within 1 hour. The best tolerated doses are those of 5.0 to 7.5 mg, given three or four times daily. Cevimeline HCl is another parasympathomimetic agonist that is EDA approved for the treatment of symptoms of oral dryness in Sjögren's syndrome.

Y	• Yellow Bone Marrow

YELLOW BONE MARROW

Bone marrow is a general term for soft tissue that occupies the medullary cavity of a long bone, the spaces amid the trabeculae of spongy bone and the larger central canals. There are three kinds of marrow—red, yellow and gelatinous. We can best appreciate their differences by considering how marrow changes over a person's lifetime.

In a child, the medullary cavity of nearly every bone is filled with **red bone marrow (myeloid tissue).** This is a *hemopoietic* tissue—that is, it produces blood cells. Red bone marrow looks like blood but with a thicker consistency. It consists of a delicate mesh of reticular tissue saturated with immature blood cells and scattered adipocytes. In young to middle-aged adults, most of this red marrow turns to fatty **yellow bone marrow,** like the fat at the center of a hambone. Yellow bone marrow no longer produces blood, although in the event of severe or chronic anemia, it can transform back into red marrow. In adults, red marrow is limited to the vertebrae, ribs, sternum, part of the pelvic (hip) girdle and the proximal heads of the humerus and femur. By old age, most of the yellow bone marrow has turned to a reddish jelly called **gelatinous bone marrow.**

Z	• Alzheimer's Disease

ALZHEIMER'S DISEASE

Alzheimer's disease is the most common cause (50% of cases) of slowly progressive dementia over several years. The mental symptoms and signs precede the physical signs by several months to years. Nearly all patients are over 60 years of age and it is estimated that 5–10% of people over 65 are affected. Pathologically, there are characteristic senile plaques, neurofibrillary tangles and amyloid angiopathy. In addition to ageing, other risk factors include a family history of the disease, head injury, low educational achievement and Down's syndrome. The most common presentation is with a loss of recent memory, often associated with a personality change, apathy and antisocial behavior followed by focal signs such as dysphasia, dyslexia, dyspraxia, agnosia and later loss of sphincter control. Sleep disturbance is common. Disturbance of gait reduces mobility, but in the later stage patients are inclined to wander, especially at night and may injure themselves by falling. The end result is that patients become bed-bound and incontinent.

16

Index

- **Medical Dictionary**
- **Abbreviations**
  - **Equivalents**
  - **Domestic Measures**
  - **Metric Weight and Volume**

a

Abscess A localized pocket of purulent exudates surrounded by inflammation.

Acetylcholine (ACh) A neurotransmitter.

Acidosis An increased number of hydrogen ions; a blood pH of less than 7.4.

Acute A disease with sudden onset of signs and short course.

Adhesion A band of fibrous scar tissue forming an abnormal connection between two surfaces or structures, e.g. binding two loops of intestine together.

Adrenergic Related to the sympathetic nervous system transmitters, norepinephrine (noradrenaline) and epinephrine (adrenaline).

Afferent Toward the center; e.g. afferent nerves carry impulses toward the central nervous system.

Albumin A plasma protein responsible for maintaining osmotic pressure of the blood.

Aldosterone A mineralocorticoid hormone that increases the reabsorption of sodium and water in the renal tubules.

Alkalosis A decreased number of hydrogen ions; a blood pH greater than 7.4.

Allergen An antigen that can initiate an allergic reaction.

Amenorrhea The absence of menstrual periods.

Amnesia Loss of memory.

Amputation The removal of a body part, often a limb or part of a limb, to remove a tumor, prevent spread of infection, or relieve pain.

Anabolism The building up or synthesis of complex compounds from simple molecules.

Anaerobic Metabolism and function without oxygen.

Analgesic A substance that relieve pain.

Anaphylaxis A life-threatening systemic allergic or hypersensitivity reaction, with rerspiratory obstruction and decreased blood pressure.

Anaplasia Undifferentiated primitive cells of variable size and shape, associated with cancer.

Anastomosis Is connection between two blood vessels or tubes.

Anemia A decrease in circulating hemoglobin and oxygen-carrying capacity in the blood because of decreased erythrocyte production, decreased hemoglobin production, excessive hemolysis, or loss of blood.

Anesthetic A substance that reduces sensation, locally or systemically.

Aneurysm An outpouching or abnormal dilated area in a blood vessel.

Angiogenesis Is the development of new capillaries.

Angiography An examination of blood vessels using radiographs with a contrast medium.

Angioplasty Repair of a blood vessel.

Angiotensin-converting enzyme (ACE) An enzyme that converts angiotensin I to angiotensin II, a potent general vasoconstrictor and stimulus for aldosterone secretion.

Anion A negatively charged ion such as chloride, Cl.

Ankylosis Fixation or immobility at a joint.

Anomally An abnormal structure, often congenital.

Anorexia Loss of appetite.

Antagonism Opposing action.

Antibiotic A substance derived from microorganisms that is used to treat infection.

Antigen A substance that causes the production of antibodies.

Antimicrobial An agent that kills or inhibits growth and reproduction of microorganisms.

Antimicrobial An agent that kills or inhibits growth and reproduction of microorganisms.

Antineoplastic A substance or process that destroys neoplastic cells.

Antioxidant A substance such as vitamin E that reduces oxygenation and production of damaging free radicals during cell metabolism.

Antiseptic Reduces the number of microorganisms on the skin.

Anuria Absence of urine production.

Aphasia Loss of the ability to communicate, to speak coherently, or to understand speech.

Apnea Lack of breathing.

Apoptosis Normal programmed cell death in tissues.

Arrhythmia Loss of normal heart rate and rhythm; dysrhythmia.

Arteriosclerosis Hardening and loss of elasticity of the arterial wall with narrowing of the lumen.

Arthroscopy Examination and possible treatment of a joint through insertion of a small instrument.

Ascites Abnormal accumulation of fluid in the abdominal cavity.

Asepsis The absence of pathogens.

Aspiration Inhaling liquid or solid material into the lungs or withdrawing fluid or tissue from a cavity or organ.

Asymptomatic No signs or symptoms.

Ataxia Impaired coordination, imbalance, staggering gait.

Atherosclerosis Development of obstruction by cholesterol plaques and thrombus on the walls of large arteries.

Atrophy Degeneration and wasting of tissue, organs, or muscle due to decrease in size.

Auscultation Listening for sounds, perhaps with a stethoscope, within the body, e.g. lungs, heart, intestine.

Autoclave An appliance to sterilie instruments or materials with steam at high temperature and pressure.

Autoimmune The development of antibodies to self-antigens.

Autopsy An examination of part or all of a body, including organs, after death (postmortem) to determine the cause of illness and death.

b

B lymphocyte A lymphocyte that functions as an antigen-presenting cell and in humoral immunity, differentiates into an antibody-producing plasma cell; also called a *B cell*.

Bacteremia Bacteria present in the circulating blood.

Bactericidal Chemical that destroys bacteria.

Bacteriostatic Substance that reduces the growth and reproduction of bacteria.

Baroreceptor A sensory nerve receptor that is stimulated by a change in pressure, perhaps blood pressure.

Basal metabolic rate (BMR) The amount of energy (measured by oxygen requirements) to maintain essential function in the body at rest.

Basophil A granulocyte with coarse cytoplasmic granules that produces heparin, histamine and other chemicals involved in inflammation.

Benign Non-threatening mild, or non-malignant.

Bicarbonate buffer system An equilibrium mixture of carbonic acid, bicarbonate ions and hydrogen ions (H_2CO_3 = HCO_3 + H) that stabilizes the pH of the body fluids.

Bicarbonate ion An anion, HCO_3 that functions as a base in the buffering of body fluids.

Bile A secretion produced by the liver, concentrated and stored in the gallbladder and released into the small intestine; consists mainly of wastes such as excess cholesterol, salts and bile pigments but also contains lecithin and bile acids, which aid in fat digestion.

Bile pigments Strongly colored organic compounds produced by the breakdown of hemoglobin, including biliverdin and bilirubin.

Bilirubin A yellow to orange bile pigment produced by the breakdown of hemoglobin. It causes jaundice and neurotoxic effects, if present in excessive concentration.

Biopsy The removal of a small piece of living tissue for microscopic excamination to determine a diagnosis.

Blood-brain barrier (BBB) A barrier between the bloodstream and nervous tissue of the brain that is impermeable to many blood solutes and thus prevents them from affecting the brain tissue; formed by the tight junctions between capillary endothelial cells, the basement membrane of the endothelium and the perivascular feet of astrocytes.

Bradycardia Abnormally slow heart rate.

Bradykinin A chemical mediator released during inflammation causing vasodilation, increases capillary permeability and stimulates pain receptors.

Burkitt's lymphoma A malignant lymphoma, particularly of the B lymphocytes characterized by a large osteolytic lesion in the facial bones and is associated with the Epstein-Barr virus.

c

C- reactive protein (CRP) Appears in the blood with inflammation and necrosis.

Cachexia Extreme loss of weight and body wasting associated with serious illness.

Calcitonin A hormone secreted by C cells of the thyroid gland that promotes calcium deposition in the skeleton and lowers blood calcium concentration.

Calorie The amount of thermal energy that will raise the temperature of 1 g of water by 1°C. Also called a *small calorie*.

Calorigenic Heat-producing, as in the calorigenic effect of thyroid hormone.

Capillary exchange The process of fluid transfer between the bloodstream and tissue fluid.

Carbohydrate A hydrophilic organic compound composed of carbon and a 2:1 ratio of hydrogen to oxygen; includes sugars, starches, glycogen.

Carcinogen A substance that causes cancer by changing normal cells.

Cardiac output (CO) The amount of blood pump by each ventricle of the heart in 1 minute.

Cardiac reserve The difference between maximum and resting cardiac output; determines a person's tolerance for exercise.

Carotid body A small cellular mass immediately superior to the branch in the common carotid artery, containing sensory cells that detect changes in blood pH and carbon dioxide and oxygen content.

Carotid sinus A dilation of the common carotid artery at the point where it branches into the internal and external carotids; contains baroreceptors, which monitor changes in blood pressure.

Carrier A person hosting an infectious pathogen, who shows no signs of disease, but could transmit the infection to others.

Catabolism The breakdown of complex molecules into simple molecules during metabolism.

Cataract An opacity of the lens of eye.

Catecholamine A subclass of biogenic amines that includes epinephrine, norepinephrine and dopamine.

Catheter A small tube inserted into the baldder to remove urine; a tube inserted into a blood vessel or other structure to allow drainage or maintain an opening.

Cation A positively charged ion with more protons than electrons and consequently a net positive charge, such as sodium, Na^+.

Cerebrospinal fluid (CSF) A liquid that fills the ventricles of the brain, the central canal of the spinal cord, and the space between the CNS and dura mater.

Cerebrovascular accident (CVA) The loss of blood flow to any part of the brain due to obstruction or hemorrhage of an artery, leading to the necrosis of nervous tissue; also called *stroke* or *apoplexy*.

Channel protein A protein in the plasma membrane that has a pore through it for the passage of materials between the cytoplasm and extracellular fluid.

Chemoreceptor An organ or cell specialized to detect chemicals, as in the carotid bodies and taste buds, a sensory nerve receptor stimulated by chemical changes such as pH.

Chemotaxis The movement of cells toward or away from an area of the body in response to chemical signals e.g. phagocytic cells move to an area of tissue injury.

Cholesterol A steroid that functions as part of the plasma membrane and as a precursor for all other steroids in the body.

Cholinergic Pertaining to acetylcholine (ACh), as in cholinergic nerve fibers that secrete ACh, cholinergic receptors that bind it, or cholinergic effects on a target organ.

Chromatin Filamentous material in the interphase nucleus, composed of DNA and associated proteins.

Chromosome A complex of DNA and protein carrying the genetic material of a cell's nucleus. Normally there are 46 chromosomes in the nucleus of each cell except germ cells.

Chronic bronchitis A chronic obstructive pulmonary disease characterized by damaged and immobilized respiratory cilia, excessive mucus secretion, infection of the lower respiratory tract, and bronchial inflammation; caused especially by cigarette smoking. *See also* chronic obstructive pulmonary disease.

Chronic obstructive pulmonary disease (COPD) A group of lung diseases (asthma, chronic bronchitis, and emphysema) that result in long-term obstruction of airflow and substantially reduced pulmonary ventilation; one of the leading causes of death in old age.

Circulatory shock A state of cardiac output inadequate to meet the metabolic needs of the body.

Cirrhosis A degenerative liver disease characterized by replacement of functional parenchyma with fibrous and adipose tissue causes include alcohol, other poisons and viral and bacterial inflammation.

Climacteric A period in the lives of men and women, usually in the early 50s, marked by changes in the level of reproductive hormones, a variety of somatic and psychological effects and in women, cessation of ovulation and menstruation (menopause).

Coagulation The clotting of blood, lymph, tissue fluid, or semen.

Cognition Mental processes such as awareness, knowledge, memory, perception and thinking are collectively called cognition. The association areas of the cerebrum, which forms about 70% of the nervous tissue in the brain, are responsible for both cognition and the processing and integration of information between sensory input and the motor output areas.

Collagen The common protein making up connective tissue and bone.

Collagenase An enzyme that breaks down collagen fibers.

Coma Unconscious state, person cannot aroused.

Complement A series of inactive proteins circulating in the blood; when activated, they can destroy bacteria or antigens, or participate in the inflammatory response.

Complement 1. To complete or enhance the structure or function of something else, as in the co-ordinated action of two different hormones. 2. A system of plasma proteins involved in nonspecific defense against pathogens.

Computerized tomography (CT) A method of medical imaging that uses X rays and a computer to create an image of a thin section of the body.

Concentration gradient A difference in chemical concentration from one point to another, as on two sides of a plasma membrane.

Congenital Present at birth; for example, an anatomical defect, a syphilis infection, or a hereditary disease.

Contamination The presence of pathogen on a body, clothing, or inanimate object.

Contracture Shortening of a muscle or scar tissue causing immobility and deformity of a joint or structure.

Contralateral On opposite sides of the body, as in reflex arcs where the stimulus comes from one side of the body and a response is given by muscles on the other side.

Contusion Tissue injury or bruise; bleeding into tissues.

Convergent Coming together, as in a convergent muscle and a converging neuronal circuit.

Corticosteroid The steroid hormones from the adrenal cortex, including the glucocorticoids (cortisol) and minicralo-corticoids (aldosterone).

Crepitus The noise beared when the ends of a broken bone rub together or when fluid is present in the lung.

Cross section A cut perpendicular to the long axis of the body or an organ.

Culture Growth of microorganisms on a specific nutritious medium in a laboratory.

Cyanosis A bluish color of skin and mucosa that occurs when a large proportion of hemoglobin is unoxygenated.

Cyst A closed sac or capsule lined with epithelium, containing fluid.

Cytotoxic A substance that damages or destroys cells.

d

Debridement Surgical removal of dead tissue and foreign material from a wound.

Decussation The crossing of nerve fibers from the right side of the central nervous system to the left or vice versa, especially in the spinal cord, medulla oblongata, and optic chiasm.

Dehydration A deficit of water in the body.

Dementia Progressive loss of intellectual function, loss of memory, personality change.

Demyelination Loss of myelin sheath from a nerve surface, interfering with conduction.

Denude Stripping off skin, leaving bare.

Dermatome An area of skin innervated by specific spinal nerve.

Detoxification The removal of toxic or poisonous material and its effects from a person.

Diabetes Any disease characterized by chronic polyuria of metabolic origin; diabetes mellitus unless otherwise specified.

Diabetes insipidus A form of diabetes that results from hyposecretion of antidiuretic hormone; unlike other forms, it is not characterized by hyperglycemia or glycosuria.

Diabetes mellitus (DM) A form of diabetes that results from hyposecretion of insulin or from a deficient target cell response to it; signs include hyperglycemia and glycosuria.

Dialysis A procedure to remove wastes and excess fluid or adjust blood to normal values in cases of renal failure. It is the separation of some solute particles from others by diffusion through a selectively permeable membrane. Hemodialysis, the process of separating wastes from the bloodstream and sometimes adding other substances to it (such as drugs and nutrients) by circulating the blood through a machine with a selectively permeable membrane, used to treat cases of renal or hepatic insufficiency.

Diapedesis The passage of leukocytes through intact capillary walls to a site of inflammation.

Diaphoresis Excessive perspiration.

Differentiation Development of a relatively unspecialized cell or tissue into one with a more specific structure and function.

Diplopia Double vision.

Disinfectant A chemical that may destroy or inhibit the growth and reproduction of microorganisms.

Disorientation Mental confusion with inadequate or incorrect awareness of time, place and person.

Disseminated intravascular coagulation (DIC) Widespread clotting of the blood within unbroken vessels, leading to hemorrhaging, congestion of the vessels with clotted blood and ischemia and necrosis of organs.

Diuresis Excessive amount of urine.

Diuretic A chemical that increases urine output.

Dopamine An inhibitory catecholamine neurotransmitter of the central nervous system, especially of the basal nuclei, where it acts to suppress unwanted motor activity.

Dysphagia Painful or difficult swallowing.

Dysplasia Disorganized cells which may vary in size and shape with large nuclei.

Dyspnea Difficult breathing.

Dysuria Painful urination.

e

Ecchymosis Reddish blue discoloration of skin or mucosa because of bleeding.

Ectopic Away from the normal position.

Edema The accumulation of excess fluid in cells, tissue, or a cavity, resulting in a swelling.

Efferent Moving away from the center, e.g. efferent nerve fibers carry motor impulses to muscles.

Effusion The accumulation of fluid leaking from a blood vessel into a cavity or potential space.

Elastic fiber A connective tissue fiber, composed of the protein elastin, that stretches under tension and returns to its original length when released; responsible for the resilience of organs such as the skin and lungs.

Elasticity The tendency of a stretched structure to return to its original dimensions when tension is released.

Electrocardiogram (ECG) A record of conduction in the heart.

Embolus A mass, e.g. blood clot, air, fat, tumor cells, that breaks away into the circulation and obstructs a blood vessel.

Embryo A developing individual from the end of the second week of gestation when the three primary germ layers have formed, through the end of the eighth week when all of the organ systems are present. *Compare* conceptus, fetus.

Emphysema A degenerative lung disease characterized by a breakdown of alveoli and diminishing surface area available for gas exchange; occurs with aging of the lungs but is greatly accelerated by smoking or air pollution.

Encephalopathy Impaired function of the brain.

Endemic A disease that is always present in a specific region.

Endogenous Originating from within the body.

Endorphins Morphine-like substance produced in the body that block pain stimuli at sites in the brain and spinal cord.

Endoscope An illuminated optic instrument that can be inserted into a body cavity, tube, or organ to visualize any changes (bronchoscope, cystoscope, laparoscope).

Endotoxin A toxin released from the walls of certain Gram-negative bacteria following lysis.

Eosinophil A granulocyte with a large, often bilobed nucleus and coarse cytoplasmic granules that stain with eosin; phagocytizes antigen-antibody complexes, allergens and inflammatory chemicals and secretes enzymes that combat parasitic infections.

Epidemic A disease occurring in higher numbers than usual in a certain population within a given time period.

Epinephrine A catecholamine that functions as a neurotransmitter in the sympathetic nervous system and as a hormone secreted by the adrenal medulla; also called *adrenaline*.

Epitaxis Nose bleed

Erythema Redness and inflammation of the skin or mucosa due to vasodilation.

Erythrocyte sedimentation rate (ESR) The rate at which RBCs settle out of a blood specimen (containing anticoagulant); an elevation in ESR is a general characteristic of inflammation.

Estrogens A family of steroid hormones known especially for producing female secondary sex characteristics and regulating various aspects of the menstrual cycle and pregnancy; major forms are estradiol, estriol, and estrone.

Euphoria An exaggerated feeling of well-being or unrealistic relation.

Exacerbation An acute episode or increased severity of manifestations.

Exogenous Originating from outside the body.

Exotoxin Toxin excreted by a bacterium, e.g. neurotoxin, or enterotoxin.

Exudate A fluid that accumulates and may leak from tissue, e.g. a serous exudate due to allergy, a purulent exudate or pus associated with infection.

f

Fascia A layer of connective tissue between the muscles (deep fascia) or separating the muscles from the skin (superficial fascia).

Fetus The human child in utero between 8 weeks and birth. In human development, an individual from the beginning of the ninth week when all of the organ systems are present, through the time of birth. *Compare* conceptus, embryo.

Fibrinogen The plasma protein that is formed into solid fibrin strands during the clotting process.

Fibrinolysis The breakdown of fibrin.

Fibrosis Growth of fibrous or scar tissue related to collagen deposits.

Fissure A crack or split in the surface of skin or mucous membrane.

Fistula An abnormal tube or passage formed between structures, e.g. between the esophagus and trachea or between rectum and skin.

Flaccidity Lack of tone in muscle; weakness and softness.

Free radical A byproduct of cell metabolism that damages cell membranes, proteins and DNA.

Frey's syndrome Or gustatory sweating, results when parasympathetic nerves supplying the parotid or submandibular glands are cut to remove the gland. During healing, the nerves grow and may innervate the sweat gland of the overlying skin. The affected skin then sweats sometimes profusely on eating or the thought of food. This is an unpleasant and distressing complication and is difficult to control with anticholinergic drugs.

Frontal plane An anatomical plane that passes through the body or an organ from right to left and superior to inferior; also called a *coronal plane*.

Fulminant Rapid, severe, uncontrolled progress of a disease or infection.

Furuncles Staphylococcal infection produces painful pus-filled inflamed hair follicles and involves surrounding skin and subcutaneous tissue.

g

Ganglion A collection of nerve cell bodies, usually outside the central nervous system.

Gangrene Necrotic tissue infected by bacteria.

Gas gangrene The formation of gas bubbles and subsequent destruction of connective tissue and cell membranes resulting from the hydrolic enzymes produced by bacterium of the Clostridium species.

Gene A unit of DNA (a nucleic acid sequence) in a particular location on a specific chromosome.

Generalized anxiety disorder (GAD) An anxiety disorder characterized by an excessively anxious mood lasting at least 1 month that interferes with daily functioning and may be accompanied by tiredness, sweating, feeling of catastrophe concerning one's family or self and irritability.

Genetic Inherited.

Genotype The genetic makeup of a cell or individual.

Gestation The time between conception and birth.

Globulin A group of proteins in the blood.

Glucocorticoid The steroid hormones from the adrenal cortex, e.g. cortisol (hydrocortisone), that increase blood glucose levels and act to decrease inflammation and allergic reactions.

Gluconeogenesis The production of glucose from protein or fat.

Glucose A monosaccharide also known as blood sugar; glycogen, starch, cellulose and maltose are made entirely of glucose and glucose constitutes half of a sucrose or lactose molecule.

Glucose-sparing effect An effect of fats or other energy substrates in which they are used as fuel by most cells, so that those cells do not consume glucose; this makes more glucose available to cells such as neurons that cannot use alternative energy substrates.

Glucosuria Glucose in urine.

Glycogen A polysaccharide, made up of glucose molecules, stored in skeletal muscle or the liver.

Glycoprotein A combination of protein and carbohydrate.

Goiter A non-cancerous enlargement of the thyroid gland that is visible as a swelling at the front of the neck.

Gonorrhea A sexually transmitted disease caused by the bacteria gonococci that invade the mucous membranes of the genitals and urinary tract and in women the cervix, fallopian tubes and ovaries, causing chronic pelvic pain or infertility.

Gout A disorder of uric-acid metabolism that causes painful inflammation of the joints, commonly the big toe, and arthritic attacks resulting from elevated levels of uric acid in the blood and the deposition of negatively urate crystals around the joints.

Gradient A difference or change in any variable, such as pressure or chemical concentration, from one point in space to another; provides a basis for molecular movements such as gas exchange, osmosis and facilitated diffusion and for bulk movements such as blood flow and airflow.

Gram stain A stain for bacteria that differentiates the cell walls of gram-positive from that of gram-negative bacteria; used for identification and choice of drug treatment.

Granulation tissue Newly developed fragile tissue, consisting of fibroblasts and blood vessels, formed during healing.

Growth factor A chemical messenger that stimulates mitosis and differentiation of target cells that have receptors for it; important in such processes as fetal development, tissue maintenance and repair and hemopoiesis; sometimes a contributing factor in cancer.

Growth hormone (GH) A hormone of the anterior pituitary gland with multiple effects on many tissues, generally promoting tissue growth.

h

Hagemen factor (factor XII) Component of the kinin system that activates the clotting system, prekallikrein and Cl in the complement system and converts plasminogen proactivator to plasminogen activator.

Half-life (Tl/2) **1.** The time required for one-half of a quantity of a radioactive element to decay to a stable isotope (*physical half-life*) or to be cleared from the body through a combination of radioactive decay and physiological excretion (*biological half-life*). **2.** The time required for one-half of a quantity of hormone to be cleared from the bloodstream.

Hallucination A sensory perception, e.g. visual or auditory, that is not real but results from nervous system excitation.

Helper T cell A type of lymphocyte that performs a central co-ordinating role in humoral and cellular immunity; target of the human immunodeficiency virus (HIV).

Hemarthrosis Bleeding into a joint cavity.

Hematemesis Vomiting blood; may be called "coffee-grounds" vomitus because it appears brown and granular.

Hematocrit Percentage of erythrocytes in a blood sample.

Hematoma A blood clot formed following bleeding into a tissue or organ.

Hematuria Blood in the urine; may be microscopic (small amount) or gross (large amount, darkening the color).

Heme The non-protein, iron-containing prosthetic group of hemoglobin or myoglobin; oxygen binds to its ferrous ion.

Hemiparesis Weakness on one side of the body.

Hemiplegia Paralysis on one side of the body.

Hemolysis Destruction of erythrocytes with release of hemoglobin.

Hemophilia A (classic hemophilia) a genetic disorder in which a mutation in factor VIII causes prolonged clotting time, decreased formation of thromboplastin, and diminished conversion of prothrombin.

Hemophilia B (Christmas disease) Genetic disorder similar to hemophilia A in terms of symptoms but with a mutation in the factor IX gene.

Hemophilia C (Factor XI deficiency) A gene disorder characterized by a deficiency in factor XI, resulting in a mild form of hemophilia.

Hemoptysis A condition in which blood-stained sputum is spit or coughed from bronchi, larynx, trachea, or lungs. It is a manifestation of various respiratory, neoplastic or hemolytic conditions.

Hemostasis Blood clotting or controlling bleeding.

Heparin A substance present in the body to prevent blood clotting.

Hepatitis A A virus that is spread by the fecal-oral route through contaminated food and water or by close and intimate contact and results in liver inflammation, flu-like symptoms, nausea, poor appetite, abdominal pain, fatigue, yellow eyes and skin and dark urine that can last weeks to months.

Hepatitis B virus (HBV) A DNA virus that is transmitted by contaminated blood or blood derivatives in transfusion, by sexual contact, or by the use of contaminated needles and instruments and may become chronic and cause long-term damage including hepatocellular carcinoma in the liver.

Hepatitis C An RNA virus that transmitted primarily by blood and blood products and sometimes through sexual contact and may become chronic with few to no symptoms while causing long-term damage to the liver, such as cirrhosis and hepatocellular carcinoma.

Hepatomegaly Enlarged liver.

Histamine An active amine produced by mast cells and basophils during immune reactions, causes vasodilation, abnormal permeability, regulates gastric acid production in the gastrointestinal tract and bronchoconstriction and causes many symptoms of the allergic reaction.

Histamine A chemical released from mast cells.

Hodgkin lymphoma (HL) A cancer of lymphoid tissue in which the lymph nodes, spleen and liver become enlarged and is often accompanied by anemia, fever, and eventually death, if not treated at an early stage; also referred to as Hodgkin's disease.

Homeostasis A relatively stable or constant environment in the body, including blood pressure, temperature, and pH, maintained by the various control mechanisms.

Homologous **1.** Having the same embryonic or evolutionary origin but not necessarily the same function, such as the scrotum and labia majora. **2.** Pertaining to two chromosomes with identical structures and gene loci but not necessarily identical alleles; each member of the pair is inherited from a different parent.

Host cell Any cell belonging to the human body, as opposed to foreign cells introduced to it by such causes as infections and tissue transplants.

Human immunodeficiency virus (HIV) A virus that infects human helper T cells and other cells, suppresses immunity, and causes AIDS.

Hunchbacked Is a condition where the spine curves backward abnormally, usually at the thoracic level. A characteristic "hunchbacked" or "round backed" appearance results. Adolescent kyphosis is the most common form. It generally results from infection or other disturbances of the vertebral epiphysis during the active growth period. Adult kyphosis is generally caused by a degeneration of the intervertebral discs, resulting in collapse of the vertebrae, but many other factors, such as poor posture and tuberculosis of the spine, may be responsible.

Hyaline cartilage A form of cartilage with a relatively clear matrix and fine collagen fibers but no conspicuous elastic fibers or coarse collagen bundles as in other types of cartilage.

Hyaluronic acid A glycosaminoglycan that is particularly abundant in connective tissues, where it becomes hydrated and forms the tissue gel.

Hydrostatic pressure The physical force generated by a liquid such as blood or tissue fluid, as opposed to osmotic and atmospheric pressures.

Hypercapnia An excess of carbon dioxide in the blood.

Hyperemia Increased blood flow in an area, resulting in a warm, red area.

Hyperkalemia Abnormally high level of potassium ions (K⁺) in the blood.

Hypernatremia Abnormally high level of sodium ions (Na⁺) in the blood.

Hyperplasia An abnormal increase in the number of cells resulting in an increased tissue mass.

Hyertension A persistant elevation of blood pressure.

Hypertonic A solution with a greater concentration of solutes or high Cosmotic pressure than that inside the cells present in the solution.

Hypertrophy Increased size of an organ or muscle due to increased size of individual cells.

Hypoxia A decreased or insufficient level of oxygen in the tissues.

i

Icterus neonatorum (neonatal jaundice) Jaundice in newborn infants caused by functional immaturity of the liver and usually subsides within the first few days of life.

Infectious mononucleosis (IM) A disease that is caused by the Epstein-Barr virus or the cytomegalovirus that is transmitted by exchanging saliva or blood or by coughing and sneezing and acts by infecting the B cells and atypical T cells resulting in fever, sore throat and fatigue.

Innate resistance (immunity) Protection or resistance to infection by non-immune mechanisms such as natural physical, mechanical and biochemical barriers.

Insulin Protein hormone that is secreted by the beta cells of the islets of Langerhans and functions in carbohydrate and fat metabolism by increasing glucose uptake into and subsequent glycogen production in muscle and by activating adipose cells to form fat.

Intrinsic pathway A component of the coagulation cascade that causes blood clotting in response to contact with a foreign substance.

Icterus neonatorum (neonatal jaundice) Jaundice in newborn infants caused by functional immaturity of the liver and usually subsides within the first few days of life.

Infectious mononucleosis (IM) A disease that is caused by the Epstein-Barr virus or the cytomegalovirus that is transmitted by exchanging saliva or blood or by coughing and sneezing and acts by infecting the B cells and atypical T cells resulting in fever, sore throat and fatigue.

Intrinsic pathway A component of the coagulation cascade that causes blood clotting in response to contact with foreign substance.

k

Ketone bodies Certain ketones (acetone, acetoacetic acid and hydroxybutyric acid) produced by the incomplete oxidation of fats, especially when fats are being rapidly catabolized. *See also* ketosis.

Ketonuria The abnormal presence of ketones in the urine as an effect of ketosis.

Ketosis An abnormally high concentration of ketone bodies in the blood, occurring in pregnancy, starvation, diabetes mellitus and other conditions; tends to cause acidosis and to depress the nervous system.

Kilocalorie The amount of heat energy needed to raise the temperature of 1 kg of water by 1°C; (1,000 calories). Also called a *large calorie*.

l

Leukocytosis An increase in the number of leukocytes in the blood as a result of fever, inflammation, hemorrhage, infection, etc.

Leukopenia A condition in which the number of white blood cells in the blood is decreased, resulting in an increased risk for infection.

Leukotriene A mediator of the prolonged inflammatory response that acts to contract smooth muscle, increase vascular permeability and attract neutrophils.

Lichen planus A recurrent rash of small, flat-topped bumps and rough scaly patches appearing on the skin, in the lining of the mouth and in the vagina in response to inflammation or an allergy to a specific medication.

Lupus erythematosus Any of a group of autoimmune connective tissue disorders that commonly produces red scaly lesions and is accompanied by fever, malaise, myalgias, fatigue and weight loss.

Lyme disease (borreliosis) Tick-brone spirochete bacterial infection that is characterized by a rash in the area of the bite, headache, neck stiffness, chills, fever, myalgia, arthralgia, malaise, fatigue and possible development of arthritis in large joints.

Lymphadenopathy Swelling of one or more lymph nodes because of diseases such as bacterial or viral infection, Hodgkin's lymphoma, non-Hodgkin's lymphoma, or unknown cause.

Lymphocyte Non-phagocytic leukocyte of immunologically competent and serves as the precursor for B and T lymphocytes.

Lymphocytopenia A decrease in the number of lymphocytes in the blood because of diseases and conditions such as human immunodeficiency virus, severe stress, or the administration of corticosteroids, chemotherapy, or radiation therapy.

Lymphocytosis An increase in the number of lymphocytes in the blood because of infection, inflammation, or leukemia.

Lymphoma Cancer arising from cell proliferation in lymphoid tissue.

m

Macrophage Phagocyte that is produced from a monocyte and is important in cellular initiation of the inflammatory response.

Major (unipolar) depression Severely depressed mood and loss of pleasure that may begin suddenly or slowly, persists for at least 2 weeks and may recur throughout life.

Major histocompatibility complex (MHC) A set of glycoproteins found on the surface of all cells expect red blood cells and serve as markers of cell recognition for the immune system by distinguishing self from non-self.

Malignant hypertension A complication of hypertension in which blood pressure is severely elevated and organ damage occurs in the eyes, brain, lung and/or kidneys.

Malignant hyperthermia An inherited life-threatening disorder that causes muscle rigidity, a hypermetabolic stat, tachycardia, and increased body temperature in response to administration of general anesthesics.

Mast cell A cell of the connective tissue that produces substances that cause activation of the inflammatory response, vasoconstriction and muscle contraction.

Memory cell T or B lymphocyte that "remembers" a specific antigen after the initial exposure and initiates a more efficient immunologic response in response to subsequent exposures to the same antigen.

Mental retardation Impaired intellectual development as a result of congenital cause, brain injury, or disease, resulting in impaired learning, social and vocational ability.

Metabolic acidosis Decrease in pH caused by an increase in non-carbonic acids or a decrease in bicarbonate.

Metabolic alkalosis Increase in pH caused by an increase in bicarbonate ions secondary to an increase in metabolic acid loss.

Metabolic syndrome A condition of unknown cause that presents with symptoms of insulin resistance, obesity, hypertension, dyslipidemia and systemic inflammation.

Metastasis Occurs when cancer cells break a way from the original tumor, enter the systemic circulation and invade distant tissues and organs.

Migraine headache Headache that usually begins in the temporal region unilaterally after vascular changes of cranial arteries and may cause irritability, nausea, vomiting, constipation or diarrhea and photophobia.

Mitosis The process of nuclear division during which two identical nuclei are produced from one parent cell after chromosomal replication.

Mitral valve A valve in the heart that lies between the left atrium and left ventricle and functions to allow blood to flow into the left ventricle during ventricular diastole and to prevent regurgitation from the ventricle to the left atrium during systole.

Mitral valve prolapse syndrome The mitral valve cannot close properly because of one or both flaps being too large, possibly resulting in mitral valve regurgitation.

Molluscum contagiosum A viral infection of the skin occurring in young children that affects the body, arms and legs and is spread through direct contact, saliva, or shared articles of clothing and is considered a sexually transmitted disease in adults, affecting the genitals, lower abdomen, buttocks and inner thighs.

Monocyte Immature white blood cell produced in bone marrow, circulates on blood and migrates to the inflammatory site where they develop into macrophages.

Monocytopenia A decreased number of monocytes in the blood by bacteria or by administration of chemotherapy or corticosteroids.

Monocytosis An increased number of monocytes in the blood because of chronic infection, autoimmune disorder, blood disorder, or cancer.

Myasthenia gravis Neuromuscular disorder caused by an autoimmune response in which antibodies to acetylcholine receptors impair neuromuscular transmission.

Myeloma A tumor composed of cells derived from hemopoietic tissue of the bone marrow.

Myositis Inflammation of a muscle, usually a voluntary muscle, resulting in pain, tenderness and sometimes spasm in the affected area.

Myositis ossificans A condition in which bone is deposited in muscle tissue, causing pain and swelling.

Myotonia A neuromuscular disorder in which muscle relaxation after voluntary contraction is delayed.

Myxedema Cutaneous edema caused by deposition of connective tissue (e.g. glycosaminoglycans and hyaluronic acid) and associated with hypothyroidism and Graves' disease. Charactized by dry skin, pretibial myxedema, swellings around the lips and nose, mental deterioration and a decrease in basal metabolic rate.

n

Natural killer (NK) cell Lymphocyte capable of killing target by binding specific receptors with or without the aid of antibodies and by releasing chemicals toxic to the targeted cells.

Neurogenic shock A type of shock caused by the sudden loss of the sympathetic nervous system signals to the smooth muscle in vessel walls, causing the vessels to relax and a decrease in peripheral vascular resistance and blood pressure.

Naturopathic pain Chronic pain associated with nerve that is perceived as burning or pins and needles or electric shock that is produced by the stimulation of pain, touch and temperature receptors in the same area.

Neutrophil (polymorphonuclear neutrophil) (PMN) Phagocyte that destroys bacterial by phagocytosis, digestion, and secretion of bacteria killing chemicals.

Neutrophilia A condition in which the number of neutrophils, especially the younger, less mature cells in the blood is increased.

Non-Hodgkin lymphoma (NHL) A malignancy of lymphoid tissue classified as B cell, T cell and NK cell lymphomas that mimics Hodgkin lymphoma but does not produce the cells characteristic of Hodgkin lymphoma and does not have a definitive cause other than association with latent Epstein - Barr virus, AIDS, or agent orange exposure.

Nystagmus Involuntary, rapid, rhythmic movements of the eyeball in the horizontal, vertical, or rotational direction.

o

Obstructive sleep apnea syndrome (OSAS) A disorder of sleep characterized by airway obstruction and episodes of apnea accompanied by snoring.

Opsonin A molecule (e.g. C3b complement, IgG and IgA) that attaches to antigens and promotes binding to phagocytes.

Orthostatic (postural) hypotension A sudden fall in blood pressure when a person assumes a standing position, resulting in dizziness, lightheadedness, blurred vision and temporary loss of consciousness.

Osmotic pressure The hydrostatic pressure that results from the difference in solute concentration within solutions that are separated by a semipermeable membrane.

Osteogenesis imperfecta (brittle bone disease) A genetic disease in which collagen production is deficient, making the bones abnormally fragile and causing recurring fractures with only minimal trauma, deformity of long bones, a bluish coloration of the sclerae, and often the development of oteosclerosis.

Osteonectin A protein in bone that binds collagen and hydroxyapatite and links collagen to minerals in the bone matrix.

p

Phantom limb pain Pain experienced in an amputated limb after the stump has healed that may be caused by spontaneous firing of afferent pain fibers in the spinal cord that were previously associated with the limb.

Physiologic dead space The volume of air that does not participate in gas exchange or the sum of anatomic and alveolar dead space.

Plasma cell A B lymphocyte that secretes antibodies in response to local cytokines released during the primary immune response.

Plasma kinin cascade A series of events that activates the kinin system to produce bradykinin.

Plasmin A degrading enzyme associated with fibrinolysis of many proteins of blood but primarily of fibrin clots.

Plasticity The ability of nervous system pathways to change function, sensitivity and so forth in response to changes in the neural environment.

Platelet-activating factor (PAF) A mast cell-derived substance that increases vascular permeability, leukocyte adhesion to endothelial cells and platelet activation.

Pneumothorax The collapse of a lung and subsequent escape of air into the pleural cavity between the lung and the chest wall that is caused by trauma, environmental factors, or spontaneous occurrence and results in a sudden pain in the chest.

Polycythemia An increase in red blood cell mass because of a defect in the erythroid progenitor cells or an increase in circulating serum factors such as erythropoietin.

Port-wine (nevus flammeus) stain A birthmark caused by superficial and deep dilated capillaries in the skin that produce a reddish to purplish discoloration of the skin, usually the face, but can occur anywhere on the body.

Premenstrual syndrome (PMS) A group of symptoms that occur in many women from 2 to 14 days before menstruation begins, such as abdominal bloating, breast tenderness, headache, fatigue, irritability, depression and emotional distress.

r

Reflex A rapid, automatic response to a stimulus.

Reflex arc The receptor, sensory neuron, motor neuron and effector involved in a particular reflex, may include interneurons.

Refractory period Period between the initiation of an action potential and the restoration of the normal resting potential, during this period, the membrane will not respond normally to stimulation.

s

Sclerosis Hardening or stiffening of a tissue, as in multiple sclerosis of the central nervous system or atherosclerosis of the blood vessels.

Senescence Degenerative changes that occur with age. Senescence is the indetermined period when an individual is said to grow old. Senescence (senescere, to grow old). By the age of 70, height is usually a full inch less than it was in the twenties or thirties. Between 70 and 80, body strength decreases to half of what it was at 25, lung capacity decreases to half and about 65% of a person's taste buds become inactive. The nose, ears and ear lobes are longer. Life expectancy is currently 71.4 for males and 78.7 for females. Current evidence suggests that the maximum human lifespan is about 110 years.

Sensation Conscious perceptions of a stimulus; pain, taste and color, for example, are not stimuli but sensations resulting from stimuli.

Sensory nerve fiber An axon that conducts information from a receptor to the central nervous system.

Serous fluid A watery, low-protein fluid similar to blood serum, formed as a filtrate of the blood or tissue fluid or as a secretion of serous gland cells; moistens the serous membranes.

Serous membrane A membrane such as the peritoneum, pleura, or pericardium that lines a body cavity or covers the external surfaces of the viscera; composed of a simple squamous mesothelium and a thin layer of areolar connective tissue.

Serum 1. The fluid that remains after blood has clotted and the solids have been removed; essentially the same as blood plasma except for a lack of fibrinogen. Used as a vehicle for vaccines. 2. Serous fluid.

Shock 1. Circulatory shock, a state of cardiac output that is insufficient to meet the body's physiological needs, with consequences ranging from fainting to death. 2. Insulin shock, a state of severe hypoglycemia caused by administration of insulin. 3. Spinal shock, a state of depressed or lost reflex activity inferior to a point of spinal cord injury. 4. Electrical shock, the effect of a current of electricity passing through the body, often causing muscular spasm and cardiac arrhythmia or arrest.

Sinus 1. An air-filled space in the cranium. 2. A modified, relatively dilated vein that lacks smooth muscle and is incapable of vasomotion, such as the dural sinuses of the cerebral circulation and coronary sinus of the heart. 3. A small fluid-filled space in an organ such as the spleen and lymph nodes. 4. Pertaining to the sinoatrial node of the heart, as in *sinus rhythm*.

Somatic 1. Pertaining to the body as a whole. 2. Pertaining to the skin, bones and skeletal muscles as opposed to the viscera. 3. Pertaining to cells other than germ cells.

Somatic nervous system A division of the nervous system that includes efferent fibers mainly from the skin, muscles and skeleton and afferent fibers to the skeletal muscles. *Compare* autonomic nervous system.

Somesthetic 1. Pertaining to widely distributed *general senses* in the skin, muscles, tendons, joint capsules and viscera, as opposed to the *special senses* found in the head only; also called *somatosensory*. 2. Pertaining to the cerebral cortex of the postcentral gyrus, which receives input from such receptors.

Stem cell Any undifferentiated cell that can divide and differentiate into more functionally specific cell types such as blood cells and germ cells.

Stenosis The narrowing of a passageway such as a heart valve or uterine tube; a permanent, pathological constriction as opposed to physiological constriction of a passageway.

Steroid A lipid molecule that consists of four interconnected carbon rings; cholesterol and several of its derivatives.

Stimulus A chemical or physical agent in a cell's surroundings that is capable of creating a physiological response in the cell; especially agents detected by sensory cells, such as chemicals, light and pressure.

Strain The extent to which a body, such as a bone, is deformed when subjected to stress. *Compare* stress.

Stress 1. A mechanical force applied to any part of the body; important in stimulating bone growth, for example. *Compare* strain. 2. A condition in which any environmental influence disturbs the homeostatic equilibrium of the body and

stimulates a physiological response, especially involving the increased secretion of hormones of the pituitary-adrenal axis.

Synergistic An effect in which two agents working together (such as two hormones) exert an effect that is greater than the sum of their separate effects. For example, neither follicle-stimulating hormone nor testosterone alone stimulates significant sperm production, but the two of them together stimulate production of vast number of sperms.

Synovial fluid A lubricating fluid similar to egg white in consistency, found in the synovial joint cavities and bursae.

Synovial joint A point where two bones are separated by a narrow, encapsulated space filled with lubricating synovial fluid; most such joints are to the skeletal muscles. *Compare* autonomic nervous system.

†

Thrombosis The formation or presence of a thrombus.

Thrombus A clot that forms in a blood vessel or heart chamber; may break free and travel in the bloodstream as a thromboembolus.

Thymus A lymphatic organ in the mediastinum superior to the heart; the site where T lymphocytes differentiate and become immunocompetent.

Thyroid gland An endocrine gland in the neck, partially encircling the trachea immediately inferior to the larynx.

Thyroid hormone Either of two similar hormones, thyroxine and triiodothyronine, synthesized from iodine and tyrosine.

Thyroid-stimulating hormone (TSH) A hormone of the anterior pituitary gland that stimulates the thyroid gland; also called *thyrotropin*.

Thyroxine (T4) The thyroid hormone secreted in greatest quantity, with four iodine atoms; also called *tetraiodothyronine*.

Tomography A radiographic image of a plane constructed by means of reciprocal linear or curved motion of the X-ray tube and film cassette; used in producing a CT scan.

Transudate Fluid that had passed through a membrane.

Triglyceride A lipid composed of three fatty acids joined to a glycerol; also called a *triacylglycerol* or *neutral fat*.

Triiodothyronine (T3) A thyroid hormone with three iodine atoms, secreted in much lesser quantities than thyroxine.

U

Ultraviolet radiation Invisible, ionizing, electromagnetic radiation with shorter wavelength and higher energy than violet light; causes skin cancer and photoaging of the skin but is required in moderate amounts for the synthesis of vitamin D.

Umbilical 1. Pertaining to the cord that connects a fetus to the placenta. 2. Pertaining to the navel (umbilicus).

Urea A nitrogenous waste produced from two ammonia molecules and carbon dioxide; the most abundant nitrogenous waste in the blood and urine.

V

Varicose vein A vein that has become permanently distended and convoluted due to a loss of competence of the venous valves; especially common in the lower extremity, esophagus and anal canal (where they are called hemorrhoids).

Viscera The organs contained in the dorsal and ventral body cavities, such as the brain, heart, lungs, stomach, intestines and kidneys.

X

X chromosomes The sex chromosome whose presence does not determine genetic maleness, two chromosomes produce a genetic female.

Y

Y chromosome The sex chromosome whose presence indicates that the individual is a genetic male.

Yolk sac One of the four extraembryonic membranes, composed of an inner layer of endoderm and an outer layer of mesoderm.

Z

Zona fasciculata The middle and largest layer of the adrenal cortex, major source of cortisol.

Zona glomerulosa The outermost layer of the adrenal cortex, sole source of aldosterone.

Zona reticularis The inner most layer of the adrenal cortex, produces cortisol along with the zona fasciculata

ABBREVIATIONS

Listed are the commonly used abbreviations every provider should know

S.i.g. or s.i.g.n.a Directions for use.

a Before

d Day

qd or od Every day

Bid Twice daily

Tid Thrice daily

qid 4 times daily

q.h. Every hour

S.t.a.t. Immediately

ac Before meals

Pc After meals

Hs or qhs At bedtime

disp Dispense

Prn As needed

Po By month (orally)

IV Intravenous

IM Intramuscular

Stat Immediately

Sq or sc Subcutaneous

Mcg or µg Micrograms

S.O.S. If necessary

Equivalents	Domestic measures
1 liter (1) = 1.76 pints.	A standard 5 ml spoon is available.
1 kilogram (kg) = 2.2 pounds (Ibs).	Otherwise the following approximations will serve:
1 gram (g)	60 mg = 1 grain.
1 milligram (mg) (1×10^{-3} g).	1 mL= 15 – 16 drops.
1 microgram (mcg or/µg) (1×10^{-6} g).	1 tablespoonful = 14 ml.
1 nanogram (ng) (1×10^{-9}g).	1 dessertspoonful = 7 ml.
1 milliliter (ml). (1×10^{-3} 1).	
1 micrometer (µm) (1×10^{-6} meters).	

Metric weight and volume

Weight	Volume
Kilogram (kg) = 1,000 gram (gm)	Liter (L) =
10 decigram (dg)	10 deciliters (dl)
100 centigram (cg)	100 centiliters (cl)
1,000 milligram (mg)	1000 milliliters (ml)
1,000,000 micrograms (µg or mcg)	1,000,000 microliters (µl)

SUGGESTED READING

- Adams CB, Microvascular compression: an alternative view and hypothesis. *J Neurosurg* 1989; 70:1–12.
- Adams CB. Microvascular compression: an alternative view and hypothesis. *J Neurology* 1989; 70:1–12.
- Akerman S, Kopp S, Nilner M, Peters A, Rohlin M. Relationship between clinical and radiologic findings of the temporomandibular joint in rheumatoid arthritis. *Oral Surg Oral Med Oral Pathol* 1988; 66: 639–43.
- Al-Belasy FA, Amer MZ. Effect of n-Butyl-2-cyanoacrylate (histoacryl) glue in warfarin treated patients undergoing oral surgery. *J Oral Maxillofac Surg* 2003; 61:1432.
- Altay A, Nemes I Pac. M. The tigeminal foramen syndrome, *Fogorv Sz* 1997; 90(5):143-150.
- American Heart Association. Circulation 2007;115:1–17.
- AndersonVC, Berrhill PC, Sandquist MA, Ciaverella DP, Nesbit GM, Burchiel KJ: High resolution three-dimensional magnetic resonance angiography and three-dimentional spoiled gradient-recalled imaging in the evolution of neurovascular compression in patients with trigeminal neuralgia: a double-blind pilot study. *Neurosurgery*. Apr 2006; 58 (4): 666–73.
- Anthony M. Headache and the greater occipital nerve. Clin Neurol Neurosurg 1992; 94:297–301.
- Aoki KR. Evidence for antinociceptive activity of botulinum toxin type A in pain management. *Headache* 2003; 43 Suppl 1:S9-S15.
- Arnett FC, Edworthy SM, Bloch DA, et al. The American Rheumatism Association 1987 revised criteria for the classification of rheumatoid arthritis. *Arthritis Rheum* 1988;31:315–24.
- Baccaglini L, Atkinson JC, Patton LL, et al. Management of oral lesions in HIV-positive patients. *Oral Surg Oral Med Oral Pathol Oral Radiol Endod* 2007; 103(suppl):S50.
- Barker 2nd EG, Jannetta PJ, Bissonette DJ, Larkins MV, Jho HD. The long-term outcome of microvascular decompression for trigeminal neuralgia. Af *Engl J Med.* 1996; 334:1077–83.
- Bartsch T, Goadsby PJ. Increased responses in trigemino-cervical nociceptive neurons to cervical input after stimulation of the dura mater. *Brain* 2003; 126:1801–13.
- Bartsch T, Goadsby PJ. Stimulation of the greater occipital nerve induces increased central excitability of dural afferent input. *Brain* 2002; 125:1496–509.
- Bartsch T, Goadsby PJ. The trigeminal complex and migraine: current concepts and synthesis. *Current headache reports* 2003; 2:149–54.
- Bederson JB, Wilson CB. Evaluation and microvascular decompression and partial sensory rhizotomy in 252 cases of trigeminal neuralgis. *J Neurosurg.* 1089;71.
- Bederson JB, Wilson CB. Evaluation of microvascular decompression and partial sensory rhizotomy in 252 cases of trigeminal neuralgia, *J Neurosurg,* 1989; 71:359–367.
- Benz EJJ, Shattil SJ, et al (eds). *Hematology: Basic Principles and Practices,* 4th ed. Philadelphia, Elsevier-Churchill Livingstone, 2005: 2081–97.
- Biwaters EGL. Lesions of bursae, tendons and tendon sheaths. *Clin Rheum Dis* 1979; 5:883–925.
- Blackwood. HJJ Arthritis of the mandibular joint. *Br Dent J* 1963; 115:317–24.
- Blumenfeld A. Botulinum toxin type a for the treatment of headache: pro. *Headache* 2004; 44:825–30.
- Bogduk N. Greater occipital neuralgia. In Long DM (ed). *Current Therapy in Neurological Surgery II.* Philadelphia: Decker, 1989:263–67.
- Bogduk N. The anatomy of occipital neuralgia. *Clin Exp Neurol* 1980; 17:167–84.
- Bonica, (Ed), *Advances in Pain Research and Therapy,* Raven Press, New York 1983; 927–933.
- Bottler T, Kuttenberger J, Hardt N, et al. Non-HIV associated Kaposi's sarcoma of the tongue. Case report and review of the literature. *Oral Maxfac Surg* 2007; 36(12):1218–1220.
- Bovim G, Bonamico L, Fredriksen TA, Linboe CF, Stolt-Neilsen A, Sjaastad O. Topographic variations in the peripheral course of the greater occipital nerve. Autopsy study with clinical correlations. *Spine* 1991; 16:475–78.
- Breslow, A: Tumor thickness, level of invasion and node dissection in stage I cutaneous melanoma. *Ann Surg* 1975; 182:572–75.
- Brief Report: Congenital tuberculosis. *N Engl J Med* 1994; 330:1051–54.
- Broggi G, Ferroli P, Franzini A, Servello D and Dones I: Microvascular decompression for trigeminal neuralgia: comments on a series of 250 cases, including 10 patients with multiple sclerosis, *J Neuro neurosurg Psychiatry.* 2000;68: 59–64.
- Brown N. Skeletal muscle and bone: effect of sex steroids and aging. *Adv Physiol Educ* 2008, 32(2):120, .
- Brroggi G, Ferrli P, Franzini A, Servello D, Dones I. Microvascular decompression for trigeminal neuralgia: Comments on a series of 250 cases, including 10 patients with multiple sclerosis. *J Neurol Neurosurg Pscychiatry,* Jan; 2000; 68 (1): 59–64.
- Bryant D H Pepys J. Oral tuberculosis. *Brit Med J* 29: 1976.
- Center for Disease Control: Opportunistic infections and Kaposi's sarcoma among Haitians in the United States. MMWR 1982; 31:353–61.
- Centers for Disease control and Prevention (CDC). Available at: resources/factsheets/At-AGlance. htm. Accessed October 2007.
- Chabner DA: *The Language of Medicine,* 6th ed. Philadelphia, WB Saunders, 2001.
- Chalmers IM, Blair GS. Rheumatoid arthritis of the temporomandibular joint. QJ Med 1973; 166: 369–86.

- Chaudhary S, Kalra N, Gomber S. Tuberculous osteomyelitis of the mandible: a case report in a 4-year-old child. *Oral Surg Oral Med Oral Pathol Oral Radiol Endod* 2004; 97: 603–06.

- Chobanian AV, Bakris GL, Black HR, et al. Seventh Report of the joint National Committee on Prevention, Detection, Evaluation, and Treatment of High Blood Pressure. *Hypertension* 2003; 42: 1206–52.

- Chuang YC, Yoshimura N, Huang CC, Chiang PH Chancellor MB: Intravesical botulinum toxin A administration produces analgesia against acetic acid induced bladder pain responses in rats. *J Urol* 2004; 172:1529–32.

- Clinical and radiological analysis of children and adolescents with Cluff LE, Thoronton GF and Seidle LG: Studies on the epidemiology of adverse drug reactions. *JAMA.* 1964, 188: 976–983.

- Cluff LE, Thoronton GF, Seidle LG. Studies on the epidemiology of adverse drug reactions. *JAMA* 1964; 188:976–83.

- Clumeck N, Robert-Guroff M, Van de Perre P, et al. Serological studies of HTLV-III antibody prevalence among selected groups of heterosexual Africans. *JAMA* 1985; 254:2599–2602.

- Clumeck N, Sonnet J, Taelman H, et al. AIDS in African patients. *New Engl J Med* 1984; 310:492–97.

- Cohen J. Role of neurologist in the evaluation and treatment of patients with trigeminal neuralgia. *Neurosurg Focus* 2005; 18: E2.

- Cohen J. Role of the neurologist in the evaluation and treatment of patients with trigeminal neuralgia. *Neurosurg Focus* 18(2005), p. E2.

- Cruccu G, Gronseth G, Alksne J, et al., JM AAN-EFNS guidelines on trigeminal neuralgia management. *Eur J N enrol.* 2008; 15:1013–28.

- Dailey RH: Acute upper airway obstruction. *Emerg Med Clin North Am* 1983, 1–261–177.

- Dalessio DJ: Trigeminal neuralgia. A practical approach to treatment. *Drugs Sept* 1982; 24 (3): 248–55.

- Das Gupta A, Ghosh RN, Poddar AK, Mukherjee C, Mitra PK. Fine needle aspiration cytology of cervical lymphadenopathy with special reference to tuberculosis. *J Indian Pathol Microbiol* 1996; 39: 74–75.

- Delitala A, Brunori, Chiappetta F, Microsurgical posterior fossa exploration for trigeminal neuralgia: a study on 48 cases, *Minim Invasive Neurosurg* (2001) 44:152–56.

- Dimitrakopoulos I, Zouloumis L, Lazaridis N, Karakasis D, Trigonidis G, Sichletidis L. Primary tuberculosis of the oral cavity. *Oral Surg Oral Med Oral Pathol* 1991;72:712–15.

- Dinkar and Prabhudessai: Primary tuberculous osteomyelitis of the mandible: a case report. *Dentomaxillofacial Radiology* 2008; 37, 415–20.

- Dodick D, Blumenfeld A, Silberstein SD. Botulinum neurotoxin for the treatment of migraine and other primary headache disorders. *Clin Dermatol* 2004; 22:76–81.

- Dohil MA, Lin P, Lee J, et al.: The epidemiology of molluscum contagiosum in children. *J Am Acad Dermatol* 2006; 54:47–54.

- Dolly O. Synaptic transmission: Inhibition of neurotransmitter release by botulinum toxins. *Headache* 2003; 43 Suppl 1:S16–S24.

- Drummond PD, Granston A, Facial pain increases nausea and headache during motion sickness in migraine sufferers. *Brain* 2004; 127:526–34.

- Drummond PD. Photophobia and autonomic responses to facial pain in migraine. *Brain* 1997; 120:1857–64.

- Durham PL, Cady R. Cady R. Regulation of calcitonin- gene related peptide secretion from trigeminal nerve cells by botulinum toxin type A. Implications for migraine therapy. Headache 2004; 44:35–43.

- Ebenezer J, Samuel R, Mathew GC, Koshy S, Chacko RK, Jesudason MV: Primary oral tuberculosis. Report of two cases. *Ind J Dent Res* 2006; 11:41–44.

- Elias WE, Burchiel KJ. Trigeminal neuralgia and other neuropathic pain syndromes of the head and face. *Curr Pain Headache Reports* 2002; 6:115–24.

- Epstein JB, Marcoe JH. Topical application of capsaicin for treatment of for second-division trigeminal neuralgia. *Br J Anaesth.* 2006;97(4):559.

- Eramus JH, Thompson IOC, van der Westhuijzen AJ. Tuberculous osteomyelitis of the mandible: report of a case. *J Oral Maxillofac Surg* 1998; 56: 1355–58.

- Evers S, Vollmer-Haase J, Schwaag S, Rahmann A, Husstedt IW, Frese A. Botulinum toxin A in the prophylactic treatment of migraine—a randomized, double-blind, placebocontrolled study. Cephalalgia 2004; 24:838–13.

- Feller L, Wood NH, Lemmer J. HIV-associated Kaposi's Sarcoma: pathogenic mechanisms. *Oral Surg Oral Med Oral Pathol Oral RadiolEndod* 2007; 104:521–29.

- Fliss DM, Parikh J, Freeman JL: AIDS-related Kaposi's sarcoma of the sphenoid sinus. *J Otolaryngol* 1992; 21: 235-37.

- Fogele RH et al. Ovarian and androgen production in post-menopausal women. *J Cin Endocrinol Metab* 92(8):3040, 2007.

- Forbes CD, Jackson WF. *Color Atlas of Clinical Medicine* Elsevier 3rd ed. 2003.

- Formm Gh: Medical treatment patients with trigeminal neuralgia. In: G.H. Fromm and B.J. Sessle, Editors, *Trigeminal neuralgia: Current concepts regrading pathogenesis and treatment,* Butterworth-Heinemann, Boston. 1991;131–144.

- Fornatora ML, Reich RF, Gray RG, et al.: Intraoral molluscum contagiosum: a report of a case and a review of the literature. *Oral Surg Oral Med Oral Pathol Oral Radiol Endod* 2001; 92:318–20.

- Freemont AJ and Millac P. The place of peripheral neurectomy in the management of trigeminal neuralgia. *Postgrad Med J* 57;1981:75–76.

- Fromm GH, Chattha AS, Terrence CF, Glass JD. Role of inhibitory mechanisms in trigeminal neuralgia. *Neurology* 1981; 31:683–87.19 Fromm 2006; 66(1):139–41.

- Fukuda J, Shingo Y, Miyako H. Primary tuberculous osteomyelitis of the mandible. A case report. *Oral Surg Oral Med Oral Pathol* 1992; 73: 278–80.
- Fukushima T: Posterior cranial fossa neurovascular decompression (Jannetta method) for trigeminal neuralgia and facial spasm, *No Shinkei Geka* 10, 1982; 1257–61 Japanese.
- Fukushimat. Posterior cranial fossa neurovascular decompression (Jannetta mettod) for trigeminal neuralgia and facial spasm. *No Shinker Geka*. 1982:10. Japanese.
- Gartner MS, et. al. Acute HIV infection presenting with painful swallowing and esophageal ulcers. JAMA 1990; 263:2318–22.
- Gawel MJ and Rothbart PJ. Occipital nerve block in the management of headache and cervical pain. Cephalalgia 1992;12:9–13.
- GH, Chattha AS, Terrence CF and Glass JD. Role of inhibitory mechanisms in trigeminal neuralgia. *Neurology* 1981;31:683–7.
- GH, Chattha AS, Terrence CF and Glass JD. Role of inhibitory mechanisms in trigeminal neuralgia. Neurology 1981; 31:683–7. 19 *Fromm* 2006; 66(1):139–141.
- Glickmam MS and Jacobs WR: *Microbial pathogenesis of Mycobacterium tuberculosis:* dawn of a discipline. *Cell* 2001; 104:477–85.
- Gnepp DR, Chandler W and Hyams V. Primary Kaposi's sarcoma of the head and neck. *Ann Inter Med* 1984; 100:107–114:487.
- Gobel H: Botulinum toxin in migraine prophylaxis. J Neurol 2004; 251 Suppl 1:I8–I11.
- Goldman L and Ausiello D: Cecil Textbook of Medicine, 22nd ed. Philadelphia, Saunders, 2004. B, From Seidel H, Mosby's guide to Physical Examination, 4th ed. St. Louis, Mosby, 1999.
- Gould BE. Pathophysiology for the Health Profession. 3rd ed, Saunders Elsevier. 2006
- Grant's Atlas of Anatomy: Agur AMR, Lee M J. 10th ed. Lippincott Williams & Wilkins 1999.
- Gray's Anatomy: Williams PL. 38 ed. EL BS with Churchill Livingstone 1995.
- Gronseth G, Cruccs G, Alksne J et al: Practice parameter: the diagnostic evaluation and treatment of trigeminal neuralgia (an evidence-based review): report of the American Academy of Neurology and the European Federation of Neurological Societies. *Neurology,* 2008; 71:1183–90.
- Grouplille P, Fouquet B, Cotty P, Goga D J Goga D, Mateu J and Valat JP: The termporomandibular joint in rheumatoid arthritis: correlation between clinical and computed tomography features. J Rheumatol 1990; 17:1285–1289.
- Gupta KB, Manchanda M, Yadav SPS and Mittal A : Tubercular osteomyelitis of mandible. Indian J Tuberc 2005; 52:147–150.
- Guyton AC and Hall JE: Textbook of medical physiology, ed 11, Philadelphia, 2006, Elsevier Saunders.
- Gynther GW, Holmund AB, Reinholt FB and Lindblad S: Temporomandibular joint involvement in generalized osteoarthritis and rheumatoid arthritis: a clinical arthroscopic, histological, and immunohistochemical study. Int J Oral Maxillofac Surg 1997; 26:10–6.
- Hakanson S. Retrogasserian glycerol injection as a treatment of tic douloureux. In: Bonica JJ., (Ed)., *Advances in pain Research and Therapy,* Raven Press, New York.1983; 927–33.
- Hakanson S. Trigeminal neuralgia treated by the injection of glycerol into the trigeminal cistern. *Neurosurgery.* 1981; 9:638–46.
- Hamada S., Asahara H., Fukushima T. Comparison of percutaneous gasserian-ganglion glycerol injection and microvascular decompression for the management of trigeminal neuralgia, *Masui* 1985; 34:1668–72 Japanese.
- Hamlyn PJ, King TT. Neurovascular compression in trigeminal neuralgia: a clinical and anatomical study. J Neurosurg 1992; 76:948–54.
- Hampf G, Tasanen A, Nordling S. Surgery in mandibular condylar hyperplasia. *J. Maxillofac Surg* 1985; 13:74–78.
- Haslett C, Chilvers ER, Boon NA. Colledge NR. *Davidson's Principles and Practice of Medicine,* 19 ed. Livingstone C 2002.
- Headache Classification Subcommittee of the International Headache Society. The international classification of headache disorders: 2nd ed. *Cephalalgia* 2004; 24(Suppl 1): 9–160.
- Helms CA. *Fundamentals of Skeletal Radiology,* 3rd ed. Philadelphia, WB Saunders, 2005. In: Oral and Maxillofacial Pathology (2nd edn). Kundli Haryana:
- Horowitz MB, Yonas H. Occipital neuralgia treated by intradural dorsal nerve root sectioning. *Cephalalgia* 1993; 13:354–60.
- Howng SL, Chang DS: Partial sensory rhizotomy as an alternative treatment of trigeminal neuralgia. *Kaohsiung J Med Sci* 1998; 14:492–97.
- J Stewart Tepper. The New England Center for Headache, sjtepper@aol. com. January 2005 doi: 10.1111/j.1468-2982.2005.00959.x Blackwell Publishing Ltd. *Cephalalgia,* 2005.
- Jannetta PJ, McLaughlin MR, Casey KF: Technique of microvascular decompression: Technical note. *Neurosurg Focus* 18,2005; p. E5.
- Jannetta PJ: Arterial compression of the trigeminal nerve at the pons in patients with trigeminal neuralgia. *J Neurosurg* 1967; 26(Suppl): 159–62.
- K Ganda: Dentist's Guide To Medical Conditions and Complications. 2008, Wiley-Blackwell.
- Karol EA, Karol B and Larramendy M. Reducing unnecessary morbidity from percutaneous thermocoagulation in the treatment of trigeminal neuralgia: Part B: a computerized protocol for quantitative analysis of data for radiofrequency thermocoagulation with the quadripolar electrode method and technique, N enrol Res 2005; 27:571–79.
- Karol EA, Perez A, Cueto G, Karol B: Reducing unnecessary morbidity from percutaneous thermo-coagulation in the treatment of trigeminal neuralgia: Part C: a starting point

for a somatotopic map of the human Gasserian ganglion, *Nenrol Res* 2005; 27:835–42.

- Klun B. Microvascular decompression and partial sensory rhizotomy in the treatment of trigeminal neuralgia: personal experience with 220 patients, *Neurosurgery* 1992, 30:49–52.

- Lee ST, Chen JF. Percutaneous trigeminal ganglion balloon compression for treatment of trigeminal neuralgia, part II: results related to compression duration. *Surg Neurol* 2003; 60:149–53 discussion 153–54.

- Li ST, Pan Q, Liu N, Shen F, Liu Z, Guan Y. Trigeminal neuralgia: what are the important factors for good operative outcomes with microvascular decompression. *Surg Neurol* 2004; 62:400–404.

- Lovely TJ, Jannetta PJ, Microvascular decompression for trigeminal neuralgia: Surgical technique and long-term results. *NeurosurgClin N Am 1991*; 8:11–29.

- Lunsford LD, Bennett MH. Percutaneous retrogasserian glycerol rhizotomy for tic douloureux: Part 1: Technique and results in 112 patients. *Neurosurgery.* 1984; 14:424–30.

- Magnusson T, Ragnarsson T, Bjornsson A. Occipital nerve release in patients with whiplash trauma and occipital neuralgia. *Headache* 1996; 36:323–26.

- Mahadevia, Brandwein-Gensler Piot P, Taelman H, Mbendi N, et al. AIDS in a heterosexual population in Zaire. *Lancet* 1984; ii:65–69.

- Malamed S. *Medical Emergencies in the Dental Office.* 6th ed Mosby 2007.

- Mansur AT, Goktay F, Gunduz S, et al. Multiple giant molluscum contagiosum in a renal transplant recipient. *Transpl Infect Dis* 2004; 6:120–23.

- *Mariae Curie Sklodowska [Med]* 2003; 58:185–186.

- Marmor M, Laubenstein L, Wiliam DC, et al: Risk factors for Kaposi's sarcoma in homosexual men. *Lancet* 1982; i: 1083–87.

- Martini FH, Bartholomew EF, Beldsoe BE. *Anatomy and Physiology for Emergency Care.* 2nd ed. Pearson- Prentice Hall, 2008.

- Mathew NT and Kaup AO: The Use of Botulinum Toxin Type A in Headache Treatment. *Curr Treat Options Neurol* 2002; 4:365–73.

- McKinley M, O'loughlin DV: *Human Anatomy.* 2006. McGraw Hill, International Edition.

- Meaney JF, Miles JB Nixon TE, Whitehouse GH, Ballantyne ES, Eldridge PR. Vascular contact with the fifth cranial nerve at the pons in patients with trigeminal neuralgia: detection with 3D FISP imaging. *AJRAm JRoentgenol* 1994; 163:1447–52.

- Meglio M, Cioni B, Moles A, Visocchi M. Microvascular decompression versus percutaneous procedures for typical trigeminal neuralgia: personal experience. *Stereo Fact Funct Neurosurg* 1990; 54–55.

- Mense S. Neurobiological basis for the use of botulinum toxin in pain therapy. *J Neurol* 2004; 251 Suppl 1:11–17.

- Merskey H, Bogduk N: *Classification of Chronic Pain. Descriptors of Chronic Pain Syndromes and Definitions of Pain Terms.* 1994; 2nd edn. IASP Press, Seattle.

- Milburn HI: Primary tuberculosis. *Curr Opin Pulm Med* 2001;7:133–41.

- Miyazaki H, A Deveze and J Magnan: Neuro-otological surgery through minimally invasive retrosigmoid approach: endoscope assisted microvascular decompression, vestibular neurotomy, and tumor removal, *Laryngoscope.* 2005; 115:1612–1617.

- *Mosby's Paramedic Textbook* 3rd ed. St. Louis, Mosby, 2005.

- Moss JP, Gray SJ: Serial sections of the jaw of a ferret. *Lab Practice.* 1973; 22:39–42.

- MVolcy M, Tepper 31 Bartsch T and Goadsby PJ: Increased responses in trigeminocervical nociceptive neurons to cervical input after stimulation of the dura mater. *Brain* 2003; 126:1801–13.

- Nardell EA. Environmental control of tuberculosis. *Med Clin N Amer* 1993; 77(6):1315–34.

- Nelson BL, Thompson LD. Molluscum contagiosum. *Ear Nose Throat J* 2003; 82:560.

- Netter FH. Atlas of human anatomy, fourth ed., 1991

- Netter: *Netter's Atlas of Human Physiology,* by Hansen, J T & Koeppen, BM. 1991.

- Neuralgia Internat.*J Clin.Pract.*2008; 62, 2, 248–54.

- Neuralgia. *Neurology.* 2005; 65(8): 1306–08.

- Neville B, Danm DD, Alien CM, et al. *Oral and Maxillofacial Pathology,* 2nd ed. Philadelphia, Saunders, 2002.

- Neville BW, Damm DD, Alien CM, Bouqot JE: Bone Pathology. In: *Oral and Maxillofacial Pathology* (2nd edn). Kundli Haryana: Replika Press Pvt. Ltd, 2005; 581.

- Norman JE de BDJ: Post-traumatic disorders of the jaw joint. Ann. Royal Coll. Surg.Engl. 1982; 64:29–36.

- Norman JED, Bramley P: Textbook and Color Atlas of the Temporomandibular Joint, Year Book Med., Pub, Inc, 1990.

- Ogus II. Rheumatoid arthritis of the temporomandibular joint. *Br J Oral Surg.* 1975; 12: 275–84.

- Okeson JP. Management of the temporomandibular joint disorders and occlusion. St Louis: Mosby Year Book, 1993.

- Olesen J. Classification and diagnostic criteria for headache disorders, cranial neuralgias and facial pain: First edition, *Cephalalgia.* 1988;8 (Suppl 7): 1–96.

- Olesen J. The international classification of headache disorder: 2nd edition. *Cephalalgia* 2004; 24 (Suppl 1): 1–160.

- Osteomyelitis of mandible. *Indian J Tuberc* 2005; 52: 147–50.

- *Pain Syndromes and Definitions of Pain Terms.* 2nd edn. I ASP Press, Seattl Pathol 1992; 73: 278–80.

- Paul W, Ladenson MD. The Johns Hopkins University and Hospital, Baltimore MD, in Seidel HM, Ball JW, Dains JE, Benedict GW. Mosby's guide to Physical Examination, 6th ed. St. Louis, Mosby, 2006.

- Perelson HN: Occipital nerve tenderness: a sign of headache. *Soth Med* J 1947; 40:653–6. 24 Hammond SR, Danta G. Occipital Neuralgia Clin Exp Neurol 1978; 15:258–70.

- Piatt JH, Wilkins RH: Treatment of tic douloureux and hemifacial spasm by posterior fossa exploration. *Neurosurgery* 1984; 14:462–71.

- *Piatt Jr JH* and *Wilkins RH.* Treatment of tic douloureux and hemifacial spasm by posterior fossa exploration: therapeutic implications of various neurovascular relationships, *Neurosurgery*. 1984; 14:462–71.

- Pierce J, Sims SL, Holman GH. Transmission of tuberculosis to hospital workers by a patient with AIDS. *Chest* 1992; 101:581–82.

- Piovesan EJ, Kowacs PA, Oshinky ML: Convergence of Cervical and Trigeminal sensory afferents. *Current Headache Reports* 2003; 2:155–61.

- Pollock BE. Comparison of posterior fossa exploration and stereotactic radiosurgery in patients with previously nonsurgically treated idiopathic trigeminal neuralgia *Neurosurg Focus* 2005; 18: p. E6.

- Pollock BE: Comparison of posterior fossa exploration and stereotactic radiofrequency in patients with previously non surgically treated idiopathic trigeminal neuralgia. *Neurosug Focus* 2005:18.

- Poon CY: Cryotherapy in the management of trigeminal neuralgia: a review of the literature and report of three cases, *Singapore Dent J* 23 (2000), 49–55.

- Popli MB, Mehta N, Nijhavan VS, Popli V. Cngenital tuberculosis. *Australas Radiol* 1998;43:256–57.

- Prabhu SR, Sengupta SK: Bacterial infections due to mycobacteria A. Tuberculosis. In: Oral Diseases in the Tropics. Prabhu SR, Wilson DF, Daftary DK, Johnson NW. Oxford: Oxford University Press, 1993, 195–202.

- Pradel W, Hlawitschka M, Eckelt U, Herzog R, Koch K: Cryosurgical treatment of genuine trigeminal neuralgia. *British Journal of Oral and Maxillofacial Surgery* 2002; 40:244–47

- Proteous NB, Terezhalmy: Continuing education: 2 hours. Tubercolsis: Infection control/Exposure control. Issues for oral health care workers Crest- Oral B Feb 2008.

- *Quinn JH* and Weil T. Trigeminal neuralgia: treatment by repetitive peripheral neurectomy: Supplemental report,/ *Oral Surg*. 1975; 33:591–95.

- Ragon C. The general management of rheumatoid arthritis. *JAMA* 1949; 141: 124–27.

- Rahnama M, Gaweda A. Trigeminal neuralgia—own observations. *Ann Univ Mariae Curie Sklodowska [Med]* 2003; 58:185–86.

- Rapoport AM , Sheftell FD, Bigal ME. 1Botulinum toxin A for the treatment of greater occipital neuralgia and trigeminal neuralgia: a case report with pathophysiological considerations. *Cephalalgia,* Blackwell Publishing Ltd. 2005.

- Raustia AM, Pyhtinen J. Computed tomography of the masticatory system in rheumatoid arthritis. JRheumatol 1991; 18:1143–49.

- RB Tenser and Trigeminal neuralgia: mechanisms of treatment. *Neurology* 1998; 51:17–19.

- Regezi, JA, Sciubba JJ 49 Jordan RCK: *Oral Pathology Clinical Pathologic Corerelation*. SaundesElsevier 2008.

- Reid R, Roberts F. Pathology Illustrated 2005, 6th ed. *Elsevier Churchill Livingston*.

- Rudolph and Krafft. Trigeminal Neuralgia, *American Family Physician: Volume 77, Number 9, May 7, 2008.*

- Saladin: *Anatomy and Physiology: The Unity of Form and Function*. Mc-Graw-Hill Co. 3rd.ed.2003.

- Saunders BM, Cooper AM. Restraining mycobacteria: role of granulomas in mycobacterial infections. *Immunol Cell Biol* 2000;78:334–41.

- Saunders, 2004. B, From Seidel H, *Mosby's Guide to Physical Examination*, 4th ed. St. Louis, Mosby, 1999.

- Scully C, Cawson RA: *Medical Problems in Dentistry*. Elservier Churchill Livingstone, 2005.

- Seeley RR, Stephen TD, Tate P. *Essentials of Anatomy and Physiology*, 2nd ed. Mosby 1996.

- Seidel HM, Ball JW, Dains JE, et al. *Mosby's Guide to Physical Examination*, 6th ed. St. Louis, Mosby, 2006.

- Sethi A, Sareen D, Agarwal AK, Bansal R: Primary tuberculous osteomyelitis of zygoma. *Int J Oral Maxillofac Surg*. 2006; 35: 376–77.

- Shahabuddin MD and Raghuveer CV. Role of fine needle aspiration cytology in detecting extrapulmonary tuberculosis. *J Odontol Conserv* 2003; 20: 77–78.

- Shier D, Butler J, Lewis R: *Hole's Essential of Human Anatomy and Physiology,* 10th ed, McGraw-Hill- Higher 2009.

- Siebert C: Smallpox is dead. Long live smallpox. New York Times 1994 August 21; 6:31–55.

- Smith WHR, Davis D, Mason KD, Onions JP. Intraoral and pulmonary tuberculosis following dental manipulation. *Lancet* 1982; 1:842–43.

- Spatz AL, Zakrzewska JM, Kay EJ: Decision analysis of medical and surgical treatments for trigeminal neuralgia: how patient evaluations of benefits and risks affect the utility of treatment decisions. *Pain* 131; 2007: 302–10.

- Stechison MT, Moller A, Lovely TJ. Intraoperative mapping of the trigeminal nerve root: technique and application in the surgical management of facial pain. *Neurosurgery* 1996; 38:76–81.

- Stuart DM. Drug metabolism, Pharm. Index September-October, 1968.

- Sun T, Saito S, Nakai O, Ando T: Long-term results of microvascuilar compression for trigeminal neuralgia with reference of probability of recurrence. *Acta Neurochir* (Wein)1994; 126:144–48.

- Swartz MH. *Textbook of Physical Diagnosis: History and Examination, 5th ed*. Philadelphia, Saunders, 2006.

- Syrjanen SM. The temporomandibular joint in rheumatoid arthritis. *Acta Radiol Diagnosis* 1985; 26:235–43.

- Takehara T. Dentition status and temporomandibular joint disorders in patients with rheumatoid arthritis. *Cranio* 2002; 20:165–71.

- Tenser RB. Trigeminal neuralgia: mechanisms of treatment. *Neurology* 1998; 51: 17–19.

- Terzi T, Karakurum B, Sgler S, Inan LE, Tulunay C. Greater occipital nerve blockade in migraine, tension-type headache and cervicogenic headache. *J Headache Pain* 2002; 3:137–41.

- The American Heart Association: Circulation. 2007, 115:1–17.

- Thomson NC, Kirkwood EM, Levers RS. In: Thomson NC, et al (eds): *Handbook of Clinical Allergy*. Oxford, Blackwell Scientific,1990, 1–36.

- Toda K. Etiology of trigeminal neuralgia. *Oral Science International* 2007; 4:10–8.
- Toller, PA. Temporomandibular arthropathy. *Proc. Royal Soc. Med.* 1974; 67:153–59.
- Trigonidis G, Sichletidis L: Primary tuberculosis of the oral tuberculosis in Bahia, Brazil. *BJID* 2003; 7: 73–81.
- Tronnier VM, Rasche D, Hamer J, Kienle and S Kunze: Treatment of idiopathic trigeminal neuralgia: comparison of long-term outcome after radiofrequency rhizotomy and microvascular decompression. *Neurosurgery* 2001; 48:1261–67.
- UNAIDS. 2004 Report on the global AIDS epidemic July 449. Rabeneck L, Popovic.
- Van de Perre P, Lepage P, Kestelyn P, et al. AIDS in Rwanda. *Lancet* 1984; ii:62–65.
- Van Wynsberghe D, Noback CR Carola R: *Human Anatomy and physiology.* 1995.
- Venizelos I, Andreadis C, Tatsiou Z. Primary Kaposi's sarcoma of the nasal cavity not associated with AIDS. *Eur Arch Otorhinolaryngol* 2008; 265(6):717–20.
- Vickers ER, Cousins MJ. Neuropathic orofacial pain part 1. *Prevalence Pathophysiol Aust Endod J* 2000; 26:19–26.
- Vital JM, Grenier F, Dautheribes M, Baspeyre H, Lavignolle B, Senegas J, An Anatomic and dynamic study of the greater occipital nerve (n of Arnold). Applications to the treatment of Arnolds neuralgia. *Sur Radiol Anat* 1989.
- Volcy M, Tepper 31 Bartsch T, Goadsby PJ: Increased responses in trigeminocervical nociceptive neurons to cervical input after stimulation of the dura mater. *Brain* 2003; 126:1801–13.
- Von ARX, Hussain, Oral tuberculosis. *Brit, Dent, J.* 2001.190, 8.
- Wahl MJ. Dental surgery in anticoagulated patients. *Arch Intern Med*, 1998, 158:1610.
- Weitz. JI. Anticoagulant and fibrinolytic drugs. In: Hoffman R, et al (eds). *Hematology: Basic Principles and Practices*, 4th ed. Philadelphia, Churchill Livingstone, 2005.
- Welch KM. Botulinum toxin type a for the treatment of headache: con. *Headache* 2004; 44:831–33.
- Welch MJ, Purkiss JR, Foster KA. Sensitivity of embryonic rat dorsal root ganglia neurons to *Clostridium botulinum neurotoxins*. *Toxicon* 2000; 38:245–58.
- Wesley E Shankland II, DOS, MS. *The Journal of Craniomandibular Practice January* 2009, Vol 27, No. 1.
- Woolf CJ, Salter MW. Neuronal plasticity: increasing the gain in pain. *Science* 2000; 288:1765–69.
- Worth HM. Infections of the jaws. In: *Principles and Practice of Oral Radiologic Interpretation.* Chicago, IL: Year Book Medical Publishers Inc., 1975; 242.
- Yamakawa M, Ansai T, Kasai S, Ohmaru T, Takeuchi H, Kawaguchi T, Takehara T. Dentition status and temporomandibular joint disorders in patients with rheumatoid arthritis. *Cranio* 2002; 20:165–71.
- Yi-Chun L, Hsu ML, Yang JS, HauLiag T, Chou SL, Lin HY. Temporomandibular joint disorders in patients with rheumatoid arthritis. *J Chin Med Assoc* 2007; 70:527–43.
- Yoshida A, Higuchi Y, Kondo M, Tabata O, Ohishi M. Range of motion of temporomandibular joint in rheumatoid arthritis: relationship to the severity of disease. *Cranio.* 1998; 16:162–167.
- Zakrzewska JM *Insights: facts and stories behind trigeminal neuralgia.* Trigeminal neuralgia association, 2006; Gainesville.
- Zakrzewska JM, Lopez BC: Quality of reporting in evaluations of surgical treatment of trigeminal neuralgia: recommendations for future reports. *Neurosurgery* 2003; 53:110–122.
- Zakrzewska JM, Nally FF. The role of cryotherapy (cryoanalgesia) in the management of paroxysmal trigeminal neuralgia: a six year experience. *Br J Oral Maxillofac Surg.* 1988; 26:18–25.
- Zakrzewska JM, Patsalos PN: Long-term cohort study comparing medical (oxycarbazepine) and surgical management of interactable trigeminal neuralgia. *Pain* 2002; 95: 259–66.
- Zakrzewska JM, Thomas DG. Patient's assessment of outcome after three surgical procedures for the management of trigeminal neuralgia *Acta Neurochir (Wien).* 1993; 122:225–230.
- Zakrzewska JM. Consumer views on management of trigeminal neuralgia, *Headache.* 2001; 41:369–76.
- Zakrzewska JM. Diagnosis and differential diagnosis of trigeminal neuralgia. *din J Pain* 2002; 18:14–21.
- Zakrzewska JM. Surgical management of trigeminal neuralgia *Br Dent J* 1991; 170:61–62.
- Zakrzewska JM. *Trigeminal Neuralgia*, W.B. Saunders, London 1995.
- Zakrzewska JM: Trigeminal neuralgia. London: W.B. Saunder Zakrzewskas 1995.